g.uk/library

FAMILY MEDICINE

THE CLASSIC PAPERS

WITHDRAWN
FROM LIBRARY

D1333594

WITHDRAWN
FROM LIBRARY

BRITISH MEDICAL ASSOCIATION

1000641

FAMILY MEDICINE
THE CLASSIC PAPERS

EDITED BY

Michael Kidd • Iona Heath • Amanda Howe

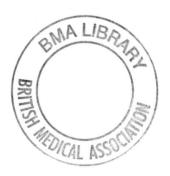

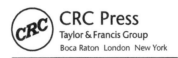

CRC Press
Taylor & Francis Group
Boca Raton London New York

CRC Press is an imprint of the
Taylor & Francis Group, an **informa** business

CRC Press
Taylor & Francis Group
6000 Broken Sound Parkway NW, Suite 300
Boca Raton, FL 33487-2742

© 2017 by Taylor & Francis Group, LLC
CRC Press is an imprint of Taylor & Francis Group, an Informa business

No claim to original U.S. Government works

Printed on acid-free paper
Version Date: 20160628

International Standard Book Number-13: 978-1-84619-994-3 (Hardback)

This book contains information obtained from authentic and highly regarded sources. While all reasonable efforts have been made to publish reliable data and information, neither the author[s] nor the publisher can accept any legal responsibility or liability for any errors or omissions that may be made. The publishers wish to make clear that any views or opinions expressed in this book by individual editors, authors or contributors are personal to them and do not necessarily reflect the views/opinions of the publishers. The information or guidance contained in this book is intended for use by medical, scientific or health-care professionals and is provided strictly as a supplement to the medical or other professional's own judgement, their knowledge of the patient's medical history, relevant manufacturer's instructions and the appropriate best practice guidelines. Because of the rapid advances in medical science, any information or advice on dosages, procedures or diagnoses should be independently verified. The reader is strongly urged to consult the relevant national drug formulary and the drug companies' and device or material manufacturers' printed instructions, and their websites, before administering or utilizing any of the drugs, devices or materials mentioned in this book. This book does not indicate whether a particular treatment is appropriate or suitable for a particular individual. Ultimately it is the sole responsibility of the medical professional to make his or her own professional judgements, so as to advise and treat patients appropriately. The authors and publishers have also attempted to trace the copyright holders of all material reproduced in this publication and apologize to copyright holders if permission to publish in this form has not been obtained. If any copyright material has not been acknowledged please write and let us know so we may rectify in any future reprint.

Except as permitted under U.S. Copyright Law, no part of this book may be reprinted, reproduced, transmitted, or utilized in any form by any electronic, mechanical, or other means, now known or hereafter invented, including photocopying, microfilming, and recording, or in any information storage or retrieval system, without written permission from the publishers.

For permission to photocopy or use material electronically from this work, please access www.copyright.com (http://www.copyright.com/) or contact the Copyright Clearance Center, Inc. (CCC), 222 Rosewood Drive, Danvers, MA 01923, 978-750-8400. CCC is a not-for-profit organization that provides licenses and registration for a variety of users. For organizations that have been granted a photocopy license by the CCC, a separate system of payment has been arranged.

Trademark Notice: Product or corporate names may be trademarks or registered trademarks, and are used only for identification and explanation without intent to infringe.

Visit the Taylor & Francis Web site at
http://www.taylorandfrancis.com

and the CRC Press Web site at
http://www.crcpress.com

Printed in Great Britain by Ashford Colour Press Ltd

FSC
www.fsc.org

MIX
Paper from
responsible sources
FSC® C011748

To our family medicine colleagues around the world who inspire us by their great work with their individual patients and communities each day, and through their service to the people who trust them for their medical care and advice.

Contents

Preface   xi

Acknowledgements   xii

1 Arthur Conan Doyle on Medical humanism and our values as
   family doctors (1894)   1
   Anna Stavdal (Norway)

2 Joseph Collings on The transformation of family medicine into a
   distinct medical discipline (1950)   7
   Michael Kidd (Australia)

3 Cees van den Dool on Anticipatory medicine – prevention as
   part of the consultation in family medicine (1970)   37
   Chris van Weel (the Netherlands)

4 Julian Tudor Hart on The Inverse Care Law (1971)   45
   Andy Haines (United Kingdom)

5 Charles Bridges-Webb on How family medicine research can
   lead to systematic understanding of health and illness within a
   local community (1973)   57
   Jane Gunn (Australia)

6 Ian McWhinney on Problem-solving and decision-making in
   family practice (1979)   69
   Roger Strasser (Canada)

7 Gayle Stephens on The intellectual basis of family practice (1982)   77
   Raman Kumar (India)

8 James W. Mold and colleagues on The shift to goal-oriented
   medical care (1991)   91
   Jan De Maeseneer (Belgium)

9 James McCormick on The place of judgement in
   medicine (1994)   101
   Iona Heath (United Kingdom)

10 Cynthia Haq and colleagues on The development of family
   medicine around the world (1995)   107
   Luisa Pettigrew (United Kingdom)

11 The World Organization of Family Doctors (WONCA) on Training
   the world's rural family medicine workforce (1995)   121
   John Wynn-Jones (Wales)

12 Ian McWhinney on The importance of being different (1996)   141
   Ruth Wilson (Canada)

13 Alastair McColl, Helen Smith and colleagues on Family doctors
   and evidence-based medicine (1998)   149
   Lubna Al-Ansary (Saudi Arabia)

14 Chris van Weel and Walter Rosser on The contribution of family
   medicine research to improving global healthcare (2004)   157
   Waris Qidwai (Pakistan)

15 Igor Švab and colleagues on Family medicine development in
   Eastern Europe (2004)   173
   Bohumil Seifert (Czech Republic)

16 John Gabbay and Andrée le May on New perspectives on
   evidence-based medicine (2004)   183
   Trisha Greenhalgh (United Kingdom)

17 Barbara Starfield and colleagues on The contribution of primary
   care to health systems and health (2005)   191
   Shannon Barkley (United States of America)

18 Julio Ceitlin on The development of family medicine in Latin America (2006)   241

Maria Inez Padula Anderson (Brazil)

19 Paul Little and colleagues on The importance of research in family medicine (2006)   249

Felicity Goodyear-Smith (New Zealand)

20 James Macinko and colleagues on Family medicine development in Brazil (2006)   259

Gustavo Gusso (Brazil)

21 Barbara Starfield on Global health, equity and primary care (2007)   269

Katherine Rouleau (Canada)

22 Harvey Chochinov on Dignity and the essence of medicine (2007)   275

Garth Manning (Thailand)

23 The World Health Organization on Primary care: putting people first (2008)   283

Antoinette Perera (Sri Lanka)

24 Kurt Stange and Robert Ferrer on The paradox of primary care (2009)   307

Andrew Bazemore (United States of America)

25 Charles Boelen and Bob Woollard on Social accountability and medical education (2009)   317

Allyn Walsh (Canada)

26 Bob Mash and Steve Reid on Family medicine in Africa (2010)   329

Shabir Moosa (South Africa)

27 Karen Barnett, Stewart Mercer and colleagues on Multimorbidity (2012)   337

Amanda Howe (United Kingdom)

28 Leiyu Shi on The impact of primary care and the importance of indicators (2012)   347

Kate Anteyi (Nigeria)

29 Iona Heath on The art of doing nothing (2012)   373

Job Metsemakers (the Netherlands)

30 The State Council of the People's Republic of China on Family medicine development in China (2013)   381

Shanzhu Zhu (China) and Donald K.T. Li (Hong Kong)

31 Amogh Basnyat on Family medicine transforming rural primary care in Nepal (2013)   405

Pratap Prasad (Nepal)

32 The World Health Organization on Family medicine development in the nations of the Middle East (2014)   413

Faisal Alnasir (Bahrain)

33 Roger Ruiz Moral and colleagues on The challenge of assisting people in improving adherence to medications (2015)   421

Christos Lionis (Greece)

Index   431

Preface

In this book we have endeavoured to collect in one place the classic papers from family medicine from around the world. This book aims to serve as a showcase of some of the most important ideas and research carried out in, or about, family medicine, demonstrate the broad scope of primary healthcare delivered by family doctors around the world, and serve as an inspiration to current family doctors as well as to doctors in training and medical students.

We have invited some of the leading family medicine experts in the world to take part in this publication by nominating the one journal article each feels has had the greatest impact on family medicine development. Some are papers describing original research, some are opinions or viewpoints; all are fascinating.

We also wanted to capture knowledge from the non-English language medical literature so you will notice papers in a number of languages.

Each chapter is based around one classic paper. The nominator has provided an outline of why she or he believes this article is important to family medicine, how it contributes to medical knowledge and the health and well being of the people of the world, why it was important when published and why it is still important now.

The nominator has also provided some details about the lead author of the nominated paper, and also a little about themselves.

We have also asked each family medicine leader to provide a few words of advice to new family medicine doctors, educators and researchers. This is something each person wishes they had been told at the start of their own career.

We hope you enjoy exploring these classic papers and receive inspiration from the wonderful concepts they outline about family medicine around the world.

We thank medical publisher Taylor & Francis for agreeing to publish this book. All royalties received by the editors will be paid to the World Organization of Family Doctors (WONCA), and the WONCA world executive has agreed to contribute the royalties towards a new fund to support research awards for new family medicine researchers from around the world.

We hope you are inspired by the papers collected in this book and the stories of the women and men who have helped shape global family medicine over the past century.

Michael Kidd, Iona Heath, Amanda Howe
November 2016

Acknowledgements

Our thanks to Gillian Nineham, formerly of Radcliffe Publishing, who, while we were sitting under the oak trees in Russell Square in London discussing possible ideas for new publications, enthusiastically supported the idea of a book bringing together some of the most important and influential papers from family medicine around the world.

Thank you to Alice Ovens at Taylor & Francis and to the many editors and publishers of medical journals from around the world who allowed us to reproduce the papers selected for this book.

Thank you to Rachel Cork at Flinders University who kept track of the development of each of the chapters of this book, and to Julie-Anne Burton for additional invaluable support.

Thank you to the secretariat staff of WONCA, the World Organization of Family Doctors, based in Bangkok, led by Dr Nongluck Suwisith, and Chief Executive Officer, Dr Garth Manning.

Thank you to each of the family medicine leaders around the world who eagerly embraced this publication and offered their recommendations of papers to be included.

Thank you to all the original authors, some no longer with us, for their contributions to the development of our discipline of family medicine, and for their pioneering work towards ensuring that high-quality medical care is available to all people in all countries of the world.

And thank you to Alastair, David and Barry, and our families, for their unflagging support, allowing us the privilege to do all that we do.

CHAPTER 1

Medical humanism and our values as family doctors

Anna Stavdal

NOMINATED CLASSIC PAPER

Arthur Conan Doyle. Behind the Times. In: *Round the Red Lamp – being facts and fancies of medical life*. Methuen & Co., London, 1894: 1–8.

Many great writers have described experiences in family medicine. This short story illustrates how continuity of care by an experienced and loyal general practitioner (GP) should be lived and carried out, illustrating the very core of the calling of the family doctor. At the time when this story unfolded, the content of the doctor's toolbox was extremely modest compared to the abundance available to medical practitioners in many parts of the world today. The expectations and hope for a favourable outcome when disease struck more often had to be left to fate and faith, rather than resulting from efficient treatment. It might be said that the choices that needed to be made and the dilemmas faced in those days were not nearly as pronounced and prominent as those confronting the doctor of the 21st century.

Dazzled by an ever-increasing flow of new tools, the modern doctor risks losing sight of a very central and essential ingredient in their toolbox, an ingredient based on the implicit contract between doctor and patient, something that is never up for sale: 'I will be there when you need me. I will make an effort to understand you, in your own context, offer cure if I can, try to alleviate your pain, always offer you comfort, and I will do my utmost never to expose you to any harm. And you should know that your secrets are safe with me.'

This short story should not be read as a nostalgic story romanticising an old country doctor. On the contrary, this is a story about a modern doctor of her time who hasn't lost sight of the core values of her profession.

ABOUT THE AUTHOR OF THIS PAPER

Sir Arthur Ignatius Conan Doyle (22 May 1859 to 7 July 1930) was a Scottish writer and physician, most noted for his fictional stories about the detective Sherlock Holmes.

He grew up in dire socioeconomic conditions, as his family became socially degraded and disadvantaged due to his father's alcohol addiction and mental health problems.

He graduated from medical school at the age of 22, starting his career as a physician working on board ships in long-haul service. Later he trained as an ophthalmologist, and set up his own practice. After suffering losses of family members, including his wife and a son, he found comfort in spiritualism.

Arthur was a fervent advocate of justice and he personally conducted investigations into two cases, which led to two men being exonerated of the felonies of which they were accused and convicted. He could draw on experience from many fields when engaging in the public debate of his time, always advocating the need for social development.

His broad perspective in life gave him a good base for his literary endeavours and, starting out from an early age, he was a prolific writer whose works include fantasy and science fiction stories, as well as plays, romances, poetry, and even non-fiction and historical novels.

ABOUT THE NOMINATOR OF THIS PAPER

Dr Anna Stavdal has worked as a general practitioner in the same area in the city centre of Oslo for the past 27 years. For almost as long, she has held a part-time post at the University of Oslo, teaching medical students. She is a past chair of the Norwegian College of General Practice, past president of Nordic Federation of General Practice, and current vice president of WONCA Europe.

> 'Search for insight, knowledge and experience from life itself. Be aware that sound patient-centred medicine presupposes deep understanding of your own self, enabling you to recognise when your own needs in the interplay with your patient, overshadow the needs of your patient. Develop your skills for self-scrutiny. Make a commitment to understand your society.'

> *Dr Anna Stavdal, Norway*

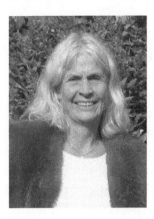

Attribution:

This short story was originally published in an anthology called *Round the Red Lamp* in 1894. We acknowledge the Conan Doyle Estate Ltd, owned by the members of the Arthur Conan Doyle family.

BEHIND THE TIMES

My first interview with Dr James Winter was under dramatic circumstances. It occurred at two in the morning in the bedroom of an old country house. I kicked him twice on the white waistcoat and knocked off his gold spectacles, while he with the aid of a female accomplice stifled my angry cries in a flannel petticoat and thrust me into a warm bath. I am told that one of my parents, who happened to be present, remarked in a whisper that there was nothing the matter with my lungs. I cannot recall how Dr Winter looked at the time, for I had other things to think of, but his description of my own appearance is far from flattering. A fluffy head, a body like a trussed goose, very bandy legs, and feet with the soles turned inwards – those are the main items which he can remember.

From this time onwards the epochs of my life were the periodical assaults which Dr Winter made upon me. He vaccinated me; he cut me for an abscess; he blistered me for mumps. It was a world of peace and he the one dark cloud that threatened. But at last there came a time of real illness – a time when I lay for months together inside my wickerwork-basket bed, and then it was that I learned that that hard face could relax, that those country-made creaking boots could steal very gently to a bedside, and that that rough voice could thin into a whisper when it spoke to a sick child.

And now the child is himself a medical man, and yet Dr Winter is the same as ever. I can see no change since first I can remember him, save that perhaps the brindled hair is a trifle whiter, and the huge shoulders a little more bowed. He is a very tall man, though he loses a couple of inches from his stoop. That big back of his has curved itself over sick beds until it has set in that shape. His face is of a walnut brown, and tells of long winter drives over bleak country roads, with the wind and the rain in his teeth. It looks smooth at a little distance, but as you approach him you see that it is shot with innumerable fine wrinkles, like a last year's apple. They are hardly to be seen when he is in repose, but when he laughs his face breaks like a starred glass, and you realise then that though he looks old, he must be older than he looks.

How old that is I could never discover. I have often tried to find out, and have struck his stream as high up as George the Fourth and even of the Regency, but without ever getting quite to the source. His mind must have been open to impressions very early, but it must also have closed early, for the politics of the day have little interest for him, while he is fiercely excited about questions which are entirely prehistoric. He shakes his head when he speaks of the first Reform Bill and expresses grave doubts as to its wisdom, and I have heard him, when he was warmed by a glass of wine, say bitter things about Robert Peel and his abandoning of the Corn Laws. The death of that statesman brought the history of England to a definite close, and Dr Winter refers to everything which had happened since then as to an insignificant anti-climax.

But it was only when I had myself become a medical man that I was able to appreciate how entirely he is a survival of a past generation. He had learned his medicine under that obsolete and forgotten system by which a youth was apprenticed to a surgeon, in the days when the study of anatomy was often approached through a violated grave. His views upon his own profession are even more reactionary than in politics. Fifty years have brought him little and deprived him of less. Vaccination was well within the teaching of his youth, though I think he has a secret preference for inoculation. Bleeding he would practise freely but for public opinion. Chloroform he regards as a dangerous innovation, and he always clicks with his tongue when it is mentioned. He has even been known to say vain things about Laennec, and to refer to the stethoscope as 'a new-fangled French toy.' He carries one in his hat out of deference to the expectations of his patients; but he is very hard of hearing, so that it makes little difference whether he uses it or not.

He always reads, as a duty, his weekly medical paper, so that he has a general idea as to the advance of modern science. He always persists in looking upon it, however, as a huge and rather ludicrous experiment. The germ theory of disease set him chuckling for a long time, and his favourite joke in the sick room was to say, 'Shut the door or the germs will be getting in.' As to the Darwinian theory, it struck him as being the crowning joke of the century. 'The children in the nursery and the ancestors in the stable,' he would cry, and laugh the tears out of his eyes.

He is so very much behind the day that occasionally, as things move round in their usual circle, he finds himself, to his bewilderment, in the front of the fashion. Dietetic treatment, for example, had been much in vogue in his youth, and he has more practical knowledge of it than any one whom I have met. Massage, too, was familiar to him when it was new to our generation. He had been trained also at a time when instruments were in a rudimentary state, and when men learned to trust more to their own fingers. He has a model surgical hand, muscular in the palm, tapering in the fingers, 'with an eye at the end of each.' I shall not easily forget how Dr Patterson and I cut Sir John Sirwell, the County Member, and were unable to find the stone. It was a horrible moment. Both our careers were at stake. And then it was that Dr Winter, whom we had asked out of courtesy to be present, introduced into the wound a finger which seemed to our excited senses to be about nine inches long, and hooked out the stone at the end of it.

'It's always well to bring one in your waistcoat-pocket,' said he with a chuckle, 'but I suppose you youngsters are above all that.'

We made him president of our Branch of the British Medical Association, but he resigned after the first meeting. 'The young men are too much for me,' he said.

'I don't understand what they are talking about.' Yet his patients do very well. He has the healing touch – that magnetic thing which defies explanation or analysis, but which is a very evident fact none the less. His mere presence leaves the patient with more hopefulness and vitality. The sight of disease affects him as dust does a careful housewife. It makes him angry and impatient. 'Tut, tut, this will never do!' he cries, as he takes over a new case. He would shoo death out of the room as though he were an intrusive hen. But when the intruder refuses to be dislodged, when the blood moves more slowly and the eyes grow dimmer, then it is that Dr Winter is of more avail than all the drugs in his surgery. Dying folk cling to his hand as if the presence of his bulk and vigour gives them more courage to face the change; and that kindly, wind-beaten face has been the last earthly impression which many a sufferer has carried into the unknown.

When Dr Patterson and I, both of us young energetic, and up-to-date, settled in the district, we were most cordially received by the old doctor, who would have been only too happy to be relieved of some of his patients. The patients themselves, however, followed their own inclinations, which is a reprehensible way that patients have, so that we remained neglected with our modern instruments and our latest alkaloids, while he was serving out senna and calomel to all the countryside. We both of us loved the old fellow, but at the same time, in the privacy of our own intimate conversations, we could not help commenting upon this deplorable lack of judgment.

'It's all very well for the poorer people,' said Patterson. 'But after all the educated classes have a right to expect that their medical man will know the difference between a mitral murmur and a bronchitic rale. It's the judicial frame of mind, not the sympathetic, which is the essential one.'

I thoroughly agreed with Patterson in what he said. It happened, however, that very shortly afterwards the epidemic of influenza broke out, and we were all worked to death. One morning I met Patterson on my round, and found him looking rather pale and fagged out. He made the same remark about me. I was in fact, feeling far from well, and I lay upon the sofa all the afternoon with a splitting headache and pains in every joint. As evening closed in I could no longer disguise the fact that the scourge was upon me, and I felt that I should have medical advice without delay. It was of Patterson naturally that I thought, but somehow the idea of him had suddenly become repugnant to me. I thought of his cold, critical attitude, of his endless questions, of his tests and his tappings. I wanted something more soothing – something more genial.

'Mrs Hudson,' said I to my housekeeper, 'would you kindly run along to old Dr Winter and tell him that I should be obliged to him if he would step round?'

She was back with an answer presently.

'Dr Winter will come round in an hour or so, sir, but he has just been called in to attend Dr Patterson.'

Arthur Conan Doyle (1894)

CHAPTER 2

The transformation of family medicine into a distinct medical discipline

Michael Kidd

NOMINATED CLASSIC PAPER

Joseph S. Collings. General practice in England today: a reconnaissance. *The Lancet*, 1950; i: 555–85.

This paper caused a storm when it was published in 1950 in *The Lancet*. It was based on a survey of British general practice conducted by a young, and somewhat cocky, Australian medical graduate, Dr Joe Collings, who was working at the time as a health services researcher at Harvard University in Boston in the United States of America, and who had been seconded by the Nuffield Trust in the United Kingdom to undertake this review.

The Lancet published Joe Collings' 30-page report in full, highlighting the poor conditions of many British general practices and the low morale of many general practitioners (GPs).

Joe Collings noted that general practice had no academic basis, with 'no real standards for general practice. What a doctor does and how he does it depends entirely on his own conscience.' He also stated that his observations, 'led me to recognise the importance of general practice and the dangers of continuing to pretend that it is something which it is not.'

Joe Collings was frank in his assessment, criticising both urban and rural general practices, and stating that inner-city practice was 'at best … very unsatisfactory and at worst a positive source of public danger'. He was not the first person to point out the deficiencies of general practice as he saw them, as George Bernard Shaw had done so 50 years earlier in his play *The Doctor's Dilemma*.

Joe Collings' paper inspired a group of concerned and responsible British GPs to join together in 1952 to form a college of general practitioners, later named The Royal College of General Practitioners (RCGP), established to provide professional leadership and to serve as an 'academic headquarters for general practice [and] to raise the standards and status of general practice'. Some 100 years earlier there had been a similar push to create a College of General Practice but the established colleges of the Physicians and the Surgeons had vetoed that at the time. The founding of the National Health Service in 1948 had brought things to a head with British GPs becoming responsible for all personal medical care and providing the gateway for access to all other health services, but without being provided with adequate physical infrastructure, resources and financial support. For the benefit of both patients and doctors, things had to change, and, thanks at least in part to Joe Collings' paper, they did.

The establishment of the College in the United Kingdom started a ripple effect around the world with colleges and societies of general practice and family medicine quickly being established in many other countries, especially among nations of the former British Empire. This effect continues to this day through the support provided to many other nations through the international programmes of the RCGP and other member organisations of WONCA (the World Organization of Family Doctors). Joe Collings' report also triggered a flood of publications on standards for general practice and the importance of the doctor–patient relationship, and contributed to the development of general practice/family medicine as a unique and distinct medical discipline.

ABOUT THE AUTHOR OF THIS PAPER

Joseph Silver Collings was born in Sydney, Australia in 1918. He graduated with degrees in agricultural science and medicine from the University of Sydney. After graduation he developed an interest in the organisation of health services, and travelled to the United States where he was appointed as a research fellow at the Harvard School of Public Health. From Harvard he was seconded to the Nuffield Trust in the United Kingdom to undertake a review of British general practice.

He returned to the United States and, in 1952, was appointed Associate Medical Director of the Health Insurance Plan of Greater New York, and was also engaged as a consultant to President Harry S. Truman's Commission on Health Needs of the Nation. He later moved back to Australia where he was appointed as Head of the Department of Physical Medicine at the Royal Melbourne Hospital. He was a Foundation Member of the Royal Australian College of General Practitioners (RACGP) and put his experiences into action by setting up a 'model' general practice in Melbourne. I am told he resigned from the RACGP in 1964 after a disagreement with the leadership of the day, which comes as no surprise. He died in Melbourne in 1971.

ABOUT THE NOMINATOR OF THIS PAPER

Professor Michael Kidd is an Australian family doctor, primary care researcher and medical educator. Following his graduation from the School of Medicine at the University of Melbourne in 1983, postgraduate training in general practice, and doctoral research at Monash University, he was appointed as Professor of General Practice at the University of Sydney in 1995, and later as Dean of the Faculty of Medicine, Nursing and Health Sciences at Flinders University in Adelaide in 2009. He was president of the Royal Australian College of General Practitioners from 2002 to 2006, and president of the World Organization of Family Doctors (WONCA) from 2013 to 2016. In 2009 he was made a Member of the Order of Australia for his contributions to healthcare and education.

> 'The story of Joe Collings, a young and passionate doctor, and his influence on the development of family medicine, serves as an example to us all. Each of us has the potential to contribute our own lasting legacy through the examples that we set through our life's work as doctors, through our vision as community leaders, and through our role as advocates who are not afraid to make our views known when we see things that should not happen that affect the health and well-being of our patients and our communities.'

Professor Michael Kidd AM, Australia

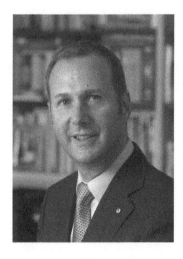

Attribution:

Reprinted with permission from Elsevier (Joseph S. Collings. General practice in England today: a reconnaissance. *The Lancet*, 1950; i: 555–85). With thanks to the National Library of Australia for archival details on Joseph Collings, to Emeritus Professor Wes Fabb AM, inaugural secretary-general of the World Organization of Family Doctors (WONCA) for his advice on background publications, and to Dr Eric Fisher AM, past president of the Royal Australian College of General Practitioners, for his personal recollections of Joseph Collings.

THE LANCET] GENERAL PRACTICE IN ENGLAND TODAY [MARCH 25, 1950 555

GENERAL PRACTICE IN ENGLAND TODAY
A RECONNAISSANCE

JOSEPH S. COLLINGS *
M.B., B.Sc. (Agr) Sydney

GENERAL medical practice is a unique social phenomenon. The general practitioner enjoys more prestige and wields more power than any other citizen, unless it be the judge on his bench. In a world of ever-increasing management, the powers of even the senior managers are petty compared with the powers of the doctor to influence the physical, psychological, and economic destiny of other people.

But unlike the manager, who exercises his controls over whole groups of society, the doctor exercises his in a microcosm and in relation to individuals ; and for this and other reasons he is largely free from the limitations which democratic principles set on the acquisition of power.

General practice is unique in other ways also. For example, it is accepted as being something specific, without anyone knowing what it really is. Neither the teacher responsible for instructing future general practitioners, nor the specialist who supposedly works in continuous association with the G.P., nor for that matter the G.P. himself, can give an adequate definition of general practice. Though generally identified with the last-century concept of " family doctoring," usually it has long ceased to be this. Nevertheless its stability and its reputation rest largely on this identification.

While other branches of medicine have progressed and developed, general practice, instead of developing concurrently, has adapted itself to the changing patterns ; and sometimes this adaptation has in fact been regression.

There are no real standards for general practice. What the doctor does, and how he does it, depends almost wholly on his own conscience.

The conduct of general practice and of the individual practitioner is inextricably interwoven with commercial and emotional considerations, which too often negate the code of medical ethics by which the public are supposedly safeguarded and from which the high reputation of medicine stems. Hence material and moral issues have become inseparable, and it is impossible to discuss general practice without discussing morals, and therefore without moralising. In this report the issues are kept separate as far as possible, but this is not very far.

Section I describes how the observations were made ; section II is an account of general practice as I found it ; and section III deals with the National Health Service in relation to general practice as I found it. I contrast this with the usual endeavour made to interpret the Act in terms of what general practice is supposed to be or what we might like to think it is.

I know well that many of my deductions rest on subjective impressions rather than objective fact, though I have tried to keep the two apart. Very little statistical evidence is used—principally because little valuable evidence of this kind is available, and secondarily because the major problems of general practice are not soluble in terms of statistics.

My observations have led me to write what is indeed a condemnation of general practice in its present form ; but they have also led me to recognise the importance of general practice and the dangers of continuing to pretend that it is something which it is not. Instead of continuing a policy of compensating for its deficiencies, we should admit them honestly and try to correct them at their source. If I do no more than convey this, I shall be satisfied.

I. SCOPE AND METHOD OF STUDY

At the outset I was advised that no accurate picture could be obtained by detailed inquiries in the London area, with its aggregation of teaching hospitals and many other complicating factors peculiar to a city of this size. I therefore decided to work outside London, in regions selected so that a mosaic might be constructed which would present the general picture. Having no knowledge of British geography or economy, I was guided by various advisers who knew the country, and eventually decided on three regions—in the north, the north-west, and the south. For purposes of comparison I also spent some time in Scotland.

Thanks to the willing coöperation of all the doctors approached, I have been able to see their work, both in their surgeries and in the homes of their patients, to become conversant with their difficulties, professional and personal, and to learn a great deal about their individual and collective attitudes to the new service.

Though others were visited, I have studied in some detail the work of 55 English practices, operated by 104 doctors. These 55 may be classified as :

Industrial	..		..	16
Urban-residential		..	..	17
Rural	..	..	..	22

The 16 industrial practices can be further divided into complete industrial 9 and " mixed " (industrial better-class residential) 7. The 22 rural practices can be divided

into rural-town 8 and isolated rural 14. Some 30 of the practices were run by individual practitioners ; the rest were partnerships or partner-assistantships with 2–6 doctors working together.

The 55 practices visited varied greatly in size (both number of patients and area) and in history and development.

Of the one-man practices some had full lists (4000) while others ranged down through 3000 and 2000 to less than 1000. Examples of different sizes were seen in all areas, though in the industrial areas only two practices were seen where the doctor's list was less than 2000, and in the rural areas only three where the lists approximated to or exceeded 3500. The partnerships and partner-assistantships studied covered much the same wide range of patient numbers, though very few had less than 2000 per partner.

In terms of area covered by a practice and accessibility of patients, conditions ranged from the most compact type of practice, in densely populated urban areas, to remote rural practices with less than 1000 patients living miles apart.

The history and development of the practices showed a similar wide range of variation. Some were over a century old ; others had been established before the war but had since been entirely re-established. Many of the industrial practices had had large " panel " and " club " lists since the early days of the old National Health Insurance scheme, and had depended on these for the greater part of the income ; but there were various gradations of the panel-private ratio through to completely private practice.

* At present research fellow, Harvard School of Public Health, Boston, Mass.

Each practice was reviewed in respect of three factors which jointly seem to determine the nature, scope, and quality of medical care :

1. The doctor.
2. The doctor's working environment :
    (a) Surgery.
    (b) Equipment.
    (c) Patient load.
    (d) Ancillary facilities.
3. The general social environment.

Of these, nos. 2 and 3 lend themselves to objective evaluation. No. 1, the doctor, is much more intangible ; but being undoubtedly the most important single unit in the whole field of medical care, he must be discussed with whatever objectivity is possible.

METHOD OF STUDY

My observations were made by " sitting in on " each practice—a term which requires careful explanation because the validity of these observations, and of some of the conclusions reached, depends on the technique adopted.

In retrospect, " sitting in on " a practice connotes to me a very wide range of behaviour ; everything, in fact, from sitting quietly in a corner trying to efface myself, while the doctor in an embarrassed and artificial way attempted to conduct his consultations, to a nearly complete identification with the doctor's work and behaviour. In the latter cases I found I was able to join in examinations, to interrogate patients, and to discuss points at issue without embarrassment to any of the parties concerned. Fortunately, as a rule the situation approximated, at least after a time, to the last-mentioned happy state of affairs. In the few cases where it did not, I have endeavoured to make allowances or write off the evidence obtained.

Similarly the domiciliary work I did with the doctors ranged from sitting in the car outside the patient's residence and discussing the case with the doctor, or being entertained by the relatives in the front parlour while he had his consultation in the bedroom upstairs, to complete and uninhibited participation in the consultation and examination. Here again the last-mentioned circumstances usually prevailed, and full allowances have been made where they did not.

The time spent " sitting in on " the work of a practice varied from one to-four or five days. It depended sometimes on advance arrangements made through a third party, but more often on a personal estimate of the value of the practice as a source of relevant information.

SELECTION OF PRACTICES

The selection of practices and practitioners to be seen was as much beyond my control as the selection of geographical areas in which to work. It was obviously not feasible to take a completely random sample, and precautions had to be taken against the selection of a whole group of " good men." Different people did the selecting in different areas. In most areas a number of people helped to make the selection ; they were asked to select some " good," some " fair," and some " bad " practices. Those usually consulted were regional medical officers who had experience of " refereeing " in the area ; consultants who knew, sometimes personally, always by repute, the practitioners in the area ; local-authority medical officers ; and in some parts of Scotland the chairman and secretary of the local medical committees. Sometimes it was possible to choose the common factors from the lists suggested by two or three people ; sometimes the choice depended partly on which practitioners were available.

The selection among the rural practitioners in the southern region was much more random. It was made by one person, who knew most of those selected by name only. They were chosen largely on geographical situation and not on reputation. In north-west Scotland

particular areas were selected and all the practitioners in them were visited.

Occasionally I was passed on from one practitioner to another ; but generally I tried to avoid this. Once I asked to see the work of a particular " group " practice. Always I was introduced to the practice concerned by a disinterested third party who was kind enough to undertake this task.

I am well satisfied that, by this diverse means of sampling, a fair and representative sample of general practice under the various environmental conditions was obtained.

In the northern and north-western regions, before any approach was made to the question of general practice, I sought information from people working for regional hospital boards, executive councils, and local authorities. In the southern region, as a rough control to any bias which might result from this sequence of activity, the general practitioners were visited before I consulted the authorities.

HOSPITALS AND GENERAL PRACTICE

Originally it was proposed that, after reviewing the work of a number of practices in a given area, observations should be made in the outpatient department of the hospitals fed by these practices. It was never intended to follow up particular cases, but to see whether the outpatient work would provide some sort of index of what was happening in a particular type of practice. It was also hoped that some statistical data might be obtained—e.g., the volume and nature of outpatient work before and after July 5, 1948—which would throw light on trends in general practice since the introduction of the service.

In some places it proved possible to do such a " follow through " ; in others, either because the practices fed too many hospitals or because the hospitals were too far away, I could not make any real correlation between the work of the practices and of the outpatient department. However, in every instance I visited some hospitals in or beside the area of study and considered what was happening in the outpatient department.

THE ACT AND THE PROBLEM

When the study began, the National Health Service had been in operation less than six months, and I recognised that it was very early to start assessing its effects on general practice. I also recognised that many of the initial difficulties, often described as " teething troubles," could obscure or complicate the picture. I have therefore tried to separate the " teething " problems from the more formidable long-term problems, and at this early stage I have concerned myself with general trends in the pattern of medical care rather than with the difficulties facing individual practitioners.

It soon became obvious that many problems which had existed for years, and were inherent in general practice as we know it, were being interpreted as results of the new National Health Service. This was very serious because it was preventing clear thought on important issues. Accordingly I decided to attempt first an assessment of general practice at this point of time, out of relation to the new Act, and secondly an interpretation of the actual and possible effects of the Act upon it.

Straight away, some very elementary questions presented. What constitutes general practice today ? What does the general practitioner do ? How does he do it ? What criteria have we for judging the quality of general practice ? How does general practice integrate with other medical services—hospital, specialist, and preventive ? To these and other apparently simple yet fundamental questions there are no simple ready-made answers. To some there are just no answers.

I shall begin, then, with a general account of what was seen in the practices studied.

THE LANCET]   GENERAL PRACTICE IN ENGLAND TODAY   [MARCH 25, 1950   557

II. THE STATE OF GENERAL PRACTICE

THREE MAIN PATTERNS

General practice is not, as generally assumed, something specific and definable. There are different patterns of practice, and I must distinguish these before describing specific examples.

From the first, I suspected that there were big differences not only in the quality of practice in different areas but also in its nature ; but I did not imagine that the differences would be so great or so basic as they proved to be. I thought, rather naïvely, that it was an easy matter to select " good," " average," and " bad " practitioners, and to identify the " good " doctor with good practice or the " bad " doctor with bad practice. I supposed that the " good " doctor would practise well in spite of the social environment in which he worked ; but this assumption likewise proved to be false.

The three main patterns of general practice are set by the social environment. They are :

1. General practice in urban industrial areas. (Henceforth called industrial practice.)

2. General practice in better-class urban residential areas. (Henceforth called urban-residential practice.)

3. General practice in rural areas. (Henceforth called rural practice.)

Industrial Practice

Industrial practice has departed a very long way from the ideal of family doctoring. The facilities for medical work are almost always unsatisfactory.

SURGERIES

Consider first the surgeries—the buildings which serve as the doctors' workshops. These are usually located in what was once a shop, or a residence above a shop, or in the downstairs rooms of a house tenanted by some person who takes care of the surgery or occasionally by the doctor himself.

The adaptation of shop or house to doctor's surgery is usually very elementary. As a rule two adjacent rooms serve as waiting and consulting rooms, and where dispensing is undertaken a third room may be set aside for this purpose. That is the basic plan, and there is very little variation from it. Where two or more doctors are working together, there may be two or even three consulting-rooms adjacent to a common waiting-room. The size and plan of the original premises largely determine any other differences between surgeries in industrial areas. I did not see a single industrial surgery which was built for its purpose.

In most cases the waiting-rooms are too small, cold, and generally inhospitable. In peak hours in big practices it is usual to see patients standing, waiting their turn to consult the doctor, and it is not uncommon to see them standing in the garden, where there is one, or queueing in the street where there is not. The comfort of patients and the needs of the sick have certainly not determined the nature of the industrial-practice type of waiting-room.

Consulting-rooms vary greatly in size and furnishings, but are generally comparable from a functional standpoint. Everything is done in this one all-purpose room. The patient is interrogated and the history taken ; if he is to be examined he removes such clothing as is necessary (or is convenient) and either hangs it on a hook or piles it on the chair on which he was previously sitting (very rarely a screen is provided, behind which he can change in relative comfort with minimum embarrassment, and very very rarely there may be a changing-room, though I have not myself seen one in an industrial practice) ; and then the examination is made, sometimes including

the collection of a specimen of urine, which is tested at a sink in the same room. It is indeed an all-purpose room.

Quite often the consulting-room is far from sound-proof and the most intimate details of a consultation can be distinctly heard in the waiting-room beside it.

The equipment contained in these consulting-rooms also varies considerably. In the sample of practices studied, the range was from satisfactory to dangerously poor—with too many approaching this last category. If we set the basic " heavy " equipment at desk, chairs, examining couch, filing cabinet, instrument cupboard, steriliser, and wash-basin with hot and cold water, and take this as a minimum level of essential heavy equipment for satisfactory practice, we immediately have to classify many industrial practices as unsatisfactory. In several of the surgeries I visited there were no examining couches ; in many there were no filing cabinets, and such records as were kept lay around the room either loose or in boxes ; in one there was a chair for the doctor only (the patient remained standing throughout consultation and examination) ; in some a saucepan on a gas-ring served as steriliser ; frequently I observed that instruments were kept in odd drawers, or on a table, window-ledge, or mantelpiece, exposed to the atmosphere ; and sometimes the doctor had to walk to another part of the premises to wash his hands.

I noted a similar range in the instruments of diagnosis and therapy with which these surgeries were provided. Always obvious were stethoscope, thermometer, tongue-depressor (sometimes of the old bone type, standing in a jar of " antiseptic "), sphygmomanometer, watch, syringes, and needles. Apart from these indispensable articles of practice, there was usually an ophthalmoscope, an auriscope set, and a variety of instruments of varying vintage and type. Proctoscope and vaginal specula were usually in evidence, although frequently there was also abundant evidence of their long disuse. Besides these, a variety of other instruments, antique or sometimes relatively modern, were often to be seen lying around as mementos of past interest in various aspects of medical work.

I have laboured these points of detail somewhat, because it is necessary to recognise the unsatisfactory nature of the doctor's workshop in an average industrial practice ; for this factor in itself sets a limit to the scope and quality of his work, to the treatment his patients receive, and to improvement of the situation. Few skilled craftsmen, be they plumbers, butchers, or motor mechanics, would be prepared to work under conditions or with equipment as bad (comparably) as that tolerated by many doctors working in industrial practices. But even more important than these material conditions is what goes on inside the surgeries and what use is made of the resources they possess.

EXAMINING THE PATIENT

The frequency with which the examining couch is used is a good index of the nature of medical practice under these conditions. I noticed on some occasions that a perfectly serviceable couch was piled with boxes and bottles ; the adherence of these articles to the leather cover showed that they had occupied this position for some time. Often I have sat on a doctor's examining couch throughout a consulting hour ; and, though many patients gave histories and presented symptoms which indicated the need for thorough examination, they left without any attempt being made to examine them or any arrangements being made for a future examination.

I particularly noted cases where, in my opinion, the history suggested an urgent need for rectal or vaginal examination ; and I had listed over forty such cases before I saw a general practitioner pull on a rubber glove and make the examination, or arrange with the patient to do so at a later date. A small proportion of these people were referred to hospital outpatient departments, on the strength of their history alone ; but the majority received reassurance and local symptomatic treatment.

In fact, under the prevailing conditions of industrial practice, anything approaching a general or complete examination is out of the question ; "examinations" are usually confined to the offending organ and even then are cursory. Certain routine procedures are followed, sometimes almost religiously : throats and tongues are looked at, pulse-rates and temperatures are taken, blood-pressures are recorded on indication, and chests are "listened to," either at the patient's request or for some specific reason. (The process of "listening to" must not be confused with a chest examination : it consists merely in applying the stethoscope to some area readily exposed by unbuttoning a shirt or pulling down an undergarment.) On urgent indication an abdomen may be palpated : I have often seen this done with the patient standing, and I have rarely seen what could be termed a thorough abdominal examination made in an industrial practice.

Once or twice I have seen a doctor, working under these conditions, take a blood sample to send to the laboratory for examination ; but as a rule, when such an investigation is thought necessary, the patient is sent in person to the hospital, without consideration for his convenience or sensitivity.

EFFECTS OF ENVIRONMENT

One could go on listing the shortcomings of general practice in industrial areas ; but it is neither my purpose nor my desire to defame the overworked and often conscientious doctor who has to suffer the indignities of this way of working.

Where these shortcomings are admitted, people are apt to attribute most of them to the volume of work which the industrial practitioner has to handle. This provides a convenient rationalisation of an otherwise embarrassing situation.

There is no doubt that the volume of work *is* too great, but this is merely a secondary factor. If the doctors' surgeries were better from a functional point of view ; if they were equipped at least to some minimum standard ; if a little order were brought into the chaos which characterises the organisation of the average practice (e.g., by employing clerical assistants) ; and if the work of the industrial practitioner were coördinated with that of other medical agencies—then the same volume of work could be handled at a much higher level and with due regard to the safety and comfort of the patient. (As I shall show later, the average industrial practitioner, though he works in close proximity to the great urban medical centres, is more isolated from the benefits these could bestow on him than is his colleague working out in the countryside.)

I found that the working environment of general practitioners in industrial areas was so limiting that their individual capacity as doctors counted for very little. In the circumstances prevailing, the most essential qualification for the industrial G.P., from the standpoint of public safety, is ability as a snap diagnostician—an ability to reach an accurate diagnosis on a minimum of evidence, objective or subjective. The skill attained in this type of diagnosis is sometimes really remarkable, but it very seldom bears any relation to our accepted ideas of "quality" as assessed by academic qualifications or conventional clinical experience. Some of the doctors with least to show in qualifications or hospital experience proved to be the best snap diagnosticians, and therefore the best and safest industrial practitioners, whom I met.

These facts have obviously affected the type of doctor who has entered the jungle of medical practice in industrial areas. Broadly speaking, I came across two types, which one might call the mercenaries and the missionaries. Among the latter are men of outstanding character, sincerity, and occasionally medical ability as displayed by qualifications and experience, who have gone into the industrial areas to "do good." Among the former are some who, by our accepted standards, are judged undesirables.

I saw and worked with some of both of these types and formed the opinion that their environment levels them to a degree where, in effectiveness, there is little to choose between them. In fact, the "mercenary" who is a good snap diagnostician may be of greater value than the "missionary" who cannot match him in this. Under the conditions of industrial practice the "good" doctor has little or no opportunity to exercise his humanistic, psychological, or educational function, which we accept as an essential and integral part of general practice.

Thus in industrial areas medical practice has moved far from the last-century concept of family doctoring ; it has not progressed in terms of modern scientific knowledge ; and it has reached a point where, despite the efforts of the most conscientious individual doctors, it is at the best a very unsatisfactory medical service and at the worst a positive source of public danger. This is no sudden or recent happening, but is the result of long neglect of the important medical and ethical principles to which we so readily pay lip service.

In 1924 Abraham Flexner [1] wrote :

"Less than half a century ago the office of an able urban practitioner consisted of two rooms, one for waiting and the other for consultation. There was little to indicate which was which beyond the ancient tilting haircloth examining chair, the wash basin, . . . a few simple instruments which, used for all sorts of purposes, were never boiled, two or three vials containing mercury or carbolic acid for local applications, and the mantelpiece strewn with proprietary preparations in dust-covered bottles. Urinalysis was employed—practically no other laboratory procedure. The doctor made up his mind on the basis of symptoms and obvious physical indications. Long experience and natural shrewdness sharpened by necessity carried the best of the old family physicians far . . . inability to penetrate beneath the surface constantly forced the practitioner to guess or fumble."

Flexner's description of medical practice in the last decades of the 19th century is almost a perfect word-picture of general practice as I found it in the industrial areas of England in 1949. This section of general practice indeed provides an example of what Mannheim has defined as "non-contemporaneous contemporaneity."

If, in the process of becoming an anachronism, this branch of medicine had retained the ideals and the human elements of the old concepts of family doctoring we might even be able to defend and applaud what has happened ; but it would be dishonest to pretend that it has.

SCOPE OF WORK

To display more fully the pattern of medical practice in industrial areas I must summarise the work done under these conditions.

Diagnosis

With limited time, facilities, and equipment, the doctor attempts to arrive at diagnoses and to refer those patients requiring more skilled attention to a place where such attention can be given. Much of this diagnostic work is empirical and some almost intuitive.

For the most part he deals with people of ages ranging from the late teens to the early sixties—the working section of the community. The school clinics and maternity and child-welfare clinics have relieved him of responsibility for caring, in a comprehensive way, for the school and preschool child, and also for the expectant

1. Flexner, A. Medical Education. London, 1925 ; p. 9.

and nursing mother. While he may attend many patients over sixty years of age, it is more a question of attending than caring for them : the time and the inclination to bring medical skills to bear on the problems of this age-group are sadly lacking.

Therapy

Treatment is even more restricted than diagnosis. Most of it is symptomatic, and nearly all of it is medicinal ; for there is neither time nor opportunity for physical therapy or psychotherapy.

Without access to hospitals, doctors working under these conditions naturally do no major surgery. Most of them do no minor surgery either. It is rare indeed to see a practitioner in an industrial area open an abscess, put in a suture, remove a fingernail, or indeed undertake any procedure requiring sterilisation of instruments.

Midwifery

Before July, 1948, most industrial practitioners had long since yielded all responsibility for midwifery to the midwives and the maternity and child-welfare clinics. The few who continued to dabble in midwifery were mostly considered by midwives and other responsible observers to be a menace, and from what I saw of the antenatal work of some of them I can endorse this opinion.

Minor Laboratory Work

This is almost confined to testing urines for albumin and sugar, and then only on specific indication (e.g., an apparent toxæmia of pregnancy as opposed to routine antenatal test). A microscope is seldom seen among the G.P.'s equipment. Estimations of hæmoglobin and sedimentation-rates, and other simple and useful tests, are seldom done ; though, as I said before, the surgery often contains odd pieces of apparatus, the instruments of such tests.

To analyse the doctor's work beyond this point is scarcely possible at present ; nor, in my opinion, is it necessary. With a problem so crude, greater detail is of little but academic interest. Time-studies, age, sex, pathological, or other breakdowns of the doctor's work are out of the question with medical records either non-existent or so superficial as to be valueless for this purpose.

The important point is that this form of practice constitutes the pattern for most industrial areas, and that the pattern is accepted by doctor and patient alike. It is far away from the ideal of family doctoring on the one hand, and of modern scientific medical practice on the other ; yet it is still wilfully identified with both of these.

Rural Practice

Rural practice is in many ways the antithesis of industrial practice ; and in judging the quality of rural medical care we have to employ different criteria.

SURGERIES

Though built to the same pattern, and functionally little different, the country surgeries I visited were much pleasanter places than their town equivalents. For the most part they were better equipped—though I did see two without an examining couch and others where this was merely an adornment. Moreover, functional imperfections in a rural surgery are less important than the same imperfections in an urban one, where time and efficiency are paramount factors in the quality of the service which can be offered. In fact, premises which would be deplorable under urban conditions may pass as interesting and quaint examples of last-century architecture and custom when they are found, say, in a small south-country village. I saw some surgeries which had served successive doctors for over a century, and they served well enough today, though they might not satisfy an efficiency expert.

In a rural town the doctor's surgery must be considered in association with the cottage hospital, as a combined unit, the one supplementing the other. In isolated rural practice, on the other hand, the doctor's surgery assumes a new importance ; it needs to be well enough equipped to enable him to meet responsibilities and demands which his colleagues nearer centres of civilisation can pass on at a moment's notice. At least by existing standards, the rural-town cottage-hospital combination is nearly always satisfactory (if we exclude the requirements for major operations) ; but the surgery of the isolated country practitioner is as often unsatisfactory in the extreme, and places him, and accordingly his patients, at a serious disadvantage.

I saw this latter point illustrated many times. For example, I have seen a patient sent many miles when a microscopical examination of urine might have confirmed a diagnosis of pyelitis rather than one of appendicitis ; but there was no microscope. Similarly the absence of a microscope necessitates more empirical diagnosis, and consequent empirical therapy, than is desirable, and causes unnecessary inconvenience, expense, and sometimes danger to patients who have to travel to the nearest hospital. The microscope, indeed, is almost indispensable to the isolated country practitioner, yet is seldom included in his equipment ; and other simple things, such as hæmoglobinometers and blood-sedimentation apparatus, are very uncommon. It is, of course, debatable how much the individual practitioner should attempt on his own ; but it is surely fair to expect him to do whatever he is able to do for the convenience and benefit of his patients.

I saw some isolated rural practices which were quite as badly equipped as the worst industrial practices I visited. But in spite of the poorness of these surgeries and equipment, and the question of how a serious emergency would be met in them, it is impossible to assess the quality of such a practice on the same basis as would be appropriate for an urban practice. Not only has the country doctor the time to examine his patients but he also has the time to know them intimately ; and his judgment is usually based on a greater knowledge and a deeper consideration, both of the person and of the ailment, than his city colleagues can compass.

This is not to say that he could not do much better work under better conditions, but rather that the good country doctor can and does overcome the obstacles of bad environment, in terms of surgery and equipment, in a way impossible for the city doctor. Furthermore, the country G.P. is fulfilling a function, in the psychological as distinct from the organic field, in a real way which again is impossible for the city doctor. A rural practitioner, who may only be " fair " so far as organic medicine is concerned, may still qualify as an excellent family doctor.

STANDARD OF WORK

Under the conditions prevailing in rural practice, the quality of the medical care is governed chiefly by the quality of the doctor himself. This is very difficult to assess but not difficult to recognise.

During my study, I met and worked with some men who could be graded, on an absolute standard, as first-class. They were good clinicians, good technicians, and fine humanists. Of the others, the majority, while belonging to the third category, rapidly fell away through fair to bad in the first and the second. Yet, as I have just said, this does not necessarily mean that they were not " good " doctors.

This again brings up the question of criteria. In seeking a sample of " good," " average," and " bad " practices, I found it hard to get people to nominate " bad " doctors in rural areas. There is a tendency to regard the country doctor as " good," if for no other reason than the urge to identify him with our concept of the ideal—the real family doctor. However, in the south, where a more or less random sample was taken,

I was better able to make an unbiased classification of the doctors I visited.

From the strictly technical standpoint many of them were " bad " : though they all had a working knowledge of the use of such modern preparations as penicillin and the sulpha drugs, their knowledge on the whole was out of date. But if the skills they exercised were very limited in any one field, they embraced many fields ; and so long as the man was a good and conscientious observer he was usually a " good " doctor in the circumstances in which he practised.

However, I worked with some who, though regarded as " good " by both the profession and the public, were in fact " bad " in absolute terms. All the men I would put in this category were well qualified from reputable medical schools ; most of them had been in practice for many years and were regarded, more or less, as " the squire." Their chief fault, as I saw it, was that they were not good or thorough observers of either organic or psychological problems, and took no pains to check their impressions and opinions by objective investigation. They worked to a routine and within limits that had long since dulled their curiosity and their sensitivity. For example :

Taking a surgery with a practitioner who enjoyed a high reputation both professionally and publicly, I saw a man come in who was icteric and almost emaciated. The object of his visit was to get a bottle of medicine for his wife. I asked, after he had gone, what was the cause of his strange colour and condition. The answer was " Oh, I don't know, there's nothing much wrong with him ; he's been like that for three years."

At another time a doctor took me to see a case of which he was particularly proud—an old man of sixty-five with a dry gangrenous leg, which had been preserved by keeping the patient in bed for twelve months since the sudden onset of the condition, still undiagnosed. The doctor visited regularly to " dress " the dead appendage, and his attitude was that here was an old man comfortable enough in bed and not requiring any active therapy.

In the same region I spent some days with a young doctor who had only a small number of patients but who tried to give a service satisfying his own high standards. As this practice was very isolated and poorly served by consultant and laboratory services, he had built his own little laboratory and fitted it with apparatus which enabled him to do many things not normally considered part of general practice. He did a lot of microscopy and such tests as blood-sugars, blood-ureas, and clotting-times ; also he had a portable electrocardiograph and other equipment which enabled him to do a most comprehensive job of diagnosis and therapy.

While I am not saying that this should be the model of general practice, or that this man was not taking on too much, I must emphasise that as an individual, looking after 1300 patients, he was exercising a wider range of skills than any other G.P. I have seen, and in my opinion exercising them within the limits of safety. Beyond dispute he was offering a quality of service far above anything his colleagues could offer. The point I want to make is that these colleagues, who had larger practices, enjoyed unassailable reputations, and had no cause for jealousy, regarded this doctor as crazy. In their unqualified opinions he was mad—merely because he endeavoured to exercise to the limit the skills of which he was capable in the interests of his patients. Because of his small practice, and in spite of his excellent work, he was suffering serious financial embarrassment, and has probably by now been forced out of his practice and into some more lucrative field.

I also came across a " group " practice, which had been operating for about eighteen years in a small village. It was run by a group of four—three partners and an assistant. Their surgery was the first and only one I saw which had been carefully planned and built as a separate working unit, and, though they would like to improve on the design, it was far better than any other surgery I visited in Great Britain.

In qualifications and experience the doctors working this group were wholly comparable with their neighbours. But, from the point of view of the patient, the service they offered was vastly superior to anything that could be provided by the surrounding doctors. They ran a highly organised group practice, and by virtue of their good organisation alone they had more time to devote to their work and interests. One was particularly interested in surgery and another in obstetrics, but they were all general practitioners in the full meaning of the term. Their records were better than any others I have seen in England (I still would not say that they were good) ; they employed clerical and nursing assistance ; and they did not share the common opinion that the expense of such assistance was unjustified or could not be carried by a practice of moderate size and income. Their whole attitude of mind was different from that of the average doctor ; they were constantly trying to improve their equipment and to widen their scope of work, and they were interested in children and old people to a degree not usual in the general practitioner.

THE RURAL PATTERN

Enough has been said to illustrate the two points I want to make at this stage :

1. That the whole pattern of practice in rural areas differs greatly from that in industrial areas.
2. That we must apply different criteria when judging the quality of medical care offered by, or possible within, these two types of practice.

For purposes of contrast I summarise the scope of work undertaken by the rural practitioner :

Diagnosis

Rural practitioners often undertake a high level of diagnostic responsibility, though some of them work in the same empirical way as their industrial colleagues and to about the same elementary level. The difference is that in the country the level usually depends on the doctor's choice and is not imposed by his environment.

With reasonable cottage-hospital facilities the rural practitioner can and often does work to much the same level as the consultant physician, with the added advantage that he knows his patients intimately and often over a long period.

He deals with people of all ages—not primarily with the working section of the community. Nevertheless, for the most part he has the same attitude as his urban colleagues towards the medical problems of his elderly or " chronic " patients.

Therapy

The therapeutic responsibility of the rural practitioner is also wide. He seldom limits himself to medicinal treatment. Physical and psychological therapy come well within his terms of reference ; minor surgical procedures are almost a daily routine ; and, where he has access to a cottage hospital, he commonly undertakes major surgery.

Midwifery

Though the trend for many years has been away from general-practice obstetrics, the country doctor still usually does some of the midwifery of his area. From such observations as I was able to make, the average rural G.P. is no obstetric paragon. However, through his association with mother and child he retains an intimacy and a bond which marks him as a family doctor.

Minor Laboratory Work

Again, the amount of minor laboratory work undertaken by the rural G.P. is determined by his own interest rather than by the circumstances which restrict the man in industrial practice. A still significant proportion of country doctors carry their side-bench work beyond casually testing an odd urine for sugar and albumin. Some do quite advanced laboratory work even within the confines of their own surgery.

THE LANCET] GENERAL PRACTICE IN ENGLAND TODAY [MARCH 25, 1950 **561**

The range of work undertaken in different practices is wide ; but it seems clear that the rural practitioner on the one hand still approximates to the ideal of the family doctor, and, on the other, at least aspires to meet the demands of modern science and procedure. It must be said, however, that over a considerable section of rural practice these aspirations do not take us very far, and that, compared with his colleagues in the industrial areas, the rural practitioner must accept a greater measure of responsibility for his own shortcomings. Conversely he is entitled to due respect for his achievements.

In the final analysis present-day rural practice remains an anachronism, though one which has retained many of the virtues of the past.

Urban-residential Practice

Urban-residential practice is dealt with out of turn because, though it is intermediate between the extremes of industrial and rural practice, it is less easily defined in terms of scope or quality. " Good " practices of this type resemble the best of rural practice, and " bad " practices the kind of thing so common in industrial areas ; yet urban-residential practice has certain features which establish a distinctive pattern.

Some of these are superficial—no more than a veneer of sophistication on the crudities of industrial practice. Others are more basic, and quite characteristic. The superficial differences are perhaps the more obvious.

SURGERIES

Take the surgeries, for example. Most of them follow the two-room design of the industrial type, but there is a world of difference in the furnishings, style, and regard for patients' comfort and tastes. A large proportion of these surgeries have been " made over " from the front rooms of a family home in much the same way as the surgeries of the industrial practitioner have been adapted from an erstwhile shop or residence. But I have been in surgeries built by the doctor for the specific purpose, and have been impressed by the fact that they too have usually followed the two-room (waiting-room and consulting-room) pattern. Evidently the belief that two rooms are all that is necessary to run a general practice is firmly rooted in the medical mind. Twice I have met doctors who at some stage were adventurous enough to build themselves three-room surgeries, but who, over the years, have reverted to type and are now working in two and using the third room for storage. There are, of course, exceptions to this rule, and some doctors have built surgeries which are excellent from the functional point of view ; but these are very definitely exceptions. One cannot suppose that the difference in capital outlay required to construct a good as opposed to an unsatisfactory surgery has been the determining factor. The designs must be primarily the result of an unquestioning acceptance of the traditions of the last century and a failure to think about general practice in contemporary and constructive terms.

The waiting-room in an urban-residential practice is in striking contrast to the waiting-rooms in industrial practice ; for the patient with more cultivated taste expects attention to the niceties. Similarly the consulting-room is of a more refined type : the basic " heavy " equipment is more attractive in appearance ; instrument cupboards, containing sometimes quite an extraordinary range of instruments, are usually in evidence ; and equipment for filing records is often an asset to the furnishings. Yet these differences in the two types of practice, impressive though they look, are actually very superficial and often make very little difference to the quality of care offered. Thus, despite the advantage of good filing equipment, I have noticed little significant

difference in record-keeping in the two types of practice. Again, except where in absolute terms he qualifies as a " good " doctor, I have seldom observed that the more abundant equipment carried by the urban-residential practitioner has been put to much significant use. I could cite numerous cases of patients presenting histories indicating the need for ophthalmoscopic examination who have left the surgery without any such examination, though an excellent and expensive ophthalmoscope lay within reach of the doctor ; and in some of the cases already mentioned, where rectal or vaginal examination seemed desirable, the patient was standing within feet of a selection of very fine specula, never called into service.

There is absolutely no cynicism about these remarks. It is perfectly natural that the demand for well-appointed waiting and consulting rooms should lead to their being supplied. But it is important that we should avoid the assumption that if a surgery is attractively appointed it is functionally good, and the further assumption that an apparently good surgery means good medical care. In the course of my study I continually found these assumptions in the minds of people from whom a more objective opinion might have been expected.

I would say that though most of the urban-residential surgeries I visited were better equipped and better appointed, they were functionally almost as unsatisfactory as their industrial-area equivalents.

NATURE OF THE WORK

In urban-residential areas the capacity of the individual doctor has more free play than in industrial areas, but usually less than in the countryside. The few doctors left with hospital privileges have much the same scope of work as the rural practitioner, and may know their patients in much the same way. The majority, however, work under greater pressure and lack these hospital privileges, and on the average they represent a rather unhappy compromise between the two extremes.

The number of patients handled by the urban-residential practitioner is very variable, and an extra 500–600 can reduce the standard of his work much more appreciably than a similar numerical increase will reduce the standard of work of the industrial practitioner.

As local-authority services do not operate to nearly the same extent in these better residential environments, the general practitioner should carry a greater responsibility, for example, in the care of mother and child. But I saw little to suggest that he does so ; and I can only conclude that in these areas the work which is done elsewhere by the local-authority clinics is usually not done satisfactorily or not done at all.

Compared with the industrial doctor, the urban-residential doctor spends a considerably longer time on each patient. But on the whole there seems to be little difference in the time spent on physical examination. There are, of course, exceptions.

The scope of the urban-residential practitioner's work has possibly undergone more change of late years than that of either of the other two groups ; and for this if no other reason it is harder to establish a pattern. The doctor's individual capacity is still reflected in his work, but to an ever-decreasing extent. He has more social contact with his consultant colleagues than doctors have in either of the other environments, but probably no more professional contact.

Urban-residential practice is certainly the most difficult to assess. It represents the transition from the ideal of family practice to the " casualty-clearing station " type of practice seen in industrial areas. While it obviously does not meet all the requirements of medical care, it is more or less immune from the contrary criticisms which can be directed against rural practice on the one hand and industrial practice on the other.

SPECIFIC EXAMPLES OF GENERAL PRACTICE

I shall now describe a few examples of practice under the various environmental conditions, including one or two which illustrate the effect of differences in the number of patients or the history of the practice.

Industrial Practice

I

Two partners and an assistant. Approximately 10,000 patients on the list. No private patients.

This practice, locally classified as " good," had been established for many years and had always had a large " panel " list under the National Health Insurance Act. The district it served was densely populated, and in area no more than a few square miles ; most of the housing was very bad, though some slum clearance had gone on at different times and there were rehousing estates of various dates. The inhabitants were largely engaged in heavy or light industry, the former predominating.

The surgery was on the ground floor of a tenement house and was difficult of access for many patients. It comprised a very small waiting-room, two consulting-rooms, and a dispensary ; and, though the site was unsuitable, it was well equipped compared with most of the other industrial surgeries I visited.

The doctors held morning and evening consulting hours six days a week, two of them working simultaneously in the surgery while the third was out on " calls." The consulting " hour " always extended to two or three hours, and they were seeing anything from 30 to 50 patients each during the consulting period. They employed a lady dispenser, who also acted as telephonist and receptionist and undertook some clerical duties.

An attempt was made to keep a file record, but this consisted mainly of a very few brief notes pertaining to the " really serious illnesses," and such letters and reports as came back from the various hospitals to which patients had been referred. A remarkably large proportion of the record cards which I saw coming out of, and going back into, the files bore nothing more than the patient's name, age, and address.

Two of the doctors undertook domiciliary midwifery ; between them they totalled about 25 cases a year.

On the occasions I attended the surgery, the waiting-room was packed and sometimes patients were standing in the front grounds. I was informed that this was not a heavy period, there being a relative absence of epidemics. The average length of a consultation was three to five minutes, whether it was a new case or a return visit ; a " serious case " or one involving some degree of physical examination would take, perhaps, ten to fifteen minutes.

It is hardly necessary to say that, in such circumstances and working to such a schedule, physical examinations were cursory and were kept to a minimum. Most examinations were made with the patient sitting or standing, and with removal of the least possible amount of clothing. The examining couch was seldom called into use. I never saw vaginal, rectal, or ophthalmoscopic examination attempted, though during my time at this surgery many patients were seen who seemed to me to require one or other of these examinations. In all such cases I asked the doctor and/or the patient whether such an examination had been made at a previous time, and the answer was always No. It must, however, be said that a proportion of these people were sent to hospital for the opinion of a specialist. Indeed in most cases where the brief histories taken, or the examination made, suggested potentially serious organic disease, the patient was referred to an outpatient department. In this particular practice a great number of patients were similarly referred for laboratory and radiological

diagnostic tests. Usually all the doctor wanted was the result of the particular test and not another opinion.

These practitioners undertook the antenatal care of their own patients. This was done in a very loose way. Inquiry was made as to how the patient felt ; blood-pressures were taken only on some specific indication ; samples of urine were brought only occasionally and then examined only if there was some special reason. In the only case of early pregnancy which came in during my stay no attempt was made to make a pelvic or general examination : the patient was told to " come back in a couple of months to be antenataled " and it was left at that. The chief purpose of the visit, so far as both patient and doctor were concerned, seemed to be the supply of certificates for the various benefits accorded to the expectant mother. No antenatal records were kept.

The treatment of the numerous children who were brought in during my time in this practice was similar to that of the adults, but on the least suspicion of serious illness they were referred to a pædiatric clinic at the local hospital.

Though this practice had run a dispensary for many years, the " bottle of medicine " mentality was not highly developed, and indiscriminate prescribing seemed to be at a minimum.

It is often very difficult to assess the legitimacy of claims made for sickness benefits and the like, but I formed the impression that these practitioners erred considerably on the side of leniency. The time and effort required to meet the demands of certification did not seem excessive.

I made a considerable number of domiciliary visits with these doctors. It was always a rush to get through the list, and the same factors as led to cursory examination in the surgery operated in home calls also. Except in special circumstances, three or four minutes sufficed for each visit.

In both surgery and domiciliary work a lack of interest in the non-acute cases was conspicuous—particularly with elderly or " chronic " patients. Though these were visited with scrupulous conscientiousness, it was apparently not thought worth bringing medical skills to bear on their problems. In fact, the over-sixties suffering from any condition resulting in long-continued immobilisation were regarded as more or less hopeless cases, worthy of pity and charity but scarcely of serious medical attention.

The many patients seen who presented themselves obviously for psychological and not for organic reasons were treated with hearty reassurance and quick dismissal.

These doctors had no hospital or nursing-home facilities for their own use. They had no visiting rights at the large general or special hospitals. They knew and were on good terms with the consultants of the district, but saw very little of them. They were very hard-working and conscientious, and, as far as one could ascertain from the limited clinical procedures they undertook, they were good clinicians, at least within the limits set by the type of work they were doing. Certainly they were highly skilled at snap diagnosis.

This was very much the picture in all the " good " industrial practices where the conditions of work were similar. The only absolute difference was that in most of them no midwifery was done. The man who, in terms of qualifications and hospital experience, was the best industrial practitioner I saw working under comparable conditions conducted his practice in just the same way. He was one of a partnership of four. In his company, I did a round which took us to 38 houses between 11 A.M. and 4.30 P.M. (with time off for lunch). There is little need to elaborate on the perfunctory nature of the visits or the effects of such a manner of practice on a man of very high clinical ability. This particular

THE LANCET]   GENERAL PRACTICE IN ENGLAND TODAY   [MARCH 25, 1950   **563**

partnership was the only industrial practice I visited where there was any significant division of the field of work. One partner had taken responsibility for the "old chronics," which not only reduced the load on his colleagues handling "acute" cases but also greatly benefited the old patients.

Throughout the "good" industrial practices visited, premises and equipment were unsatisfactory; record-keeping, at the best, was not good; antenatal work, where done at all, was casual; and the routine work of diagnosis and therapy was limited by time and circumstance much as in the practice I have described.

II

Four partners and two assistants.   Approximately 20,000 patients on the list.

This practice was of fairly long standing, and under the National Health Insurance Act had carried a very large "panel" list. It was in a densely populated area, where light industry predominated and housing conditions were deplorable; whole terraces of houses had been condemned for years, but little in the way of slum clearance had been undertaken. The boundaries of the practice encompassed several square miles, and the total mileage covered by the doctors in the year was large.

The surgery consisted of a small dilapidated waiting-room, three equally small and untidy consulting-rooms, and a kind of cupboard which served as a dispensary (the practice had always done its own dispensing). The consulting-rooms were dirty and ill equipped. There were no examining couches and no apparent means of sterilising anything; indeed, apart from a few rusty and dusty antique instruments, there was no sign of any sort of equipment. Large stock bottles were standing all over the place, and the desk and floor were littered with papers. Only one of the consulting-rooms was equipped with a hand-basin and hot and cold water.

I made my visit during an afternoon consulting hour, and found a queue of people extending about 200 yards up the street, waiting their turn to see the doctors; they were standing packed in the waiting-room and I had to force an entrance. I was made welcome "to see the procession," given a seat and a cup of tea, and invited to stay "as long as I liked." I was told, not without pride, that "we have seen 500 already today"; and I have no reason to doubt it.

During my stay of an hour and a quarter about 120 more patients came in. They were "seen" by three different doctors, who replaced one another with almost bewildering rapidity. No pretence was made at real examination of any of these patients. An occasional temperature or pulse-rate was taken; four or five times a stethoscope was applied to a point somewhere below the thyroid gland and some such utterance made as "ah, a bit chesty."

The bottle of medicine was the sine-qua-non of this practice. One small child came in requesting "a bottle for the lady over the road." He could give no further information, apart from her name and address, which obviously conveyed nothing to the doctor; but he produced a dirty-looking bottle with some dregs in the bottom, and after a glance the doctor prescribed a small something, passed it to the child, and called the next patient. Other patients came requesting "a note for bronchitis" or some similar malady. With no further formality than "name and address?" this was issued and the patient dismissed. "Notes" and "bottles" were asked for by almost everyone seen, and were supplied on request. Almost everyone seemed to have "a slight touch" of something or other; bronchitis most commonly, occasionally pleurisy, once or twice rheumatism, and once measles.

One patient produced his identity card in lieu of his medical card, to be told "this isn't your medical card." He replied without hesitation: "I know that, and I've been using it here for three months. This is the first time you've noticed."

A number of patients, either because their complaints sounded serious, or because their history was suggestive and they looked really ill, were referred to hospital. This procedure seemed to be known as "sending them through."

Around 4 P.M. the queue, still extending well up the street, was broken off and the front door was locked. I was told that sometimes the housekeeper was posted at the back gate "to stop them coming in there," and that "if we did not do this the queue would remain from 9 A.M. to 9 P.M. and we'd never get our visits done."

The visiting-list was made up, and though I did not count the number of visits to be made it was certainly most formidable. When I asked about records, the reply was: "We have no time for that sort of nonsense. However, we have a secretary who comes in two or three days a week, and makes up records from these old prescription pads. Of course she's months behind." These practitioners do a considerable amount of midwifery and, I was informed, "run our own nursing-home." When asked about antenatal work, the senior member of the firm said: "We don't have much time for that sort of thing." Unfortunately I had no opportunity to pay any domiciliary visits with these doctors, or to see their nursing-home.

The doctors themselves seemed intelligent and made no real effort to explain or excuse their way of practice. Obviously the work had been done in this way for a long time, and the method was accepted, by them and their patients at least, as satisfactory or inevitable. The younger members of the partnership with whom I talked had a high regard for their seniors and claimed that they "don't miss much." One of them, who had been in the practice for only about two years, seemed somewhat perturbed by the nature of things; but "it is all that can be done in the circumstances," he said.

I set these two examples of large industrial practice at the upper and lower limits of "ordinary" industrial practice. Doubtless examples could be found that would be better than the example cited as "good," but I did not see them in England. If better practices existed within the industrial areas studied, I fancy I would have been referred to at least one.

III

Single-handed practices.   Small patient-load.

I do not imagine that industrial areas contain many small single-handed practices; but I recall two. Practice A was run by a practitioner who had chosen to work in an industrial area and who limited his list to about 1500 patients, claiming that he could not do justice to more. Practice B was run by a practitioner who had been establishing himself before the war, but on returning from the Services had found his practice almost gone. He had had to begin again to build it up, and when I saw him he had just over 2000 patients. Obviously these two could be called special cases, and so probably could most others which would fall into this group. A few of the doctors would be young and recently started in practice.

Both the men I have mentioned had their surgeries at their homes. In both cases they had adapted two rooms, originally part of the dwelling, to their needs. Both surgeries were reasonably well equipped, that of the elder (practice A) particularly well. His waiting and consulting rooms were comfortably and tastefully furnished, and the latter was well supplied with the essential instruments of practice. This surgery was far more like the type of thing seen in the better-class residential practices than the usual industrial surgery.

The practices covered similar areas, and the housing and economic conditions in the two places were similar, housing being bad in both. There the comparison ceases, and I shall describe them separately. It should be noted that both these practices were locally described to me as " good."

Practice A.—All patients were seen by appointment ; a quarter of an hour was assigned to each, but whenever necessary more time was given. Patients on return visits requiring certificates or repeat prescriptions were asked to come at the beginning of the consulting hour, and 10–12 came within the hour. Physical examinations were thorough, and reasonably full records were kept. During my time in this practice I saw no-one referred for an opinion until the case had been investigated as far as could be done in the surgery. When necessary, urine was examined microscopically, and hæmoglobin and blood-sedimentation rates were estimated. If possible, when further laboratory tests were required, a specimen rather than the patient was sent to the hospital.

Minor surgical procedures, such as the opening of superficial abscesses, strapping of sprains, removal of fingernails, and minor sutures, were done in the surgery. Psychological problems received careful attention and a good deal of time was devoted to them when necessary. No midwifery had been done for some years, but the doctor was about to recommence booking cases, because his income had dropped appreciably since July 5, 1948.

Though this had been a dispensing practice for many years, there was no evidence of the " bottle of medicine " mentality. All claims for sickness and other benefits were examined carefully from the social and psychological angle, as well as the organic.

There was ample time for domiciliary visits, and the same thorough routine was followed in them. The doctor was on friendly terms with many of the consultants in the area, and, though he had no visiting rights in any of the hospitals, he managed to see many of his patients who had been admitted, and often did a round with one or other of the local consultants.

Practice B.—With only a small difference in the patient-load of this practice, the doctor was seeing about three times as many people at each consulting hour and making about twice as many domiciliary visits. There was no appointment system.

History-taking and physical examinations were cursory. The doctor told me that he did not attempt to do rectal examinations, but that if a case was in the least suggestive of cancer of the rectum he sent it straight to hospital. Wherever indicated, some sort of an examination was made of chest or abdomen, and if symptoms or signs were in the least suggestive of possibly serious organic disease the patient was referred to an outpatient department for another opinion. No great effort was made to define the possibilities before referring the patient.

During my stay in the practice no records were made of any of the patients seen. Files and record cards were kept on what were considered important points, but from what I saw of the cards the notes were mainly on prescriptions issued.

This doctor booked confinements and did most of his own antenatal work. He asked about the patient's health since her last visit, took her blood-pressure, and examined her urine. No records of these were kept unless there seemed to be some abnormality. None of the minor surgical procedures undertaken in the other practice were attempted here : the patient was sent to hospital.

Domiciliary visits amounted to 10–15 a day (except during epidemics, when they were considerably more numerous). This allowed the doctor to spend a reasonable time on each visit ; but the actual examinations made were of the same cursory kind as in the surgery.

Rural Practice

I

Three partners. About 10,000 patients. Good cottage-hospital facilities and three small nursing-homes.

This practice, established for almost a century in a town now having 20,000 inhabitants, had never had more than a few hundred on the " panel." There were several other doctors in the town, practising alone or in pairs.

With two senior partners and one junior, the practice served an area extending about ten miles from the surgery, with good road communications. Most of the people were engaged in farming, but the town had some light industry. Both town and countryside could be described as prosperous.

The surgery was a converted shop and residence above the shop. The waiting-room was downstairs and was adequate and well furnished. There was also a dispensary with a dispenser-receptionist working in a small room opening on the waiting-room. Upstairs there were three consulting-rooms, and an office where records were kept and other clerical work was done. A full-time male clerk lived on the premises and worked for all three doctors. The consulting-rooms were spacious and typical of the all-purpose type described previously. They were well equipped both basically and with instruments.

The cottage hospital was run by all the G.P.s in the town, but this partnership made by far the greatest use of it. It was a 50-bed unit, with both medical and surgical wards, a fairly up-to-date operating-theatre, a small department of physiotherapy, an X-ray department, and a small recently acquired department of pathology. This last, though it was not very well equipped, employed a junior and a senior technician and met most of the requirements of the hospital and the local practitioners. Consultant surgeons and physicians visited the hospital once a month, or more frequently if asked.

There were three small private nursing-homes. One was a 5-bed unit for maternity cases only ; the other two had about 10 beds each, and an operating-theatre, and took general medical and surgical cases.

To some extent the three partners divided their routine duties. One did most of the surgery, not only for his own practice but for the district ; one did some " minor " surgery, such as tonsillectomies and appendicectomies ; and the third gave most of the anæsthetics. Night-duty was worked on a roster system and they relieved one another for days off. All three did their own midwifery, which amounted to 10–30 confinements each per year. The surgeon of the partnership undertook most of the abnormal midwifery for the district, including all cæsarean sections.

There were three consulting hours six days a week, with two doctors working simultaneously at each period. No routine appointment system for consulting hours had been introduced, but special appointments would be made when patients had to come a long way, or where transport communications were bad, or when it was expected that consultation and examination would take a long time. About 15–20 patients were seen by each doctor during a consulting " hour," which sometimes lasted as long as one and a half hours ; and as much as twenty minutes would be devoted to a patient needing particular attention. If further or more detailed examination was deemed necessary he was brought back to the surgery by appointment or seen as an outpatient at the cottage hospital. Apart from simple urine-testing, all laboratory tests were done by a technician in the hospital pathology department.

THE LANCET] · GENERAL PRACTICE IN ENGLAND TODAY [MARCH 25, 1950 565

Record-keeping was unsatisfactory, even on the more important and serious cases. Antenatal work was much as described for other practices ; notes were made only if some abnormality was suspected.

At the time I was in this practice domiciliary visits were averaging some 10–20 per day per doctor—mostly nearer the lower figure—and I was told that this was usual except during winter epidemics. At this rate ample time could be devoted to those patients who required detailed attention and examination. Though the domiciliary visits involved a lot of driving, roads were good and farms and houses readily accessible, and the time spent " on the road " did not seem disproportionate.

The cottage hospital was used primarily for surgical cases, but a few beds were allotted to medical ones. Difficult surgery was undertaken by the G.P. surgeon, and as little as possible was " given away " to visiting consultants or sent to the larger city hospitals. I was told that potential cases for cæsarean section were kept in the district and admitted to the local hospital as " emergencies " rather than let the case be " lost " to a city hospital. I was also told that the figure for cæsarean sections in this area is 25 times the average figure for the United Kingdom. I have not verified this statement, but in the circumstances the rate would certainly be well above average.

The whole question of the general practitioner with cottage-hospital facilities, and the " excesses " of surgery performed under these conditions, will be considered later in this report.

Compared with those obtaining in industrial areas, the standards of physical examination in this practice were very good. If they were judged against the disciplines and routines of examination in any reasonable hospital, they would seem superficial and not too satisfactory ; but they were thorough and comprehensive enough to assure that most organic diseases would not be missed. It was evident that the doctors knew the patients intimately and were constantly watching for aberrations from the personal norm ; and within the limits set by time, equipment, and general facilities their routine work would pass as excellent. They paid serious attention to the psychological problems their patients brought them, and though they were obviously not versed in modern psychiatric theory their knowledge of the patients and their understanding of their ways and habits enabled them to give valuable help.

In short, these practitioners were " family doctoring " and at the same time aspiring to relatively good standards in organic medicine. Comparatively, if not in absolute terms, the organisational side of the practice was also good.

II

Three partners. About 10,000 patients. Fair cottage-hospital facilities.

This practice, established for many years in a town now having some 25,000 inhabitants, had also never had more than a few hundred on the " panel." Its general similarity to the one I have just described will at once be noted. Like the other, it was referred to me as a " good " practice, and I am describing it mainly to demonstrate how wide a range of medical conduct is still accepted in professional circles as within this category. The medical people I consulted about my sampling did not classify any rural practice as " bad," though they thought that some of the practitioners were doing too much surgery in the cottage hospitals.

The similarity between this and the previous practice extended beyond the broad description given above : the surgery lay-out, the staffing, and the organisation were all very much the same, except that this practice was less well equipped. But there was a big difference, I thought, in the work of the doctors. Though, like the others, they devoted ten to twenty minutes to each consultation, their standard of physical examination was about the same as I saw in the large industrial practices : it was superficial, restricted to the offending organ, or concerned with some expressed symptom. Similarly, the psychological problems were considered casually and treated by reassurance in a most empirical way. I did not myself see a single laboratory test done in this practice. A bottle of medicine was almost always prescribed, and certification for sickness benefits was generous and unconsidered. The antenatal work I witnessed consisted in a brief chat between the doctor and the expectant mother, without an examination of any kind.

In this particular practice there were many elderly patients, and they were treated with the greatest kindness—but not with medical skill. In the course of domiciliary visits I stood at the bedside of several old people suffering from congestive cardiac failure and receiving, as treatment, continuous bed rest and frequent injections of morphine. One such patient, with a generalised dropsy, had had six months' bed rest and morphine at home without investigation before being admitted to the cottage hospital, where paracentesis abdomini was performed as initial treatment. I also saw several patients who had had a mild " stroke," and they too were bed-ridden and receiving the morphine and reassurance therapy.

Bad as this account sounds, and bad as the practice in fact was, in terms of human kindliness these doctors were doing a job of " family doctoring " which, in contrast with what goes on in the industrial areas, must be considered good. Furthermore, at the more leisurely pace of work, and with some personal knowledge of their patients, I believe they were doing at least an equally good job of organic diagnosis, except for the elderly. Locally, their ability was highly regarded, primarily because they could open an abdomen and remove an acute appendix or untwist a torsion of the ovary ; and they were well liked because they were essentially kind and human.

THE VILLAGE DOCTOR

The above type of country-town cottage-hospital practice is almost as distinct from isolated individual rural practice as it is from industrial areas. In many remote areas the country doctor has not moved very far from the horse-and-buggy days ; he has learned to use some of the new drugs such as penicillin, and may have caught up on a few new techniques ; but essentially he is comparable in most respects to the old family doctor of the last century.

His surgery has often served successive doctors for many decades, and sometimes there has been little change in, or addition to, his equipment over the same period. Occasionally you find the young doctor (or once young doctor) who has started practising in a quiet country village and who has set about revolutionising the way of practice and bringing modern medicine to the villagers ; after a time these doctors usually strike a happy compromise between scientific zeal and human relations, and perhaps represent the very best of general practice.

In this realm the doctor is the absolute autocrat, and what he does and how he does it is no more and no less than a reflection of his personal capacity. So a description of this type of practice in any detail would amount to no more than a description of a number of individual men. I shall later say something about the problems which arise from such practices ; and I must point out at this stage that many of them (some enjoying excellent reputations) are so badly equipped as to be quite unable to meet a serious emergency, even by way of offering satisfactory first-aid. This in no way alters the fact that the doctors running them are often first-class family doctors. We see again how hard it is to equate the dictates of modern medicine with the essential humanism of our concept of general practice.

Urban-residential Practice

I

One doctor. About 2000 patients. Access to two small nursing-homes.

This practice, about twenty-five years old, had been run by the practitioner for fourteen years, and he had never taken " panel " patients. It was one of the few I visited where the surgery had been built for its purpose, and there were three rooms, though the third had not been used (except for storage) for many years. The waiting-room was commodious, well furnished, and altogether pleasant. The consulting-room was well laid out and well equipped.

The doctor employed no clerical or nursing assistance, but he worked to an appointment system, kept fairly good records, and displayed much better organisational ability than is usual. Appointments were set at quarter-hour intervals, but if half an hour or more was needed to complete a consultation and examination this time was taken. Physical examination was thorough, and during my stay in this practice clinical laboratory tests were undertaken whenever indicated. They were done at the local hospital, but the doctor was having increasing difficulty about this because he had lately lost his place on the hospital staff. Similarly, he had been accustomed to doing his own minor surgery at the hospital, and as his private surgery was not equipped for this purpose he now had to send patients, whom previously he would have had no hesitation in treating himself, to another doctor.

This practice provided an excellent example of the really good doctor who is suffering in every respect from the curtailment of his terms of reference. Through his past association with the hospital, he knew intimately, and was on excellent terms with, his consultant colleagues, and this long association stood him in good stead after his exclusion from the hospital staff. He also knew his patients intimately and was at great pains to handle their psychological problems as well as possible ; but at the same time he tolerated no abuse of his services and was certainly not burdened by " silly " claims on his time. He undertook no major surgery at all, but he did a good deal of midwifery and gave thorough attention to expectant mothers throughout pregnancy.

Within the present concept of individual general practice, the work here was as good as one could hope to see. But it was being done under increasing difficulties.

II

One doctor. About 2500 patients. Access to small local hospital and nursing-homes.

This long-established practice, run by the same doctor for the past dozen years, had had about 300–400 patients under National Health Insurance. The consulting-room and waiting-room were adapted from the two front rooms of the residence, and their arrangement gave no guarantee of privacy to either the patients or the doctor's family. Both rooms were tastefully and comfortably furnished, but the chaotic state of the consulting-room made smooth and efficient work very difficult. It was poorly equipped and no pretence was made of keeping records. There was no appointment system, and consultations involved a minimum of physical examination. A considerable amount of dispensing was done, and a bottle of medicine was the usual termination of a consultation.

The doctor had access to the local hospital, but he did not seem to take any great advantage of this and made very little use of the laboratory service, though

he sent many patients for radiography. He did no midwifery and apparently had very little to do with the children of the area.

Comparing this practice with the previous one, the bigger demand for service was out of all proportion to the additional 500 patients on the list. The doctor worked really hard in his endeavour to meet this demand —proportionately much harder than the first doctor. But the necessity for this hard work arose from his failure to exercise reasonable discipline with his patients. Though the two practices were both nominated as " good," the first was in fact well above the average of the practices of this type which I studied, while the second was below the average.

Symptoms and Causes

An account of some of the patients who passed through surgeries I visited would make quite dramatic reading. I could list many who gave histories suggestive of malignant disease or other obvious and readily diagnosable conditions, but who left, bearing a bottle of medicine, without having had any physical examination ; and I could tell some very sad stories of people dying in unnecessary discomfort for want (in my opinion) of a little elementary medical skill. However, I do not believe that such stories, however striking in themselves, would contribute anything to the analysis or solution of the problems of general practice. When an individual error is pointed out, the usual reply is " we can all make mistakes." This is certainly true in general practice, and the individual mistake pales into insignificance beside the predisposing factors which make serious mistakes not only possible but in some circumstances highly probable. I have concerned myself throughout with these causes and predisposing factors and not with collecting examples of errors. I regard the errors as merely symptoms of the chronic illness of general practice today.

It would be foolish, however, to examine general practice in a vacuum, and before I try to summarise its present state I must say something about the relationship of this branch of medicine with other agencies of medical care.

THE GENERAL PRACTITIONER, THE HOSPITAL, AND THE SPECIALIST

It is difficult to say very much about the general practitioner's relation to hospital and specialist services ; for, except in a remote way, he has little to do with either.

He has no direct access to the larger institutions and sees little or nothing of the people who work in them. When he refers a patient he does so either by telephone or with a written introduction outlining the case-history and stating his own opinion. In due course he gets back a written summary of the consultant's views and suggestions, or, if the patient has been admitted for treatment, a statement of the principal things that have been done, with advice about further management.

His other line of communication with the specialist is through domiciliary consultations ; but the average practitioner has few of these. Some I have talked with have as few as one or two a year, and I should think that ten or twenty would be quite a high figure.

The degree of liaison between practitioner and specialist varies from place to place. It is least in the industrial areas—i.e., in those practices closest to the large hospitals—and seems to be greatest in upper-middle-class residential areas. Of course, before the introduction of the National Health Service Act, domiciliary consultation was largely a function of the patient's ability to buy the service, and it will be interesting to note what happens now that it can be had by all. Such observations as I was able to make on this point will be discussed

THE LANCET]   GENERAL PRACTICE IN ENGLAND TODAY   [MARCH 25, 1950   567

when I come to consider the effects of the Act on general practice.

In some places practitioners and specialists move more nearly on the same social plane, which undoubtedly brings them into closer professional contact also. This was particularly noticeable in a relatively small yet highly developed northern city which I visited. There the G.P.s and the specialists are often products of the same school and are not infrequently of about the same vintage. While one may have achieved specialist status and the other has remained a G.P., they have retained mutual respect and friendship, and this is reflected in their professional relations. The same observation applies to Scotland.

In larger cities one would expect to find that at the periphery of the town, where there are large secondary hospitals, the relations between the practitioners in the area and the specialists on the hospital staff would be good; but I have not found this to be the case. Practitioners will often completely by-pass the local hospital (even when it has a good reputation and is well staffed) and send their patients longish distances to see the men they "know." The "knowing" may have been ten or twenty years ago, but loyalties and personal sentiment often seem to outweigh objective judgment. Circumstances such as this certainly do nothing to improve the liaison or relations between G.P. and specialist on a local basis.

Actually the rural G.P. often has more contact with specialists than his city colleagues do, because the specialists periodically visit the country hospitals.

I met one hospital superintendent who used to hold Sunday meetings for the G.P.s who worked in the area round his hospital. He claimed that the attendances and results were good, and knowing the man and his reputation I fully believe they were. A few others say they have tried the same thing, but the attendances and response of the G.P.s were so disappointing that the venture was dropped. Intermittent meetings of medical societies seem to be only as successful as the organising ability and leadership of the local chairman or secretary make them. The many G.P.s with whom I have talked demonstrate a fairly constant lack of interest in this sort of thing.

In brief, I find it hard to imagine any circumstances which would more effectively isolate the general practitioner from the specialists and the hospital services than the circumstances now prevailing in most of the areas I visited.

THE GENERAL PRACTITIONER AND LOCAL-AUTHORITY HEALTH SERVICES

In whatever region or district I worked, I made a point of seeing the medical officer of health, and, whenever possible, of talking with representatives of the various branches of local-authority services—doctors, midwives, nurses, and health visitors. I also saw some examples of their work. However, I was not making a study of local-authority services as such, and my attention was directed to the relationship of the local authority with the general practitioner.

In practical terms it is fair to say that such a relationship hardly exists. Often there is a mutual animosity and distrust. The idea that the local-authority services are complementary to the work of the G.P. is, in my opinion, theoretical; in fact these services are substitutes for some of the work which was once his responsibility but has long since passed from his hands.

The one possible exception to this rule is the home nursing service. The doctors are ready enough to use the nurse to give injections, to do dressings, to give enemas, and to perform other routine nursing tasks; but even so it is rather a one-way business. Except in country districts, I met very few doctors who knew their nurses or had anything to do with them beyond telephoning instructions for them to go to such and such an address and do this or that thing.

Before July 5, 1948, the midwifery and maternity and child-welfare services had in many areas relieved the G.P. of almost all responsibility for conducting confinements or taking an interest in the health and welfare of the normal mother and child. There is practically no two-way communication between the clinic and the practitioner. The clinic doctor or the midwife will inform the G.P. of any abnormalities they discover; but the practitioner seldom seems to give any information to them, or to trouble himself about what goes on at the clinics, even where his own patients are concerned.

More than once I have seen a mother come into the doctor's surgery carrying in her arms a baby three or four months old, and this was the first intimation he had ever had that the lady had so much as been pregnant.

So far as I can ascertain, efforts made to use the G.P. as a part-time worker in the maternity and child-welfare clinics have met with little success.

Some of these issues were highlighted when the Act came into operation. The uneasy equilibrium which had been established between the G.P. and the local authority was disturbed as soon as the question of certain remuneration for maternity services was raised. The doctors, who had yielded a large measure of responsibility to the midwives, now sought to re-establish themselves. They claimed that, as they were licensed to practise midwifery, they were therefore the right people to be responsible for confinements—though very many of them had not done obstetric work for years. The final compromise by which practitioners were reclassified into two classes—those worth £5 5s. and those worth £7 7s. per confinement—speaks for itself.

All the midwives, local-authority doctors, and consultant obstetricians with whom I have spoken expressed the hope that the G.P.s who are now booking midwifery cases will leave the actual work to the midwives and clinics. Many doctors are doing this, but at the same time these incidents have upset the midwives considerably, and, I am told, have had bad effects on midwife recruitment. Certainly they have not improved relations between doctor and local authority.

Many of the same remarks apply to the relationship of the G.P. and the school doctor; but unless financial issues intrude, as they have done in the midwifery services, the present equilibrium is unlikely to be disturbed.

To the average practitioner the health visitor seems to be an enigma. He regards her with something between suspicion and cynicism, and I have not heard of a G.P., on his own initiative, using the services of a health visitor. Admittedly health visitors are more than fully occupied meeting the demands of the tuberculous patients and "new" mothers; but this is not the reason for the doctor's lack of interest in them or for his not seeking their assistance.

I must repeat that the local-authority services, instead of complementing the work of the general practitioner, have in fact assumed almost complete responsibility for some of the work that was once his concern.

THE STATE OF GENERAL PRACTICE : A SUMMARY

1. General practice is a term without specific meaning or definition. There are three distinct patterns, which are determined principally by social environment. These are :

> General practice in industrial areas.
> General practice in urban-residential areas.
> General practice in rural areas.

2. The three patterns have evolved from a common parent—the family doctor of last century. Their evolution has been largely a process of adaptation to the growth and development of other medical services, such as those provided by hospitals and specialists. This process has resulted in the decline rather than the progressive evolution of general practice, and in wide departure from both the idea and the ideal of family doctoring.

3. There are no objective standards for general practice and no recognised criteria by which such standards might be established.

4. The reputation of general practice has been maintained through a continued identification with the idea and ideal of family doctoring ; but, except in certain circumstances, this reputation will no longer stand up to examination.

5. As a result of the process of adaptation, and the failure to establish and maintain standards, general practice is now worst in close proximity to large hospital and clinical centres and improves in both scope and quality almost in proportion to the distance away from those centres.

6. It follows that the worst elements of general practice are to be found in those places where there is the greatest and most urgent demand for good medical service—i.e., in areas of dense population.

7. The working conditions (surgeries and equipment, organisation and staffing) of many general practices are unsatisfactory. Some are bad enough to require condemnation in the public interest.

8. In some cases—particularly in industrial areas—the working conditions are so bad as to override the abilities and skills of the individual doctor. They tend to reduce the work of both good and bad doctors to a common level.

9. Many doctors have been isolated from hospital facilities and are now working under conditions which make useless much of their elaborate and expensive training, and negate the disciplines taught in hospital and medical school. Some conditions of general practice are bad enough to change a good doctor to a bad doctor within a very short time. These very bad conditions are to be found chiefly in industrial areas.

10. Rural practice represents the last outpost of real family doctoring, and in some respects it has gained more from modern medical knowledge and techniques than urban practice.

11. The over-all state of general practice is bad and still deteriorating. The deterioration will continue until such time as the province and function of the general practitioner is clearly defined, objective standards of practice are established, and steps are taken to see that these standards are attained and maintained.

III. GENERAL PRACTICE AND THE NATIONAL HEALTH SERVICE ACT

DIRECT IMPLICATIONS OF THE ACT

The National Health Service Act has made large and fundamental changes in both hospital and specialist services, and has considerably altered the medical responsibilities of local authorities. It has done little, in any direct or immediate way, to upset the status quo of general practice.

By extending National Health Insurance to cover 100% of the population, instead of the 40% previously covered, it has suddenly thrown a greater load (in terms of volume) on the existing structure of general practice, and by introducing new techniques for remunerating the doctors it has caused a redistribution of income within the profession. But neither of these things implies any basic or direct change in the nature of general practice.

THE GREATER LOAD

It is very difficult to assess the effects of the increased volume of work on any particular practice, or even its scale. It is certainly not possible to generalise about the over-all effects of this increase on the quality of medical care in Britain.

The weight of the patient-load depends, of course, not only on the number of patients registered with a doctor but also on the demands these patients make ; and a great deal has been made of the increase in these demands since medical care became free to the patient. On this I have collected a lot of varied opinions, but very little in the way of actual data.

I tried to correlate what was happening in hospital outpatient departments with what was happening in general practice. I thought that hospital figures for periods before and after July 5, 1948, would provide some sort of index of what was going on in general practice. But the figures were not available, and to dig them out of hospital records would have been a long and formidable job. Absolute figures, not broken down into new and return patients and into the various branches of work, are of little value here ; but, for what they are worth, those I did see indicated no significant increase in the volume of people attending outpatient departments, and this finding was usually supported by hospital superintendents, consultants, and resident staff.

Opinions collected from the same sources, when they seemed to be considered opinions, suggested that the medical character of the cases coming into outpatients had not materially altered since the beginning of the service. Considerable fuss was made about the time taken up in measuring people for appliances, but this seemed to be a matter of petty annoyance rather than serious grievance.

Opinions as to the increased demands on their time and effort since the beginning of the new service were also collected from all practitioners whom I visited. Almost without exception they said that, while they were seeing considerably more patients in the surgery (they estimated the increase at anything from 10 to 40%), their domiciliary work remained much as before. They generally agreed that in this regard the public were being very considerate, the chief complaint being of late requests to visit. Night work had not increased. Some doctors, indeed, expressed anxiety at the reluctance of patients to call them out in potentially serious cases, and one or two quoted examples of catastrophe narrowly averted.

Almost all spoke of the increased demands for spectacles, for appliances of various types, for drugs and dressings which the patient would previously have bought for himself without consulting the doctor, and for certificates. My own impression, based on all the practices I visited, was that so far as consumption of the doctor's time was concerned it was again a case of petty annoyance. The practitioners who complained most vigorously were usually those who took the line of least resistance and met almost all requests, without protest or discussion, and irrespective of the merits of the case. One doctor used to sign batches of forms certifying the need for ophthalmic tests, and put them on the waiting-room table for patients to help themselves. I saw very few who made any pretence of examining a patient's eyes, and I saw none make a physical or ophthalmoscopic examination before issuing a certificate for eye-testing. Requests for appliances of all types were usually dealt with by immediately issuing a note referring the patient to a hospital department where he could be fitted ; I never saw a G.P. " waste " his time by carefully examining before referring.

This whole question of " patient abuse " is mostly a matter of speculation. The patient's reason for consulting a doctor is his own anxiety, which nobody else may be able to assess. Nevertheless the intensity of anxiety is largely governed by understanding of its causes, and the person with the most external control over it is the doctor.

Whenever a doctor has had a practice for any length of time, and has exercised a reasonable educational and disciplinary function, he is not a victim of patient abuse ; the amount of this he suffers from is almost directly proportional to his laxity in these regards. It is interesting to contrast the current attitude of the doctors in Britain, where " patient demand " is probably now at its peak and where practitioners are beginning to appreciate the advantages of (even partial) emancipation from " patient blackmail," with that of the doctors in New Zealand, who have long since passed through this phase. I shall refer to this again in the appendix on New Zealand.

The demand for service is intimately tied up with the doctor's personal behaviour. I saw many practices where the doctor contended that the demand was very little greater than before July 5, 1948. I saw others where, though there had been little or no increase in the number of patients covered by the practice, the demand had increased so much that the quality of the work was suffering.

Apropos of this, I met a number of doctors, running practices which before the Act were mainly composed of panel patients, who were actively refusing to keep on the " good paying patients " of former days unless they would come on their N.H.S. list. The doctor's attitude was usually expressed something like this : " I didn't mind wasting my time with these people before the service started, but they're not worth it any more." Various inferences can be drawn from this, but they hardly need elaborating.

I met one practitioner who had had several years' hospital experience before going into general practice, enjoyed a considerable reputation in professional circles, and had many doctors' families on his list. The rest of his practice was 80% industrial and 20% " private," the private part being made up of schoolteachers, clerical workers, skilled artisans, and the like. From July 5, 1948, he kept careful records of the demands for service that patients in the various groups made on him. In the first nine months of the new service the ratio of demand by members of doctors' families, " private " patients, and industrial patients was about 3 : 2 : 1.

Another doctor had built up a large partnership; commencing from humble origins in an industrial centre, he had finished up with a small and select practice of " good paying patients " in a high-class residential area. There were fewer than 2000 on his books and the financial returns were good. Soon after the introduction of the service, this man closed his practice and " retired" to the industrial part of the partnership, taking on a list of about 4000.

I cite these two cases to illustrate the difficulty of estimating, either in absolute or in comparative terms, the increase of work brought by the Act, or the doctor's reactions, private and expressed, to the new circumstances. The size of the doctor's list is not a good index of what is actually happening, though of course in the upper ranges (3500 and over), with conditions of practice as they are, there is no disputing that the load is grossly excessive.

The increased load, whatever its weight and nature, has clearly demonstrated points of basic weakness in the present structure of general practice. For these weaknesses the National Health Service Act is not responsible. Blame rests on the service only in so far as it has failed to provide the means of reinforcing general practice, so that it can take the new load.

REMUNERATION

I hesitate to enter the controversy on ways and means of remunerating the doctor. All sorts of extravagant statements have been made about the intrinsic evils of the capitation system of payment. The greatest tangible evil is the fact that it puts a premium on quantity rather than quality of work. It penalises the man with a small practice doing very good work, and it pays handsomely the man with a big list, however bad his work may be. But neither here nor in New Zealand have I seen any acceptable evidence that it operates to the detriment of the doctor-patient relationship.

It is too early to say whether the various devices, such as mileage-rates, special inducement payments, and basic salaries will successfully minimise or close the gap between quantitative and qualitative reward. In any case, we should recognise that the alteration in the method of payment has not altered the structure of general practice.

The desire of the doctor to relate the size of his income, and the manner in which it is received, to " patient benefit " has led to frightful confusion. It has complicated both political and professional issues and has obscured more fundamental considerations.

INTERFERENCE ?

The establishment of executive councils as the bodies responsible for general-practitioner services could be the means of interfering with the manner of general practice or of limiting the doctor's autonomy. I found no evidence that the councils were operating in this way. All those I visited regarded their function as purely administrative.

I always asked the doctors I met or worked with whether there was any sign of interference with their clinical freedom. Only one claimed that there was, and he showed me a circular, sent out by his executive council, which said : " It is considered that all cases of ringworm of the scalp should be referred in the first instance to specialist skin clinics." This was signed by the clerk of the council. Almost certainly the suggestion, or " directive " as the doctor called it, had its genesis at a higher level than the executive council. The doctor objected not to the idea as such but to the way in which it had been put forward, and to the precedent set. He argued that if he could be told what he should do about ringworm of the scalp he could similarly be told about the rest of his work. I agree with him, and I was surprised that many other doctors I saw, who had received the same memorandum, did not draw attention to it. Probably many of them had not read it. However, this was the only instance of direct clinical interference that any doctor gave me.

The chief direct implication of the Act for general practice lies in the provision made for developing health centres. But this is a matter for the future rather than the immediate present, and I shall consider it separately.

INDIRECT IMPLICATIONS OF THE ACT

The changes just considered are responsible for many of the teething troubles of the new service. It may be hoped that time and experience will provide remedies. But while there is little doubt that the present emotional tensions will subside fairly quickly, there is no assurance —indeed no real hope—that sound solutions will be found for these problems unless a great deal of thinking and a good deal of fact-finding is undertaken.

For the future of general practice the indirect implications of the Act are much more important than the direct ones, and chief among them is the new emphasis given to hospital and specialist services.

I have already given my opinion that :

1. The G.P. surgeon is the chief target in what I term the "attack" on general practice, and there is a tendency to extend the case against him into other provinces of the G.P.'s activity.

2. Up to the present, the development of hospital and specialist services, far from assisting the G.P. to do better work, has depressed both the scope and quality of his work.

I am not suggesting that it is impossible to increase both the amount and scope of hospital and specialist services and simultaneously to upgrade the G.P.; but there is no sign that the new service is going to bring about this desirable end. On the contrary, there is some indication that it is worsening the present unsatisfactory state of affairs.

As at present conducted, the upgrading of the smaller hospital units implies exclusion of general practitioners from the staff; it further implies the employment of many junior specialists, often with no experience of general practice; and it closes the already half-shut door on the G.P.'s chance of entrance into the realm of the specialist. I have just been told of two hospitals upgraded in this way, with exclusion of the G.P. obstetricians of the area. The reason advanced for such exclusion is of course that the G.P. is not the proper person to do midwifery; and similar arguments are brought against the G.P. surgeon, the G.P. E.N.T. man, the G.P. anæsthetist, and in fact any G.P. who shows a particular interest, and attempts to develop a particular skill, in almost any branch of medicine. So long as the general practitioner's province and function is undefined, he is in no position to defend himself against those who would constrict it further.

I met a number of G.P.s, of long experience and real ability, with well-established practices, who had sons either in medical school or recently graduated. These men told me that they had planned to retire relatively early and allow their sons to succeed to the practice; but they had now given up these ideas and were encouraging their boys to seek a different kind of life in one of the specialties. They were moved to this decision not by financial dissatisfaction or fears of bureaucratic controls, but because they foresaw limitation of the scope of the G.P.'s work and responsibility.

CHILDREN

Compared with the other specialties, which concern themselves only with anatomical or physiological parts of the body, the newer specialties of pædiatrics and geriatrics bite more deeply into general practice, because they assume responsibility for whole age-groups of society.

Pædiatrics, the longer and more firmly established of the two, has gained much ground in recent years. As a new and socially conscious group, the pædiatricians have made valuable contributions to both the medical and the social welfare of children, and in a lesser degree to that of mothers. But, unlike most other specialists, the pædiatrician does not confine himself to the more difficult parts of his subject. In fact nothing seems to be too menial for him. Child health, infant feeding, and minor ailments, in which the G.P. has shown a conspicuous lack of interest, have captured the pædiatrician's imagination and have all been drawn into his net. Apart from the obstetrician, he is probably the only practising doctor who can claim to have an active interest in preventive medicine.

No-one would argue that there is no place for pædiatrics, but it is a moot point whether the pædiatrician should take so much of the responsibility for the general medical care of a whole age-group, thus further fractionating the continuity of care and relieving the G.P. of yet another part of his duties. I have observed the work in several pædiatric clinics and have been struck by the large proportion of the specialist's time which is taken up with minor matters which a good G.P. should be fully capable of handling. I would estimate these minor cases at something like 50% of those I saw passing through the clinics. In New Zealand, for example, where midwifery and what one may call the lower strata of pædiatrics form the very basis of general practice, these 50% would never get near a clinic or a specialist pædiatrician, and it is my firm opinion that the mothers and children are better off because of this.

Often I was struck by the anxiety caused to the mother by a clinic visit—I refer here to hospital outpatient clinics, not to local-authority maternity and child-welfare clinics—and also by the failure of the pædiatrician either to appreciate this anxiety or to give time to allaying it. When working in G.P.s' surgeries I was similarly impressed by the obvious anxiety caused by the suggestion of a visit to the hospital pædiatrician, and even more by the anxious state of some of the mothers returning from such visits. Usually this anxiety seemed to be accepted by the doctor as a normal part of the procedure; and again little was done to allay it.

This problem of the creation or fixation of anxiety is not peculiar to pædiatrics. I think I hardly ever sat through a consulting hour without witnessing a case where anxiety had either been created or intensified by a visit to a hospital outpatient department. For this if no other reason, the aim of any good medical service should be the minimum use of hospital outpatient departments compatible with good medical care. Yet the trend seems to be in the opposite direction.

I visited one sick children's hospital where, though the bed capacity had not changed for ten years, the medical staff had increased by 300%, and the vast majority of these doctors were engaged on routine and not research work. I also worked with some of the G.P.s in the environs of this hospital. The best of these could obviously have handled capably many of the problems which they referred almost automatically to the pædiatrician. When asked about specific cases they had referred and the reasons for referral, the answer was always the same : "The pædiatrician is there to be used. Why should we assume the responsibility for the children ?"

Thus the mere existence of the pædiatrician impels even the good G.P. to use his services. If the existing demand for pædiatricians is going to be taken as a measure of the real need for them, the figure reached is certainly going to be excessive, and ultimately the general practitioner, in towns, will be relieved of all responsibility for the care of children.

OLD PEOPLE

The position as regards geriatrics is somewhat different, though some of the same considerations apply. The problem of long-term illness in an ageing population has become very important. The G.P.'s attitude and attention to what he calls his "old chronics" is well known and has been mentioned already.

But is it certain that this problem will be best solved by having a new team of specialists, the geriatricians, and much more institutional care ? At present, because of the indifference of the G.P. to the illness of old age, it looks superficially as though geriatric units and more geriatricians are the logical, if not the only, solution. Further force is given to this argument when one considers the way in which "chronics" have been dumped on general hospitals and have lingered there indefinitely, occupying beds needed for acute illness and putting up maintenance costs.

I studied the situation in a county where the population is ageing rapidly because the young people have been drifting to the cities. Environmental conditions,

THE LANCET]   GENERAL PRACTICE IN ENGLAND TODAY   [MARCH 25, 1950 571

as represented by housing and possibly nutrition, were relatively good in this area, and there was an excellent geriatric hospital surrounded by rural practitioners, who in my estimation are the best type of G.P.s. But I was unimpressed by the attention given to the old people of the community. Working with doctors within a few miles of the geriatric hospital, I found that they knew little or nothing of its work. The contrast between the handling of a case (say a paraplegic, an arthritic, or a cardiac failure) by the G.P. and by the people in the hospital was most striking.

At first, therefore, one was inclined to say that here, in the specialised hospital, was the answer to many of the problems of old age. But on reflection it was evident that much of the benefit obtainable there could be obtained at home if only the general practitioner would exercise his medical skills on his old patients. The efforts of the hospital to convey this to the practitioners of the area had met with little success.

The important point is that, if geriatric units could be used as an instrument for educating the G.P., and if the emphasis could be put on G.P. home care rather than on specialist-hospital care, the present perspective would appreciably change, and we should need to reconsider our ideas on hospital development for the care of old people. That this could in fact be done is in my opinion beyond question ; but the work of the units would need to be oriented in this direction. Failing such action, it is almost inevitable that the success now being achieved in geriatric units will sooner or later receive the recognition it so well deserves and will set an institutional pattern for the care of the " chronic " and aged sick.

THE THREAT TO GENERAL PRACTICE

The socially conscious attitude of the pædiatricians, and latterly the geriatricians, when contrasted with the usual attitude of other branches of curative medicine, has justified their claims to work which normally would not be thought to require specialists. While this socially conscious attitude of mind is to be applauded, the consequences of making new specialties on the basis of whole age-groups of society should be watched very closely.

The current growth of pædiatrics and geriatrics represents another attempt to compensate for deficiencies in general practice in terms of more specialist and hospital care. This trend has been going on for a long time ; but if it continues it is bound to result in over-compensation, unnecessary expense, further dehumanising of medical care, and ultimately the elimination of the general practitioner as a responsible person.

The greatest single threat to the future of general practice is the gap between the general practitioner and the specialist. This gap has been widened by the impetus given by the Act to hospital development, and the simultaneous neglect of general practice as an issue of policy.

ADMINISTRATIVE AUTHORITIES AND THEIR RELATION TO GENERAL PRACTICE

THE REGIONAL HOSPITAL BOARD

At this early stage in the history of the new service it is easy to be too critical of deficiencies and weaknesses, many of which are unavoidable and will be ironed out. It is equally easy to be too tolerant and to overlook major faults which might be corrected now but which otherwise will soon be firmly fixed.

The establishment of regional hospital boards, and the granting of the powers vested in them, is probably the most revolutionary feature of the whole Act. The difficulties of staffing these boards and the various committees and subcommittees which work under them,

the difficulties of reaching a satisfactory compromise between central and peripheral control, and all the problems which arise from the assumption of new powers by new people strange to them, call for tolerance in comment and patience while early mistakes are overcome.

But the failure to provide a link between the regional hospital boards (responsible for hospital and specialist services) and the executive councils (responsible for general-practitioner services) cannot be classified as an initial or experimental error, and the lack of such a link must be regarded as a primary and serious defect in the structure of the service. The idea that members common to the two kinds of body might form the necessary liaison is not supported by the happenings to date.

The responsibility for this state of affairs rests mainly with the executive councils and others connected with general-practice policy who could take the initiative in defining the rôle of general practice in an integrated medical service. But it is hard to see how the regional hospital people can do their job properly unless they too interest themselves in this fundamental issue. Unfortunately none of the hospital-board members or executives I interviewed showed either a particular interest in, or understanding of, the problems or significance of general practice. They seemed to regard administration of hospital and specialist services as a separate task not concerning, or concerned with, the general practitioner. I do not know of any hospital board which has asked either an executive council or any other body for a statement of policy on general practice ; nor do I know of such a statement being drawn up and tendered spontaneously.

Thus hospital and specialist requirements are being worked out with no real regard to the present state, or the future development, of general practice. I saw a good example of this when I visited two hospitals, of similar size and type, which had been included in a previous hospital survey and had lately been assessed for staff and equipment. One of them worked in association with a long-established group practice and the other in association with a number of doctors working independently. The work that was being done by the group completely altered the requirements of the first of these hospitals ; yet nobody official had ever visited the group or taken any account of the things that were being done, or could be done, by it. Even in situations like this, where the whole history and development of the hospital had been in the hands of the general practitioner, the future of the hospital now seems to be considered as something apart from him. This is an extension of the attitude which has prevailed in larger hospitals for a long time—i.e., that the general practitioner has no place in hospital work and therefore merits no direct consideration in hospital planning and development.

The senior administrative medical officers hold, at least for the time being, the key position in the activities of the hospital boards. All those I met were either ex-public-health men or ex-members of the staff of the Ministry of Health. From the standpoint of administration this is probably the best background they could have ; but from the point of view of medical-care policy, particularly general-practitioner services, it is probably the worst.

Whenever general practice came up for discussion, they drew attention to the surgical crimes of the G.P. working in a cottage hospital. Most of them expressed their determination to eliminate the G.P. surgeon. This seemed to be their focal point for thinking about general practice. Their attitude to the problems presented by industrial practice was one of resignation to the inevitability of that sort of thing, of hopelessness of doing anything about it at its source, and of consequent acceptance of the need to compensate for it through the agency of hospital and specialist services.

Incidentally, as an outsider, I was struck by the paucity of field work being done by the regional hospital boards. Shortage of staff no doubt limits what is possible, but the result is that many important decisions have to be taken in committee and founded on opinion instead of on investigation. I was also impressed by the tenuousness of coördination between the regional boards and central authority at the Ministry of Health.

For all practical purposes it must be concluded that at the policy level there is no coördination between the regional hospital boards and the people responsible for general-practitioner services.

LOCAL AUTHORITY

The relationship, or rather the lack of relationship, of the individual general practitioner with the local-authority services has already been discussed.

On the introduction of the Act the local health authority, while losing control over municipal hospitals, gained new powers with regard to general practice, in that it was given the responsibility for health-centre development. Except in terms of politics it is hard to see why this responsibility for health centres was vested in local government while responsibility for general-practitioner services was given to executive councils. The failure of all parties interested in the new service to define what they meant by a health centre, and the general acceptance that it had to do with health and therefore preventive medicine, which in turn is identifiable with local-authority services and not with general practice, no doubt made it plausible to hand the responsibility to the local authorities. In Scotland, where a more realistic view was taken and the political complications were less, the Department of Health retained central responsibility for health centres, and the possibilities of fairly rapid and sound development are therefore better than they are in England.

It is natural enough that the local health authorities, having these powers with regard to health centres, should think first of all about their own services and only secondarily about medical care and the general practitioner. It is *not* natural that the G.P., who expressed real concern about health centres at the time of negotiations before July 5, 1948, and who now thinks he has been let down badly over them, and the executive councils, which reputedly look after general-practitioner services, should be taking no active interest in the efforts of local authorities or in the possible alternatives.

The fact that executive councils are confining themselves to administration makes this state of affairs more understandable; but even that does not explain the failure of local authorities to take the initiative and " tie up " with those responsible for general-practitioner services.

The local medical committees similarly show no active interest in the health-centre question. They are interested in a passive way, but they seem to have accepted the edict of " no steel, and houses before health centres " as an absolute reason for doing nothing new.

I could find no evidence that the new responsibilities of local authorities had brought them into any close coöperation or connection with the G.P. Indeed, the construction which is being put on health centres as bigger and better local-authority services, with some secondary consideration for the general practitioner, is widening the breach. The fact that a medical officer of health or a local-authority doctor sits on an executive council, or even on a local medical committee, does not seem to make any difference to the over-all relationship.

Twice I met medical officers of health whose interest was as much in medical care as in problems of public health. Both these men were trying to interest G.P.s individually, and the responsible authorities, in health centres oriented mainly towards the requirements of general practice.

They seemed to be having little success; but in both places the general relationship of the G.P.s with the local-authority services was better than I saw elsewhere.

EXECUTIVE COUNCILS

Executive councils sometimes deal in terms of policy with exigencies which crop up from time to time, but never with broad general issues. The local medical committees run a parallel course and seem to be wholly preoccupied with day-to-day affairs. There are any number of these, as can be expected in the early days of a new service, and everyone can plead lack of time to deliberate on underlying principles.

The permanent staff of most of the executive councils have been inherited from the old insurance committees of National Health Insurance, and while they are doubtless very competent to deal with the machinery of the insurance scheme, most of them seem to be well out of their depth when it comes to other matters concerning general practice. This reduces the likelihood of executive councils doing anything more than the most routine kind of job; and yet they are the only official body directly responsible for general-practitioner services.

THE DOCTOR'S ATTITUDE TO CURRENT PROBLEMS OF GENERAL PRACTICE

The British Medical Association has expressed the official attitude of doctors to the National Health Service. Just how far this attitude of organised medicine in Britain represents the summation of individual opinion is open to question. From my contacts with a large number of doctors—some approving the official attitude; some disapproving it ; .but mostly " ordinary " doctors, asking no more than to be allowed to get on with their job as they see it—I was unable to correlate the thoughtful opinions of the majority with the statements of the organisation which represents them.

It is perhaps significant that these thoughtful opinions rarely find their way into the channels of public communication. This does not imply that any censorship is exercised over them ; but they remain unexpressed through the inertia of those who hold them, through a sense of modesty, or through a feeling of the futility of individual effort in issues as vast as this.

So far as general practitioners are concerned, I believe that a feeling of futility and insecurity, more than anything else, has prevented their expressing opinion on policy. Because of this, I am sure we are missing a wealth of experience and wisdom which would be available if general practitioners were given the necessary encouragement and opportunity to put forward their views.

As things stand, general practitioners are having little share in determining their own destiny or professional future, and this is leading to a demoralisation which can only accelerate the decline and fall of general practice.

In the course of this study I sought opinion from men long established in practice and from young men trying to enter it or make their way in it. The same sense of hopelessness pervaded both generations. Some of the best family doctors whom I met were actively discouraging their sons and daughters from succeeding them in general practice : as I have already explained, they believed that the eclipse of general practice is at hand— that it is to be supplanted by more and more institutional and specialist medicine.

It is noteworthy that even these fine family doctors, who for years have acted as family counsellors as well as ministering to the organic needs of their patients, give priority of interest to the organic aspects of their work. The reason for this, I feel sure, is that, within our cultural pattern, the doctor's ability to establish rapport with his patient, and thus place himself in a position to

THE LANCET]   GENERAL PRACTICE IN ENGLAND TODAY   [MARCH 25, 1950 573

cope with psychological problems, rests largely on his ability to handle physical disease—not only the minor physical disorder but also, to a great extent, the major one. This dates from the time when patients had to rely on the family doctor for almost every kind of medical care; for many people still suppose that he carries this great burden of responsibility—which he rarely does. I have actually met doctors who believe that they must do a certain amount of major surgery or lose the respect or "faith" of their patients; and this is undoubtedly true in some degree.

While the doctors' attitude in this regard could probably be altered fairly rapidly by a reorientation of medical education, the corresponding change in the cultural pattern would probably take generations rather than merely years.

THE CONTRACTING SPHERE

This brings us back to the question of how much responsibility for medical care can be safely centred in one person.

I have drawn attention to the efforts to control the excesses of the general practitioner in surgery, and to the extension of similar empirical control (or limitation) to other parts of his work. Now, looking at the non-organic side of his activities, it is very obvious, in the light of modern psychological and psychiatric knowledge, that it is potentially dangerous to have a "half-trained" doctor handling psychological problems. Yet we are faced with a situation where he does handle them; and moreover one where—the cultural pattern being what it is—the patient accepts the ministrations of the general practitioner as orthodox, whereas he would be suspicious of the "modern heresies" of the psychologist, the psychiatrist, the psychiatric social worker, and the home visitor. So long as this is so, we cannot afford to reject the G.P. by over-curtailment of his responsibility for organic medicine, or to force the new heresies on the public in obedience to the dictates of organic statistics on the one hand and modern psychological theory on the other. The present trend towards institutional and specialist care is in fact a rejection of the general practitioner, an assault on our cultural patterns, and perhaps an indirect admission of inability to resurrect all that is good in general practice and turn it from an anachronism into a contemporary and inestimably valuable service.

Though the behaviour of the doctors I have mentioned was founded on these considerations, they did not express themselves in these words. Some saw the decline of general practice in terms only of a growing contraction of their sphere of activity in the realm of organic medicine: they resented, for example, the threat to their positions on the staff of cottage hospitals. In fact, while the consensus of opinion is that general practice is doomed, they very seldom volunteered a cogent analysis of why this is so, or what ought to be done about it. Nevertheless, once given encouragement and some sort of a lead, these same doctors, from their large personal experience, talked about general practice in a critical and constructive manner which is not often reflected in official or public utterance.

I think it highly significant that good established general practitioners should be advising the younger generation to stay out of this field, so long before their fears may become reality. It is even more significant, in view of what is said by their representatives, that none of the doctors I met expressed serious discouragement in terms of the evils of the capitation system of payment or of the bureaucratic tyrannies which are supposed to characterise the new service.

The foregoing is not an argument for stopping experiment with different kinds of medical care; nor is it a reactionary appeal on my part to retard progress in bringing modern medical knowledge and technique to those who need it. It is, however, an appeal not to throw away what is good in general practice, and relegate this part of medical care to the scrap-heap, but rather to use, reinforce, and bring up to date these good elements. General practice as we know it could, if we wished, be converted into general practice as we like to imagine it; and if this is to be our aim we must not rush too far ahead with the development of our so-called public-health services and specialist services, which are largely attempts to patch up obvious weaknesses in the provision of medical care. It is time that the cause of the weakness, rather than the symptom, received attention.

METHOD OF REMUNERATION

On the highly controversial issue of the capitation system of remuneration I found, as I have said, much less strong feeling than I had been led to expect. Those doctors who had big lists were as well off as previously, or even better off; and no serious complaints were made by this group. I met a few doctors who had previously had a small high-fee-paying clientele and who had been badly hit by the Act—particularly in urban areas where mileage-rates and special inducement payments did not function as a means of subsidy. Rural practitioners, it was argued, would fare worst; yet those with whom I came in contact were relatively unperturbed about either the method of remuneration or the size of the capitation fee. Indeed I found few doctors claiming that the different manner of remuneration had materially altered their way of practice. The few who spoke strongly about patient abuse and disturbance of doctor-patient relations since July, 1948, failed to support their statements to my satisfaction; and in most cases where such statements were made there was evidence of poorly organised and badly disciplined practice which seemed to be of more than twelve months' standing.

The attitude of some of these doctors to the various social and economic groups among their patients was interesting. Especially in the latter months of my study, I noted a growing resentment against those social groups which used to form the paying part of a given practice, with a developing interest in, and attention to, what was once the "panel" part (or its equivalent). This went deeper than a mere objection to the well-to-do patient wanting the benefits of the National Health Service. It arose chiefly from the demands of this social group for more time and attention than their less fortunate neighbours are accustomed to receive, and it was increased by the tendency of better-educated patients to question diagnosis or therapy, to seek reasons for statements and instructions, or even to challenge the doctor's edict.

One subject which cropped up continually in my talks with all manner of general practitioners was that of salaried practice: the hypothetical and real dangers of such a system, and the possibility that it would be the final outcome of the capitation service, were often discussed. I met many doctors who thought that, given reasonable guarantees of autonomy, a salaried service would be preferable to the capitation service. (Of course, emphasis was laid on the need for autonomy.) On this issue, as well as others, I found the thoughtful doctor, both in individual and group discussion, embarrassed when he was identified with the official professional attitude.

ACCEPTANCE OF BAD CONDITIONS

But my attempts to get individual doctors or groups of doctors to appraise the more basic conditions of their work met with little success. The traditional pattern of general practice—i.e., one man doing all his work in a single room with such equipment as he deems necessary or can afford—is firmly established and readily accepted as being, if not " the best of all possible worlds," at least the best attainable for the time being. The doctor who worked in an unattractive surgery almost always criticised it from the point of view of his own and his patient's comfort, but very seldom from a functional point of view. The doctor with a nicely appointed surgery, though this was functionally little or no better than the other, usually had no criticism to offer, and often took pride in an establishment which, as regards ease and efficiency of work, was indeed very bad.

This limited outlook on general practice, by the general practitioner himself, is quite as important a factor in retarding health-centre development as is his expressed disinclination to sink his individuality or independence in the coöperative effort of a group. The one bright spot in this otherwise gloomy sky is the fact that, once shown possibilities beyond the present narrow and ever-narrowing limits of general practice, he exhibits a latent enthusiasm, and often a breadth of vision, not to be suspected from his normal conduct and attitudes.

The lack of critical faculty among doctors is curious. A well-trained man will throw over the hard-won disciplines of clinical training, and accept the stultifying limitations of general practice within its present concepts ; a really good doctor will divide his working time between a well-equipped, well-run cottage hospital, and a poorly equipped, badly run surgery, without apparently noticing his changing environments of work. Such acceptance of bad conditions has a deadening effect.

REFRESHER COURSES

Efforts have long been made to help the general practitioner to keep abreast of modern knowledge and technique, and to encourage him to maintain standards of work. The so-called refresher courses have been the means mainly used for doing this, and there is much discussion about providing more of them and about ways of freeing the doctor from duty so that he may attend them. But many of the more thoughtful practitioners are sceptical about their value. My own opinion is that, with conditions of practice as they are, these refresher courses do the general practitioner about as much good as an injection of adrenaline does a patient with terminal heart-failure.

AID FROM SPECIALISTS

The attitude of the general practitioner to the specialist naturally varies from doctor to doctor and from circumstance to circumstance ; but several points about it need to be noted. At the higher levels of work, exemplified by advanced surgery or medicine as practised in large hospitals, the respect of the G.P. for the good specialist is absolute and unqualified. But at the lower levels of work, as represented by domiciliary and some aspects of outpatient consultations, he does not show the same confidence. And it is at the domiciliary level that practitioner and specialist have most contact.

The line of demarcation between the patient who can be treated at home and the patient who requires hospital care is fairly clear so far as acute diseases are concerned. Hence the general practitioner rarely wants what one may call an emergency domiciliary consultation—his view being that anything as serious as this is not a matter to be debated in the bedroom. It is chiefly in the case of long-term or chronic illness, where there is no clear line of demarcation, that he needs the specialist's help in the homes of his patients. But as, on the whole, both G.P. and specialist lack interest in the chronic medical diseases, particularly those of old age, the demand for domiciliary consultation is not very great.

Thus the good general practitioners whom I met made little use of, and felt little need for, specialist assistance in the home. Many of them said that they have no more

than three or four such consultations in a working year, and sometimes not that ; and in retrospect they doubted the need for even these few. The specialists whom they called in could not help them much, they thought, with illness in old age. Indeed, so far as these good general practitioners are concerned, the chief reason for calling a consultant is to relieve the anxiety of relatives or the patient ; they seldom expect any help for him physically. Such practitioners have made little or no more use of domiciliary consultation since the Act made it generally available.

One good practitioner with whom I worked used the domiciliary consultation for purposes of personal tuition : he collected a number of interesting cases and then arranged for one or more specialists to see them and discuss them with him on some suitable afternoon. While such an arrangement carries obvious benefit to both G.P. and specialist (and probably to the patient), it is perhaps an unnecessarily expensive mode of instruction, and something of an abuse of the system.

In the whole course of my study I did not attend any domiciliary consultations, and I had difficulty in ascertaining how this service is being used. Some practitioners spoke of checking their therapy in chronic or long-term cases (particularly cardiac) ; but they added that in fact they got very little useful assistance from the specialists. A few expressed satisfaction at being able to call in a specialist in cases involving children— particularly an otologist in cases of otitis media and possible mastoid. But I think the object of the consultation, as they saw it, was to relieve the parents' anxiety as much as to confirm their own opinion.

The relief of genuine anxiety in the patient or his relatives is certainly a very good reason for a domiciliary consultation ; but I doubt whether this was the purpose for which the service was provided. The point that impressed me most was that the really good G.P. had, or believed he had, little need to call the specialist to the home, and little (or infrequent) desire to do so. On the other hand, the G.P. of lesser quality could legitimately call in specialists much more often than they were really needed.

On three occasions I met general practitioners who, in all good faith, were calling in young consultants in order to help them financially and get them established. This kindly personal gesture was, of course, billed back to the taxpayer. There was never any question of dichotomy.

From my observations and questions I can only conclude that the good doctor felt little need for specialist assistance in his everyday work as at present constituted, and had little faith in the specialist's ability to do more than he could himself. The less good general practitioner, if self-assured, took the same line as his more competent colleagues ; if not self-assured, he used the specialist to compensate for his own weakness.

With general practice as it is today, there is little likelihood of domiciliary consultation being applied properly : indeed until the province and function of general practice has been determined, and real standards have been established, it is useless to speculate on the proper relations between the specialist and the general practitioner in domiciliary work. Both in money and in time, domiciliary consultation is a very expensive means of compensating for weaknesses in general practice ; and in present circumstances it is a very dubious means of trying to correct these weaknesses at their source. Perhaps the greatest benefit is to the specialist, who is brought out of his world of institutional medicine and into the world of his patient.

THE PRESENT AND THE FUTURE

In general, I found the attitude of the established practitioner to the new health service only a pale reflection of the vehement stand taken by organised medicine on

THE LANCET] GENERAL PRACTICE IN ENGLAND TODAY [MARCH 25, 1950 575

his behalf. His views have been severely limited by the political and emotional considerations which have governed professional policy since the Act was first mooted, and in another way even more severely limited by the deeply rooted traditions of the British " family doctor." But I found that whenever these considerations could be temporarily laid aside, and he could be induced to think critically, he had a valuable contribution to make to the whole field of thought on medical care.

The attitude of the young doctor to general practice is of special importance for the future. Medical education at present tends to direct the student away from general practice, and it is certainly not designed to equip him fully for this type of work. Before the introduction of the Act, economic and social pressures obliged a large proportion of medical students to accept general practice as the easiest way to a reasonable livelihood within a reasonable period of time. Nobody would suggest that this was a good means of recruiting general practitioners, but at least it was a means. Today, however, the National Health Service Act has lessened the economic pressure which previously kept some people out of the specialties, and has added few if any inducements for the young doctor to go into general practice. Over and above this, it has put new obstacles in his way.

Even in the hypothetical under-doctored areas, of which the Medical Practices Committee has published long lists, vacancies by death and retirement are few ; and sometimes the circumstances in which they have been filled have been such as to discourage candidates from trying again. At the moment the one easy way into general practice is to secure an assistantship in a busy urban practice with the possibility of later partnership. But in the circumstances prevailing in this type of practice it is a shame to see potentially good doctors entering through this channel, since their chances of improving the bad conditions to which they are going are very slim, while the chances of their own retrogression are very great.

The attraction of an apprentice appointment with an approved established practitioner is not really very strong, and so far few such appointments have been made.

The very few young doctors I met who had entered general practice at or about the time the Act came into force were in difficult circumstances and looking for a way out. In section II I described the case of a very able young practitioner who, because he tried to exercise a wide range of medical skills, was regarded as a professional oddity, and who was facing financial disaster because of the limited nature (volumetrically) of his practice. He is perhaps an extreme example, but still an example, of the difficulties and the discouragement which confront anyone with a genuine interest in this type of work. Another illustration is provided by a doctor in a large city where one would imagine that establishment in practice was much easier. He had a senior qualification (M.R.C.P.) and a very strong desire to make his career in general practice. At the time I saw him and witnessed his quite superior work he had been in practice for about eighteen months. He then had some 800 patients on his list, a considerable overdraft at the bank, and a family to support. He had set his own deadline at 1500 patients on his panel by early 1950, failing which he would retreat from general practice into some form of specialist work which offered an assured future and less financial worry.

To the young doctor, as to the old, the promise of health centres as at present conceived is almost meaningless, though to the young perhaps it is not quite the same bogy. The new ideal certainly does not permeate back into the years of undergraduate training, and it is unlikely to have any appreciable effect on recruitment to general practice in the foreseeable future. And it is these fore-seeable years ahead which are going to determine the patterns, quality, and nature of medical care for a long time to come.

I cannot report that I found any more spontaneous constructive criticism of general practice among young doctors than among old. Unless they are given a lead, it is useless to look to the latest generation to advance the field of general practice in any radical or fruitful way. They are as closely bound by tradition and the status quo as the generations preceding them ; and, though they may resent the present nature of general practice, they tend either to accept it philosophically or to escape into other branches of medicine.

Nevertheless, I found many significant inconsistencies between the opinions of a large number of individual doctors and their opinion as represented by the spokes-men of the profession. More important, I found that, given encouragement, these same doctors, who apparently had nothing more to say than has been said officially, were ready to make a contribution to the planning of both their own future and the future of the medical service as a whole. It is to be hoped that they will be given the opportunity.

HEALTH CENTRES

Both before and after the introduction of the National Health Service, the promise of health centres repre-sented the chief hope of the general practitioners for a " new deal." But though there was much talk about health centres for the future, this future has since been defined as the time when we have more steel, more building materials, more labour, and more money. Many practitioners now regard the promise of health centres as a political trick, designed to gain their support at the time of the negotiations, or at least as an unful-filled promise whose fulfilment is now unlikely. There are still the optimists who see the health centre as the panacea for all the disorders of general practice ; but few of this group can explain what they mean by a health centre, much less show the way to translate it into reality.

Apart from recent deliberative work by the Health Centre Committee of the Central Health Services Council, the only positive steps towards development of health centres have been taken by local authorities. This is natural in so far as responsibility for health centres has been vested in local government ; but it has led to an interpretation of the health centre primarily as a large building in which to house the personal preventive health services—maternity and child welfare, health visiting, school medicine, &c.—with only secondary and small consideration for the work of the general practitioner.

Whatever the value of such a health centre may be, it will do little or nothing to improve the standards of general practice. Moreover, general practitioners may refuse to work in a centre of this kind. The vast majority of them are prejudiced against, and suspicious of, local-authority services, even at their present level of develop-ment, and for this if no other reason few doctors already established in practice will want to submerge their independence and individuality, as they see it, in the larger machinery of new local-authority health centres. Also there are more material objections—notably the benefits of tax allowances while they remain in their own surgeries.

Many local authorities have been very active in plan-ning health centres, and have committed large and expensive schemes to paper. Perhaps fortunately, however, the great majority have been deterred by shortage of money and materials from proceeding at once with their projects. While they are held up there is time to think again about health centres and to define and design some functional units which might set the course for a better comprehensive medical service.

WHAT KIND OF MEDICAL CARE ?

The health centre is merely a mechanism, a means to an end and not an end in itself ; and unless we can define the end we may as well forget about the means.

If I am correct in setting down the three determining factors of the quality of general medical care as

1. The general social environment
2. The doctor as an individual
3. The immediate environment in which the doctor works

and in claiming that (3) is the only immediate variable and one which can greatly influence (2), then health centres can become the chief factor in raising the quality of general medical care.

As these three factors are by no means constant, there can be no absolute definition of a health centre : the needs of different environments will have to be met in very different ways. Nevertheless it should be possible to establish some criteria for what one might call a theoretical optimum health centre, and then to adapt this to different places and conditions. If we are to do this, we must clear our minds of two ideas :

1. That general practice, as it exists at present, is good or even good enough to meet the needs of any community.
2. That health centres are concerned primarily with preventive medicine as we recognise it at present.

We must then reverse our thinking on hospital and specialist services (medical and ancillary) : instead of considering how far we can build these up, we must consider how far we can dispense with them. For both human and economic reasons, we should work from two premises :

1. That as many people as possible should be kept *out* of hospitals—whether as inpatients or as outpatients.
2. That the medical care of the patient should be integrated, not fractionated.

On this basis the optimum health centre must be, first and foremost, a high-grade diagnostic and therapeutic centre ; which implies good (if necessary elaborate) equipment and all the people necessary to use it. Continuity of responsibility for medical care of a patient cannot be achieved unless the general practitioner assumes high-level responsibility in a wide range of activities. It is true that there is virtually nothing in his work which some specialist cannot in theory do better ; but we must firmly resist the conclusion that therefore we must keep on fractionating and specialising.

Admittedly, general practitioners working with limited equipment and in isolation can easily become dangerous through taking on too much responsibility, but in a health centre well staffed and well equipped it should be possible to minimise such dangers and ascertain by experiment the level of responsibility which suits practitioner and patient best.

APPLYING THE PRINCIPLES

There are very few places in England where the establishment of an " optimum " health centre is possible : except perhaps in rapidly expanding towns, medical services cannot be planned entirely afresh. So we must think mainly in terms of adaptations of the " optimum " which will fit in with the services already provided by the general practitioner, the hospital, and the local authority.

Our object will be to change the working environment of the G.P. and make it possible for him to do better work and to retain, instead of discarding, the good disciplines of medical school and hospital. If this one thing can be done, a lot of other difficulties should be overcome with relative ease. The schism between hospital-specialist and G.P. services will narrow rapidly instead of widening as at present, and the relationship—or rather the balance of power—between local-authority services and general practice should improve.

Though, in my opinion, it is impossible to draw up a blueprint for a widely applicable prototype health centre, we can set down some indispensable requisites—namely

1. Separate and private units for consultation and examination by each doctor working in the centre.
2. Adequate personal equipment for each doctor.
3. Such nursing staff as is needed to relieve the doctor of unnecessary and time-consuming duties.
4. Such clerical staff and office equipment as are needed for proper organisation, running, and record-keeping.

To these, various additions (differing in different circumstances) will be necessary. For example

1. Laboratory facilities and technicians.
2. Radiological facilities and technicians.
3. Physiotherapeutic facilities and physiotherapists.
4. Rooms for visiting specialists or consultants.

To this medical-care nucleus can be added offices for local-authority services and personnel, and for such welfare functions as may be considered desirable in given circumstances.

In the present situation, both medical and economic, priorities of attention must be allotted. Number 1 priority should go to general practice and not (as now) to local-authority services, and it should go to the worst part of general practice—i.e., general practice in dense urban areas.

In these industrial areas, where the level of general practice is low and where hospital and local-authority services are highly developed, it is unrealistic to think in terms of elaborate health centres. It is equally unrealistic to set out to duplicate an already existing service : for example, in a health centre adjacent to a large hospital unit it would be silly to have expensive diagnostic equipment. Nevertheless the health centre will fail in its purpose unless the necessary facilities are made available to the people working in it.—And I do not mean available in the sense they are available already, when a G.P. can send his patient to a hospital outpatient department and in course of time get back a brief report on what ought to be done (or what has been done) for the patient. The G.P. must have open access to these diagnostic facilities and to the specialists and consultants who are nowadays working in isolation from him.

The health centre should very largely replace the outpatient department. This does not merely imply changing the venue of the department ; if it did, no useful purpose would be served. It implies cutting out the episodic care which characterises present outpatient work, by bringing the specialist into the health centre, where he should do the equivalent of his outpatient consultations in the presence of the G.P. concerned with the particular case. The G.P. would then be responsible for coördinating the efforts of the various specialists who handle the patients and for the continuity of care. More than anything else, this is a problem of organisation—and not a particularly difficult one. If the work and responsibility of the G.P. is upgraded and his facilities are improved, the volume of outpatient department work (or its equivalent in the health centre) will be considerably reduced (vide Appendix II).

In large urban health centres a good case can now be made out for the full-time employment of a consultant physician, who would be continuously accessible to all the G.P.s working the centre and who could follow up all cases which interested him. If a consultant physician, to remain at consultant level, must have hospital beds and inpatients, that could be arranged ; but the bulk of his time should be devoted to work within the health centre and domiciliary work associated with this.

In the " optimum " health centre similar arguments can be adduced for full-time radiologists, pathologists, &c., working in the centre ; but, as I have said, there will be little call for the " optimum " type.

THE LANCET] GENERAL PRACTICE IN ENGLAND TODAY [MARCH 25, 1950 577

The relationship of local-authority services with such a centre must be considered very carefully. Where such services are functioning even reasonably well, even under makeshift conditions, no elaborate provision should be made for them, in the first instance, within the health centre. Offices should be provided in the health centre for representatives of various branches of local-authority services (e.g., home nursing, midwifery, and health visiting), and the work of these people should be coördinated with that of the doctor working in the centre, who should in turn be encouraged to use these services to the full. Once equilibrium and understanding have been established between the G.P.s and the local-authority personnel—by no means a forlorn hope, given these conditions—the question of shifting the local-authority clinic into the health centre can be considered realistically instead of theoretically.

INDIVIDUAL AND GROUP

The ideal of "family doctoring" is still an excellent, desirable, and probably attainable ideal. However, the horse-and-buggy days are far behind, and it is absurd to try to recapture the 19th-century concept of the benign old doctor in his frock coat and silk hat sitting through the night, awaiting the pneumonia crisis or the delayed arrival of the first-born. Our task is rather to resynthesise all that is good in this concept and discard all that is anachronistic.

In this modern age such a resynthesis implies teamwork between doctors, nurses, social workers, and technicians, with the general practitioner as the coördinating agent of the team. My own belief is that, as obstacles to such team-work, the so-called rugged individualism of the average doctor, and his antipathy to any form of organisation or imposed discipline, are much overrated. The general practitioner has acquired a position of great personal power, and naturally he is not prepared to yield any of it without adequate compensation. By this I do not mean merely financial compensation. The kind of compensation I chiefly have in mind is the opportunity to do better, more useful, and more satisfying work.

Our task, as I see it, is to re-establish general practice and make it the basis of a positive preventive programme. And I suggest that, as a first step, we should form "basic group-practice units" which could be developed quickly and become the nucleus of future health centres.

THE BASIC GROUP-PRACTICE UNIT

The primary consideration is personnel, not buildings. In the first instance any shell which could be renovated and adapted might serve to house the unit.

The number of doctors who would work together would be determined by population density and the nature of communications to the site. I picture small units of 6–10 doctors, looking after 15,000–25,000 people. The unit would be fully staffed with nurses, clerical assistants, and some form of all-purpose technician who could undertake urinalysis, blood hæmoglobins, sedimentation-rates, and the like. It would be furnished with all the equipment necessary for a good G.P. service.

The crucial question is, how can the incumbents of existing general practices be enticed to coöperate in these circumstances? And now that responsibility for health centres has been vested in local authorities, how can such a programme be made to work?

If conditions for doing good work are offered, and if assurances of professional autonomy can be given, I believe that the problem of recruitment will largely solve itself. The individual doctor, apart from running his car, should have no overhead expenses to bear; he should certainly not be charged even the non-economic rent which is at present mooted. (I found the idea of even a small rental charge a positive deterrent to coöperation in any such project—quite apart from the negative deterrent of loss in tax-rebates for the doctor who gives up all his private practice.) Under such an arrangement very good terms of service should be possible. For example, it would be practicable to offer good and regular vacation and study periods. (The present offer of refresher courses, even with the provision of paid locums, is merely pie in the sky so far as many general practitioners are concerned.) These inducements, once made realities, would strongly attract both present and future practitioners to the "basic group-practice unit."

I have suggested units of 6–10 doctors looking after 15,000–25,000 people. This sets an average of 2500 patients, instead of the permissible 4000, on any one doctor's list. But with the removal of all overhead expenses, and with the other inducements offered, the financial return from this number should be enough to attract anyone except perhaps those whose lists are at present full; and we should further be able, under these conditions, to recruit young doctors in large enough numbers to maintain a ratio of one doctor to 2500 patients.

Group practice is sometimes commended on the ground that it enables the good G.P. to do specialised work and thus make his way into a specialty. But if the conditions of general practice are made sufficiently satisfying, the desire to be a specialist may lessen, and general practice may then compete for the very best medical graduates.

At the "basic group-practice unit" level of development it will certainly be possible to integrate the general-practitioner services with the hospital and specialist services, and there will be no difficulty in bringing the specialist into the unit. (At present this cannot be done.) But, for emotional and political reasons if for no others, it will be necessary to go warily with the introduction of local-authority services, and at the outset no local-authority clinics should be brought into the unit, though, as I have said, an initial liaison should be formed by providing offices for representatives of the local-authority agencies most closely allied to general practice—e.g., home nursing, health visiting, and midwifery. From this liaison the more comprehensive type of health centre should eventually develop.

The capital expense of setting up such units should not be great; but in the circumstances it is hardly a burden to be carried by local authority. The most satisfactory solution would seem to be grants-in-aid from central funds to the local authority, to be spent within the terms set down.

ADVANTAGES

Only on some such basis as this is there a chance of correcting the paradox that general medical care is at its worst in closest proximity to the large clinical centres—at its worst not only for organic reasons but equally for human and psychological reasons. Again on this basis it should be possible to remove much of the empiricism, in diagnosis and therapy, at present prevalent in general practice, and to begin the development of some effective clinical and human research, which in itself would do much to raise the status of such practice.

There is also the question of the doctor as a teacher. He is potentially perhaps the most important of all teachers: he can and often does influence individual and family conduct to a much greater extent than all the other agencies of health education put together. Yet the approach of the average doctor to this part of his responsibility is even more empirical than is his approach to organic medicine. The same factors in a basic group-

578 THE LANCET] GENERAL PRACTICE IN ENGLAND TODAY [MARCH 25, 1950

practice unit which would allow the G.P. wide diagnostic and therapeutic responsibility, while simultaneously creating safeguards against excesses, would tend to operate also in relation to his educational function.

That the group-practice health centre would improve medical care is almost self-evident. To bring together a number of people working on different aspects of a common problem, to provide them with facilities and conditions better than those they have had previously, and to offer them professional incentives to improvement—all this seems bound to result in a better deal for doctor and patient alike. But there are many sceptics, and the only way to satisfy them is by practical demonstration—I mean really practical demonstration in which the sceptics themselves have the opportunity to participate.

AN EXISTING GROUP

In section II I described the only real group practice I visited in England.

The doctors had designed and built their own clinic, which was extremely well equipped, and they employed nursing and semi-trained technical staff as well as clerical assistants. They claimed that their overhead was in no way incompatible with their income from an average of 2500 patients per head. The range of work of the four practitioners and their trainee assistant was comparable to that described for good G.P.s in New Zealand, and though they undertook obstetrics and a large amount of surgery (against which a strong case could be made) they were by no means overburdened. The record-keeping was comparatively good, and the standards and thoroughness of physical examination as high as any I saw in Britain. The head of the group told me that they had not suffered from " patient abuse "

since the introduction of the new service, and it was obvious that their ways of practice had not been altered by the terms of the Act.

Judged on premises, equipment, and record-keeping, which can be assessed objectively, this practice was in advance of anything else I saw; and my subjective impression of the standards of work led me to think of it as a beacon in the darkness. Yet in its eighteen years of existence it has received no official or professional attention, and, as I have mentioned, the survey committee which looked at the cottage hospital where these doctors work did not so much as call at the " group clinic " to see what went on there. Fearing that they will in the long run be eliminated from this hospital, at least one of the group contemplates turning to a specialty.

THE FIRST STEP

Though I heard of other such groups existing in various parts of the country, I did not have the opportunity to visit any. But I have no doubt that even the most simply organised group offers an overwhelmingly better medical service than that of individual practitioners.

Even the most elementary steps towards organising the present chaos of individual general practice must result in improved medical service and a fairer deal for doctor and patient, and I am sure that these elementary steps should be taken before any grandiose or idealistic experiments in health-centre development are attempted.

The future of general practice depends on our ability to give definition to a concept which is at present nebulous. Having designed our ends, we must design means to achieve them and to maintain them. The " basic group-practice unit " is the first and most urgent necessity.

IV. CONCLUSIONS AND RECOMMENDATIONS

Conclusions

1. The present state of general practice is unsatisfactory. Its defects existed before the National Health Service Act, and arise from failure to define general practice and to establish and maintain standards. For several decades general practice has adapted itself to the growth and development of hospital, specialist, and other medical services ; but it has not developed concurrently.

2. The National Health Service Act has done nothing immediately or directly to disturb the structure of general practice.

3. The extension of National Health Insurance has increased the load on general practice, and at some points this has caused serious strain or near-breakdown.

4. It is difficult either to confirm or to deny the claims made that this increased load has seriously depressed the quality of medical care. It is very evident, however, that many of the shortcomings attributed directly to the Act are the result of basic weaknesses in general practice which have merely been intensified by the additional load.

5. The claims that new methods for remunerating the doctor have seriously upset the doctor-patient relationship are similarly difficult to confirm or deny, but I found little evidence that they have done so.

6. The indirect effects of the Act on general practice are much more fundamental than the direct effects, around which most of the controversy has centred.

7. The impetus which the Act has given to development of hospital and specialist services has accentuated the defects outlined in (1) above.

8. Through the agency of the regional hospital boards, decisions of policy and principle relating to hospital and specialist services are being taken. No similar decisions are being taken on general practice, and the regional

boards' decisions are reached with little or no regard to the problems of general practice.

9. The executive councils responsible for general-practitioner services are fully occupied with day-to-day administration and are not working or thinking at the level of policy.

10. There is little or no coördination of the work of the executive councils and the regional hospital boards. This is not merely an administrative defect : until the executive councils take policy decisions, or have them taken for them, there is nothing of importance to coördinate.

11. For similar reasons, there is very little coördination of general-practitioner services and local-authority personal health services.

12. Hence the future of general practice is largely being determined without deliberate consideration of its problems. It is being determined mainly by the people responsible for hospital and specialist development, and in terms of compensation for recognised, or half-recognised, deficiencies, instead of the correction of these deficiencies.

13. Now that local authorities hold responsibility for health-centre development, one would expect them to be closely interested in the future of general practice. I found little evidence that this was so or was likely to become so quickly. The health centre is being considered primarily as an instrument of local-authority personal health services. Such consideration as general practice is receiving in this regard is more or less nullified by the failure to define its future province and function and to recognise it for what it really is.

14. The best elements of general practice are under attack (e.g., rural practice with cottage-hospital facilities), while the bad elements are being largely disregarded.

THE LANCET]   GENERAL PRACTICE IN ENGLAND TODAY   [MARCH 25, 1950 579

(e.g., industrial practice). This is the result of the widening schism between the specialist and the general practitioner, and inability to see beyond the practitioner's few but dramatic sins of commission (e.g., surgical) to his many more serious, if less obvious, sins of omission (e.g., missed or mistaken diagnosis).

15. With increased inducements for the young doctor to enter the specialties, and a decreasing scope for work in general practice, the latter is becoming an unattractive proposition. Furthermore, it is difficult for the young doctor with a genuine interest in this field to find a satisfactory way into it. The easiest way is through busy urban practice, and under prevailing conditions this is the least satisfactory way.

16. Unless these conditions are changed, potentially good doctors will be devalued without elevating the quality of practice. Similarly, any hope that financial reward alone will attract good senior practitioners back to these bad conditions is illusory : the good doctor will only be attracted into industrial practice by providing conditions which will enable him to do good work.

17. This question of terms and conditions of practice is of primary importance. The defects of general practice cannot fairly be attributed to the defects of medical education. However inadequate may be the teaching of social and psychological medicine, the teaching of clinical disciplines is good ; and bad conditions of practice can, do, and will continue to negate the most conscientious teaching efforts in the newer and more abstruse field of social and psychological medicine.

18. Against this background the few inducements— such as refresher courses with paid locums, and traineeships—are of very little value either as attractions or as a means of raising standards.

19. The present conditions of general practice, and the gloomy outlook for the future, have produced demoralisation in many thoughtful members of the profession. The ideas, ideals, and real dissatisfactions of a considerable number of doctors are not reflected fairly or fully by organised medicine, which has fought so vigorously for what have been called terms of service. With opportunity and encouragement, general practitioners could make a valuable contribution towards planning as well as operating the medical services.

20. If the present trend towards more and more hospital and specialist care continues, it must result in

(a) The elimination of general practice as an effective agency of medical care.

(b) The substitution of hospital, specialist, public-health, industrial-health, and similar less personal services.

(c) The breaking of the one remaining link which gives the patient some continuity of care, and the removal of a focal point for dealing with the non-organic problems—the psychological, economic, and social worries of the people.

Quite apart from human values, it is doubtful whether the policy of concentrating on hospital and specialist care is economically justifiable or even possible, and its hazards will certainly not be lessened by drifting into it.

Recommendations

In spite of this grim analysis of the present position and future prospects, the opportunity to re-establish general practice is still open.

First, an attempt should be made to define the future province and function of general practice within the framework of the National Health Service. This deliberative task should, in the first instance, be undertaken by the people most concerned—namely, " ordinary" general practitioners.

Secondly, basic group-practice units, such as I have described, should be formed as soon as possible. There is real urgency about launching this experimental work ; for relatively soon the new patterns of hospital and specialist care will be firmly established and everything will be fitted into them. If that happens it will then be virtually impossible to do very much about general practice.

APPENDICES

I. GENERAL PRACTICE IN SCOTLAND

In the absence of recognised criteria it is very difficult to draw comparisons between practice in one place and practice in another. But after examining practice in Scotland, by methods similar to those I used in England, I came away with the firm impression that, all in all, its quality is higher than that of the English equivalent. I do not claim that the best English practice is not at least as good as the best Scotland can show ; but if one can admit an average for the diverse types which go to make up what we call general practice, then in my opinion Scotland is in front.

A DIFFERENT ATTITUDE ?

The attitude of most general practitioners to both local and central authority, as represented by city and county health departments and the Department of Health for Scotland, seemed more reasonable and coöperative than that of English doctors to the corresponding authorities here. Though it could not be said that the relationships were by any means ideal, for the most part they were at least workable.

In England any association, real or imaginary, between my survey work and local or central authority militated against good relations and created obvious suspicion. In Scotland, on the other hand, wherever I went I found I could use either a local authority or the Department of Health as a means of introduction to general practice, without embarrassment and without arousing any serious misgivings. Indeed in one part of Scotland I actually travelled with an officer of the Department, who accompanied me into the various practices I visited ; and the doctors were quite as frank in his presence as if I had been alone. In England, on the few occasions when I was introduced by such an officer, I found relations with the doctors strained until I had explained my association with, and established my independence of, officialdom.

The explanation that has been offered me for this difference—that it is merely a matter of the size of the community—is not good enough. The relationships even in country towns in England are often worse than comparable relationships in big cities in Scotland. There is a basic difference in attitude of mind.

This difference in attitude is reflected in other ways. In England discussion with general practitioners on the new health service usually centred on the size of capitation fees, the number of patients on the list, mileage-rates, basic salaries, and so on, until it was steered into professional as distinct from commercial channels. In Scotland I found much more spontaneous interest in professional issues such as the quality of medical service, the relation of general practice to hospital and specialist services, and the development of health centres.

I do not want to give the impression that I am attributing all good to the Scottish doctor and all bad to the English. This is not the case at all. But there is an appreciable difference.

Anticipatory medicine – prevention as part of the consultation in family medicine

Chris van Weel

NOMINATED CLASSIC PAPER

Cees van den Dool. Surveillance van risicogroepen; anticiperende geneeskunde (English: Surveillance of risk groups; anticipatory medicine). *Huisarts en Wetenschap*, 1970; 13: 59–62 (published in Dutch).

Shortly after its publication, I stumbled across this paper about anticipatory medicine in the university library in Leiden in the Netherlands. As a medical student, I was intuitively interested in general practice but, given the medical school curriculum of that time, I was not receiving much support in that direction. My decision to become a general practitioner (GP) and combine this work with research was finalised there and then in the library. The concept of anticipatory medicine triggered the decisive moment with its focus on caring for individuals and communities. Anticipatory medicine went on to be the theme of my first-ever presentation and publication and subsequently of my PhD.

In this paper, Cees van den Dool proposed an operationalisation of personal prevention as part of regular consultations. The paper opens with a reference to the mission statement of the Dutch College of General Practitioners, the Woudschoten Declaration that had been published just 10 years earlier. Prevention was one of the tasks set out in that Declaration, but there were clear signs that Dutch GPs felt overwhelmed by it.

The paper claimed that GPs were excellently positioned to promote secondary prevention, when using their regular consultations with their patients, and applying a high-risk approach. This was followed by an extensive review, placed in a large table, of available secondary preventive interventions, listed across the medical life history of patients – from surveillance of psychomotor development of newborns, through pulmonary function and blood pressure measurement in middle age, to assessing hearing and vision in the elderly – and specified for gender with cervical smears and breast (self) examination for women and prostate examination in men.

In this overview, the author made a distinction between interventions that should be routinely applied and those depending on individual circumstances, and clarified which interventions could be done by nurses, practice assistants or laboratory personnel. This latter was stressed in response to GPs' claims of lack of time, with the explanation that changing the prevailing single-handed practices into partnerships with multidisciplinary teams would enable a broader range of interventions – including secondary preventive – to be undertaken.

There were two caveats added to this. The first was the importance of understanding each patient's reasons for each visit, since, while every patient might benefit from anticipatory secondary prevention, not all consultations are appropriate to introduce this. The second reflected on the apparent dominance of physical health problems, and made the point that consultations could, and should, serve as opportunities to also explore psychosocial problems.

At first sight this paper reads as yet another opinion-based paper, but nothing is further from the truth. The author developed his concept of anticipatory medicine – devoting part of the consultation to addressing the patient's needs unrelated to their actual reason for the consultation. This is the evidence base of the concept and the scientific core of the paper; the *format* of presenting this concept in a rather subdued way is a reflection of the norms when it was published. But that takes nothing away from the scientific *content*, which was based on research of the process and outcome of a series of preventive investigations conducted with his practice population over a number of years.

This practice-based research found that preventive investigations did reveal a lot of pathology, but that in subsequent preventive investigations, the same abnormalities were found again in the same patients, despite the fact that they had been advised to make an appointment and consult their GP. This cast doubt on the value of stand-alone preventive investigations and from the empirical data in this population-based longitudinal study of his own practice, the author built his visionary concept of anticipatory medicine as presented in this paper.

Published in Dutch, in the Journal of the Dutch College of General Practitioners, *Huisarts en Wetenschap* (*General Practitioner and Science*), this paper stood little chance of reaching beyond its circle of Dutch and Flemish GP readers. But the global impact of anticipatory medicine became substantial, facilitated through the author's collaboration with Julian Tudor Hart, who applied the concept in his own practice in the village of Glyncorrwg in Wales.

The lasting value of this paper is the development of the concept of a population-based approach to promote health through regular person-centred consultations in general practice. There is also lasting value in the practice-based evidence that informed this seminal concept. Both are as relevant for primary healthcare today as they were at the time of publication in 1970.

ABOUT THE AUTHOR OF THIS PAPER

C.W.A. (Cees) van den Dool was born in 1921 in Goes, in the Netherlands, and studied medicine in Leiden and Amsterdam. He entered general practice as a locum, before military service as a physician in, at that time, Dutch New Guinea (now West Papua in Indonesia). He settled as GP principal in Krabbendijke (1950–1953) then in Stolwijk (1953–1976), a village between Utrecht and The Hague with 3000 inhabitants. He was among the first GPs in the Netherlands to reform their single-handed practice into a group practice and health centre.

Cees was a founding member of the Dutch College of General Practitioners in 1956, serving on the research and practice management committees. In 1969 he joined the staff of the Utrecht University Department of General Practice registrar training programme, in combination with hosting medical students in his own practice.

In 1960 he defended his university thesis, *Early search for chronic diseases: some possibilities for the GP*, based on research carried out in his practice. Following this, he organised and evaluated a number of preventive investigations, leading to this seminal paper on anticipatory medicine.

This research brought him to the International Hypertension Congresses, where he met British GP Julian Tudor Hart, which led to global awareness of his concept of anticipatory medicine and began a lifelong friendship.

ABOUT THE NOMINATOR OF THIS PAPER

Professor Chris van Weel was born in The Hague in the Netherlands and studied Medicine at Leiden University. He worked as a GP in Rotterdam from 1973 to 1985, and completed his PhD at Erasmus University in 1981. He was Professor of General Practice at Radboud University from 1985 to 2012, and Professor of Primary Health Care Research at the Australian National University from 2013 to 2015. He served as world president of the World Organization of Family Doctors (WONCA) from 2007 to 2010. He was made an Officer of the Order of Oranje-Nassau in 2007.

'My advice to young GPs, educators and researchers is to seek inspiration from experience in clinical practice and research in making your final decision about the direction of your future career. Inspirational work, as carried

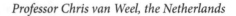

out by Cees van den Dool, is available virtually everywhere in the world. But you need to look for it – and to have the good fortune to stumble upon it at the right time.'

Professor Chris van Weel, the Netherlands

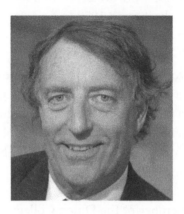

Attribution:

We attribute the original publication of *Surveillance van risicogroepen; anticiperende geneeskunde* to *Huisarts en Wetenschap*. We thank Dr Cees van den Dool for permission to reprint this paper, and Dr Just Eekhof, Editor in Chief of *Huisarts en Wetenschap*.

Surveillance van risicogroepen; anticiperende geneeskunde

DOOR DR. C. W. A. VAN DEN DOOL, HUISARTS TE STOLWIJK

Het is voor ons huisartsen, vooral wanneer wij soms aan ons bestaansrecht mochten twijfelen, zeer inspirerend om de deeltaken van de huisarts, zoals deze op de Woudschoten conferentie zijn geformuleerd en door de Commissie Wetenschappelijk Onderzoek (C.W.O.) nader zijn uitgewerkt, te herlezen (*Vroege*).

Van deze twaalf deeltaken – apotheekhoudende artsen hebben er dertien — heeft de tiende betrekking op preventie. Onder preventie rekenen wij alle maatregelen die ertoe kunnen bijdragen dat het gezondheidsniveau van onze patiënten zich niet in ongunstige zin wijzigt. Nu is het mogelijk om vrijwel alle energie en tijd op deze deeltaak te richten, maar dat moet dan tot een tekortschieten ten aanzien van andere deeltaken leiden. Een compromis zal nodig zijn. Geen enkele huisarts zal in staat zijn om alle deeltaken maximaal te vervullen. Wij zullen onze tijd en aandacht moeten verdelen. Daarbij moet worden geprobeerd met de beschikbare tijd en energie een optimum te bereiken.

Hoe kan dit ten aanzien van de preventie? Ik wil mij hier beperken tot de zogenaamde secundaire preventie, een niet voor ieder geheel duidelijk begrip, waaronder ook niet steeds hetzelfde wordt verstaan. Met secundaire preventie wordt bedoeld het zo vroegtijdig mogelijk opsporen van chronische ziekten met de gedachte dat een adequate therapie zodoende tot een betere prognose leidt dan wanneer wordt gewacht tot de zieke zich met klachten tot de arts wendt. Overigens is bekend hoe men in dit opzicht op teleurstellingen moet zijn voorbereid, vooral aan het carcinoomfront, cervixcarcinoom stadium 0 uitgezonderd.

Het ongerichte preventief geneeskundige onderzoek en de multiple screening – het sorteringsonderzoek – vormen twee mogelijkheden om tot secundaire preventie te komen. „Volledig" periodiek geneeskundig onderzoek is slechts door een klein aantal artsen inderdaad periodiek te realiseren (*Ten Cate*). Multiple screening onder leiding van de huisarts is in kleine plaatsen wel uitvoerbaar, maar zulks zal in grote praktijken organisatorische bezwaren geven (*Beek*).

In mijn vorige artikel (*Van den Dool*, 1969) kwam ik na de bespreking van de verschillende bevolkingsonderzoekingen in Stolwijk gedurende de afgelopen tien jaar tot de conclusie dat van de onderzochte mogelijkheden welke de huisarts tot zijn beschikking heeft een goed onderzoek van de patiënten die hem consulteren de beste methode lijkt, mits de huisarts deze gelegenheid aangrijpt om periodiek aan dit consult een aantal onderzoekingen te verbinden die niet met de actuele klacht van de patiënt in verband staan. Dergelijke onderzoekingen kunnen dan leiden tot opsporing van aandoeningen waarvan men – op grond van ervaring met preventief geneeskundig onderzoek – kan verwachten, dat er inderdaad een verhoogde kans bestaat op het ontdekken van deze aandoeningen. Genoemde pogingen om chronische ziekten op te sporen staan bekend als surveillance (bewaking). Daar de huisarts jaarlijks met 60 tot 80 procent van zijn patiënten in contact komt (*Van der Hoeven*), beschikt hij over vele mogelijkheden om op deze, meest natuurlijke wijze, bij patiënten die zich met klachten tot hem wenden, secundair preventief werkzaam te zijn.

Om geen energie te verspillen zal hij zich hierbij tot die groepen van patiënten moeten richten, die een duidelijk verhoogde kans hebben op het ontwikkelen van bepaalde aandoeningen of die daaraan mogelijk reeds lijden, hetzij zonder klachten, hetzij met zulke geringe klachten dat daarvoor nog geen medische hulp werd ingeroepen. De kennis van deze risicogroepen („high risk groups") is voor de huisarts bijzonder belangrijk, trouwens ook buiten het kader van de surveillance. Onze ervaring, het tijdrovende prospectieve onderzoek, de continue morbiditeitsregistratie met inschakeling van de computer en bestudering van de literatuur kan onze kennis hierover vermeerderen. Een nauwkeurig begrip over de mate waarin het risico in een bepaalde groep is verhoogd, blijkt vaak nog niet aanwezig. Toch zou zulks voor ons zeer belangrijk zijn, omdat wij dan beter in staat zouden zijn deze surveillance met een optimaal rendement te bedrijven. Per definitie is immers in een risicogroep een hoger rendement gewaarborgd.

Wanneer wordt getracht een aantal risicogroepen te omschrijven, dan kan dat worden gedaan door middel van bepaalde kenmerken zoals leeftijd, geslacht, aantal kinderen, gewoonten, beroep, sociale omstandigheden, hoeveelheid lichaamsbeweging, familiaire factoren, aangeboren kenmerken, chronische ziekten en verworven aandoeningen, waaronder operaties. Het valt niet moeilijk om voor elk kenmerk een of enkele voorbeelden te noemen.

Leeftijd: cervixcarcinoom bij vrouwen van 30 tot 50 jaar; glaucoom boven 50 jaar.

(1970) huisarts en wetenschap *13*, 59

Geslacht: hartinfarct bij mannen; anemie tengevolge van ijzertekort bij vrouwen.

Aantal kinderen: cervixcarcinoom bij moeders van grote gezinnen.

Gewoontes: longcarcinoom tengevolge van sigaretten roken; cervixcarcinoom tengevolge van slechte seksuele hygiëne.

Beroep: blaascarcinoom bij arbeiders in anilineindustrie.

Sociale omstandigheden: depressies bij crisissituaties, verlies van echtgeno(o)t(e).

Lichaamsbeweging: meer kans op hartinfarct bij weinig lichaamsbeweging.

Familiaire factoren: ulcuslijden, galsteenlijden, apoplexie.

Aangeboren kenmerken: meer maagcarcinoom bij personen met bloedgroep A; meer kans op nephritis bij rood haar(?).

Verworven kenmerken: meer maagcarcinoom bij pernicieuze anemie; meer kans op anemie tengevolge van ijzertekort na maagresectie (*Hofmans*).

Op grond van literatuurstudie (*Fuldauer, Wilson, Hodgkin, U.I.C.C.*) en eigen ervaring (*Van den Dool*, 1960) is thans voor de verschillende leeftijdscategorieën voor beide geslachten een surveillanceschema op te stellen. In het kader hiervan lijken 26 onderzoekingen geschikt. Het aantrekkelijke van deze tests is, dat 21 daarvan niet door de arts zelf behoeven te worden verricht, maar door hulpkrachten – assistente, laborante, wijkverpleegster – kunnen worden uitgevoerd (*tabel 1*).

Het schema is samengesteld uit een gedeelte A met 17 onderzoekingen en een gedeelte B met negen laboratoriumtests. Alleen het fysische onderzoek, het rectale en vaginale toucher en de inspectie van de huid dienen door de huisarts zelf te worden uitgevoerd, terwijl voor het elektrocardiogram en de tonometrie de hulp van een cardioloog en een oogarts zo nodig kan worden ingeroepen. De + tekens in het schema geven aan dat het onderzoek bij die bepaalde categorie van belang kan zijn. Dit wil uiteraard niet zeggen dat buiten deze categorieën een onderzoek niet geïndiceerd kan zijn, maar het valt dan buiten het kader van de surveillance. De volgorde van genoemde onderzoekingen en tests is zodanig dat hun plaats in het schema hoger is naarmate zij op jeugdiger leeftijd zinvol kunnen worden uitgevoerd. De frequentie waarmede men een bepaald onderzoek eventueel zal doen hangt — behalve van de mogelijkheden welke men ter beschikking heeft — af van de mate waarin het risico van de betreffende patiënt is verhoogd.

Zoals uit het schema blijkt valt de nadruk volledig op het somatische aspect van de gezondheid. Via de anamnese-vragenlijst is het echter zeer wel mogelijk om psycho-sociale problematiek aan de orde te stellen. *Bergsma* heeft dit in zijn onder-

zoek met succes gedaan. Daar uiteraard de psycho-sociale problematiek voor de verschillende leeftijden en seksen verschillend is, zou hiervoor een apart surveillanceschema zijn op te stellen, met voor elke categorie aangepaste vragen.

Het signaleren van deze problematiek is een belangrijke taak voor de huisarts. Met een surveillanceschema voor psycho-sociale problematiek, waarbij eveneens wordt rekening gehouden met zogenaamde risicofactoren, zou deze taak beter bespreekbaar worden. Dit schema zou dan bij voorkeur moeten worden opgesteld door huisartsen en

Onderzochte personen	Zuigelingen	Kleuters	School-kinderen
Leeftijdsgroepen	0 tot 1 man en vrouw	1 tot 5 man en vrouw	5 tot 15 man en vrouw
Tests			
A. 1 Fysisch onderzoek	+	+	+
2 Lengte	+	+	+
3 Gewicht	+	+	+
4 Gehoor	+		+
5 Visus: verzien lezen			+
6 Bloeddruk			+
7 Mantoux			+
8 „Peak flow" meting			+
9 Vitale capaciteit			
10 Thorax röntgen			
11 Rectaal toucher + prostaatonderzoek			
12 Vaginaal toucher + uitstrijk			
13 Mamma palperen (zelf)			
14 Anamneselijst			
15 Elektrocardiogram			
16 Tonometrie			
17 Inspectie huid			
B. 18 Fenylketonurie	+		
19 Hemoglobine	+	+	+
20 Albuminurie			+
21 Bakteriurie			+
22 Cholesterol			
23 Bloedsuiker			
24 Glucosurie			
25 Ureum			
26 Urinezuur			

Het uitvoeren van bovenstaande onderzoekingen dient men verhogende factoren, waardoor de diagnostiek gericht wordt

(1970) huisarts en wetenschap 13, 60

diegenen met wie hij op het brede terrein van de geestelijke volksgezondheid kan samenwerken. Dit is vooral gewenst omdat het pas verantwoord is iets te gaan opsporen, wanneer tevens ook de mogelijkheid van behandelen aanwezig is.

Door de surveillance van risicogroepen is men in staat om anticiperende diagnostiek te bedrijven, zelfs anticiperende geneeskunde. Het gaat dan dus om een diagnostiek en een geneeskunde die is gericht op mogelijke – meer waarschijnlijke – aandoeningen en ontwikkelingen.

Als somatisch voorbeeld zou de volgende ziektegeschiedenis kunnen dienen. Een 56-jarige man met een administratieve functie komt, nadat hij zijn huisarts in twee jaar niet heeft geconsulteerd op het spreekuur met cerumen in het oor. De prop wordt verwijderd. De assistente controleert gewicht, hemoglobinegehalte, gehoor, visus en bloeddruk. Zij verzoekt hem tevens urine van anderhalf uur na de maaltijd, in te leveren. De bloeddruk blijkt licht verhoogd (175/110 mm Hg); in de urine bevindt zich $1/2$ procent glucose. De glucose tolerantietest wijst op een lichte diabetes. Vanwege de zittende levenswijze en de glucosurie behoort de patiënt tot de risicogroep voor „ischaemic heart disease" (I.H.D.); een elektrocardiogram is derhalve op zijn plaats, ook al als document. Tevens is een cholesterolbepaling van belang, opdat daaraan zo nodig

Tabel 1. Surveillanceschema en praktijkpopulatie

JONGE VOLWASSENEN		VOLWASSENEN		OUDEREN		BEJAARDEN		Door wie? Assistente (Ass.) Verpleegster (Verpl.) Laboratorium (Lab.)	Motivering
15 tot 30 man	15 tot 30 vrouw	30 tot 45 man	30 tot 45 vrouw	45 tot 65 man	45 tot 65 vrouw	> 65 man	> 65 vrouw		
Militaire keuring	Alléén op indicatie							Arts	Diverse chronische ziekten
+	+	+	+	+	+	+	+	Ass. - Verpl.	Groeicurve
+	+	+	+	+	+	+	+	Ass. - Verpl.	Vetzucht/ondergewicht
				+	+	+	+	Ass. - Verpl.	Doofheid
+	+	+	+	+	+	+	+	Ass. - Verpl.	Onvoldoende visus
+	+	+	+	+	+	+	+	Ass. - Verpl.	Hypertensie
								Ass.	Tuberculose
+	+			+	+			Ass.	Astma, emfyseem
+	+			+	+			Ass.	CARA, cardiale aandoeningen
+	+	+	+	+	+	+	+	Team of bureau	Tuberculose, Besnier, Boeck, longcarcinoom, hartafwijkingen
		+		+		+		Arts	Rectumaandoeningen, prostaathypertrofie, prostaatcarcinoom
			+		+			Arts	Erosies, tumoren, cervixcarcinoom
			+		+		+	Instructie door wijkverpl.	Mammatumoren, waaronder carcinoom
		+	+	+	+	+	+	Ass. - Verpl.	Diverse chronische ziekten en psychosociale gegevens
		+		+	+	+	+	Ass. Cardioloog	Ischemie en dergelijke
				+	+	+	+	Ass. Oogarts	Glaucoom
						+	+	Arts	Huidcarcinoom
								Wijkverpl.	Idiotie, frequentie 1 op 10 347 tot 1 op 20 000
+	+	+	+	+	+	+	+	Ass.	Anemie, ijzertekort, pernicieuze anemie, carcinoom
	+	+	+	+	+	+	+	Ass. - Verpl.	Nephritis, nefrose, urineweginfecties, orthostatische albuminurie
+	+	+	+	+	+	+	+	Ass. - Verpl.	Urineweginfecties
				+				Lab.	Risicofactor I.H.D.
	+			+				Lab.	Diabetes
		+	+	+	+	+	+	Ass. - Verpl.	Diabetes
				+	+	+	+	Lab.	Chronische nephritis
					+	+	+	Lab.	Jicht

n afhankelijk te stellen van de aanwezigheid van risico-
t op meer waarschijnlijke ontwikkelingen (anticiperende diagnostiek).

(1970) huisarts en wetenschap *13*, 61

consequenties kunnen worden verbonden. Daar patiënt tevens hypermetroop is, zal een drukmeting van het oog van belang zijn, omdat vier risicoverhogende factoren voor het ontwikkelen van glaucoom aanwezig zijn (hypermetropie, leeftijd, hypertensie, diabetes).

Anticiperende geneeskunde zal zeker geen vermindering van het totale werk van de huisarts met zich brengen, wel een verschuiving. Een voordeel is dat zeer veel van het extra onderzoek door hulpkrachten kan worden gedaan. Bij nieuwbouw of verbouwing van de praktijkruimte zal dit consequenties kunnen hebben. Een aparte kaart – passend achter de N.H.G.-kaart met de 26 tests vóór in de marge – waarop in de verschillende datumkolommen de uitslagen kunnen worden vermeld, zal van veel nut kunnen zijn en tot een verbetering van de gehele praktijkvoering kunnen leiden.

Optimale secundaire preventie door middel van surveillance van risicogroepen – anticiperende geneeskunde – lijkt vooralsnog door gebrek aan hulpkrachten en een tekort aan huisartsen niet haalbaar. En dan wordt er nog niet eens aan de hoeveelheid werk gedacht die in het psycho-sociale vlak ligt te wachten wanneer wij systematisch via de anamnesevragenlijst klachten op dit gebied zouden introduceren. Afspraakspreekuren, groepspraktijken en het aantrekken van meer hulppersoneel zullen de mogelijkheden in deze kunnen vergroten.

Toch zal het waarschijnlijk geen enkele huisarts gelukken om geheel volgens het surveillanceschema te werken. Hij zou in dat geval – door overwaardering van een deel van een deeltaak – waarschijnlijk ook geen goede huisarts kunnen zijn.

Wanneer het principe echter juist is, kan het toch van nut zijn om af en toe aan een en ander te denken en bewust ernaar te handelen.

Beek, A. De uitvoerbaarheid van periodiek geneeskundig onderzoek in de huisartspraktijk. Van Gorcum, Assen, 1966.

Bergsma, J. J. Preventief geneeskundig onderzoek in een huisartspraktijk. Academisch proefschrift, Nijmegen, 1966.

Cate, R. S. ten (1966) huisarts en wetenschap 9, 106.

Dool, C. W. A. van den. Enige mogelijkheden tot het vroegtijdig opsporen van chronische ziekten door de huisarts. Academisch proefschrift, Leiden, 1960.

Dool, C. W. A. van den. (1969) huisarts en wetenschap, 12, 3.

Fuldauer, A. Bejaardenonderzoek in een huisartspraktijk. Academisch proefschrift, Leiden, 1966.

Hodgkin, K. Towards Earlier Diagnosis. A Family Doctors Approach. Sec. ed., Livingstone LTD, Edinburgh and London, 1966.

Hoeven, J. van der en H. H. W. Hogerzeil (1965) huisarts en wetenschap 8, 168.

Hofmans, A. (1968) huisarts en wetenschap 11, 255.

U.I.C.C. Cancer Detection. Monograph Series vol 4, Springer Verlag, Berlin, 1967.

Vroege, N. H. (1966) huisarts en wetenschap, 9, 372-385.

Wilson, J. M. G. en G. Junger. Principles and Practice of screening of disease. Public Health Papers no. 34, World Health Organization, 1968.

CHAPTER 4

The Inverse Care Law

Andy Haines

NOMINATED CLASSIC PAPER
Julian Tudor Hart. The Inverse Care Law. *The Lancet*, 1971; 297(7696): 405–12.

The Inverse Care Law was a compelling analysis of the central importance of inequalities in health and wealth to the healthcare professions and how improving the access to high quality primary care can help address these inequalities. Although its focus is on the United Kingdom (UK), and particularly South Wales, its implications are international.

The paper marshalled contemporary evidence that poor populations experienced higher levels of morbidity and mortality than wealthy populations and received lower-quality care. It also provided a cogent analysis of why market-based approaches cannot deal effectively with the challenges of providing healthcare to whole populations, because they accentuate existing inequalities. It addressed the need for adequate funding of health services, noting that even at that time, some politicians believed that the ceiling for tax-based funding of health services had been reached and that additional funds should be sought by out-of-pocket payments. This proved incorrect and expenditure on healthcare from taxation has increased in many countries, thus avoiding the regressive effects of charging for healthcare at the point of use.

Julian Tudor Hart argued for greater recruitment of medical students from non-professional backgrounds and from state rather than private schools, reasoning that students from such backgrounds were more likely to have social ties in deprived communities and thus more likely to be committed to working in them. He bemoaned the fact that in 1971 the majority of medical schools 'do not have serious departments of general practice and community medicine', a deficiency that, in the UK at least, has been largely addressed but is still a challenge in many countries. His overview of the dramatic changes in healthcare following the introduction of the National Health Service (NHS) in the UK in 1948 should be illustrative to readers living in low/middle income countries that are now increasingly moving towards universal health coverage (UHC) and facing many challenges similar to those encountered during the transition to the NHS in the UK. Indeed, this paper can be seen as visionary in its articulation of why UHC is an imperative for all countries which in 2015 was embodied in the Sustainable Development Goals as part of Goal 3 to 'Ensure healthy lives and promote well-being for all at all ages'.

ABOUT THE AUTHOR OF THIS PAPER

Julian Tudor Hart worked as a general practitioner in the mining community of Glyncorrwg in South Wales for 30 years. He is an inspirational thinker and writer about how to provide humane, effective care funded and delivered by the public sector. His practice was the first research practice recognised by the UK Medical Research Council and it pioneered many major studies. He is particularly known for his work integrating the principles of epidemiology with clinical practice in primary care, exemplified by his seminal paper 'Semi-continuous screening of a whole community for hypertension', published in *The Lancet* in 1970, and a 21-year follow-up of screen-detected hypertension in people under 40, published in the *British Medical Journal* in 1993.

Julian was the first to demonstrate rigorously the feasibility of measuring blood pressure in a whole population, capitalising on the opportunities provided by the consultation to provide 'anticipatory care'. He had the courage and integrity to expose his own practice to scrutiny in his paper 'Be your own coroner: an audit of 500 consecutive deaths in a general practice', published in the *British Medical Journal* in 1987.

Julian Tudor Hart is an exceptional example of how commitment to clinical practice in a deprived community can be combined with powerful advocacy for social justice and innovative research.

ABOUT THE NOMINATOR OF THIS PAPER

Professor Andy Haines was a trainee and research assistant in Julian Hart's practice, an epidemiologist with the Medical Research Council and subsequently an inner-city academic general practitioner in London for 20 years. He was also the Professor of Primary Health Care at University College London (UCL) and was then appointed as Dean, subsequently Director, of the London School of Hygiene and Tropical Medicine (LSHTM) for nearly 10 years. He is currently Professor of Primary Care and Public Health at LSHTM, where his focus is now on global environmental change and health.

'Keep an open mind, do not be afraid to question orthodoxy but build your criticisms on strong evidence. Do not restrict your research to merely describing problems but attempt to develop solutions and evaluate them rigorously. If your proposed interventions do not have the desired effect, do not be discouraged; learning what doesn't work can be as important as knowing what does. Do not tie yourself to a single discipline, forge transdisciplinary collaborations and learn from different perspectives.'

Professor Sir Andy Haines, United Kingdom

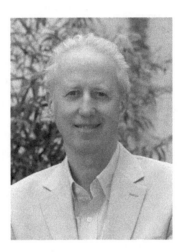

Attribution:

We attribute the original publication of *The Inverse Care Law* to *The Lancet*. With thanks to Lakshmi Priya at Elsevier.

The Lancet · Saturday 27 February 1971

THE INVERSE CARE LAW

JULIAN TUDOR HART

Glyncorrwg Health Centre, Port Talbot, Glamorgan, Wales

Summary   The availability of good medical care tends to vary inversely with the need for it in the population served. This inverse care law operates more completely where medical care is most exposed to market forces, and less so where such exposure is reduced. The market distribution of medical care is a primitive and historically outdated social form, and any return to it would further exaggerate the maldistribution of medical resources.

Interpreting the Evidence

THE existence of large social and geographical inequalities in mortality and morbidity in Britain is known, and not all of them are diminishing. Between 1934 and 1968, weighted mean standardised mortality from all causes in the Glamorgan and Monmouthshire valleys rose from 128% of England and Wales rates to 131%. Their weighted mean infant mortality rose from 115% of England and Wales rates to 124% between 1921 and 1968.[1] The Registrar General's last Decennial Supplement on Occupational Mortality for 1949–53 still showed combined social classes I and II (wholly non-manual) with a standardised mortality from all causes 18% below the mean, and combined social classes IV and V (wholly manual) 5% above it. Infant mortality was 37% below the mean for social class I (professional) and 38% above it for social class V (unskilled manual).

A just and rational distribution of the resources of medical care should show parallel social and geographical differences, or at least a uniform distribution. The common experience was described by Titmuss in 1968:

" We have learnt from 15 years' experience of the Health Service that the higher income groups know how to make better use of the service; they tend to receive more specialist attention; occupy more of the beds in better equipped and staffed hospitals; receive more elective surgery; have better maternal care, and are more likely to get psychiatric help and psychotherapy than low-income groups—particularly the unskilled."[2]

These generalisations are not easily proved statistically, because most of the statistics are either not available (for instance, outpatient waiting-lists by area and social class, age and cause specific hospital mortality-rates by area and social class, the relation between ante-mortem and post-mortem diagnosis by area and social class, and hospital staff shortage by area) or else they are essentially use-rates. Use-rates may be

interpreted either as evidence of high morbidity among high users, or of disproportionate benefit drawn by them from the National Health Service. By piling up the valid evidence that poor people in Britain have higher consultation and referral rates at all levels of the N.H.S., and by denying that these reflect actual differences in morbidity, Rein[3,4] has tried to show that Titmuss's opinion is incorrect, and that there are no significant gradients in the quality or accessibility of medical care in the N.H.S. between social classes.

Class gradients in mortality are an obvious obstacle to this view. Of these Rein says:

" One conclusion reached . . . is that since the lower classes have higher death rates, then they must be both sicker or less likely to secure treatment than other classes . . . it is useful to examine selected diseases in which there is a clear mortality class gradient and then compare these rates with the proportion of patients in each class that consulted their physician for treatment of these diseases. . . ."

He cites figures to show that high death-rates may be associated with low consultation-rates for some diseases, and with high rates for others, but, since the pattern of each holds good through all social classes, he concludes that

" a reasonable inference to be drawn from these findings is not that class mortality is an index of class morbidity, but that for certain diseases treatment is unrelated to outcome. Thus both high and low consultation rates can yield high mortality rates for specific diseases. These data do not appear to lead to the compelling conclusion that mortality votes can be easily used as an area of class-related morbidity."

This is the only argument mounted by Rein against the evidence of mortality differences, and the reasonable assumption that these probably represent the final outcome of larger differences in morbidity. Assuming that " votes " is a misprint for " rates ", I still find that the more one examines this argument the less it means. To be fair, it is only used to support the central thesis that " the availability of universal free-on-demand, comprehensive services would appear to be a crucial factor in reducing class inequalities in the use of medical care services ". It certainly would, but reduction is not abolition, as Rein would have quickly found if his stay in Britain had included more basic fieldwork in the general practitioner's surgery or the outpatient department.

Non-statistical Evidence

There is massive but mostly non-statistical evidence in favour of Titmuss's generalisations. First of all there is the evidence of social history. James[5] described the origins of the general-practitioner service in indus-

THE LANCET, FEBRUARY 27, 1971

trial and coalmining areas, from which the present has grown:

" The general practitioner in working-class areas discovered the well-tried business principle of small profits with a big turnover where the population was large and growing rapidly; it paid to treat a great many people for a small fee. A waiting-room crammed with patients, each representing 2s. 6d. for a consultation . . . not only gave a satisfactory income but also reduced the inclination to practise clinical medicine with skilful care, to attend clinical meetings, or to seek refreshment from the scientific literature. Particularly in coalmining areas, workers formed themselves into clubs to which they contributed a few pence a week, and thus secured free treatment from the club doctor for illness or accident. The club system was the forerunner of health insurance and was a humane and desirable social development. But, like the ' cash surgery ', it encouraged the doctor to undertake the treatment of more patients than he could deal with efficiently. It also created a difference between the club patients and those who could afford to pay for medical attention . . . in these circumstances it is a tribute to the profession that its standards in industrial practices were as high as they were. If criticism is necessary, it should not be of the doctors who developed large industrial practices but of the leaders of all branches of the profession, who did not see the trend of general practice, or, having seen it, did nothing to influence it. It is particularly regrettable that the revolutionary conception of a National Health Service, which has transformed the hospitals of the United Kingdom to the great benefit of the community, should not have brought about an equally radical change in general practice. Instead, because of the shortsightedness of the profession, the N.H.S. has preserved and intensified the worst features of general practice. . . ."

This preservation and intensification was described by Collings [6] in his study of the work of 104 general practitioners in 55 English practices outside London, including 9 completely and 7 partly industrial practices, six months after the start of the N.H.S. Though not randomly sampled, the selection of practices was structured in a reasonably representative manner. The very bad situation he described was the one I found when I entered a slum practice in Notting Hill in 1953, rediscovered in all but one of five industrial practices where I acted as locum tenens in 1961, and found again when I resumed practice in the South Wales valleys. Collings said:

" the working environment of general practitioners in industrial areas was so limiting that their individual capacity as doctors counted very little. In the circumstances prevailing, the most essential qualification for the industrial G.P. . . . is ability as a snap diagnostician—an ability to reach an accurate diagnosis on a minimum of evidence . . . the worst elements of general practice are to be found in those places where there is the greatest and most urgent demand for good medical service. . . . Some conditions of general practice are bad enough to change a good doctor into a bad doctor in a very short time. These very bad conditions are to be found chiefly in industrial areas."

In a counter-report promoted by the British Medical Association, Hadfield [7] contested all of Collings' conclusions, but, though his sampling was much better designed, his criticism was guarded to the point of complacency, and most vaguely defined. One of Collings' main criticisms—that purpose-built premises and ancillary staff were essential for any serious up-

grading of general practice—is only now being taken seriously; and even the present wave of health-centre construction shows signs of finishing almost as soon as it has begun, because of the present climate of political and economic opinion at the level of effective decision. Certainly in industrial and mining areas health centres exist as yet only on a token basis, and the number of new projects is declining. Aneurin Bevan described health centres as the cornerstone of the general-practitioner service under the N.H.S., before the long retreat began from the conceptions of the service born in the 1930s and apparently victorious in 1945. Health-centre construction was scrapped by ministerial circular in January, 1948, in the last months of gestation of the new service; we have had to do without them for 22 years, during which a generation of primary care was stunted.

Despite this unpromising beginning, the N.H.S. brought about a massive improvement in the delivery of medical care to previously deprived sections of the people and areas of the country. Former Poor Law hospitals were upgraded and many acquired fully trained specialist and ancillary staff and supporting diagnostic departments for the first time. The backlog of untreated disease dealt with in the first years of the service was immense, particularly in surgery and gynæcology. A study of 734 randomly sampled families in London and Northampton in 1961 [8] showed that in 99% of the families someone had attended hospital as an outpatient, and in 82% someone had been admitted to hospital. The study concluded:

" When thinking of the Health Service mothers are mainly conscious of the extent to which services have become available in recent years. They were more aware of recent changes in health services than of changes in any other service. Nearly one third thought that more money should be spend on health services, not because they thought them bad but because ' they are so important ', because ' doctors and nurses should be paid more ' or because ' there shouldn't be charges for treatment '. Doctors came second to relatives and friends in the list of those who had been helpful in times of trouble."

Among those with experience of pre-war services, appreciation for the N.H.S., often uncritical appreciation, is almost universal—so much so that, although most London teaching-hospital consultants made their opposition to the new service crudely evident to their students in 1948 and the early years, and only a courageous few openly supported it, few of them appear to recall this today. The moral defeat of the very part-time, multi-hospital consultant, nipping in here and there between private consultations to see how his registrar was coping with his public work, was total and permanent; lip-service to the N.H.S. is now mandatory. At primary-care level, private practice ceased to be relevant to the immense majority of general practitioners, and has failed to produce evidence of the special functions of leadership and quality claimed for it, in the form of serious research material. On the other hand, despite the massive economic disincentives to good work, equipment, and staffing in the N.H.S. until a few years ago, an important expansion of well-organised, community-oriented, and self-critical primary care has taken place, mainly through the efforts of the Royal College of General Practitioners;

the main source of this vigour is the democratic nature of the service—the fact that it is comprehensive and accessible to all, and that clinical decisions are therefore made more freely than ever before. The service at least permits, if it does not yet really encourage, general practitioners to think and act in terms of the care of a whole defined community, as well as of whole persons rather than diseases. Collings seems very greatly to have underestimated the importance of these changes, and the extent to which they were to overshadow the serious faults of the service—and these were faults of too little change, rather than too much. There have in fact been very big improvements in the quality and accessibility of care both at hospital and primary-care level, for all classes and in all areas.

Selective Redistribution of Care

Given the large social inequalities of mortality and morbidity that undoubtedly existed before the 1939–45 war, and the equally large differences in the quality and accessibility of medical resources to deal with them, it was clearly not enough simply to improve care for everyone: some selective redistribution was necessary, and some has taken place. But how much, and is the redistribution accelerating, stagnating, or even going into reverse ?

Ann Cartwright's study of 1370 randomly sampled adults in representative areas of England, and their 552 doctors,[9] gave some evidence on what had and what had not been achieved. She confirmed a big improvement in the quality of primary care in 1961 compared with 1948, but also found just the sort of class differences suggested by Titmuss. The consultation-rate of middle-class patients at ages under 45 was 53% less than that of working-class patients, but at ages over 75 they had a consultation-rate 62% higher; and between these two age-groups there was stepwise progression. I think it is reasonable to interpret this as evidence that middle-class consultations had a higher clinical content at all ages, that working-class consultations below retirement age had a higher administrative content, and that the middle-class was indeed able to make more effective use of primary care. Twice as many middle-class patients were critical of consulting-rooms and of their doctors, and three times as many of waiting-rooms, as were working-class patients; yet Cartwright and Marshall[10] in another study found that in predominantly working-class areas 80% of the doctors' surgeries were built before 1900, and only 5% since 1945; in middle-class areas less than 50% were built before 1900, and 25% since 1945. Middle-class patients were both more critical and better served. Three times as many middle-class patients were critical of the fullness of explanations to them about their illnesses; it is very unlikely that this was because they actually received less explanation than working-class patients, and very likely that they expected, sometimes demanded, and usually received, much more. Cartwright's study of hospital care showed the same social trend for explanations by hospital staff.[11] The same study looked at hospital patients' general practitioners, and compared those working in middle-class and in working-class areas: more middle-class area G.P.s had lists under 2000 than did working-class area G.P.s, and fewer had

lists over 2500; nearly twice as many had higher qualifications, more had access to contrast-media X-rays, nearly five times as many had access to physiotherapy, four times as many had been to Oxford or Cambridge, five times as many had been to a London medical school, twice as many held hospital appointments or hospital beds in which they could care for their own patients, and nearly three times as many sometimes visited their patients when they were in hospital under a specialist. Not all of these differences are clinically significant; so far the record of Oxbridge and the London teaching hospitals compares unfavourably with provincial medical schools for training oriented to the community. But the general conclusion must be that those most able to choose where they will work tend to go to middle-class areas, and that the areas with highest mortality and morbidity tend to get those doctors who are least able to choose where they will work. Such a system is not likely to distribute the doctors with highest morale to the places where that morale is most needed. Of those doctors who positively choose working-class areas, a few will be attracted by large lists with a big income and an uncritical clientele; many more by social and family ties of their own. Effective measures of redistribution would need to take into account the importance of increasing the proportion of medical students from working-class families in areas of this sort; the report of the Royal Commission on Medical Education[12] showed that social class I (professional and higher managerial), which is 2·8% of the population, contributed 34·5% of the final-year medical students in 1961, and 39·6% of the first-year students in 1966, whereas social class III (skilled workers, manual and non-manual), which is 49·9% of the population, contributed 27·9% of the final-year students in 1961 and 21·7% of the first-year in 1966. The proportion who had received State education was 43·4% in both years, compared with 70·9% of all school-leavers with 3 or more A-levels. In other words, despite an increasing supply of well-qualified State-educated school-leavers, the overrepresentation of professional families among medical students is increasing. Unless this trend is reversed, the difficulties of recruitment in industrial areas will increase from this cause as well, not to speak of the support it will give to the officers/other ranks' tradition in medical care and education.

The upgrading of provincial hospitals in the first few years after the Act certainly had a geographical redistributive effect, and, because some of the wealthiest areas of the country are concentrated in and around London, it also had a socially redistributive effect. There was a period in which the large formerly local-authority hospitals were accelerating faster than the former voluntary hospitals in their own areas, and some catching-up took place that was socially redistributive. But the better-endowed, better-equipped, better-staffed areas of the service draw to themselves more and better staff, and more and better equipment, and their superiority is compounded. While a technical lead in teaching hospitals is necessary and justified, these advantages do not apply only to teaching hospitals, and even these can be dangerous if they encourage complacency about the periphery, which is all too common. As we enter an era of scarcity in medical staffing and

THE LANCET, FEBRUARY 27, 1971

austerity in Treasury control, this gap will widen, and any social redistribution that has taken place is likely to be reversed.

Redistribution of general practitioners also took place at a fairly rapid pace in the early years of the N.H.S., for two reasons. First, and least important, were the inducement payments and area classifications with restricted entry to over-doctored areas. These may have been of value in discouraging further accumulation of doctors in the Home Counties and on the coast, but Collings was right in saying that " any hope that financial reward alone will attract good senior practitioners back to these bad conditions is illusory; the good doctor will only be attracted into industrial practice by providing conditions which will enable him to do good work ". The second and more important reason is that in the early years of the N.H.S. it was difficult for the increased number of young doctors trained during and just after the 1939–45 war to get posts either in hospital or in general practice, and many took the only positions open to them, bringing with them new standards of care. Few of those doctors today would choose to work in industrial areas, now that there is real choice; we know that they are not doing so. Of 169 new general practitioners who entered practice in under-doctored areas between October, 1968, and October, 1969, 164 came from abroad.[13] The process of redistribution of general practitioners ceased by 1956, and by 1961 had gone into reverse; between 1961 and 1967, the proportion of people in England and Wales in under-doctored areas rose from 17% to 34%.[14]

Increasing List Size

The quality and traditions of primary medical care in industrial and particularly in mining areas are, I think, central to the problem of persistent inequality in morbidity and mortality and the mismatched distribution of medical resources in relation to them. If doctors in industrial areas are to reach take-off speed in reorganising their work and giving it more clinical content, they must be free enough from pressure of work to stand back and look at it critically. With expanding lists this will be for the most part impossible; there is a limit to what can be expected of doctors in these circumstances, and the alcoholism that is an evident if unrecorded occupational hazard among those doctors who have spent their professional lives in industrial practice is one result of exceeding that limit. Yet list sizes are going up, and will probably do so most where a reduction is most urgent. Fry[15] and Last[16] have criticised the proposals of the Royal Commission on Medical Education[17] for an average annual increase of 100 doctors in training over the next 25 years, which would raise the number of economically active doctors per million population from 1181 in 1965 to 1801 in 1995. They claim that there are potential increases in productivity in primary care, by devolution of work to ancillary and paramedical workers and by rationalisation of administrative work, that would permit much larger average list sizes without loss of intimacy in personal care, or decline in clinical quality. Of course, much devolution and rationalisation of this sort is necessary, not to cope

with rising numbers, but to make general practice more clinically effective and satisfying, so that people can be seen less often but examined in greater depth. If clinically irrelevant work can be devoluted or abolished, it is possible to expand into new and valuable fields of work such as those opened up by Balint and his school,[18] and the imminent if not actual possibilities of presymptomatic diagnosis and screening, which can best be done at primary-care level and is possible within the present resources of N.H.S. general practice.[19] But within the real political context of 1971 the views of Last, and of Fry from his experience of London suburban practice which is very different from the industrial areas discussed here, are dangerously complacent.

Progressive change in these industrial areas depends first of all on two things, which must go hand in hand: accelerated construction of health centres, and the reduction of list sizes by a significant influx of the type of young doctor described by Barber in 1950[20]:

" so prepared for general practice, and for the difference between what he is taught to expect and what he actually finds, that he will adopt a fighting attitude against poor medicine—that is to say, against hopeless conditions for the practice of good medicine. The young man must be taught to be sufficiently courageous, so that when he arrives at the converted shop with the drab battered furniture, the couch littered with dusty bottles, and the few rusty antiquated instruments, he will make a firm stand and say ' I will not practise under these conditions; I will have more room, more light, more ancillary help, and better equipment.' "

Unfortunately, the medical ethic transmitted by most of our medical schools, at least the majority that do not have serious departments of general practice and community medicine, leads to the present fact that the young man just does not arrive at the converted shop; he has more room, more light, more ancillary help, and better equipment by going where these already exist, and no act of courage is required. The career structure and traditions of our medical schools make it clear that time spent at the periphery in the hospital service, or at the bottom of the heap in industrial general practice, is almost certain disqualification for any further advancement. Our best hope of obtaining the young men and women we need lies in the small but significant extent to which medical students are beginning to reject this ethic, influenced by the much greater critical awareness of students in other disciplines. Some are beginning to question which is the top and which the bottom of the ladder, or even whether there should be a ladder at all; and in the promise of the Todd report, of teaching oriented to the patient and the community rather than toward the doctor and the disease, there is hope that this mood in a minority of medical students may become incorporated into a new and better teaching tradition. It is possible that we may get a cohort of young men and women with the sort of ambitions Barber described, and with a realistic attitude to the battles they will have to fight to get the conditions of work and the buildings and equipment they need, in the places that need them; but we have few of them now. The prospect for primary care in industrial areas for the next ten years is bad; list sizes will probably continue

THE LANCET, FEBRUARY 27, 1971

to increase, and the pace of improvement in quality of primary care is likely to fall.

Recruitment to General Practice in South Wales

Although the most under-doctored areas are mainly of the older industrial type, the South Wales valleys have relatively good doctor/patient ratios, partly because of the declining populations, and partly because the area produces an unusually high proportion of its own doctors, who often have kinship ties nearby and may be less mobile on that account. (In Williams' survey of general practice in South Wales 72% of the 68 doctors were born in Wales and 43% had qualified at the Welsh National School of Medicine.[21]) On Jan. 1, 1970, of 36 South Wales valley areas listed, only 4 were designated as under-doctored. However, this situation is unstable; as our future becomes more apparently precarious, as pits close without alternative local employment, as unemployment rises, and out-migration that is selective for the young and healthy increases, doctors become subject to the same pressures and uncertainties as their patients. Recruitment of new young doctors is becoming more and more difficult, and dependent on doctors from abroad. Many of the industrial villages are separated from one another by several miles, and public transport is withering while as yet comparatively few have cars, so that centralisation of primary care is difficult, and could accelerate the decay of communities. These communities will not disappear, because most people with kinship ties are more stubborn than the planners, and because they have houses here and cannot get them where the work is; the danger is not the disappearance of these communities, but their persistence below the threshold of viability, with accumulating sickness and a loss of the people to deal with it.

What Should Be Done ?

Medical services are not the main determinant of mortality or morbidity; these depend most upon standards of nutrition, housing, working environment, and education, and the presence or absence of war. The high mortality and morbidity of the South Wales valleys arise mainly from lower standards in most of these variables now and in the recent past, rather than from lower standards of medical care. But that is no excuse for failure to match the greatest need with the highest standards of care. The bleak future now facing mining communities, and others that may suffer similar social dislocation as technical change blunders on without agreed social objectives, cannot be altered by doctors alone; but we do have a duty to draw attention to the need for global costing when it comes to policy decisions on redevelopment or decay of established industrial communities. Such costing would take into account the full social costs and not only those elements of profit and loss traditionally recognised in industry.

The improved access to medical care for previously deprived sections under the N.H.S. arose chiefly from the decision to remove primary-care services from exposure to market forces. The consequences of distribution of care by the operation of the market were unjust and irrational, despite all sorts of charitable modifications. The improved possibilities for constructive planning and rational distribution of resources because of this decision are immense, and even now are scarcely realised in practice. The losses predicted by opponents of this change have not in fact occurred; consultants who no longer depend on private practice have shown at least as much initiative and responsibility as before, and the standards attained in the best N.H.S. primary care are at least as good as those in private practice. It has been proved that a national health service can run quite well without the profit motive, and that the motivation of the work itself can be more powerful in a decommercialised setting. The gains of the service derive very largely from the simple and clear principles on which it was conceived: a comprehensive national service, available to all, free at the time of use, non-contributory, and financed from taxation. Departures from these principles, both when the service began (the tripartite division and omission of family-planning and chiropody services) and subsequently (dental and prescription charges, rising direct contributions, and relative reductions in financing from taxation), have not strengthened it. The principles themselves seem to me to be worth defending, despite the risk of indulging in unfashionable value-judgments. The accelerating forward movement of general practice today, impressively reviewed in a symposium on group practice held by the Royal College of General Practitioners,[22] is a movement (not always conscious) toward these principles and the ideas that prevailed generally among the minority of doctors who supported them in 1948, including their material corollary, group practice from health centres. The doctor/patient relationship, which was held by opponents of the Act to depend above all on a cash transaction between patient and doctor, has been transformed and improved by abolishing that transaction. A general practitioner can now think in terms of service to a defined community, and plan his work according to rational priorities.

Godber [23] has reviewed this question of medical priorities, which he sees as a new feature arising from the much greater real effectiveness of modern medicine, which provides a wider range of real choices, and the great costliness of certain forms of treatment. While these factors are important, there are others of greater importance which he omits. Even when the content of medicine was overwhelmingly palliative or magical —say, up to the 1914–18 war—the public could not face the intolerable facts any more than doctors could, and both had as great a sense of priorities as we have; matters of life and death arouse the same passions when hope is illusory as when it is real, as the palatial Swiss tuberculosis sanatoria testify. The greatest difference, I think, lies in the transformation in social expectations. In 1914 gross inequality and injustice were regarded as natural by the privileged, irresistible by the unprivileged, and inevitable by nearly everyone. This is no longer true; inequality is now politically dangerous once it is recognised, and its inevitability is believed in only by a minority. Diphtheria became preventable in the early 1930s, yet there were 50,000 cases in England and Wales in 1941 and 2400 of them died.[24] I knew one woman who buried four of her children in five weeks during an outbreak of

THE LANCET, FEBRUARY 27, 1971

diphtheria in the late 1930s. No systematic national campaign of immunisation was begun until well into the 1939–45 war years, and, if such a situation is unthinkable today, the difference is political rather than technical. Godber rightly points to the planning of hospital services during the war as one starting-point of the change; but he omits the huge social and political fact of 1945: that a majority of people, having experienced the market distribution of human needs before the war, and the revelation that the market could be overridden during the war for an agreed social purpose, resolved never to return to the old system.

Perhaps reasonable economy in the distribution of medical care is imperilled most of all by the old ethical concept of the isolated one-doctor/one-patient relationship, pushed relentlessly to its conclusion regardless of cost—or, to put it differently, of the needs of others. The pursuit of the very best for each patient who needs it remains an important force in the progress of care; a young person in renal failure may need a doctor who will fight for dialysis, or a grossly handicapped child one who will find the way to exactly the right department, and steer past the defeatists in the wrong ones. But this pursuit must pay some regard to humane priorities, as it may not if the patient is a purchaser of medical care as a commodity. The idealised, isolated doctor/patient relationship, that ignores the needs of other people and their claims on the doctor's time and other scarce resources, is incomplete and distorts our view of medicine. During the formative period of modern medicine this ideal situation could be realised only among the wealthy, or, in the special conditions of teaching hospitals, among those of the unprivileged with " interesting " diseases. The ambition to practise this ideal medicine under ideal conditions still makes doctors all over the world leave those who need them most, and go to those who need them least, and it retards the development of national schools of thought and practice in medicine, genuinely based on the local content of medical care. The ideal isolated doctor/patient relation has the same root as the 19th-century preoccupation with Robinson Crusoe as an economic elementary particle; both arise from a view of society that can perceive only a contractual relation between independent individuals. The new and hopeful dimension in general practice is the recognition that the primary-care doctor interacts with individual members of a defined community. Such a community-oriented doctor is not likely to encourage expensive excursions into the 21st century, since his position makes him aware, as few specialists can be, of the scale of demand at its point of origin, and will therefore be receptive to common-sense priorities. It is this primary-care doctor who in our country initiates nearly every train of causation in the use of sophisticated medical care, and has some degree of control over what is done or not done at every point. The commitment is a great deal less open-ended than many believe; we really do not prolong useless, painful, or demented lives on the scale sometimes imagined. We tend to be more interested in the people who have diseases than in the diseases themselves, and that is the first requirement of reasonable economy and a humane scale of priorities.

Return to the Market ?

The past ten years have seen a spate of papers urging that the N.H.S. be returned wholly or partly to the operation of the market. Jewkes,[25] Lees,[26] Seale,[27] and the advisory planning panel on health services financing of the British Medical Association [28] have all elaborated on this theme. Their arguments consist in a frontal attack on the policy of removing health care from the market, together with criticism of faults in the service that do not necessarily or even probably depend on that policy at all, but on the failure of Governments to devote a sufficient part of the national product to medical care. These faults include the stagnation in hospital building and senior staffing throughout the 1950s, the low wages throughout the service up to consultant level, over-centralised control, and failure to realise the objective of social and geographical equality in access to the best medical care. None of these failings is intrinsic to the original principles of the N.H.S.; all have been deplored by its supporters, and with more vigour than by these critics. The critics depend heavily on a climate of television and editorial opinion favouring the view that all but a minority of people are rich enough and willing to pay for all they need in medical care (but not through taxation), and that public services are a historically transient social form, appropriate to indigent populations, to be discarded as soon as may be in favour of distribution of health care as a bought commodity, provided by competing entrepreneurs. They depend also on the almost universal abdication of principled opposition to these views, on the part of its official opponents. The former Secretary of State for Social Services, Mr. Richard Crossman, has agreed that the upper limit of direct taxation has been reached, and that " we should not be afraid to look for alternative sources of revenue less dependent on the Chancellor's whims. . . . I should not rule out obtaining a higher proportion of the cost of the service from the Health Service contribution."[29] This is simply a suggestion that rising health costs should be met by flat-rate contributions unrelated to income—an acceptance of the view that the better-off are taxed to the limit, but also that the poor can afford to pay more in proportion. With such opposition, it is not surprising that more extravagant proposals for substantial payments at the time of illness, for consultations, home visits, and hospital care, are more widely discussed and advocated than ever before.

Seale [27] proposed a dual health service, with a major part of hospital and primary care on a fee-paying basis assisted by private insurance, and a minimum basic service excluding the " great deal of medical care which is of only marginal importance so far as the life or death or health of the individual is concerned. Do those who want the Health Service to provide only the best want the frills of medical care to be only the best, or have they so little understanding of the nature of medical care that they are unaware of the existence of the frills ?" Frills listed by Seale are: " time, convenience, freedom of choice, and privacy ". He says that " it is precisely these facets of medical care—the ' middle class ' standards—which become more important to individuals as they become more prosperous ". Do they indeed? Perhaps it is not so much that they (and other frills such as courtesy, and willingness to listen and to explain, that may be guaranteed by payment of a fee) become more important, as that they become accessible. The possession of a new car is an index of prosperity; the lack of one is not evidence that it is not wanted. Real evidence should be provided that it is possible to separate the components of medical care into frills that have no bearing on life, death, or health, and essentials which do. Life and happiness most certainly can hang on a readiness to listen, to dig beneath the presenting symptom, and to encourage a return when something appears to have been left unsaid. And not only the patient—*all* patients—value these things; to practise medicine without them makes a doctor despise his trade and his patients. Where are the doctors to be found to undertake this veterinary care? It need not be said; those of us who already work in industrial areas are expected to abandon the progress we have made toward universal, truly personal care and return to the bottom half of the traditional double standard. This is justified in anticipation by Seale:

" some doctors are very much better than others and this will always be so, and the standard of care provided by them will vary within wide limits . . . the function of the State is, in general, to do those things which the individual cannot do and to assist him to do things better. It is not to do for the individual what he can well do for himself. . . . I should like to see reform of the Health Service in the years ahead which is based on the assumption of individual responsibility for personal health, with the State's function limited to the prevention of real hardship and the encouragement of personal responsibility."

Lees'[26] central thesis is that medical care is a commodity that should be bought and sold as any other, and would be optimally distributed in a free market. A free market in houses or shoes does not distribute them optimally; rich people get too much and the poor too little, and the same is true of medical care. He claims that the N.H.S. violates " natural " economic law, and will fail if a free market is not restored, in some degree at least, and that in a free market " we would spend more on medical care than the government does on our behalf ". If the " we " in question is really all of us, no problem exists; we agree to pay higher income-tax and/or give up some million-pound bombers or whatever, and have the expanding service we want. But if the " we " merely means " us " as opposed to " them ", it means only that the higher social classes will pay more for their own care, but not for the community as a whole. They will then want value for their money, a visible differential between commodity-care and the utility brand; is it really possible, let alone desirable, to run any part of the health service in this way? Raymond Williams[30] put his finger on the real point here:

" we think of our individual patterns of use in the favourable terms of spending and satisfaction, but of our social patterns of use in the unfavourable terms of deprivation and taxation. It seems a fundamental defect of our society that social purposes are largely financed out of individual incomes, by a method of rates and taxes which makes it very easy for us to feel that society is a thing that con-

tinually deprives and limits us—without this we could all be profitably spending. . . . We think of ' my money ' . . . in these naive terms, because parts of our very idea of society are withered at root. We can hardly have any conception, in our present system, of the financing of social purposes from the social product. . . ."

Seale[31] thinks the return to the market would help to provide the continuous audit that is certainly necessary to intelligent planning in the health service:

" In a health service provided free of charge efficient management is particularly difficult because neither the purpose nor the product of the organisation can be clearly defined, and because there are few automatic checks to managerial incompetence. . . . In any large organisation management requires quantitative information if it is to be able to analyse a situation, make a decision, and know whether its actions have achieved the desired result. In commerce this quantitative information is supplied primarily in monetary terms. By using the simple, convenient, and measurable criterion of profit as both objective and product, management has a yardstick for assessing the quality of the organisation and the effectiveness of its own decisions."

The purposes and desired product of medical care are complex, but Seale has given no evidence to support his opinion that they cannot be clearly measured or defined; numerous measures of mortality, morbidity, and cost and labour effectiveness in terms of them are available and are (insufficiently) used. They can be developed much more easily in a comprehensive service outside the market than in a fragmented one within it. We already know that we can study and measure the working of the National Health Service more cheaply and easily than the diverse and often irrational medical services of areas of the United States of comparable population, though paradoxically there are certain techniques of quality control that are much more necessary in America than they are here. Tissue committees monitor the work of surgeons by identifying excised normal organs, and specialist registration protects the public from spurious claims by medical entrepreneurs. The motivation for fraud has almost disappeared from the N.H.S., and with it the need for certain forms of audit. A market economy in medical care leads to a number of wasteful trends that are acknowledged problems in the United States. Hospital admission rates are inflated to make patients eligible for insurance benefit, and, according to Fry[32]:

" In some areas, particularly the more prosperous, competition for patients exists between local hospitals, since lack of regional planning has led to an excess of hospital facilities in some localities. In such circumstances hospital administrators are encouraged to use public relations officers and other means of self-advertisement. . . . This competition also leads to certain hospital ' status symbols ', where features such as the possession of a computer; the possession of a ' cobalt bomb ' unit; the ability to perform open-heart surgery albeit infrequently; and the listing of a neurosurgeon on the staff are all current symbols of status in the eyes of certain groups of the public. Even small hospitals of 150–200 beds may consider such features as necessities."

And though these are the more obvious defects of substituting profit for the normal and direct objectives of medical care, the audit by profit has another and much more serious fault; it concentrates all our attention on tactical efficiency, while ignoring the

412

THE LANCET, FEBRUARY 27, 1971

need for strategic social decisions. A large advertising agency may be highly efficient and profitable, but is this a measure of its socially useful work ? It was the operation of the self-regulating market that resulted in a total expenditure on all forms of advertising of £455 million in 1960, compared with about £500 million on the whole of the hospital service in the same year.[33] The wonderfully self-regulating market does sometimes show a smaller intelligence than the most ignorant human voter.

All these trends of argument are gathered together in the report of the B.M.A. advisory planning panel on health services financing,[28] which recommends another dual service, one for quality and the other for minimum necessity. It states its view with a boldness that may account for its rather guarded reception by the General Medical Services Committee of the B.M.A.:

" The only sacrifice that would have to be made would be the concept of equality within the National Health Service . . . any claim that the N.H.S. has achieved its aim of providing equality in medical care is an illusion. In fact, absolute equality could never be achieved under any system of medical care, education or other essential service to the community. The motives for suggesting otherwise are political and ignore human factors."

The panel overlooks the fact that absolute correctness of diagnosis or absolute relief of suffering are also unattainable under any system of medical care; perhaps the only absolute that can be truly attained is the blindness of those who do not wish to see, and the human factor we should cease to ignore is the opposition of every privileged group to the loss of its privilege.

The Inverse Care Law

In areas with most sickness and death, general practitioners have more work, larger lists, less hospital support, and inherit more clinically ineffective traditions of consultation, than in the healthiest areas; and hospital doctors shoulder heavier case-loads with less staff and equipment, more obsolete buildings, and suffer recurrent crises in the availability of beds and replacement staff. These trends can be summed up as the inverse care law: that the availability of good medical care tends to vary inversely with the need of the population served.

If the N.H.S. had continued to adhere to its original principles, with construction of health centres a first priority in industrial areas, all financed from taxation rather than direct flat-rate contribution, free at the time of use, and fully inclusive of all personal health services, including family planning, the operation of the inverse care law would have been modified much more than it has been; but even the service as it is has been effective in redistributing care, considering the powerful social forces operating against this. If our health services had evolved as a free market, or even on a fee-for-item-of-service basis prepaid by private insurance, the law would have operated much more completely than it does; our situation might approximate to that in the United States,[34] with the added disadvantage of smaller national wealth. The force that creates and maintains the inverse care law is the operation of the market, and its cultural and ideological superstructure which has permeated the thought and directed the ambitions of our profession during all

of its modern history. The more health services are removed from the force of the market, the more successful we can be in redistributing care away from its " natural " distribution in a market economy; but this will be a redistribution, an intervention to correct a fault natural to our form of society, and therefore incompletely successful and politically unstable, in the absence of more fundamental social change.

I am grateful to Prof. W. R. S. Doll, F.R.S., for advice and criticism; to Miss M. Hammond, librarian of the Royal College of General Practitioners; and to the clerks of the Glamorgan and Monmouthshire Executive Councils for the National Health Service for data on recruitment of general practitioners in their areas.

REFERENCES

1. Hart, J. T. *J. R. Coll. gen. Practnrs* (in the press).
2. Titmuss, R. M. Commitment to Welfare. London, 1968.
3. Rein, M. *J. Am. Hosp. Ass.* 1969, **43**, 43.
4. Rein, M. *New Society*, Nov. 20, 1969, p. 807.
5. James, E. F. *Lancet*, 1961, i, 1361.
6. Collings, J. S. *ibid.* 1950, i, 555.
7. Hadfield, S. J. *Br. med. J.* 1953, ii, 683.
8. Family Needs and Social Services. Political and Economic Planning, London, 1961.
9. Cartwright, A. Patients and their Doctors. London, 1967.
10. Cartwright, A., Marshall, J. *Med. Care*, 1965, **3**, 69.
11. Cartwright, A. Human Relations and Hospital Care. London, 1964.
12. Report of the Royal Commission on Medical Education 1965–68; p. 331. London, 1968.
13. Department of Health and Social Security, Annual Report for 1969. London, 1970.
14. General Practice Today. Office of Health Economics, paper no. 28, London, 1968.
15. Fry, J. *J. R. Coll. gen. Practnrs*, 1969, **17**, 355.
16. Last, J. M. *Lancet*, 1968, ii, 166.
17. Report of the Royal Commission on Medical Education, 1965–68; p. 139. London, 1968.
18. Balint, M. The Doctor, his Patient, and the Illness. London, 1964.
19. Hart, J. T. *Lancet*, 1970, ii, 223.
20. Barber, G. *ibid.* 1950, i, 781.
21. Williams, W. O. A Study of General Practitioners' Workload in South Wales 1965–66. Royal College of General Practitioners, reports from general practice no. 12. January, 1970.
22. *J. R. Coll. gen. Practnrs*, 1970, **20**, suppl. 2.
23. Godber, G. *ibid.* 1970, **20**, 313.
24. Morris, J. N. Uses of Epidemiology. London, 1967.
25. Jewkes, J., Jewkes, S. The Genesis of the British National Health Service. Oxford, 1961.
26. Lees, D. S. Health through Choice. An Economic Study of the British National Health Service. Hobart paper no. 14, Institute of Economic Affairs, London, 1961.
27. Seale, J. *Br. med. J.* 1962, ii, 598.
28. Report of the Advisory Panel of the British Medical Association on Health Services Financing. B.M.A., London, 1970.
29. Crossman, R. H. S. Paying for the Social Services. Fabian Society, London, 1969.
30. Williams, R. The Long Revolution. London, 1961.
31. Seale, J. *Lancet*, 1961, ii, 476.
32. Fry, J. Medicine in Three Societies. Aylesbury, 1969.
33. *Observer*, March 19, 1961.
34. Battistella, R. M., Southby, R. M. F. *Lancet*, 1968, i, 581.

" Nearly half the hospital beds in the National Health Service are in mental or mental-handicap hospitals where the conditions are utterly disgraceful. Everyone admits this but no one is willing to find the relatively small amount of cash required to start putting things right. Public indifference to this mass suffering was bad enough in 1948 when the National Health Service took these hopelessly antiquated institutions over from the old Poor Law and the local authorities. It is intolerable that a quarter of a century later such asylums (though the name has been changed) still house up to 2,000 or even 3,000 inmates herded into dormitories with no room even for a locker between the beds and stripped of self-respect along with their personal property and clothes."—*New Statesman*, Feb. 19, 1971, p. 225.

CHAPTER 5

How family medicine research can lead to systematic understanding of health and illness within a local community

Jane Gunn

NOMINATED CLASSIC PAPER

Charles Bridges-Webb. The Traralgon Health and Illness Survey: method, organisation and comparison with other Australian studies. *International Journal of Epidemiology*, 1973; 2: 63–71.

This 1973 paper stands out as one of the foundational research papers of Australian primary care. It was written by Charles Bridges-Webb, a rural general practitioner (GP) who was spearheading the development of a systematic understanding of health and illness within a local community, at a time when this field was in its infancy worldwide. The paper provides a realistic and inspiring account of how he undertook research of international significance from a small practice in rural Australia. It also demonstrates a great collaboration between a GP and a primary care nurse.

The conceptual thinking behind the study demonstrates the importance of social and environmental factors upon health and their influence on the subjective experience of illness. This interest is still central to family medicine today. Charles Bridges-Webb used both interviews and health service record review to gather information from a broad range of health services including pharmacies, maternal and child health nurses, telephone helplines, relationship counselling services, and meals on wheels; this was an approach well ahead of its time. His decision to sample families as well as individuals, and the longitudinal nature of elements of the data collection, provided a rich and diverse data set that went on to provide crucial knowledge about what family doctors do and the complex community context in which they deliver healthcare.

The different perspectives included in the study provide valuable information about the visible and invisible ties that bind family medicine to the myriad of other services also operating in the community. The way in which this study collected data that generated knowledge about prevalence of illness, both acute and chronic, and the frequency with which people seek medical care, as well as the impact that illness had on people's ability to work, provide us with a wonderful insight into the health and illness patterns that make up the work of family medicine.

ABOUT THE LEAD AUTHOR OF THIS PAPER

Charles Bridges-Webb was a medical graduate of the University of Melbourne. He worked as a rural general practitioner in the Australian rural town of Traralgon, Victoria, from 1960 for 15 years, until he was appointed the Foundation Professor of Community Medicine at the University of Sydney in 1975.

Charles lived a full and rewarding life. He played important roles in the Royal Australian College of General Practitioners and was the chair of the International Classification Committee of the World Organization of Family Doctors (WONCA) from 1991 to 1999.

Charles was known for his *organised curiosity* and his painstaking approach to careful research, both of which are on full display in this paper.

Charles was an inspiring mentor to many primary care researchers and his research led to the establishment of the influential Bettering the Evaluation and Care of Health (BEACH) research programme still under way at the Family Medicine Research Centre at the University of Sydney. He wrote an autobiography, *To Travel Hopefully*, which I recommend to any family doctor looking for inspiration about how to combine a good life with research and clinical work.

ABOUT THE NOMINATOR OF THIS PAPER

Professor Jane Gunn is the Chair of Primary Care Research and Head of the Department of General Practice at the University of Melbourne. She is known for her work on depression in primary care and is one of the Expert Primary Care Advisors of the World Organization of Family Doctors (WONCA) to the World Health Organization's Mental Health Gap Action Programme.

> 'Family medicine is a great career. To make the most of it, work in a variety of practices and roles. Develop and maintain a role in medical education and research – it will keep you young and interested. Join a practice-based research

group. Learn mindfulness. Keep fit and have a hobby. Attend an international conference. Read.'

Professor Jane Gunn, Australia

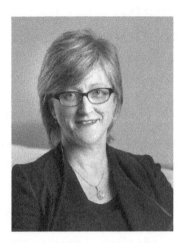

Attribution:

We attribute the original publication of *The Traralgon Health and Illness Survey: method, organization and comparison with other Australian studies* to the *International Journal of Epidemiology*. With thanks to Louise Eyre at Oxford University Press.

International Journal of Epidemiology
© Oxford University Press 1973

Vol. 2, No. 1
Printed in Great Britain

The Traralgon Health and Illness Survey; Method, Organization and Comparison with other Australian Surveys

C. BRIDGES-WEBB[1]

Bridges-Webb, C. (Dept. Social and Preventive Medicine, Monash University, Deakin Street Clinic, Traralgon 3844, Australia). The Traralgon Health and Illness Survey and comparison with other Australian surveys. *Int. J. Epid.* 1973, **2**: 63–71.
The methods and techniques used in the Traralgon Health and Illness Survey are presented in detail and compared with a number of other Australian health surveys. The importance of methodology in relation to the results of health and illness surveys is discussed using some results from Australian surveys as examples to provide further evidence of the slowly emerging picture of health and illness in Australia.

INTRODUCTION

The need to supplement data relating to mortality with data relating to morbidity as an index of sickness and health, and the importance of pre-symptomatic illness and of recognized but untreated illness, particularly chronic illness, in the community, is being increasingly recognized. Community surveys are necessary to supplement information about patients who currently use available health care services.

The Traralgon Health and Illness Survey was commenced in order to provide information about a community whose demographic, social and geographic circumstances were satisfactorily defined and not particularly atypical of communities in Australia, and in which the background and facilities for such research were available.

Since the evaluation of the information obtained in health surveys depends so much upon the methods and definitions which are used, and in accordance with the recommendation of the World Health Organization Expert Committee on Health Statistics (1) that in the publication of survey results due attention be given to describing the survey methods used, this report deals largely with the method and organization of the Survey and relates them and some general results to other Australian health surveys. Further detail is available from the author on request. Other reports dealing with the results of the survey are in preparation.

[1] Research Fellow, Royal Australian College of General Practitioners; Research Associate, Department of Social and Preventive Medicine, Monash University, Deakin Street Clinic, Traralgon 3844, Australia.

THE TRARALGON HEALTH AND ILLNESS SURVEY

The aims of the Survey were to study such social and environmental factors in health and illness in the City and Shire of Traralgon as age, place of birth, housing, occupation, climate, and urban or rural background; to obtain information about illness behaviour and health care use; and to evaluate the effectiveness of different methods of obtaining information with relation to different kinds of health and illness data.

The Traralgon Community

Traralgon is a country town in Gippsland, Victoria, 100 miles East of Melbourne, population 15,500. It is on the edge of the Latrobe Valley industrial complex where the main industries are electricity generation and paper manufacture, and has some light industry of its own. It is also a commercial and retail centre for a considerable rural district.

All categories of occupational status are represented in the community. However, compared with the Victorian population, professional, clerical, sales and service workers are somewhat under-represented whilst tradesmen and labourers are over-represented.

Eighty-four per cent of the population was born in Australia, 8 per cent in Britain and 8 per cent in other countries. Housing standards are good and the majority of families occupy their own home. Social amenities are good and include adequate kindergartens and schools, an elderly citizens' club and a civilian widows' club, and excellent and varied sporting facilities.

Medical facilities are provided by two group general practices in the town, each with five general practitioners; full-time consultant surgeons are available and other specialists are available on a visiting basis. Central Gippsland Hospital provides comprehensive hospital facilities and diagnostic services. The Hobson Park Psychiatric Hospital is the centre of the regional psychiatric service.

Method and organization

The director of the research project continued to work half-time in one of the general practice groups and half-time on the project.

Sister L. Sivertsen, a trained nursing sister, was employed full-time as research assistant. She undertook a course in medical sociology and interviewing techniques and was responsible for all interviewing and for maintaining liaison with the continuous recording families. A secretary provided part-time secretarial help as necessary.

The survey was conducted for a twelve-month period from 1 July 1970 to 30 June 1971. Information was obtained from three main sources. Firstly, a group of families recorded daily on a diary card the presence of all symptoms and illness, and all contacts with medical, nursing and paramedical personnel, for the full twelve months. Secondly, a random sample of the population was interviewed throughout the year. Thirdly, information about illness requiring medical, hospital or other attention was obtained from records kept by the appropriate health care agency. This included morbidity recorded in general practice and hospital practice, social and medical problems presented for attention to chemists, infant welfare sisters, social worker, clergy, Lifeline telephone counselling service, and the Marriage Guidance Council, and the use of municipal immunization sessions, meals on wheels, home help, district nurse, day hospital, physiotherapist, occupational therapist, and ambulance service.

Before and during the survey it was given generous cover by local newspapers, radio and television and it was obvious that these media had brought it to the attention of a large cross-section of the community.

Continuous recording families

A random sample of families was selected from the records of one of the two groups of general practitioners in Traralgon. Basic information about the family was obtained by means of the same questionnaire which was also used for interviewing

the interview households during the Survey (see below), and they were asked to record illness and health care data daily on special record cards for a period of one year, during which they were visited monthly by Sister Sivertsen.

Eighty-one families, comprising 272 persons, commenced recording. Larger and more stable families of Australian origin were over-represented in the group, while smaller families or individuals without a family attachment, more socially mobile families and individuals, and migrant families, were under-represented. Children and young people were under-represented, and middle-aged and elderly persons over-represented.

Of the 272 persons in 81 families who commenced recording, 29 (10·6 per cent) ceased recording at some time during the survey, involving a loss of 8·0 per cent of possible person weeks of recording (Table I).

TABLE I
Response of continuous recording families

	Families	Persons	Person weeks
Commenced	81	272	14,144
Ceased	13*	29 (10·6%)	1,131 (8·0%)
Unreliable recording	29*	243	13,013
		72 (29·6%)	2,182 (16·7%)
Omissions detected		171	10,831
		26 (15·2%)	
No error or omission	28 (34·6%)	145 (53·2%)	7,540 (53·5%)

* Families involved (not usually the whole family).

Of the remainder a further 72 persons (29·6 per cent) recorded unreliably in that they did not record on a day-to-day basis for all or part of the time and this resulted in unreliable recording for 16·7 per cent of the possible person weeks. A further 26 persons (15·2 per cent) produced records in which details about illness or consultations known from practice records were found to be omitted. Thus, over all, there were 145 persons (52·2 per cent) in 28 families (34·6 per cent) who recorded reliably and without any obvious error for a total of 7,540 person weeks (53·5 per cent of the possible total), while 243 persons (89·4 per cent) produced usable records for 13,013 person weeks (92 per cent of possible).

Most of the persons who ceased recording did so because they left Traralgon and these were mainly young people taking up occupations else-where. Three persons died during the survey year; two men and one woman. All were elderly and died of coronary artery disease.

Interview families

A random sample of addresses in the City and Shire of Traralgon was selected and all permanent residents at these addresses interviewed. Inter-viewing was conducted continuously throughout the year of the Survey, about eight families being interviewed each week.

Of the 434 families selected for interview, 371 (88 per cent) were successfully interviewed. Fifteen (4 per cent) could not be contacted despite several visits, and 38 (8 per cent) declined to be interviewed. There were no significant differences in the response rate in any of the four quarters of the survey year.

The families comprised 1,250 persons, an average of 3·37 persons per family. Their age and sex distribution and occupational category were not significantly different from that of the Traralgon population.

Details relating to the family or families and individuals at each address were obtained by com-pletion of a standard questionnaire (available from the author on request). Whenever possible informa-tion about adults was obtained from the person concerned but if they were not present information was accepted by proxy from an adult relative since it was not practicable to make many return visits. However, information was not accepted by proxy for non-related members of households, who were regarded as a separate family; nor for related persons who were not living and eating together with the persons interviewed and who were also regarded as a separate family. Information about children was accepted from mother or father or both. All available members of each family were interviewed together.

The questionnaire sought information about family size, number of recent changes of address, and general standard of housing and housekeeping. Personal information about individuals included age, sex, occupation, place of birth, and smoking habits. Information was obtained about all current illnesses or injuries, all medical, paramedical or social care received, all medication taken, and time lost from work or school, during the two weeks prior to interview; all in-patient hospital care during the three months prior to interview; and all chronic illness present. The check list of chronic conditions and the check list of impairments used in the United States National Health Survey were

read out to each family to probe for information regarding these conditions.

Information from health care agencies

Information about conditions requiring medical, hospital or other attention was obtained from the appropriate helping agency.

General practice. Information about general practice morbidity in Traralgon was obtained from all general practitioners who recorded all morbidity seen for one week each quarter. Each doctor working in general practice recorded on a different week, and doctors from each of the two groups recorded on alternate weeks. The order in which doctors from each group recorded during the first quarter was randomly selected. This order was then repeated in each of the subsequent quarters. If a doctor was absent during any or all of a recording week he recorded for the nearest full week he was present. If a doctor left permanently his replace-ment recorded, or if there was no replacement there was no recording during that week.

General practitioners recorded the age, sex and diagnosis or diagnoses relating to all patients whom they saw during the recording week at their surgery or in the patient's home, but not in hospital. They also recorded in relation to each diagnosis whether this was the first consultation for that episode of illness or a subsequent consultation. Illnesses were classified in terms of the Royal Australian College of General Practitioners List of Causes of Morbi-dity in General Practice. It was not possible to exclude patients who lived outside the boundaries of the City and Shire of Traralgon, so that the general practice morbidity refers to morbidity seen by doctors practising in Traralgon whose popula-tion base would include approximately 3,000 people not living within the City and Shire of Traralgon.

Hospital morbidity. The age, sex, diagnosis and duration of hospital stay, relating to all patients living within the survey area for each admission to Central Gippsland Hospital during the survey year were recorded on special record forms with the help of the medical records librarian at the hospital.

Chemists. All five chemists in Traralgon co-operated in recording for one week every six weeks (that is, two weeks per quarter) details relating to all episodes of illness or disability about which they or their staff were asked for advice. Details were not recorded in relation to requests for specific medica-tion but were recorded only in those cases in which advice was sought regarding the treatment of a complaint. In these cases the approximate age of the person concerned, sex, diagnosis and whether the chemist referred the matter to anyone else, for example a doctor, was recorded.

Other health care agencies. The two infant welfare sisters in Traralgon recorded details of the age and sex and diagnosis relating to all children about whose condition their advice was asked. This did not include normal well child supervision but included social and medical conditions about which advice was sought.

Similar information was recorded about new contacts with the social worker, all the clergy, Lifeline, the Marriage Guidance Council and the ambulance service, coming from people living within the survey boundary. The total work load of the district nurse, day hospital, meals on wheels and home help service was made available.

RESULTS

The overall community response to the survey was one of acceptance. Individual response varied from apathy to willing involvement, but there was little actual antipathy.

The acceptance of and co-operation with the survey by professional people and organizations in the town was equally as good. Co-operation was readily obtained from all doctors, from hospital staff and committee of management, from all chemists and both infant welfare sisters, the ambulance service and social worker. Information was also made available from the clergy, Lifeline and the Marriage Guidance Council, although it was less easy for those working in these less well-structured fields to know exactly what information was required. The scope of the information obtained is shown in Table II.

TABLE II
The scope of Traralgon Health and Illness Survey (one year)

	Families	Persons	Attendances	Approximate size of sample
Interview survey	371	1,250		8%
Continuous recording	81	272		2%
Health care agencies:				
Hospital admissions	—	—	2,226	100%
G.P. attendances (b)	—	—	4,923 (2,538)	8%
Chemist advice	—	—	663	15% (?)
Ambulance services	—	—	325	100%
Infant welfare advice (a)	—	—	234	100%
Church help (a)	—	—	145	(?)
District nurse (b)	—	—	250 (83)	100% (?)
Lifeline (a)	—	—	43	100%
Social welfare worker (a)	—	—	39	100%
Marriage guidance (a)	—	—	4	100%

(a) First attendances for new problems only.
(b) First attendances for new problems in brackets.

Some results of the survey are set out in Table III for the initial interview of families who were to record continuously throughout the year, and for each of the four quarters of the interview survey.

TABLE III

Some results of the Traralgon Health and Illness Survey

	Continuous recording families initial interview July 1970	Interview families				
		Quarter				
		First: Winter	Second: Spring	Third: Summer	Fourth: Autumn	Total
Number of families	81	97	99	89	86	371
Number of persons	272	323	347	304	275	1,250
Current illness in two weeks:						
% persons	53·7	66·6	61·7	62·5	66·9	64·2
Per person	0·64	0·81	0·82	0·83	0·88	0·83
Chronic illnesses per person	0·79	1·03	1·09	1·13	1·12	1·09
% reporting no illness	22·2	12·1	14·6	12·5	16·7	13·9
% of illness receiving medical care	26·2	20·1	17·5	16·2	14·4	17·4
Consultations per person per year	5·4	4·6	4·4	3·6	3·7	4·14
Days work loss per year (males aged 15–64)	11·3	12·5	6·9	1·5	10·2	7·6

It is noteworthy that each of the three measures of illness reported (the percentage of persons having current illness and the number of current illnesses per person, the number of chronic illnesses per person, and the percentage of persons reporting any illness) is considerably reduced in the continuous recording families who were interviewed first. Thereafter the differences between each quarter are relatively small. It is unlikely that this difference reflects a true difference in the illness experience of the continuous recording families but rather that it reflects the inexperience of the interviewer at this stage, despite the fact that some twenty families in another town had been previously interviewed in a pilot survey. Perusal of the original questionnaires demonstrates the increasing amount of information obtained in later interviews with this group of eighty-one families. It is also noteworthy that the more salient and less easily overlooked measurements relating to illness receiving medical care, medical consultations and work loss, were not reduced in this group. Apart from this evidence of the influence of interviewer experience, the results are remarkably consistent throughout the four quarters of interviewing, with a small reduction in current illness in summer compared with winter and a larger associated reduction in the consultation rate and rate of work loss, whilst the prevalence of chronic illness remained relatively constant.

Results relating to medication have been previously reported (2) and show a high prevalence of medication taking, associated with the high prevalence of recognition of illness demonstrated by this survey.

OTHER AUSTRALIAN HEALTH SURVEYS

A previous survey of 56 families in Traralgon in 1967 (3) was conducted using methods similar to those used in the current survey for the continuous recording families. However, families were not randomly selected. Other Australian health surveys have used basically different methods, usually depending upon multiple student interviewers and conducting the survey over a relatively short period of time.

In 1964 a community health survey of the rural town of Heyfield, Victoria, was undertaken by the Mental Health Research Institute and the Melbourne University Department of Medicine of St. Vincent's Hospital (4). Twenty-four medical students conducted interviews with the whole population over a three week period during summer, and achieved interviews with 97·5 per cent

of the population. The interviews were largely unstructured, although reported on structured pro formas, in order to obtain maximum rapport and co-operation. There was no physical examination but access to general practitioner and hospital records provided complementary data.

In 1967 a similar survey of Prahran, a defined metropolitan area of Melbourne, was undertaken jointly by workers from the Mental Health Research Institute and the three Victorian universities (5). A stratified random sample of addresses was used and interviews achieved with 66·2 per cent of families approached.

In 1966 the Busselton Community Health Survey was undertaken by the Royal Perth Hospital, the Western Australian Medical School, Busselton District Hospital and Busselton family doctors (6). This survey aimed to include all adults over the age of 21 and, as well as an interview, special tests of biochemical and physiological factors were included. Interviews were conducted by a team of doctors. A response of 91 per cent of the population was achieved.

In 1970 a survey of medical care in a defined metropolitan area of Western Sydney was undertaken (7). A 2 per cent random sample of households in the area were interviewed by a group of specially trained medical students, and a 75 per cent response was achieved.

In 1970 a survey of disability associated with chronic illness was undertaken in the metropolitan area of Brisbane using a similar method, and an 83 per cent response rate was achieved.

Since 1969 the Royal Australian College of General Practitioners has been conducting an ongoing morbidity survey with the participation of several hundred general practitioner recorders each year (8, 9). This provides comprehensive information about morbidity presented for medical attention but cannot be related to a known population base.

Some results of the Traralgon surveys compared with other Australian surveys are shown in Table IV.

DISCUSSION

Traralgon was chosen for this survey because it is a reasonably circumscribed community whose geographical, social and demographic circumstances are satisfactorily defined, it is not particularly unrepresentative of communities in Australia, and the available background and facilities for research made it feasible and practical.

The involvement and participation of the Research Director and Research Assistant with and in

68   INTERNATIONAL JOURNAL OF EPIDEMIOLOGY

TABLE IV

Some results of a number of Australian health surveys

	Traralgon		Heyfield	Prahran	Busselton	Sydney	Brisbane
	1970	1967	1964	1967	1966	1970	1970
Households interviewed	371	56	501	814	—	1,420	2,433
Persons interviewed	1,250	258	1,929	2,163	3,410	5,343	8,538
Response (%)	88	—	97·5	66·2	91	75	83
No current illness reported (%)	35·8	33·3	32·1	41·9	—	—	—
% population receiving medical care in given period	14·0	72·0	25·0	68·7	—	40·9	—
	(2 wks)	(1 yr)	(4 wks)	(1 yr)		(8 wks)	
% population in hospital per year	10·9	12·4	—	12·0	—	14·8	—
						(2 yrs)	
Annual consultation rate	4·14	—	—	—	—	3·09	—

the community at large was of great help in ensuring the enthusiastic co-operation of both lay and professional people and organizations. It ensured that the survey was conducted from a viewpoint within the community and to this extent the results may be somewhat more subjective than would have been provided by an outside research source. However, it is thought that the advantage gained in more complete and comprehensive information outweighs the unknown bias which has been thus introduced. Nor can surveys originating outside the community to be studied claim not to influence the community under surveillance.

The influence of community rapport on the response rate was demonstrated in the Australian health surveys by a better response rate in Busselton, Heyfield and Traralgon compared with Brisbane, Prahran and Sydney. The former are all country towns in which some or all of the survey personnel lived and were well known, whereas in the metropolitan areas the survey teams had much less community affiliation. However, as country communities are not necessarily adequately representative of the metropolitan communities in which the majority of the Australian population lives, and in which further health surveys are most necessary, greater attention should be paid to methods by which community participation and response can be maximized. This includes publicity through the mass media and through local community organizations and groups, involvement of local personnel and community groups in the survey, and emphasis on the relationship between the survey and continuing health and welfare activities of the community.

Since the aim of the Traralgon survey was to obtain information about the subjective experience of illness in the community and behaviour based

upon this, it was essential that the survey be comprehensive, representative and feasible. The use of a group of families recording continuously on a day-to-day basis and visited regularly over a twelve month period was an attempt to obtain the most comprehensive information with the least reliance upon the vagaries of memory. Similar methods of obtaining reliable and comprehensive information have been used and discussed by Dingle *et al.* (10), Hope-Simpson (11) and Sutton (12, 13). Frequent visiting without a daily record has been used even more often by Sydenstricker (14), Van Volkenberg and Frost (15), Doull (16), Downes (17) and Spence *et al.* (18).

A long-term longitudinal survey requires a degree of continuing interest and persevering recording by the participants which is hard to achieve and is expensive to supervise, and which is only justified by obtaining information not attainable by static surveys. Such information about the symptomatology of respiratory infections was obtained in a survey of selected families in Traralgon in 1967 (3). The use of families with young children, selected for their stability and likelihood of continuing participation, then resulted in 97 per cent of person days being recorded. In the present survey it was important that the sample should be more representative of the whole community and, since the families from one medical practice who could be selected for continuous recording were not necessarily representative, the concurrent interview survey was planned to obtain concurrent, less comprehensive, but more representative information. In fact the information obtained proved nearly as comprehensive and the longitudinal survey provided better data on only a few points. The continuous recording families turned out to be less than adequately representative of the community—not because they were selected from patients of one medical group and therefore omitted patients of other doctors and persons who have no current contact with doctors, but because it was the larger and more stable families of predominantly Australian origin who were willing to participate. Moreover, the accuracy, reliability and perseverance of their recording was not enough to justify the greater effort (by survey team and participants) and expense of this method compared with the static interview.

The concurrent recording of information obtained from medical and other services was undertaken because often such information is all that is available, and it was thought necessary to take the infrequently available opportunity of comparing it with information obtained directly from persons in the community. It also had the added advantage of informing and involving all professional workers in the community.

The effect of surveying patients rather than a sample of the community is demonstrated by the increased annual consultation rate of the continuous recording families compared with the interview families (Table III). This difference between patients and the total community as a base is particularly important in Australia where general practitioners do not have a defined list of patients. The results of morbidity surveys from general practice can therefore be related only to all current patients rather than to the whole community.

Households selected for the questionnaire survey were designed to provide a random representative sample of feasible size. The good publicity achieved in the community and the approach to the families by letter prior to being visited made the interviewer's reception and task much easier. Many of the 8 per cent of households who did not co-operate were most apologetic and the commonest cause for refusal was inability to arrange a convenient time for interview. In a few cases language difficulties prevented interview and only a small minority of people expressed lack of interest.

The use of a nursing sister with special training in interview techniques and survey methods had the advantage of providing an interviewer with a medical background who was, nevertheless, approachable and with whom those being interviewed could establish good rapport. There was the added advantage of having the one interviewer throughout in standardization of the methods of presentation of the questionnaire. Even so, the improvement in the completeness of information about illnesses obtained during the first batch of

interviews was quite marked. Subsequently there was internal evidence of very uniform interviewing technique and results. This suggests that pilot surveys for training interviewers should be of more than nominal size, even where there has been adequate theoretical preparation. The results of this survey suggest that at least 50 trial interviews are necessary. The use of a single interviewer over a period of a year rather than multiple interviewers during a shorter period has considerable advantages. The interviewing technique can be better standardized as long as there is adequate preparation and the extra ability and confidence of the interviewer results in better rapport and more comprehensive information. Since there may be considerable seasonal variation in the incidence and prevalence of acute illness, the use of medical and social care, and the social results of illness, as evidenced by the seasonal differences shown in the Traralgon survey (Table III), there are advantages in spreading interviewing throughout all seasons. It is suggested that the current tendency to emphasize surveys of relatively short duration using multiple interviewers, perhaps largely because of short-term availability of numbers of students to act as interviewers, might well be considered more critically and perhaps there is a need to evaluate the methods by a controlled trial.

The questionnaire used was based very considerably on the principles, and in many cases the detail, of that used in the United States National Health Interview Survey (19), since this provided a useful basis of comparison from a country with similar standards of living and medical services. However, all illness was recorded in the current survey, not (as in the United States) only that causing disability or receiving medical advice. The recall period of two weeks provides the best compromise between obtaining enough information about current illnesses and injuries and loss of accuracy due to the vagaries of memory. A longer recall period is necessary for information about less frequent events such as hospitalization, and since these more salient events are less liable to be overlooked, there is less loss of accuracy due to faulty memory. However, to minimize this in the current survey the recall period for hospitalization was only three months, and this did not in fact provide adequate data from the size of sample. In retrospect it was a mistake not to have conformed with the twelve-month recall period for hospitalization as used in the United States National Health Interview Survey.

The importance of definition and standardization of the recall period for information about illness and medical care is demonstrated by the information about medical care obtained from several Australian health surveys (Table III). The recall periods vary from two weeks to one year and comparison of the data is therefore of only limited value. Since the United States National Health Surveys are the most comprehensive and well founded sources of information about English-speaking communities it would be well for surveys to use their definitions and techniques whenever possible.

The check lists relating to chronic illness and disability were the same as those used in the United States survey. The use of questions as posed was very necessary in order to relate the results to the exact techniques used, since technique and results are so closely related. The attempt to interview all adult respondents personally was tempered by the practical need to obtain information from related proxy respondents for those adults who could not be present at the interview, because of the inability to programme repeat interviews within the time available. The questions relating to medication were exactly the same as those asked of respondents in the Heyfield and Prahran surveys (4, 5), again in an attempt to standardize methods whenever possible.

The response to the survey, with 88 per cent of selected families interviewed, compares favourably with other similar surveys in Australia (Table III) and other countries. The United States National Health Interview Survey achieved a 95 per cent response. Roghmann (20) achieved an 82 per cent response in New York in a survey involving day-to-day recording for a one month period, and in the Tecumseh Survey involving interview and examination an 88 per cent response was obtained (21). The importance of achieving a high response rate relates to the confidence with which the sample can be expected to be representative of the whole community and to the degree to which non-respondents may be a special group with their own particular characteristics of health, illness and use of health and welfare services. It must be remembered that not only may a high response rate reflect good survey technique but it may also be related to a more homogeneous population. This might well account for some of the differences in response rate in more circumscribed country communities compared with large metropolitan populations.

In comparing some results of different Australian health surveys (Table III), in the light of this discussion about methodology, it is obvious that the differences shown (in as far as they are at all comparable) are not very great and to this extent suggest a certain uniformity in the health and illness experience of a variety of different Australian communities. This is a common finding in health and morbidity surveys, which tend in general to be less than adequately sensitive to measure health status except in general terms which do not discriminate the relatively small differences which occur in reasonably homogeneous communities. This problem has recently been discussed by the World Health Organization Expert Committee on Health Statistics (1).

ACKNOWLEDGEMENTS

The Traralgon Health and Illness Survey has been supported by a grant from the National Health and Medical Research Council during 1970, 1971 and 1972.

I wish to acknowledge the help and support of the Research Committee of Council, Royal Australian College of General Practitioners, and Professor Hetzel and members of the Department of Social and Preventive Medicine, Monash University.

Sister Lois Sivertsen's excellent interviewing, which depended greatly on the help given by Mr. J. Brehaut of the Department of Anthropology and Sociology, Monash University, and the Traralgon families who so willingly submitted to interview and kept records, were responsible for much of the information in the survey. Traralgon doctors, hospital staff, and other professional, social welfare and medical workers in the community, readily gave their time in recording for the survey. Mrs. Brenda Libbis and Mrs. Ricki Dargavel efficiently managed the secretarial work involved. To them all I am extremely grateful.

REFERENCES

(1) World Health Organization: *Technical Report Series*, No. 218. Expert Committee on Health Statistics, Seventh Report, 1961.
(2) Bridges-Webb, C.: Drug medication in the community. *Med. J. Aust.* 1: 675, 1972.
(3) Bridges-Webb, C.: *A Study of Morbidity in Traralgon, Victoria*. M.D. Thesis, Monash University, 1971.
(4) Krupinski, J., Stoller, A., Baikie, A. G., and Graves, J. E.: *A Community Health Survey of the Rural Town of Heyfield, Victoria*. Mental Health Authority Special Publication No. 1, Melbourne, 1970.
(5) Krupinski, J., and Stoller, A.: *The Health of a Metropolis*. Melbourne: Heinemann Educational Australia, 1971.
(6) Curnow, D. H., Cullen, K. J., McCall, M. G., Stenhouse, N. S., and Welborn, T. A.: Health and disease in a rural community—a Western Australian study. *Aust. J. Sci.* 31: 281, 1969.

(7) Adams, A., Chancellor, A., and Kerr, C.: Medical care in Western Sydney. *Med. J. Aust.* **1**: 507, 1971.

(8) Hutchinson, J. M.: The Australian morbidity survey. *Annals of General Practice* **16**: 68, 1971.

(9) Bridges-Webb, C.: Respiratory diseases in the Australian morbidity survey, 1969–1970. *Med. J. Aust.* **2**: 1175, 1971.

(10) Dingle, J. H., Badger, C. F., and Jordan, W. S.: *Illness in the Home*. Cleveland: The Press of Western Reserve University, 1964.

(11) Hope-Simpson, R. E.: The epidemiology of non-infectious diseases. *Roy. Soc. of Health J.* **78**: 593, 1958.

(12) Sutton, R. N. P.: A family study of respiratory illness. *J. Coll. Gen. Pract.* **4**: 597, 1961.

(13) Sutton, R. N. P.: Minor illness in Trinidad: a longitudinal study. *Trans. Roy. Soc. Trop. Med. Hyg.* **59**: 212, 1965.

(14) Sydenstricker, E.: Study of illness in a general population group. *Pub. Health Report*, p. 2069, 1926.

(15) Van Volkenburgh, V. A., and Frost, W. H.: Acute minor respiratory diseases prevailing in a group of families in Baltimore. *Amer. J. Hyg.* **17**: 122, 1933.

(16) Doull, J. A., Herman, N. B., and Gafafer, W. M.: Minor respiratory disease in a selected adult group. *Amer. J. Hyg.* **17**: 536, 1933.

(17) Downes, J.: The longitudinal study of families as a method of research. *Millbank Mem. Fund Quart.* **30**: 101, 1952.

(18) Spence, J. C., Walton, W. A., Miller, F. J. W., and Court, S. D. M.: *One Thousand Families in Newcastle-upon-Tyne*. London: Oxford University Press, 1954.

(19) U.S. National Centre for Health Statistics: *Health Survey Procedures: Concepts, Questionnaire Development, and Definitions in the Health Interview Survey, 1964*. U.S. Govt. Printing Office, Series 1–2.

(20) Roghmann, K. J., and Haggerty, R. J.: The diary as a research instrument in the study of health and illness behaviour: experiences with a random sample of young families. Personal communication, 1970.

(21) Napier, J. A.: Field methods and response rates in the Tecumseh community health study. *Amer. J. Pub. Health* **52**: 208, 1962.

(revised version received 12 December 1972)

CHAPTER 6

Problem-solving and decision-making in family practice

Roger Strasser

NOMINATED CLASSIC PAPER

Ian McWhinney. Problem-solving and decision-making in family practice. *Canadian Family Physician*, 1979; 25: 1473–77.

When I first read this paper, I found it enormously helpful both in my approach to patient care as a clinician and also as a teacher and researcher of family medicine. The paper demonstrates well Ian McWhinney's remarkable ability to distil key concepts and to articulate his insights in ways which are accessible to novice and experienced family physicians alike.

Within this paper, Ian McWhinney provides great insight into the nature of family practice. Specifically he emphasises the centrality of patients in clinical decision making, weighing up the risks and benefits to patients through the problem-solving process. This paper places the hypothetical-deductive model of clinical problem solving and decision making in the family practice context.

In the first part of the article, Ian McWhinney crystallises the distinctive features of family medicine with emphasis on the ongoing patient–doctor relationship and on understanding patients' concerns in their family/social context. The second part of the paper focuses on clinical decision making in family practice, emphasising that, although the diagnosis may be part of the process, the goal is to make management decisions which are right for each patient. He provides criteria for assessing information derived from history taking, physical examination and special tests, including the potential value of time as a diagnostic tool.

In many ways, this paper presents the foundation for the patient-centred clinical method which Ian McWhinney and the team at Western University in Canada developed during the two decades following publication of this paper.

For me, this article by Ian McWhinney is a 'must read' for anyone interested in family medicine as it provides a conceptual framework for much of our work as family physicians engaging in our daily activities of clinical practice, as well as for understanding and researching the discipline of family medicine.

ABOUT THE AUTHOR OF THIS PAPER

I agree with others who have described Ian McWhinney as a 'father of family medicine' and 'social philosopher and naturalist who had a great influence on the development of family medicine'.

For me, though, Ian McWhinney was a mentor and personal friend whom I came to know when I moved to Canada in 1983 to undertake academic training in family medicine at the University of Western Ontario where he was the founding Chair. Studying the 'Foundations of Family Medicine' with Ian was truly exciting and opened my eyes and mind to the great potential of research in family practice.

Over time, I came to realise that Ian's insights were drawn not only from his own clinical practice experience, but also from observations of other family doctors, beginning with his own father, as well as from his eclectic reading of a broad literature. Ian McWhinney showed the way for us all with his insistence that family medicine should be learned in the family practice setting taught by family physicians.

Although he was quietly spoken and self-effacing, it was important to listen carefully and reflect on every word and every phrase Ian McWhinney spoke as they often provided extraordinary wisdom about family medicine.

ABOUT THE NOMINATOR OF THIS PAPER

Professor Roger Strasser is Professor of Rural Health, Dean and Chief Executive Officer at the Northern Ontario School of Medicine of Lakehead and Laurentian Universities in Canada. He was appointed Dean of the Northern Ontario School of Medicine in 2002. Prior to that Roger was Head of the Monash University School of Rural Health in Australia. He was Chair of the WONCA Working Party on Rural Practice from 1992 to 2004.

> 'I encourage you to read and reflect on this seminal article by Ian McWhinney. It provides you with a clear sense of direction and purpose for your interactions with patients, as well as a recognition that there is much more to family practice than the diagnosis and treatment of disease.'

Professor Roger Strasser AM, Canada

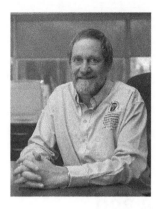

Attribution:

We attribute the original publication of *Problem-solving and decision-making in family practice* to *Canadian Family Physician*. With thanks to the members of the McWhinney family and to Peter Thomlison, Publisher, *Canadian Family Physician*.

I. R. McWhinney

Problem-Solving and Decision-Making in Family Practice

SUMMARY

The problem-solving strategies of family physicians have evolved in response to six features of family practice: the pattern of illness; the undifferentiated and unorganized nature of conditions seen; the early stage at which illness is seen; the family physician's unconditional commitment to patients; his continuing relationship with his patients, and the time pressure under which he works. The effect of these influences is described in terms of the model of the diagnostic process formulated by Elstein et al.[2] (Can Fam Physician 25:1473-1477, 1979).

Dr. McWhinney is professor and chairman of the Department of Family Medicine at the University of Western Ontario. Reprint requests to: Dept. of Family Medicine, University of Western Ontario, London, ON. N6A 5C1.

ALTHOUGH THE general principles of problem-solving are the same in all branches of medicine, each discipline has its own way of applying them. The differences between disciplines are due to differences in the problems they encounter and to differences of role within the health care system. The problem-solving strategies of primary and family physicians have evolved in response to six special features of family practice.

1. The pattern of illness approximates to the pattern of illness in the community. This means that there is a high incidence of acute, short term illness, much of it transient and self-limiting; a high prevalence of chronic illness, and a high prevalence of behavioral problems. Contrary to conventional wisdom, patients do not present with *either* physical *or* behavioral problems: they come with prob-

lems which are often a complex mixture of physical, psychological and social elements.

To deal successfully with this pattern of problems, family physicians' problem-solving strategies must be specially adapted for two purposes:

—They must be capable of separating, in the early stages of illness, the serious and life-threatening diseases from the transient and minor. Since the serious diseases come in the midst of the more common minor and transient illnesses, and since the symptoms are often very similar, this is no easy task.

—They must be capable of teasing out the physical, social and psychological elements of a patient's problem.

2. The illness is undifferentiated, i.e. it has not been previously assessed by any other physician. Because of this, the illness presented to family physicians is often in an *unorganized* state. The concept of unorganized illness is an important one for family medicine. What does it mean? When a patient first tells a physician about his problems and symptoms, he does so with little insight into their nature or cause. A patient who has had malaise,

anorexia and discolored urine for five days, and fatigue, depression and headaches for three months, does not know that in the physician's mind these add up to two clusters of symptoms: one suggesting hepatitis, the other depression. When he presents his problems for the first time, they will not usually come out in an orderly sequence which reflects a clear concept of their nature and cause. He may, of course, have his own ideas about the significance of his symptoms, but this will often be very different from the assessment made by the physician. The way the symptoms are presented will also be strongly influenced by the patient's fears and anxieties and by his ability to express his sensations in words.

Once the patient has been through the process of assessment by a physician, all this changes. He learns that the malaise, anorexia and discolored urine are not isolated phenomena, but a cluster of symptoms associated with hepatitis. He learns that his tiredness is related to his feeling of depression, that his headaches are tension headaches, and that these are quite separate problems from the hepatitis. If we now imagine that his hepatitis becomes worse and he is admitted to hospital, it is not difficult to see that the history he gives to the intern will be quite different from the one he gave to the family physician. It will be "organized" around the concepts of infective hepatitis and depression.

In summary, five factors contribute to the lack of organization in the data presented to the family physician:

- Patients often present more than one problem at the same visit. In one study,[1] the average number of problems was 2.54.
- The problems are often not presented in order of priority. The most serious problem may be left until last—or not even mentioned.
- The most sensitive problems may be expressed in indirect or metaphorical language.
- The problem is not necessarily the same as the disease.
- Much of the information presented is "noise", i.e. it is not useful in solving the patient's problems. At this stage, the patient usually has little insight into the significance of the data he is presenting.

3. Disease is often seen early, before the full clinical picture has developed. Information on which to base a precise diagnosis—the kind of information discussed in textbooks—is often not available to the family physician when he first sees the patient. Decisions have to be taken, therefore, with fewer cues than are available in the later stages of disease. They also have to be taken with different cues: symptoms change as an illness ad-

vances. Symptoms having diagnostic value in the early stages may be quite different from those which have diagnostic value in the later stages.

4. Since the family physician is available for all types of problem, he can make no prior assumptions about the type of problem likely to be encountered. His problem-solving methods must therefore be adaptable enough to deal with any problem. Since his commitment to patients is unconditional, he cannot make the categorization "my problem/not my problem," made by organ and system specialists.

5. The family physician's relationship with patients is continuous, transcending individual episodes of illness. This has two important consequences. Since the relationship is open-ended, the physician need be in no hurry to solve all the patient's problems. Observation over time can be used as a method for testing hypotheses—provided, of course, that there is no risk attached to waiting. Since the relationship is often a close one, the physician can use his personal knowledge of patients in formulating hypotheses, assessing probabilities and understanding the context of problems.

6. Since the family physician is directly available to patients, his workload can be predicted and planned to only a limited extent. This means that his decisions often have to be made under pressure of time. To be an effective decision-maker under these conditions the family physician must be particularly skilled in:

—ascertaining at an early stage what the patient's main problem is.

—formulating a strategy for dealing with the problem in the time available; focusing on the decisions which have to be taken at this visit; selecting the most efficient strategy for arriving at these decisions; formulating a plan for the longer term assessment and management of the problem.

—putting other problems in a priority order and formulating a plan for their longer term assessment and management.

The Problem Solving Process

Figure 1 shows a model of the clinical problem-solving process which applies to all fields of medicine. The model is based on the work of Elstein et al,[2] and Barrows et al.[3] When presented with a problem, the clinician responds to cues by forming one or more hypotheses about what is wrong with the patient. He then embarks on a search (the history, examination and investigation) to test the hypothesis. In the course of the search he looks for positive (confirming) and negative (infirming) evidence. If the evidence infirms the hypothesis it is revised and the search begins again. As indicated by the feedback loop in Figure 1, the process is a cyclical one, the clinician constantly revising and testing his hypothesis, until he has refined it to the point at which he feels justified in making management decisions. Even after this point, the clinician must still be prepared to revise his hypothesis if the progress of the patient is not as predicted.

Figure 2 illustrates the variety of hypotheses formed by family physicians. Besides the conventional clinical hypotheses, the family physician has to formulate hypotheses about such questions as why the patient has come, what his chief problem is and what kind of communication he is using. As indicated in the diagram, these do not follow each other in stages. The physician may have a clinical and behavioral hypothesis at the same time, or may move from one to the other and back again, wherever the evidence leads.

Cues

I define a cue as "an item of meaningful information". When a patient presents his problems, the family physician is confronted by a mass of data of varying value from the highly significant to 'noise'. Out of this mass of

Fig. 1
The Diagnostic Process

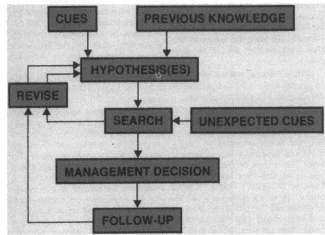

data he responds to *cues* which have meaning for him because they give him an idea about what is wrong with the patient.

Cues may point to certain or probable diagnoses. A cue may enable the physician to say with certainty what is wrong with the patient; this is usually what we mean by a spot diagnosis. These cues are unfortunately rare in family practice, as they are in most fields of medicine. Most cues indicate a number of different diseases with varying probabilities. The physician can then only formulate hypotheses, which have to be tested by a search for further information.

Of all the cues presented to family physicians, symptoms are the most important. In the early stages of illness, and in the varieties of illness seen by the family physician, signs are less frequently available. The family physician is especially concerned with two aspects of a symptom:
1. Its capacity to bring the patient to see him (i.e. its significance for the patient). Feinstein called this the "iatrotrophic stimulus".[4] For example, hemoptysis has a greater value as an iatrotrophic stimulus than cough.
2. Its sensitivity, specificity and predictive value in the early stages of illness.

Cues to the early detection of serious and life-threatening illness are of especial importance for the family physician. Even though he may see only one every ten years, he must still know how to separate the patient with subarachnoid hemorrhage from the thousands presenting with headache. He does this by recognizing key discriminating symptoms, described by Williams[5] as "red flags", which alert him to danger.

Hypotheses

Investigators of the clinical process have found consistently that clinicians form their first hypotheses very early in the process, very soon after the patient has presented his complaints. This is contrary to the orthodox view—often conveyed to medical students—that physicians collect a large body of data before formulating their hypotheses. Of course, medical students have to begin by going through a rather laborious routine, but this is because they do not yet have the knowledge and experience from which to generate useful hypotheses.

The clinician usually has between two and five hypotheses at any one

time. To handle more than six is difficult for the human brain. The hypotheses are placed in ranking order, based on two main criteria: probability and pay-off.

Probability

Given the available data, the clinician estimates the probability that the patient is suffering from disease A, disease B, disease C, and so on.

This estimation has a mathematical basis—Bayes' theorem.[6] If we have accurate information about the incidence of the symptoms and diseases in question, we can calculate the probability of a disease, given the presenting symptoms. Before doing this, however, the clinician has first to go through the crucial step of deciding what weight to give to the patient's symptoms. The family physician's personal knowledge of his patients makes this a very important step. There has been little study of the contribution of personal knowledge to decision-making in family practice, but experience suggests that it may be the most important distinguishing feature.

How much does the ranking order of hypotheses matter? It matters because the order of hypotheses determines the search strategy. I heard a physician quoted as saying that he was "tired of admitting women to hospital with fatigue, doing hundreds of dollars worth of investigations, then finding that they were depressed and unhappily married." This is an example of a faulty search strategy based on an ordering of hypotheses not based on probabilities. The generation of depression as a first-ranking hypothesis would in these cases have led to a search strategy designed first to collect evidence in favor of the hypothesis, then to exclude other causes of fatigue with a few simple tests.

Before leaving the question of probability, two fallacies must be mentioned. The first is that the family physician always thinks of common diseases first. This is not necessarily so: it depends entirely on the cue. If the cue is a highly probabilistic one, like fatigue, this will hold true. If, on the other hand, the cue indicates a rare disease with relative certainty, this will be the physician's first hypothesis. If a hypertensive patient complains of attacks of sweating and flushing, for example, his first hypothesis may be pheochromocytoma, even though he may see only one case in his whole lifetime.

The second fallacy is that diagnosis in family practice is different from diagnosis in other fields of medicine because it is probabilistic. All clinical diagnosis is probabilistic: where family practice differs is in the relatively low levels of probability at which many decisions have to be made.

Pay-off

This indicates the consequences of diagnosing or not diagnosing a disease. The more serious the disease, and the more amenable to treatment, the greater the positive pay-off of making the diagnosis and the greater the negative pay-off of missing it. If a disease has a high pay-off it may be ranked high even though it has a low probability. In a child with abdominal pain, for example, acute appendicitis may be ranked high—even though of low probability—because of the high expected value of an early diagnosis.

The Search

The purpose of the search is twofold: to test and validate the physician's hypothesis(es), and to bring to light new and unexpected cues. These purposes are fulfilled respectively by the directed and the routine search.

The Directed Search

Since its purpose is to test the physi-

Fig. 2.
Variety of Hypotheses Formed by the Family Physician

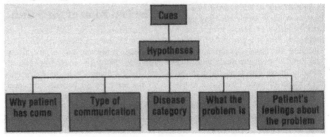

cian's initial hypothesis, the search strategy will vary with the hypothesis. In selecting a search strategy, the family physician has to make two kinds of choice: the choice of tests he will use and the extent of the search.

Choice of Tests. I use the term tests here to include history questions and items of physical examination, as well as pathological and radiological investigations.

Tests are chosen according to two kinds of criteria: sensitivity, specificity and predictive values, and calculations of risk/benefit.

Sensitivity, specificity and predictive value all measure the usefulness of a test in separating patients who have one disease from those with other diseases, or from those who are healthy. Galen and Gambino describe how these indices are applied in clinical diagnosis.[7] Two facts about the indices are significant for family physicians:

1. The predictive value of a test is strongly influenced by the incidence and prevalence of the disease. Since the incidence and prevalence of disease in a general practice population is very different from those in a hospital or clinic population, the predictive value of tests varies widely between family practice and other types of practice. Unfortunately, the advice given to family physicians by specialists is often based on experience with selected clinic populations. To learn family practice one must learn the symptoms and tests which have the highest sensitivity and predictive value *for a family practice population.*

2. Since the sensitivity of tests varies widely at different stages of a disease, and since he has a special responsibility for early diagnosis, the family physician must be particularly conversant with the sensitivity of tests in the early stages of disease. Most textbooks are written about the later stages of disease and do not describe tests in terms of their sensitivity, specificity and predictive value.

The extent of the search is a question of when to stop collecting positive and negative evidence to test the hypothesis. This is a particularly difficult decision in family practice, because the family physician deals with illness ranging in severity from upper respiratory infections and furuncles, to myocardial infarcts and carcinomata. His search strategies must therefore be flexible enough to deal with any presenting problem.

In family practice, the extent of the search is determined chiefly by the seriousness of the presenting complaint. A simple sore throat will normally require no examination beyond the head and neck. A cue to infectious mononucleosis, however, will indicate a more extensive search. A mild intercostal muscle pain will normally require no more than examination to elicit local tenderness. Tight substernal pain, on the other hand, will indicate an extensive search. Another factor influencing the extent of the search is the physician's knowledge of the patient. A patient who tends to deny illness will warrant a more extensive search than suggested by the presenting complaint.

The routine search (routine systems enquiry and physical examination).

The chief aims of the routine part of the search are to bring to light cues which have not emerged in the directed part of the search; to collect baseline and background data on the patient, and to screen for symptomless conditions like hypertension.

The routine search is sometimes referred to as a "complete history and physical". This is a misnomer, for even the routine search is a selection from a much larger number of possible tests. As in the directed search, the tests are selected for their usefulness in achieving the objective. Internists would probably include ophthalmoscopy in their routine, but not laryngoscopy—for the very good reason that ophthalmoscopy has a higher utility for generating new cues in patients seen by internists. For similar reasons, otolaryngologists would probably make the opposite choice.

For two reasons, the family physician tends to use routine searches less than some other clinicians:

1. Since the patient is usually well known to him, he may already have all the baseline data he needs.

2. In minor and transient disorders, little in the way of a routine search is required.

The End Point of the Search

Traditionally, the end point of the search has been a diagnosis. In family practice, however, this is not always realistic, because many illnesses do not have a diagnosis in the strict sense of the term. In all patients, however, decisions have to be taken, even if no diagnosis is possible. It is more helpful, therefore, to describe the end point in terms of a decision. The end point

of the search on any particular occasion is the point at which enough information is available to make an informed decision without avoidable risk to the patient.

In family practice, end points are often different from those in referral specialties. A consultant seeing a referred patient will probably feel the need to make a definitive diagnosis before referring the patient back to his own physician. A family physician is not under the same constraint. The continuing relationship with patients means that all problems do not have to be solved immediately. Since the relationship itself has no formal end point, the search can be discontinued and resumed according to need. In this sense, there is no final end point, since the family physician should always be ready to revise his hypothesis if new evidence comes available.

The family physician, because of his role, makes two types of decisions which do not often arise in other branches of medicine:

1. *The decision to wait.* In making this decision, the physician is using the evolution of the illness over time as a test of his hypothesis. Obviously, he has also decided that no extra risk will be incurred by waiting. The use of time to validate hypotheses in this way can make many investigations redundant. One example of this decision is the *eliminative diagnosis*[8, 9] in which the physician decides that the illness is transient and minor, then waits for his hypothesis to be verified.

2. *The decision to refer.* The endpoint of a search may be the decision to consult with or refer to another physician. This decision may have to be taken before a definitive diagnosis can be made, for example, with a severely ill baby or a patient with an acute abdomen. It is clear that the objective of the family physician in these cases is different from that of the referral specialist. The family physician has fulfilled his obligation if he has decided to refer the patient in time for him to receive effective treatment. He has failed to fulfill his obligation if he has worsened the outcome of the illness by delaying referral in the interests of providing a diagnostic label.

Management Decisions

Diagnosis, in the usual sense of the term, is a categorizing process. Its end point is a probabilistic statement about what is wrong with the patient. A decision, on the other hand, cannot be probabilistic. A clinician cannot "probably" prescribe an antibiotic or "probably" refer a patient. Management decisions have to be either/or. When he makes such a decision, the clinician takes the probabilistic statement and integrates it with a large number of other variables, many of them unique to the patient. Whereas diagnosis is a reductive, generalizing process, decision-making is a synthesizing, individualizing process. Among the variables which the clinician must take into account are:

—the diagnosis of the patient's main problem.

—other problems he may have.

—the prognosis.

—the personality and life situation of the patient.

—the risks and benefits of the decision alternatives.

—the patient's wishes.

—the family's wishes.

—ethical issues.

So complex are these interacting variables that two patients with the same diagnosis may be managed in different ways. Given the family physician's knowledge of his patients and their backgrounds, this may well be, as Stephens[10] has maintained, "the quintessential skill of clinical practice and the ground of what family physicians know that is unique." ◉

References

1. Bentsen BG: The accuracy of recording patient problems in family practice. J Med Educ 51:311-316, 1976.

2. Elstein AS, Shulman LS, Sprafka SA: Medical Problem Solving: An Analysis of Clinical Reasoning. Cambridge, Harvard University Press, 1978.

3. Barrows HS, Feightner W, Neufeld YR, Norman GR: Analysis of the Clinical Methods of Medical Students and Physicians. Report to the Province of Ontario Department of Health and Physicians' Services Incorporated Foundation, McMaster University, Hamilton, ON., 1978.

4. Feinstein A: Clinical Judgment. Baltimore, Williams & Wilkins, 1967.

5. Williams T: A strategy for defining the clinical content of family medicine. J Fam Pract 4:497-499, 1977.

6. Lusted LB: An Introduction to Medical Decision-Making. Springfield, IL., Thomas, 1968.

7. Galen RS, Gambino SR: Beyond Normality, The Predictive Value and Efficiency of Medical Diagnoses. New York, John Wiley, 1975.

8. Crombie DL: Diagnostic process. J Coll Gen Pract 6:579, 1963.

9. Crombie DL: General practice today and tomorrow X.—Diagnostic methods. Practitioner 191:539, 1963.

10. Stephens GG: Intellectual basis of family practice. J Fam Pract 2:423-428, 1975.

CHAPTER 7

The intellectual basis of family practice

Raman Kumar

NOMINATED CLASSIC PAPER

G.G. Stephens. *The intellectual basis of family practice.* Winter Publishing Company, Tucson, Arizona, 1982: 3–13.

This paper has been hailed as one of the most influential works ever written about family medicine. The recognition and establishment of family medicine has faced more challenges around the world, compared to many other medical specialties, often due to political tensions among professional societies within organised medicine. In this paper, Dr G. Gayle Stephens undertakes the historical obligation of defining the intellectual and academic basis of family medicine as a specialty and knowledge domain.

This paper examines the fallacies, the incorrect and deceptive arguments, which often pose a challenge to defining an academic discipline. The paper also examines beliefs that are so deeply embedded in intellectual science and modern medicine that they are almost unquestionable. Dr Stephens then tests family medicine against five criteria for intellectual respectability in any field of study, as put forward in 1965 by philosopher Mortimer Alder. He concludes that family medicine education qualifies as a legitimate academic discipline on all five counts.

The paper also describes the distinctiveness of family medicine and elaborates upon comprehensive patient management as the constant skill for family physicians.

The theories and the arguments put forward in this paper were formative for the specialty of family medicine. Physicians deal regularly with problems of life or death that require higher levels of abstraction, such as will, motivation, passion, justice and mercy. These cannot be expected to yield to persistent technological research. As the world and society change rapidly around us, there is tremendous opportunity to explore new avenues of research in family medicine as an extension of this classic work.

ABOUT THE AUTHOR OF THIS PAPER

G. Gayle Stephens (1928–2014) is considered a poet laureate of family medicine. He was a prolific writer, and left behind an extensive body of written work. He explained how family medicine was a counterculture within medicine, manifested in personal relationship and social change. His grasp on philosophy, history, religion and psychiatry enabled him to provide much-needed intellectual leadership that profoundly affected the development and establishment of family medicine as a specialty.

Born in Pike County in Missouri, Gayle is regarded as one of the founders of family medicine in the United States of America. He pioneered one of the first family medicine residency programmes in the country in Wichita, Kansas, and was instrumental in the formation of the family medicine residency programme at the University of Alabama in Huntsville. He served as the president of Society of Teachers of Family Medicine from 1973 to 1975. In addition to his institutional leadership, textbooks, scientific articles, essays, visiting professorships, and invited lectures, Gayle initiated an invitational conference known as The Keystone Conference. His literary and scientific works remain guiding tools for academicians involved with family medicine programmes around the world.

ABOUT THE NOMINATOR OF THIS PAPER

Dr Raman Kumar is a first-generation residency-trained family physician in India. He has a long-standing interest in the development of academic family medicine in his country. He, along with other young colleagues, is credited with founding the Academy of Family Physicians of India, the *Journal of Family Medicine and Primary Care*, and the National Conference of Family Medicine and Primary Care in India. He has served as the young doctor movement representative on the executive board of the World Organization of Family Doctors (WONCA). He is based in Delhi in India.

> 'Family medicine is a relatively new specialty and is still evolving in many parts of the world. We are faced with the challenge of defining the discipline of family medicine. As practising professionals, we often have limited exposure to details about the history of family medicine. Many debates, discussions and controversies with regards to family medicine have already been settled in the

past. We need to look forward and work on new models of service delivery, based on the concepts of family medicine, rather than putting ourselves on the wheel of reinvention.'

Dr Raman Kumar, India

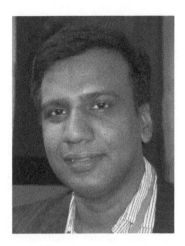

Attribution:

We attribute the original publication of *The intellectual basis of family practice* to Winter Publishing Company, and the American Academy of Family Physicians Foundation. With thanks to Jo A. Griffith, President of Winter Publishing Company, and Don Ivey, Manager of the Center for the History of Family Medicine at the American Academy of Family Physicians Foundation.

CHAPTER 1
The Intellectual Basis of Family Practice

We are still defining the family physician six years after the establishment of the American Board of Family Practice. But a shrewd observer would detect significant shifts in this process over the years. Initially, we were trying to define ourselves to others, such as other specialties, other professional societies, the federal government, and medical school deans. Now, the efforts at definition are largely internally directed. There are enough of us now to exhibit diversity; we are finding that we are not a homogeneous group. As in all reforms, there are revisionists among us, of both reactionary and radical persuasions.

In this paper, I will present some of my reflections about the intellectual and academic base of family practice. Although I cannot expect to resolve all the issues, perhaps I can clarify some of the questions. First, we need to clear away some debris. There are a number of fallacies, delusions, and phony issues which must be exposed and rejected before we can see the real ones.

Phony Issues

We should first recognize that none of the certifiable medical specialties were established on epistemological grounds. Most of them sprang up like Topsy and exist by virtue of political, economic, and technological factors that have little to do with a theory of knowledge. Most of them can be classified under the following headings:
- Characteristics of patients (Pediatrics, Obstetrics/Gynecology)
- Parts of the body (Dermatology, Orthopedics)
- Diseases or conditions (Allergy)
- Techniques of treatment (Surgery, Psychiatry)
- Relation to special machines (Radiology, Clinical Pathology)

None of these represent primary epistemological categories. All of medicine is derivative, secondary, and applied. In this respect, family practice is no more obligated to define itself than internal medicine, pediatrics, or psychiatry. All medical vocations are constantly shifting their territories, and there are many local variations on a theme decided by the political machinations of medical school departmental chairmen or hospital medical staffs.

So the first bit of debris to discard is our masochistic need to reach a degree of epistemological and intellectual purity that is not only unrealistic but also unnecessary. Let's stop hitting our thumbs with hammers! We should stop trying to solve political problems among medical specialists as though they were knowledge problems. They aren't! And I put all the problems and conflicts related to the performance of technical procedures in this category, whether the issue is surgery, obstetrics, needle biopsy, or cardioversion. All efforts to define family practice or the family physician in terms of technical procedures the physician may or may not perform will fail if approached as a rational problem of knowledge. These are problems of political relationships among professional societies within organized medicine and have more to do with hospitals, lawyers, and insurance companies than with knowledge.

A Quartet of Fallacies

The next bit of debris is a quartet of fallacies about the generalist's role and the intellectual challenge of medicine. Webster defines fallacy as "deception" but also as "an argument failing to satisfy the conditions of valid or correct inference." The following are four common but incorrect arguments which have nothing to do with defining a discipline, but which are often used in a discouraging manner.

1. *A misunderstanding about omniscience.* It is assumed, incorrectly, that a generalist is required to know too much. This takes the conversational form of: "Nobody can know everything"; "I have enough trouble with one field, I don't see how anyone can keep up with several (or all)"; or patronizingly as, "I admire you as a general practitioner. I'm not smart enough to do it."

Each of these statements reveals an assumption that anyone engaged in a field that cuts across disciplinary lines is bound to be intellectually cuckolded by one discipline or another. Those who share this point of view fail to understand the selectivity required by the generalist. Neither the word "general" nor the word "comprehensive" (as applied to health care) imply knowing everything about everything. They do indicate a range of interest and a level of expertise that is broad but not inclusive. One can only guess at the numbers of medical students frightened or shamed out of a generalist career by the fear of omniscience as a requisite.

2. *The confusion of information with knowledge.* This confusion is usually stated in terms of an overload. There is simply too much to be learned. There are too many books and journals, too many conferences and meetings. Wolf (1974) addressed this problem cogently in an editorial. He quoted a statement from Weiss (1969) as follows:

> My assessment clearly disavows the contention that we are in the midst of a "knowledge explosion." The semblance of a knowledge explosion has come from using the wrong yardstick. No doubt there has been a "data explosion," liberally equatable with an "information explosion," although not all of the collected data are truly informative. Furthermore, we are also faced with a "publication explosion." But "knowledge explosion"? Not by criteria of measurement on a scale of relevance.

4

Wolf uses the distinction between growth and obesity as a metaphor for the relation between knowledge and data. Data must be processed by human knowers who place them in relation to other information; i.e., give meaning. The one thing that facts cannot do is speak for themselves.

3. *Uncertainty and ambiguity can be eliminated by fragmentation.* How many students have succumbed to this most seductive of fallacies— that if one reduces the scope of one's field of interest, one can escape uncertainty? In medical practice, this argument takes the form of "How do I feel about myself when I look in the mirror? Am I a good doctor? Am I doing all that can be done for my patients? Is there someone else who can do more and better?" This may become a mistaken rationale for specialization, but problems of identity, confidence, and honesty are rarely settled by changing fields. These are not knowledge problems.

Identifying what can be known completely is unimportant. Pieces of knowledge can never be separated from the whole without a "reductio ad absurdum." All knowledge that keeps its relationship to the whole continues to exhibit ambiguity, uncertainty, and some degree of incomprehensibility.

Cox (1973) has written about specialization in his own field of theology. He sees a belief in fragmentation of knowledge as a way of giving oneself permission to ignore what is presumed to be "outside one's field." It is a "compulsion to master and a tendency to criminal negligence" which never quite works. "Superspecialization," he writes, "is psychologically—and therefore physiologically—pathogenic." It is also politically dangerous, for it leads to an abdication of responsibility for everything outside one's field and, in fact, necessitates hierarchy, bureaucracy, and vertical authority. The superspecialist almost always relinquishes control over how his knowledge will be used. In the Manhattan Project of the 1940s, only those at the top knew what it was all about, and it remained for a nonspecialist to make the political decision about the use of the atomic bomb. These are not arguments against a division of labor or the development of special interests or skills; they are arguments against the notion that certainty is attainable through fragmentation.

4. *Knowledge is linear or cumulative.* It is a cruel education that allows a student to suppose that he must learn all that was known in the past in addition to what is known now and what must be known for the future, as though these are steadily growing quantifiable sums. The truth is that original thought has a simplifying, clarifying effect. History is replete with examples of how men have debated endlessly while knowing nothing. Intellectual controversies tend to become obsolete and pass away.

This idea has been satirized quite effectively in a book entitled *The Saber-Tooth Curriculum* (Peddiwell, 1939), which recounts the imaginary educational foibles of a paleolithic tribe. The survival skills necessary to this tribe and taught in their schools were: (1) fish-grabbing with the bare hands, (2) woolly-horse clubbing, and (3) saber-toothed tiger scaring with fire. When a new glacial age changed the living conditions of the tribe by muddying their stream, causing the woolly horses to migrate, and giving pneumonia to the tigers, the tribe had to adapt technologically by inventing a fish net, a snare to catch antelopes, and a pit in which to trap ferocious bears. This precipitated an educational crisis. Net-making, snare-setting, and pit-digging threatened the old curriculum and a long controversy ensued about what constituted real education. The traditionalists could not give up teaching the old skills, while the radicals wanted to focus exclusively on the new ones.

The refutation of fallacies does not establish the academic role of family practice, but it is a necessary preliminary step because of the persistent nature of the fallacies.

A Trio of Delusions

articles of faith

More serious than the fallacies, which are rather easy to expose, are a trio of beliefs so deeply embedded in the intellectual tradition of modern science and modern medicine that they are almost unquestionable. These beliefs have the character of "articles of faith" which support much of the scientific enterprise but, on careful examination, they cannot be shown to satisfy the criteria of the scientific method they supposedly support.

1. *To know an object best, one must know it in its smallest dimensions.* Under most circumstances, this means that you must take the object apart. In a living system, you have to kill it, so that the philosopher Hans Jonas (1966) says that "the lifeless has become the knowable par excellence." Our knowledge of life is derived from death, a curious paradox to say the least.

2. *All complicated systems eventually can be reduced to physics and chemistry.* In medicine, this means that sociology is reducible to psychology which is reducible to biology which is reducible to molecular chemistry. This seductive and pervasive belief has recently been challenged by Krebs (1971) in an article entitled, "How the Whole Becomes More than the Sum of Its Parts." Krebs does not turn vitalistic, to be sure, but he does show how the dynamics of macromolecules and enzymes lend characteristics to living systems which are missed when one is preoccupied with the chemistry of elements or simple compounds. Hilary Putman (unpub. ms.), a philosopher of science, has made a more vigorous attack on the reductionist hypothesis, which he terms a fallacy, by asserting that there are categories of human behavior for which molecular biology is simply irrelevant.

3. *In principle, all human problems have a technological solution.* Medawar (1975) has recently argued this point quite effectively in an editorial entitled, "Some Follies of Prediction," in which he described how people have erred in the past by too easily giving up the search for technological solutions. Many problems thought to be impossible in medicine and surgery have yielded to persistent technological research. These successes, however convincing, do not prove that all problems are of this class. Physicians deal regularly with problems of life or death that require higher levels of abstraction, such as will, motivation, passion, justice, and mercy. These cannot be expected to yield to research in biology; as a matter of fact, some of these problems may even be created by technological advances. Iatrogenesis has become a major contribution to epidemiology.

Adler's Five Conditions

Now let me turn from the negative side of the debate to the positive aspects of developing a foundation for a branch of knowledge and an intellectual discipline. I take my cue from Mortimer Adler (1965), who described criteria for intellectual respectability in any field of study. His particular concern was the field of philosophy, but he stated that the following conditions "are requirements which any mode of inquiry must satisfy to be respectable. They are generic conditions, applicable to all specific branches of knowledge, among which science is only one."

First Condition: The field in question "must be a mode of inquiry that aims at, and results in, the acquisition of knowledge which is characteristically different [from knowledge provided by other fields]." This requirement is not a demand for knowledge in an absolute sense. It is more moderate, calling for knowledge which is (a) testable by reference to evidence, (b) subject to rational criticism, and (c) either corrigible or falsifiable.

Second Condition: The field in question "must be capable of being judged by appropriate criteria of goodness; i.e., criteria of truthfulness, beauty, or usefulness." We must be able to make judgments about relative goodness of data or propositions that emerge from inquiries in the field, and we must be able to subject any such judgments to tests which give evidence for or against. While no knowledge may ever be said to have been completely and finally verified, some knowledge has a higher order of certainty because it has repeatedly resisted efforts to disprove it; i.e., falsify it.

Third Condition: The field in question must "be conducted as a public enterprise." Anyone who wishes to participate in the study of a given field may do so if he is willing to try to answer common questions, to avoid appeals to private information or opinion, to share findings with others, and to subject disagreements to judgment by commonly accepted standards.

Fourth Condition: Not only must the discipline meet the first condition of distinctiveness but it must also have some degree of independence and autonomy. That is, it must have "some questions of its own to answer—questions which it can answer without reference to results obtained by any other discipline. And, on the procedural side, it must have a method of its own for answering whatever questions are proper to it."

Fifth Condition: The field must be concerned about substantial and realistic objects of study; i.e., the natural universe or the human condition. In Adler's terms, the knowledge sought "must be primarily questions about that which is or happens in the world or about what men should do and seek."

It is my contention that family practice education can qualify as a legitimate academic discipline on all five counts. It qualifies not only in a general sense as medical science but also in a special sense as a discipline within medicine.

The Distinctiveness of Family Medicine

I want to develop and defend the thesis that patient management is the quintessential skill of clinical practice and is the area of knowledge unique to family physicians. Family physicians know their patients, know their patients' families, know their practices, and know themselves. Their role in the health care process permits them to know these things in a special way denied to all those who do not fulfill this role. The true foundation of family medicine lies in the formalization and transmission of this knowledge. I would now like to try to substantiate these claims.

trail of casualties

Each of us who practices medicine has a trail of casualties among our patients which is not the result of neglect, ignorance, or professional malpractice. We have patients whom we did not manage well for a host of reasons having little to do with our knowledge of disease. We have overlooked diagnoses we are perfectly capable of making, overdiagnosed conditions that did not exist, delayed treatment, or overtreated. We have become inappropriately involved with patients who made us angry, became too dependent upon us, or did not follow instructions, and who ultimately got ejected from our practices, either formally or informally, or—ungrateful wretches—died for the wrong reasons. All of us can empathize with the bitter words of the physician quoted below (Houston, 1938):

> I suppose that I am particularly bitter about the people whom we may as well call neurotics, who as you say, take up so much of an internist's time. They are the people who drove me out of practice. I never could see any sense in paying any attention to them because . . . they have neither sense, nor gratitude, nor any idea of cooperation, nor any qualities that might endear them to man, woman, or child.

> I cannot understand why those of us who have trained ourselves to take care of people who have organic disease can't be allowed to take care of organic disease. Why won't people take our word for it that there is nothing the matter with them and let it go at that? I suppose I have as many somatic sensations as anybody on earth, but I explain them to myself in a physiological way. Why can't an intelligent neurotic take the same sort of advice that I give myself? There seems to be no way of handling them except that sort of semiquackery that some highly respectable members of our fraternity are able to get away with so successfully.

Let it be clear that, in speaking of patient management, I mean something considerably more comprehensive than treatment. Treatment, whether specific or nonspecific, is only a part of management which, among other things, includes a decision of whether or not to treat and the assumption of responsibility for that decision. I am not limiting the concept of management only to those patients who think they are sick, who fear being sick, or, in some cases, who wish to be sick. What I have in mind are the ideas expressed so convincingly by Tumulty (1973) in his chapter, "What is a Clinician, and What Does He Do?"

> Thus, a clinician is not someone whose prime function is to diagnose or to cure illness, for in many cases, he is not able to accomplish either of these.

> A clinician is more accurately defined as one whose prime function is to manage a sick person with the purpose of alleviating most effectively the total impact of illness upon that person.

Before you dismiss me as embarrassingly sentimental or hopelessly anti-intellectual, let me try to be more specific about the types of clinical problems and conditions which require a therapeutic relationship with a physician. Obviously, a great deal of medical care can be provided in a routine, dispassionate way by anonymous doctors to anonymous patients. Much of this can be delegated to co-professionals or allied health persons following diagnostic and treatment protocols. There are particular circumstances, however, which require more. Meyer (1951) wrote about those conditions which the physician cannot treat *without knowing the patient's name.* This idea has long intrigued me. What does it mean to know the patient's name? At the least, it means acquaintance, but more than that, it means knowing about a patient's life experience, something so unique that only the patient's name can symbolize it. The patient is a "series of one" and his particular biography is clinically important. Whitehorn (1961) wrote about those conditions in which man becomes pathogenic for himself—"a begettor of disease and death." Even if we could magically eliminate all known diseases, physicians would be kept busy with clinical problems arising out of man's individual and group behavior.

The following conditions and complaints seem to me to require the unique managerial skills of a wise and compassionate physician.
- Complaints which are obscure, vague, or undifferentiated.
- Complaints which arise from life-threatening disease.
- Complaints which seem out of proportion to physical or laboratory findings.
- Complaints which are unusual, bizarre, nonphysiologic, or nonanatomical.
- Complaints which are persistent and disabling.
- Complaints associated with marked anxiety or mood change.
- Complaints which result from life change, conflict, or stress.
- Complaints which may require risky diagnostic and therapeutic procedures.
- Complaints arising from conditions which may be managed electively.
- Conditions which are incurable.
- Conditions involving habits and the lifestyle of the patient.
- Conditions which require moral or ethical decisions.

All of these require something more on the part of the physician than a "standard operating procedure" or a cookbook approach to diagnosis and therapy.

Patient Management as a Science

Feinstein (1970) asserts that doctors make two basic kinds of clinical decisions, explanatory and managerial. He states, "The explanatory decisions lead to intellectual conclusions about ideas such as diagnosis, and pathogenesis of disease; the managerial decisions lead to therapeutic actions in which the patient is treated to thwart what might happen or to remedy what has occurred."

Explanatory decisions are inferential in character and are supported by our knowledge of the basic medical sciences and by data derived from the clinical laboratory. Managerial decisions, on the other hand, are not nearly so well supported by information from the traditional basic medical sciences. They may require data from "nonmedical" disciplines or even data that have yet to be collected and interpreted. Feinstein further states:

> The consequences of this scientific underdevelopment are the massive therapeutic controversies that exist in every branch of medicine and surgery today. There are controversies about such routine daily problems as the best way to treat a cold, set a fracture, relieve a backache, or deliver a baby. And there are controversies about such major dilemmas as the optimal management of diabetes mellitus. The diet, drugs, or surgery to be used for peptic ulcer, the desirability of rigorous treatment for essential hypertension, the value of anticoagulants in myocardial or cerebral infarctions, and the choices of radical surgery versus simple surgery versus radiotherapy versus chemotherapy for cancer. . . . Physicians have developed a splendid clinical science for explanatory decisions, and a magnificent technologic armamentarium of therapy, but our managerial decisions generally continue to be made as doctrinaire dogmas, immersed in dissension and doubt.

Feinstein goes on to list the specific areas in which more information is needed to bolster the reliability and predictability of managerial decisions: (1) observer variability, (2) criteria for interpreting primary data, (3) quantification of prognosis, (4) quantification of therapy, and (5) taxonomies for patients and their clinical management. He suggests that help may be obtained from the fields of linguistics, logic, psychology, statistics, and computer sciences. He deplores the practice of tinkering with medical school curricula merely in order to include the socioeconomic aspects of health care delivery. This is inadequate for the intellectual tasks facing modern medicine. Improving the bases for our managerial decisions is one dimension of patient management which requires an additional intellectual orientation for medical education and provides us with an investigative agenda for the future.

Patient Management as Art

Houston (1938) and Balint (1957) discuss another dimension of patient management that has a long and honored history but which has fallen on hard times in recent years. It is the notion that the personal characteristics of the physician and the quality of communication between the patient and the physician are important variables in determining the outcome of patient management. Houston and Balint, whose work and writings are separated by 20 years, arrived at the same conclusion from different perspectives. Houston, writing from the viewpoint of internal medicine, spoke of the "doctor as a therapeutic agent." Balint, from the perspective of a psychoanalyst studying general practitioners, spoke metaphorically of the doctor as a drug. He states in the introductory chapter of his book, "by far the most frequently used drug in general practice was the doctor himself; i.e., that it was not only the bottle of medicine or the box of pills that mattered but the way that the doctor gave them to his patient— in fact, the whole atmosphere in which the drug was given and taken."

doctor as a drug

10

Balint goes on to inquire into those situations in which the drug "doctor" does not work or may have undesirable side effects, and his book is an inquiry into the pharmacology of the doctor as therapeutic agent. Houston notes that the placebo has always been a norm of medical practice, yet much more is involved in the use of the placebo than an attitude of expectancy or credulity on the part of the patient. He says, "the doctor's attitude toward the patient is perhaps more fundamental than the patient's attitude toward the doctor. . . . The faith that heals, heals not through argument but by contagion."

It has become easy in recent times to derogate the physician's role as healer as doctors became a little "heady" with the marvels of biomedical technology. The art of medicine is often seen as a substitute for knowledge and as the stock-in-trade of pretenders and exploiters. I have found medical students, residents, and younger physicians to be quite skeptical about the art of medicine.

I am not defending the art of medicine in a trivial sense as representing courtesy, grace, or style. There is much to be said for these secondary virtues, but they do not reflect the cognitive elements of art. Art is a way of perceiving and representing reality and, in medicine, the art is a way of knowing as well as of feeling. It is an art for the physician to understand the existential dimensions of life, his own as well as those of his patients; and to communicate effectively at the personal level. Medicine not practiced at the personal level is vulnerable to a dimension of evil that can only be called demonic. Witness the separation of art from science which occurred in the Third Reich—euthanasia became training for extermination.

Patient management is the major task of clinical practice, and the skills of patient management are only partly based on education in the natural sciences. The personality of the physician and the relationship that develops between the physician and the patient are important variables in the effectiveness of patient management. It is necessary for the physician to learn how to use himself and his relationships on behalf of his patients.

objective therapeutics

The art of medicine has never been more important. I am concerned that medicine is moving towards an "objective" therapeutics which is basically technological and which separates the treatment from the therapist. The therapist may thereby become a dispassionate and relatively homogeneous vehicle through which the treatment is given; he may become more a technician than a professional. Recent developments in physician accountability, such as peer review, medical audit, recertification, and litigation against physicians are focused almost entirely on the technical and economic aspects of practice. Most of these developments are inimical to the role of the physician as healer. We are developing an erroneous assumption that health care is a product and that the health problems of the population are remediable by medical technology. These trends could lead to the establishment of a mediocre therapeutics in which the physician's role is progressively deprofessionalized. The physician may thus be separated from primary patient contacts, and his communicative skills could well atrophy as his function is more and more controlled by protocols.

11

On Teaching and Learning Patient Management

What is required to learn patient management? Certainly a great deal more than an introduction to psychiatry. While psychiatry aids our understanding of human behavior and interpersonal relationships, it is basically a consulting discipline that per se has a rather narrow application to the crucial encounters of clinical medicine. Further, psychiatrists themselves may be infected with the same biases of scientism to which I have already alluded. In addition, they may not have resolved the human issues of practice better than the rest of us. This is not to deny, however, that certain psychiatrists may be of inestimable help to fellow physicians, if a proper format for giving that help can be arranged. There are other professionals who can also help. The critical factor is not academic background but, rather, the personal characteristics of the individual and his experience with sustained therapeutic relationships.

details of clinical encounters

The key to learning patient management is appropriate supervision of the learner's interactions with patients. This may be done in individual or group settings with supervisors. The details of clinical encounters are exposed and reflected upon in a constructive manner over an appropriate period of time. What do the "details" include? Anything that happens between the doctor and the patient: the words of conversation, the behavior of each party, the feelings, the style, and the unspoken assumptions. All of these need to be brought to levels of awareness in a nonthreatening way, so that meaning can be ascribed and tested in the crucible of ongoing clinical relationships.

Each of us brings to medical school, and then to our practice, some intellectual and emotional "baggage." We have notions of what it means to be a doctor, what it means to be a patient, and how these two roles should interact. We have notions of justice, morality, and propriety. We have needs for control, for rewards, and for self-fulfillment that may never have been subjected to critical reflection. We use all this baggage in our clinical practice, and this matrix of personal characteristics in which our scientific information and skill is embedded is often as crucial to the help we are able to give patients as is our scientific information itself. It often determines and limits what we are able to see and hear and what we are willing and able to do. It sets the tone and style of our professional lives in such a way that Balint (1957) refers to it as our "apostolic function"; i.e., our natural, commonsense approach to practice to which we oblige our patients to conform if they want our help.

Now, I am not suggesting that there is some homogeneous ideal to which we all should conform, nor that all physicians need personal psychotherapy. But I am saying that through education of the proper sort, we can broaden the spectrum of people and conditions we are able to deal with effectively. Self-understanding and human communicative skills materially affect the way we practice medicine—our uses of drugs, laboratory tests, x-rays, hospitals, operations, and consultants. In short, they affect how we manage everything—not only our patients and our practices, but our time, our money, our families, and our lives.

12

CONCLUSION

This, then, is the intellectual and academic basis for family practice. This is our field for inventiveness and discovery. This is our agenda for research. To be sure, the family physician may borrow a great deal of information and knowledge from other disciplines. Such borrowings constitute a variable and will not be the same in all areas of the country or in all settings. But *the constant is the skill of patient management.* One cannot be a family physician without highly developing this skill. One's bag of technical tricks will change from time to time. One may or may not deliver babies or perform surgery. Whether one does or not depends largely on personal preference and local conditions, but the sine qua non is the knowledge and skill that allows a physician to confront relatively large numbers of unselected patients with unselected conditions, and to carry on therapeutic relationships with patients over time. This is what we should be teaching and learning and practicing. Everything else is secondary.

REFERENCES

Adler, M.M. *The Conditions of Philosophy.* New York: Atheneum, 1965.

Balint, M. *The Doctor, His Patient and the Illness.* New York: International Universities Press, 1957.

Cox, H. *The Seduction of the Spirit: The Use and Misuse of People's Religion.* New York: Simon & Schuster, 1973.

Feinstein, A.R. "What kind of basic science for clinical medicine?" *N. Engl. J. Med.* 283:847, 1970.

Houston, W.R. "The doctor himself as a therapeutic agent," *Ann. Intern. Med.* 11:1416, 1938.

Jonas, H. *The Phenomenon of Life.* New York: Harper & Row, 1966.

Krebs, H.A. "How the whole becomes more than the sum of its parts," *Perspect. Biol. Med.* 14:448, 1971.

Medawar, P.B. "Some follies of prediction," *Hosp. Prac.* 10:73, 1975.

Meyer, A. In *Collected Papers of Adolph Meyer* (E. Winters, ed.) Baltimore: Johns Hopkins Press, 1951.

Peddiwell, J.A. *Saber-Tooth Curriculum.* New York: McGraw-Hill, 1939.

Tumulty, P.A. *The Effective Clinician.* Philadelphia: Saunders, 1973.

Weiss, P.A. "Living nature and the knowledge gap," *Saturday Review,* November 29, 1969.

Whitehorn, J.C. "The doctor's image of man," *N. Engl. J. Med.* 265:301, 1961.

Wolf, S. "The real gap between bench and bedside," *N. Engl. J. Med.* 290:802, 1974.

13

CHAPTER 8

The shift to goal-oriented medical care

Jan De Maeseneer

NOMINATED CLASSIC PAPER

James W. Mold, Gregory H. Blake, and Lorne A. Becker. Goal-oriented medical care. *Family Medicine*, 1991; 23(1): 46–51.

The importance of the paper cannot be overestimated. It marks an important paradigm shift from 'problem/disease orientation' towards 'goal orientation', focusing on the goals that are defined by the patient in terms of quantity and quality of life.

This paper was published one year before Gordon Guyatt and colleagues published their own landmark paper on evidence-based medicine (EBM), another paradigm shift in the approach to the practice of medicine. EBM started to be successfully translated into guidelines, and family medicine was in the forefront of this development. However, as David Sacket and colleagues warned us in 1996, EBM is not a cookbook approach, and it is important that patient values are integrated into our clinical decision making. This reinforces the importance of goal-oriented medical care.

At Ghent University, we immediately integrated this seminal paper into our course on family medicine and primary healthcare in our university's undergraduate medical curriculum. We have further developed these ideas, realising that healthcare outcomes are decided by how the patient and the doctor perceive health and disease, and this perception needs to shift from problem orientation to goal orientation. Moreover, we recognised the importance of complementing 'medical evidence' with 'contextual evidence' and 'policy evidence'.

In recent years, the challenge of multimorbidity has led to further interest in 'goal-oriented care'. In each consultation, a clear exploration of the goals of the patient is mandatory in order to explore what really matters for the patient. Very often our patients' goals are related to being able to function and to social participation. Good medicine must involve accommodating the preferred outcomes of each of our patients as individuals.

ABOUT THE LEAD AUTHOR OF THIS PAPER

James W. Mold is a Professor and Director of the Research Division in the Department of Family and Preventive Medicine, and Adjunct Professor in the Department of Geriatrics, at the University of Oklahoma Health Sciences Center in the United States of America. He is founder and a member of the Board of Directors of the Oklahoma Physicians Resource/Research Network, a large regional primary care practice-based research network. He has substantial experience in primary care practice-based and implementation research.

James has pioneered approaches to re-engineering primary care practices to facilitate the delivery of evidence-based preventive services effectively and economically, including the use of practice facilitators. He has championed a new conceptual model of primary care, called goal-directed healthcare.

His ideas and research methods have received funding from a wide range of national and local agencies and organisations, including the National Institutes of Health. In 2008, he was elected to the Institute of Medicine.

ABOUT THE NOMINATOR OF THIS PAPER

Professor Jan De Maeseneer is a family physician and head of the Department of Family Medicine and Primary Health Care at Ghent University in Belgium. He works as a family physician in the Community Health Centre in Botermarkt. He has been involved in research on healthcare access, quality of care and health professional education, and in the development of family medicine education and training around the world, especially in Africa. In 2004, he was the inaugural recipient of the World Organization of Family Doctors (WONCA) 5-Star Doctor Award for Excellence in Health Care.

> 'New family medicine doctors, educators and researchers, actively integrating the concepts of person- and people-centred care, should try to understand how the daily interaction with individual patients can be better contextualised in global societal developments, focusing care on the goals of equity, solidarity and sustainability.'

> *Professor Jan De Maeseneer, Belgium*

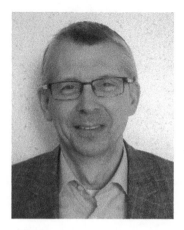

Attribution:

We attribute the original publication of *Goal-oriented medical care* to *Family Medicine*. Reprinted with permission from the Society of Teachers of Family Medicine (www.stfm.org), with thanks to Jan Cartwright and Traci Nolte.

46 January 1991 *Family Medicine*

Special Article

Goal-Oriented Medical Care

James W. Mold, MD; Gregory H. Blake, MD; Lorne A. Becker, MD

ABSTRACT

The problem-oriented model upon which much of modern medical care is based has resulted in tremendous advancements in the diagnosis and treatment of many illnesses. Unfortunately, it is less well suited to the management of a number of modern health care problems, including chronic incurable illnesses, health promotion and disease prevention, and normal life events such as pregnancy, well-child care, and death and dying. It is not particularly conducive to an interdisciplinary team approach and tends to shift control of health away from the patient and toward the physician. Since when using this approach the enemies are disease and death, defeat is inevitable.

Proposed here is a goal-oriented approach that is well suited to a greater variety of health care issues, is more compatible with a team approach, and places a greater emphasis on physician-patient collaboration. Each individual is encouraged to achieve the highest possible level of health as defined by that individual. Characterized by a greater emphasis on individual strengths and resources, this approach represents a more positive approach to health care. The enemy, not disease or death but inhumanity, can almost always be averted.

(Fam Med 1991; 23:46-51)

During most of this century, modern medical care has been oriented toward the identification and correction of health related problems. A variety of well-established strategies have risen from this model, including the problem-oriented medical record, the International Classification of Diseases (ICD-9) used for insurance reimbursement, the Diagnostic and Statistical Manual (DSM-IIIR) of psychiatric diseases, and Diagnosis-Related Groups (DRGs). Essential to the problem-oriented medical model are the following principles:

From the Department of Family Medicine, University of Oklahoma Health Sciences Center, Oklahoma City (Dr. Mold), the Family Practice Residency Program, University of Mississippi, Jackson (Dr. Blake), and the Department of Family and Community Medicine, Toronto Hospital, University of Toronto, Canada (Dr. Becker).

Address correspondence to Dr. Mold, Department of Family Medicine, University of Oklahoma Health Sciences Center, PO Box 26901, 800 NE 15th Street, Room 503, Oklahoma City, OK 73190.

1. There exists an ideal "health" state which each person should strive to achieve and maintain. Any significant deviation from this state represents a problem (disease, disorder, syndrome, etc.).
2. Each problem can be shown to have one or more potentially identifiable causes, the correction or removal of which will result in resolution of the problem and restoration of health.
3. Physicians, by virtue of their scientific understanding of the human organism and its afflictions, are generally the best judges of their patients' fit with or deviation from the healthy state and are in the best position to determine the causes and appropriate treatment of identified problems.
4. Patients are generally expected to concur with their physicians' assessments and comply with their advice.
5. A physician's success is measured primarily by the degree to which the patients' problems have been accurately and efficiently identified and labeled and appropriate medical techniques and technologies have been expertly applied in an effort to eradicate those problems.

This conceptual model is ideally suited to the understanding and management of acute and curable illnesses. It has also been extremely important for clinical research. However, acute and curable illnesses represent a smaller and smaller proportion of current medical practice, and research methods may not always be applicable to patient care.

A problem-oriented approach is not as useful in the following situations: 1) when the "problem" is normal physiology (eg, pregnancy, health promotion); 2) when the process of reaching or assigning a diagnosis may cause more harm than benefit to the patient (early diagnosis of incurable cancer); 3) when the doctor and patient disagree about whether there is in fact a problem that should be solved; 4) when the doctor and patient disagree about the utilities of different solutions (eg, "tight control" of diabetes mellitus); 5) when restoration of the ideal health state is impossible (eg, chronic or terminal illnesses); 6) when the solution is more in the hands of the patient than the doctor (eg, obesity); and 7) when the solution creates new problems equal to or greater than the original problem (eg, treatment of asymptomatic arrhythmias) or when increasingly aggressive attempts to resolve a problem, fueled by physician and patient anxiety, lead to a clinical cascade of adverse consequences.[1]

There is a need for an approach that is more applicable to the care of patients with chronic incurable illnesses, that

Original Contributions   *Vol. 23, No. 1   47*

more comfortably includes the principles of health promotion and disease prevention, that is better suited to interdisciplinary teamwork, and that allows for increased involvement of patients in their own health care. There is increasing sentiment that the time has come to examine fundamental beliefs about medical care and to propose alternative approaches which might be more useful to clinicians dealing with current health care issues.[2] This article proposes an alternative conceptual model that could open a door to new methods for dealing with a variety of modern health care concerns.

The assumption that problem solving is both necessary and sufficient for the restoration and maintenance of health allows physicians and their patients to proceed to act without ever establishing the real goals of therapy. As physicians have become more and more adept at identifying problems, armed with a greater array of powerful weapons with which to abolish them, there is an increasing need to establish the purpose of these activities (so as to not win battles while losing wars). In addition, there is the assumption that health represents the absence of disease with no positive attributes of its own. This is clearly a pessimistic perspective. With advancing age it becomes increasingly difficult to maintain health according to this definition. As stated most eloquently by Dubos:

> What is health? Theoretically, health is the complete absence of organic and mental disease. But for most of us, health is the ability to function. To be healthy does not mean that you are free of all disease; it means that you can function, do what you want to do and become what you want to become.[3]

We propose that problem solving is only one of many strategies useful for the achievement of health-related goals. Because of this, we believe that the process of establishing goals and determining strategies for achieving them, not the identification and resolution of problems, should direct health care. We will refer to this approach as goal-oriented medical care. The purpose of this paper is to introduce and explain some of the advantages and implications of a goal-oriented approach to health care without attempting to describe its practical implementation. However, some of the significant obstacles to implementation will be briefly mentioned.

The Basics of a Goal-Oriented Model

The basic assumptions of a goal-oriented approach to health care, as contrasted with the problem-oriented approach, would include the following:

1. Health must ultimately be defined by each individual and therefore will be different for different individuals and at different points in time. (An individual's definition of health might therefore differ from that of the physician).
2. An individual's health goals can best be determined through the combined efforts of that individual and his or her health care provider(s) using the special information each brings to the relationship.
3. The construction of health-related goals requires an assessment of individual strengths and resources, interests and needs, and personal values in addition to the traditional (and still very important) determination of problems.

4. Final decisions regarding prioritizing an individual's health-related goals and the amount of effort to be expended achieving them are and ultimately should be made by each individual, even if the physician is in disagreement with these decisions. Clarification of goals allows all involved parties to decide whether the relationship is likely to be beneficial and whether they want to participate in it.
5. Success for both the individual and the health care provider(s) is best measured by the degree to which the individual's health-related goals are achieved. It therefore depends on the construction of goals and strategies that are both acceptable and realistic.

A basic tenet of the goal-oriented approach is that the missions of health care (at the level of the individual physician-patient relationship) are to improve the quality and/or increase the quantity of life of individuals. Health-related goals must then relate directly to the achievement of one or both of these missions. The more clearly the goals are defined, the less likelihood there will be for misunderstanding, and the easier it will be for patient and physician to determine potentially useful strategies. Goals, particularly long-term goals, should be quantified whenever possible (based on available experimental and epidemiologic data as well as the individual judgments of physician and patient) and measureable so that progress toward achievement can be monitored. For example, an appropriate long-term goal statement might be: "Reduce my risk of heart attack by X% and thereby increase my quality-adjusted life expectancy by Y years, as determined by the QRS health-risk appraisal instrument."

The diagnosis or resolution of a problem would often (but not always) be important as an objective or strategy but would rarely if ever represent a goal. Thus, the reduction of serum cholesterol by Z% could be an objective related to the above goal, and dietary modification, smoking cessation, and medications could be potential strategies for accomplishing it. This distinction is more than a semantic one. If the most realistic estimates of life prolongation for an individual patient through reduction of identified risk factors for heart disease were only one month, and if this were included in the goal statement, the patient might decide that other goals had higher priority. On the other hand, if normalization of an elevated serum cholesterol was under-

---

Table 1

Possible Goals Related to Acute Illness

1. Learn what to do to increase the rate of recovery from this illness.
2. Suppress symptoms now, even if the duration of the illness is a bit longer.
3. Learn as much as possible about the potential complications of this illness.
4. Learn how to prevent occurrence of similar illnesses in the future.
5. Learn what to do if similar problems occur in the future.
6. Learn how to prevent others from getting my illness.
7. Return to work as soon as possible.
8. Obtain a note to remain out of work.

48   January 1991   *Family Medicine*

Table 2

Comparison of Principles of Problem-Oriented and
Goal-Oriented Approaches to Health Care

	Problem-Oriented	*Goal-Oriented*
Definition of Health	Absence of disease as defined by the health care system	Maximum desirable and achievable quality and/or quantity of life as defined by each individual
Purposes of Health Care	Eradication of disease, prevention of death	Assistance in achieving maximum individual health potential
Primary Methods	Diagnostic process, application of specific corrective measures, patient education	Definition of health goals, determination and implementation of strategies, encouragement, advocacy, empowerment
Enemies	Disease, death	Inhumanity
Measures of Success	Accuracy of diagnosis, appropriateness of treatment, eradication of disease, prevention of death	Achievement of individual goals
Evaluator of Success	Physician	Patient
Data Required	Medical history, physical exam, lab and X-ray results	Medical history, physical exam, lab and X-ray results; assessment of values, strengths, and resources; interests and needs; expectations
Conceptual Framework	Disease oriented, objectivistic, generalized, negative (correcting defects), applied science	Person oriented, constructivistic individualized, positive (achieving goals), adult education, rehabilitative

stood to be the goal, the same individual might feel compelled to achieve it in an attempt to regain health by correcting an identified problem.

Using a different kind of example, if one of the primary goals of treatment of an elderly patient with pneumonia is the restoration of a certain level of function (quality of life), the avoidance of secondary disabilities becomes an appropriate objective, and important strategies would include early mobilization, fall prevention, and nutritional support. When cure of the pneumonia is the primary goal which directs therapy, then the administration of antibiotics in addition to standard nursing care might appear to be necessary and sufficient strategies.

Health goals can be long term or short term, complex or simple. The occurrence of a minor acute deterioration of health would still be a common impetus for patients to seek health care. Table 1 lists some possible goals relevant to an acute illness. The following is an example of a patient with a relatively simple short-term goal relating to a chronic problem.

A 38-year-old man (Mr. R.) was seen for chronic right shoulder pain. Examination revealed that he probably had a chronic rotator cuff injury. Since he had already tried oral medications, injections, and various physical modalities without much benefit and was not interested in an operation, there seemed to be little that could be done. Further diagnostic tests and/or referral to an orthopedist were discussed. However, when asked what he would like to be able to do that

he could not as a result of the shoulder problem, he said that he really was not bothered much by the pain except when bow hunting. His goal was to be able to go bow hunting again. In discussing strategies to reach this goal, Mr. R. volunteered that with a doctor's note, he could hunt with a crossbow and that this might not cause a problem for his shoulder. The note was written, and his goal was achieved.

It should be pointed out that in many cases the proposed goal-oriented approach and the traditional problem-oriented approach would be perfectly congruent. In young and healthy individuals, near perfect health is often achievable, and the eradication of acute problems as they occur may be the best strategy. Even in these cases, however, viewing health in the broader sense as the goal and eradication of the acute disease as but one strategy could stimulate consideration of other strategies, such as education regarding ways to avoid similar problems in the future or reframing the illness event as an opportunity for personal growth and development.

Physician-Patient Interaction

The acknowledgement that patients ultimately decide the state of their own health, their prioritized goals regarding health, and the strategies they are willing to implement to achieve them does not imply that physicians should withdraw from participation in these decisions. On the contrary, physicians must, because of the expertise and objectivity they bring to the physician-patient relationship, be involved

Original Contributions

Vol. 23, No. 1   *49*

through active listening, patient education, recommendation and negotiation, and then encouragement and advocacy. In fact, we agree compeltely with Ingelfinger:

> A physician who merely spreads an array of vendibles in front of the patient and then says, "Go ahead and choose, it's your life," is guilty of shirking his duty, if not of malpractice. The physician, to be sure, should list the alternatives and describe their pros and cons, but then, instead of asking the patient to make the choice, the physician should recommend a specific course of action.[4]

Interaction oriented to goals, which are in theory equally understandable to both patient and physician since they relate to quantity or quality of life, would allow the patient to feel more capable of participating in the decision-making process. The process would, however, be less a search for truth than a joint effort to construct a useful reality. That is, it would be constructivist rather than objectivistic.[5] A comparison of the characteristics of goal-oriented and problem-oriented approaches is shown in Table 2.

Assessment of Results

A problem orientation depends on a carefully constructed problem list that uses both subjective and objective data. The construction of goals would also necessitate an accurate determination of problems, but in addition would require an equally comprehensive assessment of strengths and resources, needs and interests, expectations, and values. The lack of practical methods for assessment within these areas argues most persuasively that physicians are not already using a goal-oriented approach.

Decision analysts have developed techniques for assessing individual utilities in specific situations, but these methods would require considerable modification before they would be useful for more general values assessment. Social and behavioral scientists have tested a variey of methods for evaluating family and social support. However, none has so far gained wide clinical use. Psychologists and other behavioral scientists often spend weeks or months assessing needs and expectations. Developing the methods to effectively and efficiently collect these kinds of information and to incorporate them into the decision-making process would be a challenging but not impossible task.

Adult educators have moved toward goal-directed approaches to adult learning, recognizing that achievement of personal goals is often a more powerful motivator for learning than is the remediation of teacher-identified deficiencies. Individual self-directed, goal-oriented educational strategies enhance individual potentials rather than ensuring minimal competencies.[6] They build on the strengths and interests of the learner at each point in time, while still providing direction to the process. Inasmuch as learning is a prerequisite for behavioral change, the principles of adult education should be entirely appropriate and applicable to medical treatment where changes in health behavior are so often required.

Geriatricians have learned that an approach which emphasizes attainment of functional goals is in many cases more optimistic and rewarding than the traditional disease-oriented approach. Eradication of all identified health problems is often not possible. Maximization of function and independence is of greatest importance to quality of life. The increasing uniqueness of individuals as they age, as well as the greater frequency of chronic illness, disabilities, and interactive biologic, psychologic, and social problems, suggest an individualized, team-oriented approach to geriatric health care. In fact, geriatrics may be the field of medicine with the most urgent need for a new conceptual approach.[7,8]

Operating within a problem-oriented framework, pregnancy has come to be viewed as an abnormal state or, if not, as a set of problems waiting to happen. The physician's job is primarily to detect and treat problems, not to help everyone involved get the greatest possible benefit from the positive experience of pregnancy and childbirth. This task has in recent years been adopted by nurses, midwives, patient educators, and lay instructors who sometimes find themselves in direct conflict with physicians. Within a goal-oriented model, normal physiology does not preclude the need for heatlh care since health-related goals are not necessarily tied to the solution of problems.

As testing methodologies become increasingly sophisticated, the definition of normalcy (a prerequisite for the problem-oriented paradigm) will undoubtedly become even more problematic. Individual genetic patterns, for example, will undoubtedly be discovered to be adaptive in some ways and maladaptive in others. A classic example is the protective effect of sickled red blood cells against the malaria parasite. It is not unreasonable to think that because of advances in genetic mapping, it will become possible to construct extensive problem lists for infants shortly after or even before birth.

In addition, people not infrequently report that the occurence of a serious illness or other catastrophic event was overall a very positive occurrence in their lives, leading them to discover what was truly important and giving them a renewed sense of purpose. If personal strength and adaptability are goals, pain and adversity may be both positive and necessary ingredients for its achievement.

Hypercholesterolemia may be an example of this sort of complexity. While there is good evidence now that lowering serum cholesterol levels can reduce the risk of development of coronary artery disease morbidity and mortality, treatment can be unpleasant and expensive, and there is at least some evidence that it may result in increased deaths from noncardiovascular causes such as accidents, homicides, suicides, and certain types of cancer.[9-11] Nevertheless, upper levels of normal have now been established, and many hundreds of thousands of people have been informed that they have a serious medical problem requiring treatment. The role of the physician should be to help each individual assess the available information regarding cholesterol and determine whether cholesterol reduction is a strategy that should be applied to the achievement of the patient's health goals, taking into account individual values, beliefs, and tolerance for that individual's risks as well as biomedical factors.

The problem-oriented approach to disease prevention tends to be fairly rigid. Specific unhealthy life style factors are targeted for change whenever they are detected, as are the results of screening laboratory tests which fall beyond an arbitrary threshold value. Practitioners involved in developing new approaches to health promotion and disease prevention have already begun to embrace the principles of a goal-oriented approach and have demonstrated greater degrees of behavior change in patients with defined goals. Alexy, for example, found significantly greater success with weight reduction, reduction of alcohol intake, use of seat belts, and increased exercise levels by patients with specified goals in comparison with patients given information and advice only.[12]

Applications in Chronically Ill Patients

The diagnostic process can sometimes cause more harm than benefit. Reuben has pointed out that making a diagnosis is sometimes counterproductive even when using a problem-oriented approach.[13] Haynes demonstrated that diagnosing hypertension in factory workers can result in increased absenteeism from work, decreased marital satisfaction, and decreased income during the subsequent year.[14] Mental health professionals have observed and reported that labeling a person schizophrenic sometimes results in depersonalization and worsening of symptoms.

The care of patients with chronic illnesses is one of the greatest challenges of modern medicine. A problem-oriented approach suggests that when a cure is not possible, every effort should be made to control the abnormal manifestations of the condition. It is generally assumed that patients are in agreement with this goal. However, as pointed out by Marteau et al, in the case of the parents of children with diabetes, large discrepancies may exist between physicians' goals and those of their patients (or in this case, those of the patients' parents).[15] Work by Hefferin suggests that when patients participate in the goal-setting process, they are more likely to achieve positive changes in health status.[16]

One of the authors (L.B.) was the primary physicians of a 55-year-old woman (Mrs. S.) with Type II diabetes mellitus. Mrs. S. consistently reported home blood glucose values in the normal or near normal range, while fasting office measurements were consistently in the mid-200s. All attempts by Dr. B. to bring her serum glucose into the normal range were unsuccessful. During a hospitalization for another problem, Mrs. S. told the admitting resident that Dr. B. "preferred to keep her blood sugar a little on the high side." She had obviously decided at what level she wanted to keep her blood sugar, knew that her doctor's goals were different, and had developed a way of dealing with the medical system to avoid confrontation and yet accomplish her goal.

Dying patients often feel abandoned by their physicians once it is clear that all available medical treatments have failed. However, it could be argued that some of the most important health-related goals of an individual's life pertain to the circumstances associated with the dying process. Physicians ought to be in a unique position to offer guidance, support, and palliation to their patients as they struggle to achieve these often difficult goals.[17-19]

While most medical interventions require the active participation of the patient (exceptions being very ill or comatose adults or small children), physicians usually feel a measure of control over the process. However, some problems depend so heavily on the individual's ability and willingness to solve them that intervention by the physician may be completely ineffectual or even counterproductive. For example, while obesity represents a serious health problem for many people, a physician can do little to cure it without a major comitment on the part of the overweight person. In fact, by pointing out the problem repeatedly to a person who is, for whatever reasons, unable to lose weight, the physician may adversely affect that person's self-esteem, thus reducing his or her overall health. In some cases the physician's admonitions to lose weight may actually lead an obese individual, also in search of control, to gain

additional weight. This principle has been demonstrated most clearly in spousal relationships[20,21] but probably applies equally well to the physician-patient relationship. In such cases, a goal-oriented approach might be more productive.

The concept of compliance is less applicable to a goal-oriented health care model. Instead, this model would assume that individuals would be more or less successful at carrying out proposed strategies and that modifications might or might not be required of either the goals or the strategies based on that information. The physician's role would change from instructor and enforcer to collaborator and advocate, and the flavor of the interaction would shift from correction of deficiencies to encouragement of success.

Physician and Patient Roles

Sometimes the strategies employed by physicians seem to be directed more toward anxiety reduction (physician anxiety, patient anxiety, or anxiety in a larger system, eg, the hospital staff) than toward any overall health benefit for the patient. Aggressive attempts by physicians to gain control over anxiety-provoking situations sometimes result in more anxiety and less control. This decision-making pattern often results in clinical cascades in which one event leads to another and that to another, leaving the participants increasingly powerless to arrest the process.[1] One of the most consistent features of clinical cascades is that the participants either fail to clarify or lose track of their original goal(s) and as a result end up missing the mark quite badly. The most effective way to prevent cascades is to set appropriate and realistic goals and to keep them in mind at all times when decisions are being made.

Within the scientific problem-oriented paradigm, physicians, as the most highly trained applied scientists, are clearly the most influential members of the health care team. Using a goal-oriented approach, not only would the goals of treatment be clearer to all, an essential requirement for teamwork, but professionals other than physicians could be expected to take larger roles in the care of patients. In fact, it is becoming clear that the knowledge and skills of physicians are inadequate to deal with the health concerns of an increasing number of people. As a result, an interdisciplinary team approach has become essential in rehabilitation, geriatrics, home health care, and long-term care, to name only a few examples. Successful teamwork requires clarification of goals and objectives, coordination of strategies. and mutual respect.[22,23] Interestingly, nurses and many allied health care professionals already espouse a goal-oriented approach.

A goal-oriented approach to health care would probably be as difficult initially for patients as for their health care providers. The process of realistic goal setting is not currently being taught or even encouraged by most educational institutions. Grading and correction of deficiencies are the predominant motivational strategies in primary, secondary, university, and most professional schools. Most people find it much easier to identify and criticize faults than to reward achievements. Although adults are by nature goal-oriented, the ability to set realistic goals using complete information would require considerable training and practice for both patients and physicians.

At an institutional level at least some of the systems are

procedures that were put into place to facilitate the problem-oriented model would be inappropriate and would represent obstacles to the implementation of a goal-oriented approach. DRGs, for example, would be less applicable to the new paradigm. A more appropriate cost-containment system, if one were deemed necessary, might be based on the goals for the hospitalization and the anticipated/average/appropriate costs of the strategies propsed to achieve them. In a recent article, Steffen pointed out the advantages of a goal-oriented approach for measurement of quality of medical care:

> For the physician and the patient, quality of medical care can be defined as that care that has the capacity to achieve the goals of both the physician and the patient.[24]

A goal-oriented approach would probably result in a much closer physician-patient relationship. In dealing with information concerning personal strengths, needs, and expectations, physicians would be forced to respect patients as individual human beings. The discussion of personal values and beliefs would require a level of intimacy that can be more easily avoided in an applied science model. In fact, we contend that the problem-oriented approach is one way that physicians (healers) have been able to successfully distance themselves from patients (the sick ones). This defense against emotional attachment with its attendant risk of increased anguish would probably have to be dealt with in other ways (perhaps physician support groups) if a goal-oriented approach were to be adopted. The process of goal setting would also bring into brighter focus situations in which the differences between physician and patient are great enough that the relationship should be dissolved.

Conclusion

An extremely important issue at a sociopolitical level is the need for societal health care goals that may at times conflict with the goals of individuals. It is our belief that a process of goal setting should be followed at each level, but that individual physicians working with individual patients should not be concerned with societal goals except to the extent that their decisions are limited by ethics or law. For example, physicians and their patients should base decisions regarding the use of expensive technology on the applicability of that technology to the achievement of the goals which they have set, not on the perceived cost to society. The sociopolitical system, on the other hand, must look at its available resources and compose guidelines for their equitable distribution, which may then limit the options available to individual physicians and their patients.

The goal-oriented health care model which we have attempted to describe incorporates a broad and flexible definition of health, individual goals and strategies, greater involvement of patients in their own health care, a stronger physician-patient relationship, and potentially increased interdisciplinary teamwork within the health care system. It is as applicable to chronic illness and disability, terminal illness, preventive medicine, and health education as to acute disease. While it might appear to increase the burdens of already overburdened physicians, in fact it might very well do the opposite.

The process of goal setting should make it possible to more clearly define the appropriate roles of physician, patient, and other members of the health care team. Physicians would then be able to concentrate on those activities for which they have been trained, such as the diagnosis and pharmacologic treatment of disease, while counting on other members of the team to contribute in other equally important ways.

It is our contention that primary care physicians should be major participants in the goal-setting process. This will, as stated previously, require that they receive specific training not currently offered in most medical schools and residency programs.

Acknowledgements

The authors wish to thank Howard F. Stein, PhD, Jeffrey Steinbauer, MD, and Christian Ramsey, Jr., MD, for their insightful comments regarding content, Laine McCarthy for reviewing the manuscript for readability, and Debbie Isham for its preparation.

References

1. Mold JW, Stein HF. The cascade effect in the clinical care of patients. N Engl J Med 1986; 314:512-4.
2. McWhinney IR. Changing models: the impact of Kuhn's theory on medicine. Fam Pract 1983; 1:3-8.
3. Dubos R. Personal interview. Modern Maturity 1981 Aug-Sept:35.
4. Ingelfinger FJ. Arrogance. N Engl J Med 1980; 303:1507-11.
5. Berger PL, Luckman T. The social construction of reality: a treatise in the sociology of knowledge. New York: Doubleday, 1966.
6. Knowles MS. Self-directed learning: a guide for learners and teachers. New York: Cambridge Books, 1975.
7. Williams ME, Hadler NM. The illness as the focus of geriatric medicine. N Engl J Med 1983; 308:1357-60.
8. Becker PM, Cohen HJ. The functional approach to the care of the elderly: a conceptual framework. J Am Geriatri Soc 1984; 32:923-9.
9. Lipid Research Clinics Program. The Lipid Research Clinics coronary primary prevention trial results: I. Reduction in incidence of coronary heart disease. JAMA 1984; 251:351-64.
10. Frick MH, Elo O, Haapa K, et al. Helsinki Heart Study: primary prevention trial with gemfibrozil in middle-aged men with dyslipidemia. N Engl J Med 1987; 317:1237-45.
11. Isles CG, et al. Plasma cholesterol, coronary heart disease, and cancer in the Renfrew and Paisley survey. Br Med J 1989; 298:920-4.
12. Alexy B. Goal setting and health risk reduction. Nurs Res 1985; 34:283-8.
13. Reuben DB. Learning diagnostic restraint. N Engl J Med 1984; 310:591-3.
14. Haynes RB, Sackett DL, Taylor DW, Gibson ES, Johnson AL. Increased absenteeism from work after detection and labeling of hypertensive patients. N Engl J Med 1978; 299:741-4.
15. Marteau TM, Johnston M, Baum JD, Bloch S. Goals of treatment in diabetes: a comparison of doctors and parents of children with diabetes. J Behav Med 1987; 10:33-48.
16. Hefferin EA. Health goal setting: patient-nurse collaboration at the Veteran's Administration facilities. Milit Med 1979; 144:814-22.
17. Wanzer SH, et al. The physician's responsibility toward hopelessly ill patients: a second look. N Engl J Med 1989; 320:844-9.
18. Kohn M, Menon G. Life prolongation: views of elderly outpatients and health care professionals. J Am Geriatr Soc 1988; 36:840-4.
19. Benfield DG. Two philosophies of caring. Ohio State Med J 1979; 75:508-11.
20. Pearce JW, LeBow MD, Orchard J. Role of spouse involvement in the behavioral treatment of overweight women. J Consult Clin Psychol 1981; 49:236-44.
21. Hoebel FC. Family-interactional therapy in the management of cardiac-related high-risk behaviors. J Fam Pract 1976; 3:613-8.
22. Rothberg JS. The rehabilitation team: future direction. Arch Phys Med Rehabil 1981; 62:407-10.
23. Wise H, Rubin I, Bechard R. Making health teams work. Am J Dis Child 1974; 127:537-42.
24. Steffen GE. Quality medical care: a definition. JAMA 1988; 260:56-61.

CHAPTER 9

The place of judgement in medicine

Iona Heath

NOMINATED CLASSIC PAPER

James McCormick. The place of judgement in medicine. *British Journal of General Practice*, 1994; February, 44(379): 50–51.

This paper was written more than 20 years ago and was remarkably prescient. James McCormick quite clearly saw dangers looming for medicine that are only now being generally acknowledged. In this short editorial, he insisted on the enduring importance of wisdom and the necessity of judgement in clinical medicine.

Whenever scientific discoveries derived from the study of populations are applied to unique individuals, the outcome will always be uncertain to a greater or lesser degree and hence the enduring necessity of pragmatic, iterative, clinical judgement. In this context, James insisted that, 'Wisdom and judgement are close friends. Both rely on adding weight to the imponderable, value to that which cannot be quantified.' He understood the dangers of the burgeoning belief that 'medicine can be practised by some form of rule book' and anticipated the myriad ways in which algorithms and guidelines have led to over-testing, overdiagnosis and overtreatment across the globe, causing disturbing amounts of waste and harm. He urged everyone to be more honest about the limitations of medicine and its inherent risks.

The 1998 world conference of the World Organization of Family Doctors (WONCA) was held in Dublin and was memorable partly because of the bizarre nature of the venue. The building of the promised new conference centre had not been completed in time so most of the conference sessions were held in an enormous partitioned tent with totally inadequate sound insulation between competing presenters. Everybody had to shout and the resulting cacophony evoked a vision of Babel relocated to a Dublin pub. Yet this was the setting for one of the most marvellous sessions I have ever attended. As I remember, it was billed as a Q&A session with James. It was packed – with most of the audience sitting on the floor. I remember him telling us that scepticism is a moral imperative and that sentiment informs all his writing.

ABOUT THE AUTHOR OF THIS PAPER

James McCormick (1926–2007) was Professor of Community Health at Trinity College Dublin from 1973 to 1991 and, from 1974 to 1979, he also served as Dean of the School of Physic. As his successor Professor Tom O'Dowd wrote in his obituary in the *British Journal of General Practice*: 'He was sceptical of the population approach to health and feared coercion of the individual by forces hell-bent on doing good.' His writings are always provocative and always worth reading. In 1984 he was joined at Trinity by Petr Skrabanek who shared his commitment to scepticism and who was to become his principal ally. Together they published the now classic *Follies and Fallacies in Medicine* in 1989. In the acknowledgements for his later book *The Death of Humane Medicine*, Skrabanek wrote 'Professor James McCormick has been more to me than a close friend … he has been a permanent source of wise counsel and an oasis of calm when things got rough.' There are many others who would echo these words and who miss him still.

ABOUT THE NOMINATOR OF THIS PAPER

Iona Heath worked as an inner-city general practitioner in London for almost 35 years. She served as a nationally elected member of the Council of the Royal College of General Practitioners for 20 years from 1989, and in 2009 was elected President of the College for a three-year term. She served as Member at Large on the executive board of the World Organization of Family Doctors (WONCA) from 2007 to 2013.

'Listen, learn and love.'

Dr Iona Heath CBE, United Kingdom

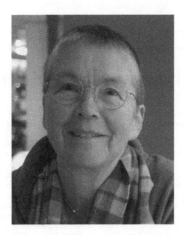

Attribution:

We attribute the original publication of *The place of judgement in medicine* to *British Journal of General Practice*. With thanks to Professor Roger Jones and Moira Davies.

EDITORIALS

The place of judgement in medicine

'The patient may well be safer with a physician who is naturally wise than one who is artificially learned.'[1]

'Working to rule can do even more harm in medicine than it does in industry. The practice of medicine requires a fresh judgement for every patient.'[1]

THESE quotations come from Theodore Fox's article 'Purposes of medicine', published in 1965. Since then there has been little emphasis upon the need for wisdom or judgement in medicine.

Despite the efforts of academic general practice, graduates from our medical schools seem to have been persuaded that medicine can be practised by some form of rule book. If the recommended procedures are followed the right diagnosis and appropriate treatment will almost automatically ensue and there should be no room for uncertainty. As a result they find the inevitable uncertainties of hospital medicine and even more those of general practice hard to cope with.

The practice of medicine is risky and difficult. Risk taking is necessary because the price of being on the safe side is often intolerable. Being on the safe side leads to waste of resources and iatrogenic harm. When the prior probability of disease is low investigations lead to large numbers of false positives which prompt further investigation and spurious diagnoses. Using drugs to lower blood pressure exposes the person, recategorized as a patient, to their side effects and to the consequences of perceiving themselves to have a life threatening disorder. While prophylactic mastectomy diminishes the possibility of death from breast cancer, it must usually be judged that the price of safety is too high.

Wisdom and judgement are close friends. Both rely on adding weight to the imponderable, value to that which cannot be quantified. Unfortunately, judgement has been mocked by the tautologous addition of 'value' to the word. Tautologous because judgement is about adding values and weights to probable consequences of action. Alas, it is easier to criticize folly than to extol wisdom. Wisdom and judgement seem to be hard to grasp, nebulous virtues which may appear to be the prerogative of the aged, if not the senile.

There is little or no obvious recognition of the value of wise judgement. Occasionally one reads in the obituary columns of somebody whose curriculum vitae was not outstanding but who was seen as a 'doctors' doctor'. It would not be a wild guess that such physicians were valued by their colleagues, not because of their learning or their skill, but because their actions were tempered by wise judgement.

Even the most apparently straightforward consultation requires the exercise of judgement in order to make wise decisions. How certain is the diagnosis? What information should the patient be given? Should uncertainty be shared? What are the consequences to the person of the disease label? What is the probability that investigation will clarify rather than confound? What are the risks of missing the diagnosis of a serious disorder at this stage of the illness? What are the costs, risks and potential benefits of treatment? What prompted the decision to consult — pain, anxiety about the meaning of symptoms or the need to take up the 'sick role'? As a general rule reliable and proven answers to these questions do not exist, yet they cannot be ignored if doctors are to offer wise advice.

The first requisite for wise judgement is appropriate knowledge. This extends beyond knowledge of those symptoms and signs which indicate disease, to include knowledge of prior probabilities. These prior probabilities are very different for general practice patients and those patients referred to hospital. Judgement requires the ability to distinguish between those things which are relatively certain and those things which are matters of opinion. It needs to be underpinned by that healthy scepticism which offers the possibility of setting a limit to error.[2] Scepticism which provides some protection against fashion, some protection against accepting the received wisdom of superiors, teachers, consensus and the written word.

Experience contributes to judgement and is of two kinds. Some experience is generic, that is it refers to patients in general rather than in particular. 'In my experience such cases do well on...' Such experience may be a fallacious guide and do little more than allow the repetition of the same mistakes with increasing confidence. It is certainly no substitute for the randomized controlled trial.

The other sort of experience is patient specific and relies on knowledge of the individual. It is much more a characteristic of general practice than of hospital medicine as it is based upon continuity of care and observations made over a number of episodes of dis-ease and over time. A recent paper has demonstrated that such knowledge substantially improves the doctor's ability to predict the presence of urinary tract infection.[3] Knowledge of the people who may have disease is sometimes as important as knowledge of the disease which people have.

'Doctors, like other people are "hot for certainties in this our life", and, like other people, they would welcome any commandment that could not be questioned and thus absolved them from painful decision.'[1] The exercise of judgement, no matter how wise, is a risk taking behaviour and discomfits those who are 'hot for certainties'. As consensus statements, guidelines, advice about accepted practice and statements about quality assurance multiply, those who do not follow not only feel that they may be in error but also that they may, in the event of misadventure, be at risk of medico-legal proceedings. For example, it is difficult to ignore the guidelines recently promulgated by the British Hypertension Society which suggest a more aggressive approach to drug treatment in elderly people than in the relatively young.[4] I believe these guidelines to be based on a false premise but should I choose to ignore them and my patient suffers a stroke I can imagine being arraigned in court. On the other hand if I treat and the person has a stroke it will be ascribed to an act of god. Yet such guidelines are based upon evidence which overvalues improvements in the prevention of morbidity and undervalues the consequences of labelling and the side effects of treatment. They oversimplify the complex and suggest that data derived from populations are applicable to every individual who seeks help.

Doctors, by a person's decision to seek advice, are given a mandate to exercise judgement on that person's behalf. This, at least to some extent, flies against the popular movement to grant patients full autonomy and the right to share. If the doctor decides that it is inappropriate to mention the distant possibility that the symptoms might betoken multiple sclerosis he or she is guilty of a degree of paternalism. Doctors cannot ask those who have cancer if they want to know the truth, doctors must exercise judgement as to the gains and benefits of such disclosure and face the possibility that their judgement will be wrong.

The exercise of judgement in medicine is analogous to the exercise of judgement in the courts of law. Having heard or collected the evidence the physician reaches a decision which is a probability statement which in the absence of certainty carries the possibility of error.

There is a place for rules in medicine, rules which can only be broken in exceptional circumstances and which if ignored carry the possibility of grave harm. Such rules can only properly exist when there is good evidence of their value. For the most part good rules are concerned with potentially life threatening situations, in which failure to make an appropriate response may have serious consequences. In a sense these are simple situations in which there can be no difference of opinion about the immediate necessities.

Such simple situations are the exception and the notion that rules can be devised for medicine as a whole carries the danger of great harm. As knowledge grows rules become more appropriate. Because the nature of a car engine is well understood it is easy to devise rules for detecting faults. Because of our ignorance it is impossible to devise rules which will always apply to the individual who seeks our help.

There is a growing tendency, prompted by a desire to improve standards in medicine, to promulgate guidelines and consensus statements. This is potentially dangerous as it attempts to simplify situations which are inherently complex and not amenable to management by rule. As a result physicians may be forced to act in ways which will harm their patients in order to protect themselves from possible action in the courts.

Most decisions in medicine are not simple and straightforward but require the exercise of judgement to advise the best option for each patient. Attempts to oversimplify, even from the best of motives, carry the danger of widespread iatrogenic harm. We must take care that guidelines remain just that, and are not taken to describe accepted and desirable practice. We need to cultivate judgement and come to accept that its inherent risks are in the best interests of our patients.

JAMES McCORMICK
Fellow emeritus, Trinity College, Dublin

References

1. Fox T. Purposes of medicine. *Lancet* 1965; **2:** 801-805.
2. Skrabanek P, McCormick J. *Follies and fallacies in medicine.* 2nd edition. Glasgow: Tarragon Press, 1992.
3. Nazareth I, King M. Decision making by general practitioners in diagnosis and management of lower urinary tract symptoms in women. *BMJ* 1993; **306:** 1103-1106.
4. Sever P, Beevers G, Bulpitt C, *et al.* Management guidelines in essential hypertension: report of the second working party of the British Hypertension Society. *BMJ* 1993; **306:** 983-987.

Address for correspondence

Professor J McCormick, University of Dublin, Department of Community Health and General Practice, 199 Pearse Street, Dublin 2, Ireland.

CHAPTER 10

The development of family medicine around the world

Luisa Pettigrew

NOMINATED CLASSIC PAPER

Cynthia Haq, William Ventres, Vincent Hunt, Dennis Mull, Robert Thompson, Marc Rivo, Philip Johnson. Where there is no family doctor: the development of family practice around the world. *Academic Medicine*, 1995; 70(5): 370–80.

This paper, for the first time ever, mapped the global status of family medicine. The authors build a powerful argument for the need to strengthen family medicine worldwide and of the role of family doctors as cornerstones in the delivery of comprehensive primary healthcare. They highlight the then emergent epidemiological shift from acute to chronic diseases for which broadly trained family doctors are a necessity. Recognising that while the skills required by family doctors may vary according to population needs, health facilities and resources available, they emphasise that the principles of family medicine are universal. The authors identify 10 barriers to the global development of family medicine and propose 10 strategies to overcome them. The paper includes case examples of the development of family medicine in South Korea, Venezuela and Pakistan.

The paper was a milestone in the global development of family medicine and a seminal publication describing the history and logic for training family doctors. It was published at a time when many countries did not yet consider family medicine a legitimate medical specialty. The content caught the attention of medical educators and provided a rationale for the global expansion of the specialty. It served as the basis for the original 2002 Guidebook on the contribution of family medicine to improving health systems by the World Organization of Family Doctors (WONCA), and for further collaboration with the World Health Organization. It provided evidence for renewed emphasis on human resources and primary healthcare as critical components of successful health systems.

So, 21 years on, has family medicine come of age? Undoubtedly there are new case studies that could be generated to update the original paper. However, there are still many places where access to comprehensive primary healthcare and well-trained family doctors remains a distant reality. The barriers identified in 1995 resonate with the challenges numerous countries still face to train and retain sufficient numbers of family doctors who can provide comprehensive care, and provide that missing link across various levels of health and social care settings. Likewise, most of the strategies proposed for the successful development of family medicine are still applicable in many settings. This makes this paper as relevant now as it was when first published.

This paper confirmed that the principles and challenges of family medicine are universal. It helped inspire the global expansion and increased numbers of family doctors who now contribute to primary healthcare and the well-being of people throughout the world.

ABOUT THE LEAD AUTHOR OF THIS PAPER

Cynthia Haq is Professor of Family Medicine and Community Health at the University of Wisconsin in the United States of America, and a champion for primary healthcare and medical education to promote health equity.

Cynthia received her medical degree at Indiana University. Early in her career she served as medical director for a rural health centre in Kasangati, Uganda where she learned the importance of primary healthcare, community and public health. She has served as a Fulbright Scholar at the Aga Khan University in Karachi, Pakistan, worked at the faculty of Makerere University, Uganda, and at Addis Ababa University in Ethiopia to introduce and strengthen family medicine. She co-authored the first edition of the WONCA Guidebook on the contribution of family medicine to improving health systems. She has served as a consultant for various national and international organisations, has published widely, and has won multiple awards for her achievements.

Cynthia practised full-scope family medicine in rural Wisconsin from 1989 to 2008. She now leads a programme to prepare students for working with urban medically underserved populations and continues global health collaborations. She is also the proud mother of four children.

ABOUT THE NOMINATOR OF THIS PAPER

Dr Luisa Pettigrew currently works as a family doctor in London and a research fellow at the London School of Hygiene and Tropical Medicine. She is passionate about the contribution of primary healthcare and family medicine to global health. Luisa serves as an elected member-at-large of WONCA's global executive committee and as WONCA's liaison person to the World Health Organization.

'Step off the medical training treadmill when you can. Seize opportunities to immerse yourself in other cultures; do so thoughtfully. Learn from different health systems and develop friendships with international colleagues. It can surprise, inspire and enthuse. It may give you a new perspective of your own health system and of how you could contribute to better health globally.'

Dr Luisa Pettigrew, United Kingdom

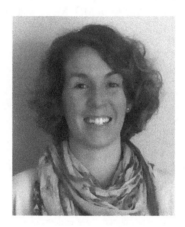

Attribution:

We attribute the original publication of *Where there is no family doctor: the development of family practice around the world* to *Academic Medicine*. With thanks to the authors of this paper, to David P. Sklar, MD, Editor-in-Chief, and to Mary Beth DeVilbiss, Managing Editor.

QUARTERLY FEATURE

INTERNATIONAL MEDICAL EDUCATION
Arthur Kaufman, MD, Associate Editor

Where There Is No Family Doctor: The Development of Family Practice around the World

*Cynthia Haq, MD, William Ventres, MD, MA, Vincent Hunt, MD, Dennis Mull, MD, MPH,
Robert Thompson, MD, Marc Rivo, MD, MPH, and Philip Johnson, MD*

Abstract: Family physicians are generalists trained at the postgraduate level to address the majority of primary care needs of patients of all ages in communities they serve. Throughout the world there is a need for family physicians to serve as cornerstones of comprehensive health care systems that provide high-quality, cost-effective medical and public health services to the entire population. To meet this need, each country must value and adequately finance essential medical and public health services and must provide family physicians with a thorough education focused on the relevant health care problems of the population being served. The authors present an overview of the status of this training throughout the world, outline challenges to the development of such training, and suggest strategies for successful development accompanied by illustrative case studies from South Korea, Venezuela, and Pakistan.
Acad. Med. 70(1995):370–380.

The recent debate on health care reform has brought to the forefront the need for well-trained generalist physicians in the United States. Physicians and policymakers have focused attention on training more family and other primary care medical practitioners to provide high-quality accessible medical care.[1,2] These concerns are not confined to the United States; recently, there has been a global call for expanded training of primary care physicians.[3]

Primary medical care is the field of medicine that provides first-contact, comprehensive, curative, and preventive health care services. These services are delivered by primary health care teams that include physicians, community health nurses, village health workers, and other health professionals. Primary care or generalist physicians in the United States include family physicians, general internists, and general pediatricians. Family physicians are the only generalist physicians trained to care for patients of all ages. Because of their ability to provide comprehensive, continuous care to patients of both sexes and all ages, and to cost-effectively integrate preventive and curative care, family physicians are well suited to address comprehensive primary health care needs of people in developed and developing nations.

Family physicians are generalists trained at the postgraduate level to address the majority of primary health care needs of patients of all ages in the communities they serve. Training and terminology for these physicians vary throughout the world. For example, in the United States and Canada, such physicians are called family physicians and their academic specialty is called family medicine; in Great Britain and other Northern European countries, the most common terms are general practitioner and family practice. In this paper, we use the term family practice to describe this medical specialty designed to provide comprehensive care for patients of all ages and both sexes. We use the term family medicine when that is the formal name for the specialty or department in a particular country or school.

While "the principles of family medicine are universal,"[4] the skills required of family physicians to adequately address the primary health care needs of the patients and communities they serve vary, depending on location of the practice, the diseases prevalent in the region, the resources available, and the proximity to other health care services. In some countries family physicians are active in the care of hospitalized patients (Canada, United States, Nepal), while elsewhere they are based almost exclusively in ambulatory care settings (United Kingdom, Latin America). In most countries, family doctors work as integral members of primary health care teams along with other allied-health professionals.

Even though family practice is expanding throughout the world, many countries still do not have family doctors, due to conceptual, political, financial, and professional barriers. We present strategies to address these barriers and promote successful family practice development.

THE INTERNATIONAL NEED

Since 1978, when the World Health Organization (WHO) began its Health for All program,[5] primary health care has figured prominently in the development plans of government agencies, international donor groups, and nongovernmental voluntary organizations. These organizations have concentrated on promoting both comprehensive and selective primary health care, with an emphasis on public health programs, while focusing limited attention on the appropriate roles of medical care, the physician workforce, and medical education. Today, much of the world's population still lacks access to comprehensive primary care services. This need is most striking in developing nations, but it is also present in many developed countries, where imbalances in the training and distribution of physicians result in shortages of generalist physicians, especially in rural and inner city areas.

In order to address primary health-care needs in developing countries in a cost-effective fashion, many countries have trained cadres of community health workers to implement UNICEF's GOBI–FF (growth monitoring, oral rehydration, breast feeding, immunizations, fertility control, and female education) strategies.[6] These interventions have been important and have been shown to reduce infant mortality by more than half in many communities.[7] However, improvements in infant survival rates have leveled off in these communities, and there have been fewer positive changes in adult morbidity and mortality.

In addition, developing countries show shifts in the patterns of diseases observed over time. An initial preponderance of infectious diseases is shifting to a preponderance of chronic illnesses coupled with an increase in diseases related to behavior and the environment.[8] In most developing countries, infectious diseases are the leading causes of child deaths, while chronic diseases are the leading causes of adult deaths.[9] Practitioners in developing countries may face concurrently high infant mortality and expanding aging populations with their burden of chronic disease. These changes necessitate services considerably beyond the capabilities of the community health worker and call for a more sophisticated and broadly trained family physician.

While changes within the public health sphere have been under way, changes have occurred within medical education that have produced a worldwide consortium of community-oriented medical schools[10] and a call for academic medical centers to assume responsibility for population-based health care.[11] The 1993 World Summit on Medical Education, at-

tended by 240 medical educators from 80 countries, called for "doctors to promote health, prevent illness, palliate disability, become health team managers, advocates for communities, and providers of primary care."[3] The World Health Organization has called for a "paradigm shift in medical education, challenging universities to leave their cloistered environment, assume responsibility for the health of local populations, and to develop curricula that engage faculty and students in population-based medical education."[12] These and other proposed models for community-responsive medical education, while focusing on the importance of restructuring the academic environment, have given less emphasis to the establishment of a viable and functioning generalist-physician work force.

The quality of training for generalist physicians varies throughout the world. In many countries, general practitioners are simply non-specialists who receive limited to no postgraduate training in the provision of primary care. Typically, in these countries medical students have little contact with ambulatory patients and limited instruction in primary care and prevention. As a result, these students fail to gain the skills necessary to function as competent generalist physicians.

Concerns about the relevance, quality, cost–effectiveness, and equity of medical care are growing in importance internationally and focusing renewed attention on the important role of the well-trained generalist physician. Studies demonstrate that residency-trained family physicians provide high-quality, cost-effective care for a broad range of problems at the entry-point of a health care system.[13–15] Furthermore, the quality of care provided by family physicians has been found comparable to that of other specialists in a variety of areas, including uncomplicated obstetrics and perinatal outcomes,[16–18] congestive heart failure,[19] and critical care.[20] The continuity and comprehensiveness of care provided by well-trained family physicians are closely linked with improved quality. Franks and colleagues reviewed eight studies that correlate these characteristics with improved outcomes for patients of all ages, including higher birthweight, reduced morbidity in children, and reduced hospitalization of the elderly.[21]

Today, many individuals and organizations throughout the world are working to increase the relevance of medical practice and medical education and to enhance the role of the general practitioner in health care delivery. In October 1993, the Health Resources and Services Administration (HRSA) and Brown University School of Medicine cosponsored the International Conference on the Education of Family Physicians at the National Institutes of Health. A manual is being developed from this conference to assist those family medicine educators asked to serve as international consultants for developing family practice training programs.[22] In June 1994, the first Global Conference on International Collaboration in Medical Education Reform met in Rockford, Illinois. Cosponsored by the WHO and the University of Illinois College of Medicine at Rockford, the conference helped launch a global network of community-oriented medical schools to collaborate on new models of population-based medical education.[23] In November 1994, the WHO and the World Organization of Family Doctors (WONCA) cosponsored in London, Ontario, a global strategic action forum, "Making Medical Practice and Medical Education More Responsive to Public Need: The Role of Family Doctors." Subsequently, the WHO and the WONCA collaborated on an action plan for achieving the "Health for All" goals, aimed at enhancing the relevance of medical practice and medical education and emphasizing the role of general practitioners in health care delivery. In January 1995, the WHO's executive board formed a resolution developed from the recommendations of the WHO–WONCA report[24] and recommended that it be adopted at the 49th World Health Assembly in May 1995.

THE CURRENT GLOBAL STATUS OF FAMILY PRACTICE

The map (Figure 1) summarizes the information we have gathered regarding the training of family physicians around the world at this time. For simplicity and for the sake of comparison, we delineate three levels of the status of family practice:

I. No identified system of postgraduate training of family physicians

II. Postgraduate training programs being developed for family physicians

III. Established postgraduate training programs for family physicians

The data presented were gathered from a number of sources, including reports in the WONCA News over the last six years,[25] personal files, reviews,[26–28] and preliminary results of a comprehensive survey of postgraduate generalist training in member countries of the WONCA. The latter survey was

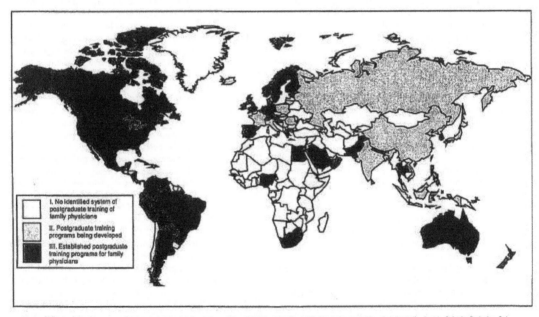

Figure 1. Status of family practice training around the world. **Countries with established family medicine programs:** Argentina, Australia, Austria, Bahrain, Barbados, Belgium, Bolivia, Brazil, Canada, Colombia, Costa Rica, Croatia, Cuba, Denmark, Dominican Republic, Ecuador, Egypt, England, Estonia, Finland, Germany, Greece, Hong Kong, Ireland, Israel, Jamaica, Lebanon, Macau, Malta, Mexico, Nepal, Netherlands, New Zealand, Nicaragua, Nigeria, Norway, Oman, Pakistan, Panama, Paraguay, Peru, Philippines, Portugal, Saudi Arabia, Scotland, Singapore, Slovenia, South Africa, South Korea, Spain, Sri Lanka, Sweden, Switzerland, Taiwan, United States, Venezuela. **Countries with developing family medicine programs:** Chile, China, Czech Republic, France, Guatemala, Hungary, India, Indonesia, Italy, Japan, Jordan, Lithuania, Malaysia, Poland, Romania, Russia, Slovakia, Uruguay.

an extensive cross-sectional study conducted by the Department of Family Medicine at Brown University and HRSA. A 30-page, self-administered branching questionnaire was mailed to 130 persons in 66 countries identified as key individuals from the WONCA directory. Sixty-seven individuals representing 52 countries from all continents responded.

The map is intended to provide an approximate indication of the progress of family practice throughout the world. Because of the difficulty in defining terms and obtaining accurate data for countries in transition, some level I countries may have training programs that we were not able to identify. The situation is also changing rapidly as many countries begin to plan or implement training programs for family physicians. Furthermore, countries indicated at the same level are not necessarily identical in their development of family practice. Some level III countries may have only one certified training program for family physicians, while others may have hundreds. There are considerable differences among countries in requirements for certification, requirements for accreditation, continuing medical education, and the percentages of postgraduate-trained generalists providing care. Data from the WONCA survey and other sources suggest that at least 56 countries have postgraduate training programs in family practice. Of note, half the programs were established after 1970, an indication of the rapid growth and relevance of the specialty and of the need to enhance training for general practitioners.

NORTH AMERICA, THE CARIBBEAN, CENTRAL AND SOUTH AMERICA

Many stages of family practice development are evident in the Americas. Family practice is well established in Canada, where all 16 medical schools have departments of family medicine. Family physician faculty are actively involved as teachers in the undergraduate medical curriculum, and about half of medical school graduates pursue careers in family practice. In the United States, since its designation as a specialty in 1969, family medicine has grown to include over 400 residencies. Approximately 14% of 1994 medical school graduates entered these programs, and 90% of medical schools have departments or divisions of family medicine. Family physicians in the United States represent 12.7% of all non-federal MDs engaged in patient care.[29]

Cuba has developed a comprehensive program of family physician training and placement designed to provide health coverage for all of its citizens.[30] The situation in other Latin American countries is more fluid. Whereas Argentina has many programs, most Latin American countries have limited numbers of residencies with minimal medical school involvement. In the 1970s and early 1980s, family medicine expanded rapidly in Mexico, but recently the number of training centers has decreased considerably.[31] Nevertheless, a cadre of dedicated and committed family physicians is being trained throughout Latin America with encouragement and leadership from several organizations.

EUROPE

Postgraduate training programs for family physicians (referred to as general practitioners in Europe) are well established in the United Kingdom, Ireland, Denmark, The Netherlands, Scandinavia, Portugal, and Spain. Training is less developed in the Southern European countries. Many Eastern European countries are now developing pilot programs. The evolution of family practice in Europe has been affected by the increasing unity of European nations and the breakdown of communist Eastern and Central Europe. For instance, 12 countries of the European Economic Community (EEC) have agreed to the minimum requirement that all generalists receive two full years of postgraduate training, including six months in an approved practice. The European Academy of Teachers of General Practice has been established, as has a European Center for Research and Development in Primary Health Care, with the intention of disseminating information on research and development initiatives in general practice/family medicine within Europe.

AFRICA, MIDDLE EAST, ASIA, AND AUSTRALIA

Family practice training is established in South Africa, Nigeria, and at the Suez Canal University in Egypt. Other African countries have no training or training programs in early stages. In the Middle East, vocational training for generalists is well established in Israel, where all four medical schools have departments of family medicine. The American University of Beirut initiated the first family medicine training program in the Arab world in 1979, followed within months by Bahrain in the Arabian Gulf. Postgraduate training programs are functioning in Saudi Arabia, Kuwait, Oman, and, most recently, in Jordan. An Arab Board of Family Practice sets standards for training programs throughout the Arab world. Also, 14 Asian Pacific countries have agreed upon a common core curriculum in family practice that is flexible and adaptable to local circumstances. Among these countries, family practice has been established in Taiwan, the Philippines, Hong Kong, Malaysia, and Singapore, and throughout South Korea. Family practice training has begun in Pakistan and Sri Lanka, and pilot programs are in progress in China, Russia, and India. Australia and New Zealand have well-developed postgraduate training programs.

CHALLENGES TO THE DEVELOPMENT OF FAMILY PRACTICE

There are many challenges to producing adequate numbers of appropriately trained family physicians internationally. While these challenges present barriers to the establishment

List 1

Barriers to the Global Development of Family Practice
1. Failure to appreciate that family medicine is a specialty
2. Failure to understand the need to integrate clinical and community health skills and services
3. Failure to understand the need to integrate preventive with curative care
4. Preference for selective over comprehensive care
5. Historical trends toward medical subspecialization
6. Increased dependence on tertiary care technologies
7. Disproportionate funding of tertiary care
8. Preference for urban versus rural health development
9. Low intra-professional status of family physicians
10. Limited training opportunities in primary care
11. Lack of family practice leadership and role models
12. Medical education biased toward subspecialty training in hospital settings
13. Lack of commitment to comprehensive, accessible, primary health care

of family practice in developed countries, they form serious impediments to the introduction of well-trained family physicians within primary health care systems of developing countries. These challenges are summarized in List 1.

Even in countries where family practice has been established for many years, there is a prevailing view that it is not possible to produce broadly trained generalists who can practice high-quality, cost-effective primary health care. Advances in medical knowledge and technological developments have created the perception that it is too difficult to keep abreast of the broad scope of family practice. This misconception results from the failure to appreciate that family practice is a specialty whose breadth is appropriate for addressing the majority of health needs in the primary care setting. Effectively integrating hospital, clinical, and community skills presents additional challenges to family practice.

Since World War II, the model of subspecialized, technologically-dependent medical care, increasingly dominant in the United States, has been exported to developing countries. This emphasis on subspecialty care spurred an increase in health-care financing for tertiary care. In most countries, hospitals now consume the bulk of public spending on health care, and in developing countries hospitals may consume up to 80% of government health budgets.[32] In only a few countries that provide universal access to primary medical care have sufficient funds been allocated for the development of strong primary care programs with adequate personnel and funding.[33,34] In large part due to the high proportion of spending for subspecialized, tertiary care, the funds available in most countries for the support of primary care training or primary care clinical infrastructure develop-

ment are limited.

Not surprisingly, primary care physicians throughout the world have endured a lower professional status than their subspecialist counterparts. They usually receive less pay than subspecialty physicians and their working conditions are frequently difficult, with numerous patients to be seen, few diagnostic resources available, and professional isolation from colleagues. Family practice has commonly had difficulty obtaining acceptance within the medical hierarchy as a legitimate specialty, and even in countries where family medicine is recognized, family physicians have had to work hard to establish their domain of medical care and obtain appropriate hospital privileges.

Given these factors and the limited exposure to primary care in medical school, in many countries few students choose to enter generalist careers except by default. Often there are no opportunities to pursue postgraduate training in family practice, as many countries have no such programs.

The political forces that determine medical education and public health policy in many countries frequently do not advocate for the establishment of family practice. There may be conflict between policy-making bodies such as governmental organizations, academic medical centers, and medical associations regarding the balance of medical providers needed and their training requirements. There are usually few advocates for family practice specialists in decision-making positions, especially in countries where a strong system of primary care is not already developed. In such countries, this lack of clinical and academic role models is a serious handicap for development of the field. Additionally, many countries have historically separated the provision of clinical and public health services. Clinicians in these systems often have limited experience integrating the provision of preventive care with clinical services, which is a major goal in family medicine.

PROPOSED STRATEGIES

The effective promotion of family practice internationally will require a series of independent yet coordinated efforts from local communities to international organizations. Here we describe strategies relevant to the items in List 2, followed by case studies from three different countries that illustrate their applications.

Obtain political and financial support. National political and financial support for universal access to primary care is critical for securing adequate resources and for developing a system that values primary care. Without this support, educational reform will have limited impact.

Integrate public health and medical care. Community health education lies at the heart of any effective system of primary health care. This includes education of community members about disease prevention, hygiene, common health

List 2

Strategies for Successful Global Development of Family Practice

1. Obtain political and financial support for universal access to primary care
2. Integrate public health and medical care
3. Upgrade the status of general practitioners
4. Develop family physician faculty and clinician role models
5. Develop undergraduate (medical school) curriculum
6. Develop postgraduate (residency) curriculum
7. Engage subspecialists in training and work with family physicians
8. Develop organizations of family physicians
9. Establish specialty board certification with national medical society status
10. Encourage governments to take a more active role
11. Involve leadership of international health organizations
12. Work with leadership of international family medicine organizations

problems, and when and how to access the health care system. While many primary care initiatives have used community health workers to address these needs, in order to be most effective these workers must be adequately backed up by primary care physicians who are trained to care for more complex problems over the broad range of primary health care issues. Education of community members regarding the need for a system of locally accessible, comprehensive primary care that includes family physicians can aid community health development, provide pressure for legislative change, and support the recruitment and retention of such physicians.

Upgrade general practitioners. By upgrading their abilities through competency-based continuing education and professional certification, currently practicing generalists who have not received postgraduate training can improve their capabilities to provide quality primary care at the same time as they enhance their status and contribute to the growing support for and presence of family practice. In addition, national and international journals targeted at generalist physicians are important for sharing professional information, keeping practitioners informed of new developments, and communicating expectations for high standards.

Develop family physician faculty. Strong leaders are needed who can demonstrate excellence in clinical skills as well as effectively teach the principles of family practice. The involvement of primary care physicians familiar with local disease patterns, cultural patterns, and community needs is crucial to assure that training programs are relevant to local needs. In countries without established training for family physicians, leaders can be exemplary local general practitioners, subspecialists who support generalist training, local physicians who have completed postgraduate training

out of their native countries, or expatriate family physicians. In countries that have few family physicians, providing these physicians with adequate opportunities to balance patient care with teaching is essential to expanding the field. Fellowship opportunities are available for visiting faculty at selected institutions in the United States, but costs limit out-of-country training opportunities.[35]

Develop undergraduate and postgraduate curricula. Undergraduate programs should provide all medical students with knowledge of community health problems and experience in ambulatory care. These fundamental components of family practice are most effective when taught longitudinally, beginning in the first year of medical school. Early exposure to a generalist curriculum increases the chances of students' choosing generalist careers.[2] Family practice concepts should occupy a position of highest importance in the curriculum, using family physicians or other leaders in primary care as prominent faculty members and role model clinicians. Schools dedicated to producing adequate numbers of family physicians may devote 25% of curriculum time to this effort.

Residency education typically lasts two to three years, depending on local needs. It should be as rigorous as subspecialty training and carefully evaluated to be sure that it prepares graduates to provide comprehensive primary care with competence in managing problems prevalent in their communities. An examination-based program of certification, followed by requirements for continuing medical education and recertification, assures that practitioners meet quality standards and remain abreast of new developments.

Ultimately, the ability to attract students to careers in family practice depends on a curriculum that emphasizes primary care during medical school, exposure to family physician role models during clinical training, quality postgraduate training opportunities, and career opportunities with attractive salaries following training. Unless there is a differential in pay between the general practitioner with no postgraduate training and the residency-trained specialist in family practice, there will be little incentive for medical school graduates to invest additional years in residency training. In developed countries, the differential allocation of rewards based on length of training is accomplished by insurance companies and hospital medical staff regulations. In developing countries, governmental policy can be just as influential. For example, in Mexico, the social security system, the principal health care delivery system for salaried employees, preferentially hired residency-trained family physicians and caused a shift in career aspirations of medical students.[36]

Engage subspecialists. Subspecialists can play a critical role in providing family physicians with a disciplined approach to clinical decision making, recognition of patients with problems that need referral, and stabilization of critically ill patients for transfer. Subspecialists' skills can be most effectively utilized when they work in a coordinated fashion with family physicians and other primary care providers who care for common problems and refer to them patients with more complex diseases. In this manner subspecialists maintain expertise consistent with their training, experience, and orientation.

Create national specialty certification and organizations. Specialty boards set standards for training, define the scope of specialty practice, and define the requirements for examination of new and recertifying members. Specialty certification not only assures a minimum standard of quality, but allows for recognition of standards of practice by patients and other medical practitioners. Without standardized training or certification requirements, there will be wide variations in the practice patterns of self-designated family physicians and the qualities of the care they provide, and the specialty will have limited credibility. Officially recognized organizations of family physicians can play a major role in establishment and enforcement of standards of certification.

Involve government. Governments play a large role in the financing of medical education. In many countries they also determine the number of medical graduates and the number of specialty training positions available and their geographic locations. In order to assure that adequate numbers of family physicians are trained, governments must take active roles to redirect funds and address imbalances that have produced surplus subspecialists and shortages of appropriately trained family physicians. In countries that have national health systems committed to providing universal primary health care to all inhabitants, about half of all physicians are generalists who work primarily in ambulatory care settings.[33] In countries whose resources are very limited, primary health care teams with adequate numbers of well-trained non-physician providers (village health workers, traditional birth attendants, community health nurses, physician's assistants or nurse practitioners) supported by family physicians provide the most cost-effective primary health care for all.

Involve international health organizations. The World Health Organization (WHO), has served as an important leader in international public health developments, defining important standards of health for all and outlining methods by which all countries can work toward these goals. These standards have been used by organizations such as the World Bank, the International Monetary Fund, and the U.S. Agency for International Development to determine funding priorities for international development efforts. The WHO has articulated the need for generalist physicians throughout the world.[37] This call for action will need broad support in order to be realized.

Work with family medicine organizations. Several medical societies exist that promote both the exchange of ideas among family physicians from different countries and the training of family physicians throughout the world. The

WONCA promotes the training of family physicians around the world. The International Center for Family Medicine (ICFM), based in Argentina, promotes training of family physicians in Latin America. Members of several national organizations of family physicians or general practitioners have worked actively to promote the development of family medicine in other countries. These organizations have included the Royal College of General Practitioners (United Kingdom, Australia, and New Zealand), the Canadian College of Family Physicians, the American Academy of Family Physicians (AAFP), and the U.S. Society of Teachers of Family Medicine. The Department of Family Medicine of the University of Texas Medical Branch at Galveston provides faculty development courses to Latin American teachers of family medicine. International exchanges of family physicians and the establishment and funding of an international center for the promotion and training of family medicine could allow colleagues to learn strengths of individual programs and promote mutual development, as well as to provide faculty development and technical assistance for many countries interested in training family physicians.

CASE STUDIES

The following case studies illustrate how family practice programs have been developed in three diverse health-care systems. All of the barriers listed in List 1 were encountered in each country. The strategies used to overcome them varied according to local circumstances.

South Korea

Family medicine was introduced to South Korea in 1979. At that time, general practitioners were physicians with no postgraduate, or only internship, training, and more than 20% of specialty-trained physicians were estimated to be practicing only primary care.[38]

The first family medicine residency program was started at the Seoul National University Hospital with assistance from an American consultant. Many early graduates became directors of similar programs in other institutions in the country. Family medicine has now become the fastest growing specialty in South Korea. Over the past five years, 38 new residency programs have been established, bringing the current total to 68. In 1994, family medicine residency programs selected 253 first-year residents, second only to internal medicine. Eighteen of the 35 medical schools now have departments of family medicine.

Family physicians practice in rural and urban underserved areas more frequently than any other specialists. Furthermore, clinical preventive services, sports medicine, and behavioral medicine are practiced almost solely by family physicians. Family physicians often appear in the mass media and are viewed by the public as forceful advocates of health education. This discipline became the first specialty to send undergraduate medical students to work with community family physicians during their clerkships. Also, family physicians have worked to incorporate concepts of oriental medicine into their practices, which is especially important in a country with a strong tradition of folk medicine.

The Korean Academy of Family Medicine now represents about 2,500 board-certified family physicians, and its members play an essential role in the national and international scene. In large part through the efforts of this organization, family physicians in South Korea have come to be viewed by the general public as friendly and responsive to community needs, and under the Academy's auspices, the 1997 WONCA Asia Pacific conference will be held in Seoul.

Four circumstances have been particularly important in the remarkable development of family medicine in South Korea. First, family medicine was introduced in the country's premier medical school by a highly respected physician, Dr. Chang Yee Hong. Second, in 1985 family medicine achieved the status of board certification and became the 23rd specialty in South Korea. Third, universal medical insurance mandated by the government in 1989 required that tertiary centers could see only patients who were referred from physicians in local clinics or hospitals. Family practice centers within the tertiary care centers were exceptions and could provide direct care to patients and refer those requiring specialty services. This policy encouraged tertiary care hospitals to establish new family practice departments. Fourth, family physicians have exhibited remarkable commitment and dedication to teaching and promoting their discipline among students and residents. Additional strategies have included grassroots promotion of community health education, development of a number of vigorous training programs, and leadership in international family medicine.

Venezuela

Primarily due to its petroleum industry, for most of the twentieth century Venezuela has been the wealthiest country in Latin America. In the 1970s and into the 1980s, the government sent many physicians to the United States and Europe for training. This contributed to the country's emphasis on subspecialty and tertiary care medicine. By the late 1970s, the country sought to improve its health-care system in response to national criticism and in response to information from other countries about the concept of "primary care." Since then, several key people, strategies, and events have contributed to the development of the specialty of family medicine as a model for primary care.

In 1979, Dr. Pedro Iturbe, an influential retired Venezuelan pulmonologist, decided that the country needed a new community-oriented model for health care delivery. He in-

vited regional politicians and academic leaders to seminars about family medicine. Simultaneously, the Pan American Federation of Medical School Faculties in Caracas sent a group of health care leaders to visit the United States and Canada to learn about family medicine as a primary care model and a strategy for improving health care delivery.

With the financial support of the local government, in 1980 Dr. Iturbe recruited a Venezuelan physician and epidemiologist, Dr. Felix Gruber, to return to Venezuela after ten years of studying and teaching family medicine in the United States in order to start the country's first family practice ambulatory care center. The next year, Dr. Iturbe convinced government and private industries to underwrite the Venezuelan Foundation for Family Medicine (FUNVEMEFA), which continues to provide financial support for faculty and resident salaries, professional meetings, and publicity for the new specialty.

As Drs. Gruber and Iturbe were developing and promoting family medicine in Maracaibo, Dr. Carmen de Carpio began to promote this specialty in the capital city of Caracas, working within the Social Security Institute. In 1982, three residency programs opened simultaneously, two sponsored by state universities (in Maracaibo and Merida) and one by the Social Security Institute (Caracas). Family physicians were and continue to be trained to work in ambulatory care community-based clinics, with a specific goal of reducing the need for patients to be treated in hospitals. From the beginning, this ambulatory care focus reduced resistance from other specialties, and promoted their support of the new training programs. Mostly because of political lobbying by these three influential physicians, the Venezuelan National Medical Association formally recognized family medicine as a medical specialty in 1984.[39]

To create role model clinician–educators, five young physicians with leadership potential were sent in the mid 1980s for training in family medicine programs in Canada, Mexico, and the United States. Later, FUNVEMEFA sent 12 other Venezuelan physicians to Puerto Rico for a six-month family medicine faculty development program. Many of these 17 physicians trained outside of Venezuela continue to be influential academicians in the country. In addition, Dr. Iturbe arranged for McWhinney's text, *Introduction to Family Medicine*, to be translated into Spanish. This Canadian perspective of the family physician is reviewed in detail and debated by small groups of new residents each year throughout the country.

The development of family medicine in Venezuela provides an example of how much influence a few leaders can have. By enlisting the support of influential local physicians, courting government and private financial support, and carefully identifying and nurturing leadership potential among the earliest-trained Venezuelan family physicians, Dr. Iturbe led the development of a network of effective and stable residency programs by the time of his death in 1993. There are now 11 family practice residency programs and over 500 residency-trained family physicians in Venezuela.

Pakistan

Pakistan is a developing country characterized by high levels of poverty (mean GNP per capita 380 U.S. dollars), illiteracy (75%), annual population growth (3.2%), and infant mortality (134 deaths per 1,000 live births). Only 55% of the population of 122 million have access to adequate primary health services, and two-thirds of all deaths are due to infectious diseases.[40]

A government-sponsored national health-care system does exist, but funds are inadequate, as per capita spending on health is only about $6 per year. More than 80% of the government's health-care budget is devoted to the funding of hospitals and less than 20% to primary care. Over 90% of all medical students are trained in 18 government-funded schools, and until very recently less than 5% of the medical school curriculum was devoted to primary care.

In 1985, the Aga Khan University, a private medical college, was established in Karachi with a commitment to train physicians able to address the health-care needs of Pakistan. The Department of Community Health Sciences leads in the teaching of community medicine, which comprises 20% of the five-year medical school curriculum. The ambulatory care clinical training of students is accomplished in a system of community-oriented primary care centers. A computerized medical information system was developed to track morbidity and mortality data at the centers. Using information from this system, which describes local disease patterns, physicians in the Department of Community Health Sciences and general practitioners in the community in 1989 developed a Diploma in Family Medicine examination, offered by the College of Physicians and Surgeons of Pakistan. Through this diploma, general physicians demonstrating high standards of primary care receive official recognition by passing the specialty examination.

In 1990, the first family medicine residency program was initiated in response to the perceived need for adequately trained family physicians who could serve as clinicians and educators. Visiting family physicians from the United States worked closely with Pakistani primary care physicians to develop training criteria that would address local health needs. Efforts at the level of the community, local medical school, hospital, and National College of Physicians and Surgeons of Pakistan were necessary to gain acceptance of the new specialty. Articles were published in national medical journals, and presentations were made at national meetings.[41,42]

Initially, the residency had limited success until the specialty was accepted at a fellowship level by the Pakistan College of Physicians and Surgeons. Now residents believe there is a future for them. At a 1994 meeting on community-oriented medical education, participants called on the government to create a department of family medicine at every medical college in the country and to create positions in basic health units for diploma-level family physicians and positions in hospitals for fellowship-level family physicians.[43] An established base at a leading medical school, recognition by the National College of Physicians and the Pakistan Medical and Dental Council, and government support have all aided the early stages of family medicine development in Pakistan.

CONCLUSION

The establishment of academic departments of family medicine and of the clinical specialty of family practice is vitally important to the realization of accessible, effective, and comprehensive primary health care. In order to enhance this process, it is first necessary to establish the need for well-trained generalist clinicians among the leaders of medical education and the agencies promoting international and national health care development. Second, medical educators and health planners must understand the importance of an integrated plan for primary health care training and delivery, beginning in and extending beyond medical school into the medical workforce. Third, coordinated efforts should be made to share experiential knowledge gained from the establishment of family practice programs in other countries. Cross-national comparisons of countries facing similar concerns can be helpful. Fourth, as health care planners seek to implement the possibilities inherent in family practice they must both define the health parameters they most wish to affect by the establishment of family practice and assess how the medical and political environments within their countries can foster the development of family practice and monitor its effectiveness. In order to be most effective, family physicians must be trained to respond appropriately to the local health care needs of the patients and communities they serve. Finally, and perhaps most importantly, financing policies must value and reimburse primary and preventive care, and rewards and opportunities must be created to provide incentives for young physicians to become residency-trained specialists in family practice.

In countries where there are no family doctors, the health care systems are dominated by physicians who are poorly equipped to practice high-quality, cost-effective, comprehensive, population-based preventive and curative primary care. The result is most often a fragmented and costly health care system focused on episodic curative care. By contrast, the front-line physician of a rational health system should be a well-trained generalist whose scope of practice encompasses curative and preventive services to the individual, families, and the community. While many nations still do not recognize the specialty of family practice, the number that do is substantial and increasing. In spite of the formidable barriers, we believe that the case is strong for the establishment of family practice as the basis of primary care in medical systems around the world. Family physicians as educators and role models are crucial for developing training programs in areas where there are no family doctors.

Dr. Haq is associate professor, Department of Family Medicine, University of Wisconsin Medical School, Madison, Wisconsin; Dr. Ventres is visiting professor and Senior Fulbright Scholar, Universidad Nacional Experimental de Tachira, San Cristobal, Venezuela; Dr. Hunt is professor and chairman, Department of Family Medicine, Brown University School of Medicine, Providence, Rhode Island; Dr. Mull is professor and regional chairman, Department of Family Medicine, Texas Tech University Health Sciences Center at El Paso; Dr. Thompson is associate professor, Department of Family Medicine, University of Texas Medical School at Galveston; Dr. Rivo is director, Division of Medicine, Health Resources Services Administration, Department of Health and Human Services, U.S. Public Health Service, Rockville, Maryland; and Dr. Johnson is visiting professor and Senior Fulbright Scholar, Aga Khan University, Karachi, Pakistan.

Correspondence and requests for reprints should be addressed to Dr. Haq at the Department of Family Medicine, University of Wisconsin, 777 S. Mills Street, Madison, WI 53715, or via the internet at chaq@fammed.wisc.edu.

This article is dedicated to the memory of Dr. Christopher Krogh, who died in a plane crash on February 24, 1994, in South Dakota, while on a mission for the U.S. Indian Health Service. Dr. Krogh was a charter member of the Society for the Teachers of Family Medicine's International Committee and the International Health Medical Education Consortium. His bright vision enriched the lives of all the authors.

The authors thank the members of the Society of Teachers of Family Medicine who joined their roundtable discussions of international family medicine education at the 1993 annual meeting of the society: Kathleen Culhane-Pera, Robert Davidson, Eugene Farley, Linda French, Robert Hall, Warren Heffron, Gabriel Smilkstein, Steven Spann, and Calvin Wilson. Special thanks to Dr. Taiwoo Yoo for supplying information about family medicine in South Korea, Ms. Mary Nelson for assistance in the preparation of the manuscript, and to Beth Harris and J. Robert Lawrence for assistance with preparation of the map. Additional thanks to Dr. Dan Ostergaard for assistance with development of the survey and to Drs. Tom Gilbert and Larry Culpepper for sharing the results of the WONCA survey, which provided essential information for the map, and Dr. Carol Gleich, survey project officer. This survey was supported by a contract from the Division of Medicine of the Health Resources and Services Administration (HRSA). The contents are solely the responsibility of the authors and do not necessarily represent the views of HRSA.

REFERENCES

1. Schroeder, S. A. Training an Appropriate Mix of Physicians to Meet the Nation's Needs. *Acad. Med.* 68(1993):118–122.
2. Colwill, J. M. Where Have All the Primary Care Applicants Gone? *N. Engl. J. Med.* 326(1992):387–393.
3. World Federation for Medical Education. *Proceedings of the World Summit on Medical Education.* Henry Walton, ed. *Med. Educ.* 28, Supplement 1 (1994).
4. Medalie, J. H. Family Medicine: Principles and Applications. Baltimore, Maryland: Williams and Wilkins, 1978.
5. *Primary Health Care.* Report of the International Conference on Primary Health Care, September 6–12, 1978, Alma Ata, USSR. Geneva, Switzerland: World Health Organization, 1978.
6. World Health Organization–United Nations Children's Fund Statement. Geneva, Switzerland: World Health Organization, 1985.

7. Bryant, J. H., et al. A Developing Country's University Oriented Toward Strengthening Health Systems: Challenges and Results. *Am. J. Public Health* 83(November 1993):1537–1543.
8. Evans, J. R., Hall, K. L., and Warford, J. Shattuck Lecture—Health Care in the Developing World: Problems of Scarcity and Choice. *N. Engl. J. Med.* 305(1981):1117–1127.
9. Jamison, D. T., and Mosley, W. H. Disease Control Priorities in Developing Countries: Health Policy Responses to Epidemiological Change. *Am. J. Public Health* 81(1991):15–22.
10. Schmidt, H. G., Neufeld, V. R., Noorman, Z. M., and Ogunbode, T. Network of Community-oriented Educational Institutions for the Health Sciences. *Acad. Med.* 66(1991):259–263.
11. Showstack, J., et al. Health of the Public: The Academic Response. *JAMA* 267(1992):2497–2502.
12. Bryant, J. H. Educating Tomorrow's Doctors. *World Health Forum* 14 (1993):217–230.
13. Cherkin, D. C., Rosenblatt, R. A., Hart, L. G., and Schneeweiss, R. The Use of Medical Resources by Residency Trained Family Physicians and General Internists: Is There a Difference? *Med. Care* 25(1987):455–468.
14. Utilization of Hospital Services: A Comparison of Internal Medicine and Family Practice. *J. Fam. Pract.* 28(1989):91–96.
15. Greenfield, S., et al. Variations in Resource Utilization among Medical Specialties and Systems of Care: Results from the Medical Outcomes Study. *JAMA* 267(1992):1624–1630.
16. Franks, P., and Eisinger, S. Adverse Perinatal Outcomes: Is Physician Specialty a Risk Factor? *J. Fam. Pract.* 24(1987):152–156.
17. Kurata, J. H., et al. Perinatal Outcomes in Obstetric and Family Medicine Services in a County Hospital. *J. Am. Board Fam. Pract.* 2(1989):82–86.
18. Rosenblatt, R. A. Perinatal Outcomes and Family Medicine Refocusing on the Research Agenda. *J. Fam. Pract.* 24(1987):119–122.
19. McGann, P. K., and Bowman, M. A. A Comparison of Morbidity and Mortality for Family Physicians' and Internists' Admissions. *J. Fam. Pract.* 31(1990):541–545.
20. Hainer, B. L., and Lawler, F. H. Comparison of Critical Care Provided by Family Physicians and General Internists. *JAMA* 260(1988):354–358.
21. Franks, P., Clancy, C. M., and Nutting, P. A. Sounding Board: Gatekeeping Revisited—Protecting Patients from Overtreatment. *N. Engl. J. Med.* 6(1992):424–427.
22. Proceedings of the International Conference on the Education of Family Physicians. Bethesda, MD, October 1993. Sponsored by the Department of Family Medicine, Brown University School of Medicine, Providence, Rhode Island and the Health Resources and Services Administration's (HRSA) Division of Medicine. HRSA Contract #240-92-0051.
23. Skolnick A. First Global Conference on Medical Education. *JAMA.* 1994; 272:504–505.
24. World Health Organization. Resolution by the WHO Executive Board entitled "Changing Medical Education and Medical Practice for Health for All". Adopted on January 25, 1995 (EB95/SR/11) and submitted to the 48th World Health Assembly for adoption. Geneva, Switzerland.
25. *WONCA News.* Oxford University Press, Vol. 14–20(2), 1988–94.
26. Rae, D. W. Family Medicine: An International Perspective. In *Proceedings of the International Soviet–Canadian Seminar.* D. I. Rice and V. A. Vladimirtsev, eds. 1991:5–6.
27. General Practice in Developing Countries. *WONCA News,* 19(Sept. 1993).
28. Ceitlin, J. Primary Care Research in Latin America, Portugal and Spain. *Fam. Med.* 8(1991):161–167.
29. *Facts about Family Practice.* Kansas City, MO: American Academy of Family Physicians, 1994.
30. Perez, J. T., VonBraunmihl, J., Valencia, J. J., and Marquez, M. A. Cuba's Family Doctor Programme. Monograph published by Cuban Ministry of Pub-

lic Health, UNICEF, PAHO/WHO, UNFPA, 1991.

31. Irigoyen-Coria, A., and Gomez-Clavelina, J. F. G. Can Family Medicine Survive in Mexico? *Fam. Med.* 11(1994):162–163.

32. The World Bank. World Development Report: The International Bank for Reconstruction and Development. Oxford, England: Oxford University Press, 1993.

33. Starfield, B. Primary Care in Health: A Cross National Comparison. *JAMA* 266(1991):2268–2271.

34. Gilpin, M. Cuba: On the Road to a Family Medicine Nation. *Fam. Med.* 21(1989):405–407, 462, 464, 471.

35. Cohen, M. D., and Merenstein, J. H. The Availability of Fellowship Training for Foreign Family Physicians. *Acad. Med.* 65(1990):348–350.

36. Mull, J. D. Medicina Familiar en America Latina. *J. Fam. Pract.* 22(1986):469–470.

37. Boelen, C. Medical Education Reform: The Need for Global Action. *Acad.*

Med. 67(1992):745–749.

38. Youn, B. B. Family Medicine in Korea. *J. Am. Board Fam. Pract.* 6(1993):411–413.

39. Thompson, R., Gruber, F., and Marcano, G. Family Medicine Training in Venezuela. *Fam. Med.* 24(1992):188–190, 238.

40. United Nations Children's Fund. The State of the World's Children 1994. Oxford, England: Oxford University Press, 1994.

41. Haq, C. L., Zuberi, R. W., Quereshi, F., Inam, B., and Bryant, J. The Development of Postgraduate Training in Family Medicine in Pakistan. *Journal of the Pakistan Medical Association* 42(1992):69–73.

42. Mull, J. D. Under the Banyan Tree: Reflections on Health Care in Pakistan. *Fam. Med.* 19(1987):391–395.

43. *Augmenting Component of Community-Oriented Teaching in Medical Colleges of Pakistan.* Report of Workshop. Government of Pakistan, Ministry of Health, June 1994: 33.

CHAPTER 11

Training the world's rural family medicine workforce

John Wynn-Jones

NOMINATED CLASSIC PAPER

Policy on Training for Rural General Practice, World Organization of Family Doctors (WONCA) Working Party on Training for Rural Practice, 1995.

Rarely has one document made such a difference in the field of rural practice and rural health. More than 20 years on, academic papers on rural medical education still include the 'Policy on Training for Rural General Practice' in the list of references.

It remains as important today as when it was written because nothing existed before it and, as a consensus document, it was created by a number of motivated authors from around the world. The policy was the first piece of work undertaken by the then newly established WONCA Working Party on Rural Practice which has gone on to become a leading force in rural healthcare worldwide.

Four young disenchanted rural family doctors met by chance at the WONCA world conference in Vancouver in 1992. Despite the fact that more than half the world's population lived in rural areas where access to basic healthcare is often restricted and the recruitment and retention of health practitioners is a constant challenge, the conference had little in the way of rural content. They saw the need for a global policy document aimed at training doctors specifically for rural practice. This small group formed the core of the WONCA Working Party on Rural Practice, which was formally established three years later at the WONCA world conference in Hong Kong. Despite the vast distances separating the authors at a time before email communication became commonplace, the group developed their document by sharing drafts using fax machines.

The international distribution of the contributing authors ensured that the policy had global relevance and its recommendations could be adopted in most countries. Other policy documents have since followed but it is the *Policy on Training for Rural General Practice* that set a gold standard for rural medical practice and influenced positive change for many of those who work and live in rural areas around the world.

ABOUT THE LEAD AUTHOR OF THIS PAPER

This paper has remained relevant because it represents a global consensus by a group of contributors who had been struggling to institute change in their own countries. Coming together within a respected global professional body such as WONCA gave them the opportunity to promote a different approach to rural medical education. The subsequent impact can be seen today in the many rural education and research institutions and rural training programmes around the world.

The lead author, Roger Strasser, then based in Australia, showed immense skill in gathering such a wide range of contributing authors. Other principal authors included Ijaz Anwar (Pakistan), Bruce Chater (Australia), Robert Hall (Australia), Victor Inem (Nigeria), S.H. Lee (China), John MacLeod (Scotland), Neethia Naidoo (South Africa), Jim Rourke (Canada), and many others.

The rural family medicine movement owes a great debt to Roger Strasser for his leadership in this project. Roger was one of the world's first professors of rural health, at Monash University in Australia, and then Inaugural Dean of the Northern Ontario School of Medicine (NOSM), the first new medical school established in Canada in 30 years. Under Roger's leadership, NOSM has become a beacon for innovative approaches to rural medical education. Roger continues to champion the importance of distributed learning, community engagement, social accountability and working in partnership with individuals and communities.

ABOUT THE NOMINATOR OF THIS PAPER

Dr John Wynn-Jones has been a rural general practitioner in Wales for over 30 years, and is currently Senior Lecturer in Rural and Global Health at Keele Medical School in the United Kingdom. He founded the Institute of Rural Health in the United Kingdom and was instrumental in creating the European Rural and Isolated Practitioner's Association (EURIPA). John was one of the founding members of the WONCA Working Party on Rural Practice and took over as chair in 2013. His passion for rural practice remains unabated and he is dedicated to doing even more to reduce rural inequalities and improve the health outcomes of rural people around the world.

'Wherever you work, whatever discipline you work in, remember that this document and these doctors changed the world, and you will as well if you believe that you can. Don't wait for things to happen, because without you they may not!'

Dr John Wynn-Jones, Wales

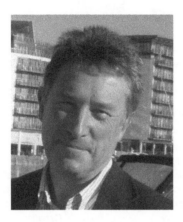

Attribution:

We thank the World Organization of Family Doctors (WONCA) for permission to include the *Policy on Training for Rural General Practice*. With thanks to Chief Executive Officer, Garth Manning.

World Organisation of Family Doctors

POLICY ON TRAINING FOR RURAL PRACTICE

Endorsed by
Wonca World Council Meeting on
9 June, 1995

This Wonca Policy on Training for Rural Practice has been prepared by the Wonca Working Party on Training for Rural Practice which was formed following the Wonca World Conference in 1992.

Original Working Party Members

Professor R Strasser (Convenor)	Australia*
Dr J Rourke	Canada*
Dr I Anwar	Pakistan*
Dr N Naidoo	South Africa*
Dr H Rabinowitz	United States of America*
Dr J McLeod	United Kingdom*
Dr P Newbery	Canada*
Dr T Aziz	Pakistan
Professor R Rosenblatt	United States of America
Professor SH Lee	China (Hong Kong)
Dr J Wynn-Jones	United Kingdom
Dr MK Rajakumar	Malaysia
Professor Gu Yuan	China
Dr B Chater	Australia
Dr T Doolan	Australia
Dr J Cowley	Ireland
Dr C Simpson	United States of America

* denotes original working party members

Enquiries regarding this policy should be directed to:

Professor Roger Strasser
Head, Monash University School of Rural Health
PO Box 424 Traralgon Victoria 3844 Australia
Telephone: + 61 3 5173 8181
Facsimile: + 61 3 5173 8182
Email: roger.strasser@med.monash.edu.au

Summary

The worldwide shortage of rural family doctors contributes directly to the difficulties with providing adequate medical care in rural and remote areas in both developed and less developed countries. Wonca believes there is an urgent need to implement strategies to improve rural health services around the world. This will require sufficient numbers of skilled rural family doctors to provide the necessary services. In order to achieve this goal, Wonca recommends:

1. Increasing the number of medical students recruited from rural areas.

2 Substantial exposure to rural practice in the medical undergraduate curriculum.

3. Specific flexible, integrated and coordinated rural practice vocational training programs.

4. Specific tailored continuing education and professional development programs which meet the identified needs of rural family physicians.

5. Appropriate academic positions, professional development and financial support for rural doctor-teachers to encourage rural research and education.

6. Medical schools should take responsibility to educate appropriately skilled doctors to meet the needs of their general geographic region including underserved areas and should play a key role in providing regional support for health professionals and accessible tertiary health care.

7. Development of appropriate needs based and culturally sensitive rural health care resources with local community involvement, regional cooperation and government support.

8. Improved professional and personal/family conditions in rural practice to promote retention of rural doctors.

9. Development and implementation of national rural health strategies with central government support.

1. Introduction

Every rural practice is unique with its own challenges and rewards. A variety of definitions is used around the world depending on local context. In Australia, the RACGP Faculty of Rural Medicine defines rural practice as medical practice outside urban areas, where the location of the practice obliges some general practitioners to have, or to acquire, procedural and other skills not usually required in urban practice.

There continues to be a worldwide shortage of family doctors (general practitioners) in rural and remote areas, and in particular doctors with the necessary skills and knowledge to work effectively and comfortably in these areas. In less well developed countries the majority of the population is located in rural areas that may lack basic health requirements such as clean water, adequate food and shelter, and where at best they have limited access to modern medical services. Developed countries also have significant shortages of rural family doctors, even in countries where there is an overall over supply of doctors.

People living in remote and rural communities require the security of ready access to medical care at times of serious illness or injury. In addition, doctors and hospitals in rural communities are important to the local economic and social fabric. Often the health status of special needs groups is worse in rural than metropolitan areas. These include the poor, the elderly, women and indigenous people. Establishment of family doctor services supported by hospitals and other health facilities provide the basis for developing primary health care and health promotion programs.

It is well recognised that the provision of medical services by broadly trained generalist family physicians is more cost effective than a range of specialist practitioners and others providing primary care. In addition, for developing countries, improvements in health status and economic development are closely linked. Consequently, it is important that all nations adopt specific policies and programs aimed at improving rural health services through increasing the numbers of broadly skilled family physicians located in rural and remote areas.

2. Advantages of Rural Practice

Rural doctors identify a series of key attractions of rural practice. First is the greater variety of practice that often includes obstetrics, surgery, anaesthetics and emergency medicine together with hospital access and care of the acutely ill. Rural practitioners are much more likely to be looking after individual patients for all of their medical problems on a continuing basis and to be caring for other family members. Thus comprehensive and continuing care are frequent realities in the country.

For many rural doctors the second great attraction of rural practice is the country environment and lifestyle which is associated with a better family life in a good place to raise children particularly in developed countries. Social satisfactions of rural practice identified by rural doctors include community standing and respect, coupled with a sense of belonging to a stable community, and enjoyment of outdoor living with many recreational opportunities. In short, rural practice can offer considerable professional rewards and satisfactions coupled with the attractions of significant social status away from the difficulties of city living.

3. Barriers to Entering Rural Practice

A number of attitudinal and perceptual barriers have been identified as discouraging medical graduates from entering rural practice. Some of these are misperceptions and others have a basis in reality. The key misperception is that rural practice is somehow "second class medical practice". Most undergraduate medical students have a city background and so have no personal experience of living and working in the country. In addition, most of the senior teachers in medical schools have an experience and view of medicine which sees teaching hospital practice as the ideal. Consequently, they assume that medical practice in rural areas without the same facilities and support as teaching hospitals is of a lesser standard.

An important attitudinal problem is that of "learned helplessness". The highest that many new medical graduates aspire to in dealing with medical problems is being able to assess to which specialist to refer the patient . Consequently, it is a frightening prospect for them to contemplate rural practice where they have to manage problems themselves without immediate access to high technology medical facilities and specialists.

There are a number of other barriers which add to the disincentives for new graduates contemplating rural practice. These include the heavy workload and long hours on call which are likely to continue while there is a shortage of doctors in the country. A lack of infrastructure and regional support is common to rural practice, especially in developing countries. Also, the relative professional isolation, which provides many challenges and rewards for rural doctors is seen as a negative factor for many students and new graduates. Often this aspect is over-emphasised within the context of urban-based training rather than the development of individual knowledge and skills required and organisational strategies to address rural health needs.

As well as the professional disincentives to rural practice, there are personal and family issues as well. Rural practice, particularly in small communities, may be difficult for the doctor's spouse. Often the spouse is treated differently from other members of the community and may become personally isolated. Employment for the spouse and education for the family are often significant problems in rural practice. Arrangement of locum relief to permit holidays and continuing education is often a major difficulty.

Even for those students and recent medical graduates who wish to enter rural practice, there are difficulties in obtaining appropriate training and ongoing educational support. Tailored training programs preparing medical graduates for rural practice are relatively few . Once in rural practice not only is continuing education difficult to arrange, but often proves to be of limited value to practising rural doctors. Generally, the knowledge and skills acquired through experience in rural practice are not given due recognition. This limits the potential for career development of doctors who choose to practice in country areas.

7

Drawing all these factors together it is not surprising that in the view of many undergraduates and new medical graduates the professional and social advantages of rural practice are overwhelmed by the disadvantages. In order to overcome these problems there needs to be developed a series of comprehensive strategies which address all the specific issues. This policy document has been developed drawing on the experience in many countries around the world and forms the framework for a comprehensive strategy plan to improve the recruitment and retention of rural family physicians.

4.   Recruitment and Retention of Rural Family Physicians

The ultimate goal of this policy is for there to be sufficient numbers of skilled doctors located in rural and remote areas to meet the health service needs of the people they serve. Although the primary focus of the policy is on education and training for rural practice, this should be seen in the wider context of recruitment to and retention of doctors in rural practice. There is a need to establish an integrated career pathway of education and training for rural practice, beginning at the pre-undergraduate level and continuing through undergraduate medical education to specific rural practice vocational training followed by appropriate continuing and university graduate education, practice structures and family supports.

Ultimately, recruitment to rural practice will only increase when students and new medical graduates see rural practice as a positive career option. The series of strategies outlined in this document are intended to bring this about through sensitising students to rural medicine early on and providing appropriate clinical teaching in the latter part of the undergraduate course and in the immediate postgraduate period.

Retention in rural practice is likely to be improved through tailored continuing education and professional development programs, and the opportunity to pursue university higher education while remaining in rural practice.

In addition to education and training issues, there are a number of other factors which require attention in any program to improve recruitment and retention to rural practice. Reasonable working conditions, including a balance between workload, on call and free time, are essential. Reliable cross coverage or locum relief is a fundamental issue. Also there needs to be appropriate financial reward for the complexity of the services provided and degree of clinical responsibility taken by the doctor. Other financial aspects include additional costs of living in rural communities with the need for transportation to larger centres for continuing education and professional development. Providing a good education for the doctor's children can be difficult and costly.

Also, retention of rural doctors depends greatly on the satisfaction of the physicians spouse and family. Often the reasons for rural practitioners returning to the city relate to spouse and family concerns. Consequently, these are given specific attention in this policy document.

5.   Undergraduate Education

Experience around the world shows that students from a rural origin are much more likely to enter rural practice after graduation. In most current medical courses, the proportion of students from a rural origin is significantly less than the proportion of the population which lives in the country. Clearly one important strategy for increasing the numbers of rural doctors involves recruitment of more medical students from a rural background.

In order for this to occur, secondary students in rural areas need to be encouraged to consider medicine as a career option and to apply for entry to medical school. Consequently there is a need for specific programs which promote medicine to rural secondary schools. In many rural areas the academic standards of the secondary schools may not be sufficiently high for their graduates to qualify for medical school entry. Thus, programs need to be developed which identify potential medical students and assist them with secondary education in preparation for medical school entry.

In order to ensure an appropriate proportion of rural origin students are recruited into medical schools, there need to be specific mechanisms included in the selection process. Criteria for selection based on marks plus other criteria are evolving.   Selection processes which include interview of applicants and give recognition and credit for rural background are to be encouraged. Specific targets for admission of students from a rural background may be needed.

After a rural background the next strongest factor associated with entering rural practice is undergraduate and postgraduate clinical experience in a rural setting. Consequently, rural exposure for all undergraduate medical students should be maximised. Early positive exposure to rural practice will encourage more students to develop an interest in rural practice as a career option and foster a better understanding of rural practice for others. All students should be introduced to rural health issues early in the medical course and have clinical rotations to rural hospitals and rural family practice later in the course.

As rural practitioners provide a wider range of services than their metropolitan counterparts, rural practice attachments provide students with the opportunity to develop a breadth of clinical skills. These include diagnostic and therapeutic procedural skills as well as skills of clinical judgement and self reliance in the practice setting. This rural experience also helps students identify their own learning needs.

In addition, students should be encouraged to undertake optional attachments and electives in rural health, ranging through rural hospital attachments, rural family practice and other rural health services.

"Rural Practice Clubs" encourage city origin students to develop an interest in rural practice and support rural background students in adjusting to the challenges of city living and university studies. Rural origin students would be assisted further through rural doctor mentor schemes whereby each student is attached to a physician practicing in the rural town or area from which the student comes.   The mentor provides the student with ongoing personal support and encouragement as well as a professional role model.

For students who indicate an early commitment to rural practice then a "rural medicine stream" in the medical school is recommended. This might take the form of one to three years of the complete medical curriculum undertaken in the rural setting, or a thread of rural attachments intertwined through the clinical components of the curriculum.

Decentralised medical schools that allow medical students to take a major part or all of their studies at centres located outside major metropolitan areas, are more likely to attract students from rural areas and be successful in producing doctors to practice in rural areas.

The development of community based family medicine curricula in medical education should be encouraged, and should include significant rural content.
Medical schools should assume a responsibility to educate appropriately trained doctors to meet the needs of their general geographic region including underserved areas. As well, they should play a key role in providing regional support for health professionals and accessible tertiary heath care. The inclusion of rural doctors as educators and researchers is integral to the development of an improved understanding of and a supportive attitude towards rural practice.

The development of undergraduate and postgraduate education and training for rural practice is greatly facilitated by the establishment of Rural Medical Education Centres. These Centres should be established in rural areas with the aim of co-ordinating undergraduate education, vocational training, continuing education and university postgraduate studies for rural doctors. An important function of these centres is to facilitate the development of reciprocal links between rural hospitals/practices and medical schools/teaching hospitals. The establishment of such Centres provides the opportunity for rural family physicians to be actively involved in teaching students and vocational trainees. They also provide a focus for other academic developments including rural health research.

6. Postgraduate Vocational Training

Rural family physicians generally provide a wider range of services than do their metropolitan counterparts. Consequently, there is a need for specific residency training programs for rural practice which prepare new medical graduates for a career in the country.

Wherever possible, training for rural practice should occur in the rural setting based at regional rural hospitals and rural family practices. In addition to standard training for family practice, rural practice vocational training requires specific emphasis on: hands-on learning of procedural skills; the spectrum of illnesses in rural and remote communities; the sociology and psychology of rural and remote communities; and professional and personal aspects of living and working in small rural communities.

Training positions for advanced rural practice skills in emergency medicine, anaesthesia, surgery, procedural obstetrics and others, need to be developed and appropriately funded. Depending on the intensity of the training program, such training may involve one to two years of additional training time over and above basic family medicine training.

Consideration should be given to recognition for rural vocational training in the form of certification in rural medicine. The opportunity to take some training in other countries can broaden experience and help develop new approaches to medical practice, medical education, and health care delivery.

7. Continuing Education and Professional Support

Most rural practitioners experience great difficulty in arranging locum relief to attend continuing education activities. Often rural family physicians find that when they do attend continuing education programs that they are of little value to them as they are not pitched at the appropriate level.

There is a need for specific tailored continuing education and professional development programs to meet the needs of rural family physicians. Generally these programs should be developed by rural doctors for rural doctors. Rural Medical Education Centres provide a very appropriate focus for developing such continuing education programs.

These programs should recognise the pre-existing knowledge and skills of rural family physicians which have often been developed through dealing with clinical problems in relative professional isolation, rather than through formal training. The programs should be responsive to the specific learning needs of the doctors which usually involves a focus that is practical, case based and problem oriented. The aim of such continuing education programs should be to empower the learner and thus extend and expand the doctors knowledge and clinical skills.

Continuing education program should also be accessible to rural practitioners which means locating them in rural regional centres rather than major cities. Also, the use of distance education methods to bring continuing education to rural practitioners is to be encouraged. This includes not only traditional published materials, but also the use of new technologies including teleconferencing, electronic mail and satellite television, and other developments in modern information technology.

Another important form of continuing education and professional development is short term hands-on clinical attachments in larger hospitals. These should be encouraged and facilitated through liaison with the specialists in these hospitals. Release from the practice maybe facilitated by rotating locum relief schemes where a group of rural practices share a rotating locum.

The opportunity to do sabbaticals or exchanges in other countries can broaden experience for practicing rural doctors and help develop new approaches to medical practice, medical education, and health care delivery.

11

8.   Higher University Studies

Currently there is no sense of career progression for doctors who go into rural practice and those who later wish to pursue an academic career are given little credit for the knowledge and experience gained while practicing in the country. There is a need to develop appropriate university postgraduate diplomas and degrees which would provide a means for career progression into education, research or administration. Also such graduate studies programs would assist in creating a pool of academically trained rural practitioners to staff Rural Medical Education Centres and other rural health academic units.

For such postgraduate studies to be of value to rural family physicians they must be offered by distance education. The use of distance education allows rural doctors to pursue higher studies while staying in their practices and towns.

9.   Financial and Material Support

As mentioned previously, practice in remote and rural areas has many financial disadvantages. In order to recruit and retain doctors in remote and rural practice these financial issues need to be addressed. This may take the form of additional payment recognising the higher level of clinical responsibility and services provided; specific incentive payments for practicing in underserved areas; financial assistance with accommodation, education and travel for the doctor and his/her family; and so on.

Another form of material support is the provision of premises and equipment for the medical practice. Many rural communities provide such facilities to assist in attracting doctors.

A physician is more likely to remain long term in a rural practice where he or she is not the sole provider of medical services. Consequently, two or three doctor group practices are to be encouraged where necessary through direct financial support so as to sustain the economic viability of the practice. In order to provide effective primary health care, rural doctors require the assistance of appropriately trained nurses and other health professionals.   Combining facilities for doctors and other health professionals in rural community health centres fosters cooperative health care delivery.

After a doctor, the next health service priority for a rural community is a hospital which provides acute medical, surgical, obstetrics and paediatric care. Many such hospitals have been constructed and equipped with considerable financial support from the local community. The hospital is important also to the economy of the town as a major employer and purchaser of goods and services within the community. Rural family doctors require facilities and privileges to provide the needed services for which they are trained and competent. Undue hardship on rural communities may result from imposition by central regulatory authorities of excessive certification or fellowship requirements for performing procedures.

Overall health care delivery may be improved by networking among doctors and sharing health care facilities and professionals between several communities. There is a role for government to ensure that the health system provides appropriate physical facilities and services to meet the needs of rural and remote communities.

10.   Family and Spouse Support

For the rural family physician, there is a major challenge in being the confidential medical adviser in the consulting room and friend in the social and recreational setting in the community. For doctors' spouses this may be more difficult as members of the community will tend to treat them differently because of the connection with the doctor. In many ways, the rural practitioner's spouse may be more socially isolated than the doctor. Consequently, there is a need for specific strategies to provide personal support for doctors spouses. Also spouses often have difficulty in obtaining employment and/or pursuing career objectives. Strategies to meet these needs must be included.

For the doctor's family, there are difficulties with education and subsequent employment. Strategies to assist with educational support and funding for going away to pursue education should be included in support programs for doctors' families.

The long periods on-call with frequent call outs lead to great family disruption such that there is a need for longer than usual periods of recreation leave for rural doctors and their families. Programs to assist must include appropriate locum relief and financial assistance to permit recreation leave away from the rural community.

11.   National Support

Central government support is essential to the provision of accessible health care particularly in rural underserved areas. National governments need to develop and implement effective national rural health strategies. This requires the cooperation of communities, doctors and other health care professionals, hospitals, medical schools, professional organisations, and governments.   Rural health care should be well resourced and funding mechanisms should be developed which meet the needs of rural populations.   Establishment of National Rural Health Research Organisations can facilitate this process.

World Organisation of Family Doctors

12. Conclusion and Recommendations

Wonca believes there is an urgent need to implement strategies to improve rural health services around the world. In order to achieve this, there needs to be sufficient numbers of skilled rural family doctors to provide the required medical services. This document has outlined a series of key issues of concern regarding training for rural practice.

It has been found that the production of more and more doctors does not lead to an overflow of physicians from the cities to the country. In order to increase the numbers and quality of rural doctors it is necessary to implement a series of strategies aimed at establishing an integrated career pathway of education and training for rural practice. In the long term, it is only this strategic approach which is likely to improve the recruitment and retention of rural family physicians.

In order to achieve this goal, Wonca recommends:

1. **Increasing the number of medical students recruited from rural areas. Strategies may include:**

    1.1 Introduction of programs promoting medicine as a career to rural secondary students.

    1.2 Establishment of scholarships and educational support programs which identify potential medical students in rural areas and assist them with secondary and tertiary education in preparation for medical school entry.

    1.3 Selection processes that encourage admission of students from rural areas.

    　　1.3.1 Selection processes including interviews should give specific recognition and credit for rural background, experience, and interest.

    　　1.3.2 Specific targets for students from a rural background may be needed.

2. **Substantial exposure to rural practice in the medical undergraduate curriculum. This may be achieved through:**

    2.1 Establishment of "Rural Practice Clubs" which encourage city origin students to develop an interest in rural practice and support rural background students in adjusting to the challenges of city living and university studies.

    2.2 Rural doctor mentor schemes which provide rural origin students with ongoing personal support and encouragement from a nominated rural family physician.

    2.3 An introduction to rural health issues early in the curriculum including specific rural practice attachments for students early in the medical course.

    2.4 Block clinical rotations to rural hospitals and rural family practice later in the course.

2.5 A rural medicine stream for a selected group of students who indicate an early commitment to rural practice. This might take the form of:

2.5.1 One to three years of complete medical curriculum undertaken in the rural setting.

2.5.2 A thread of rural attachments intertwined through the clinical components of the curriculum.

2.6 Decentralised medical schools that allow students to take most or all of their medical school education in centres outside major metropolitan areas.

3. **Specific flexible, integrated and coordinated rural practice vocational training programs. These programs should:**

3.1 Be needs driven, evidence based, and learner centred

3.2 Have appropriate faculty, hospital, and financial support

3.3 Provide particular emphasis on training in procedural skills and an appropriate core curriculum on rural practice in addition to a solid family medicine foundation

3.4 Provide a major portion of training within the rural context

3.5 Provide the opportunity and funding for advanced rural skills training in emergency medicine, anaesthesia, surgery, procedural obstetrics and others.

3.6 Provide opportunities for regular family medicine trainees to experience the joys and challenges of rural family practice

4. **Specific tailored continuing education and professional development programs whch meet the identified needs of rural family physicians.**

4.1 Continuing medical education programs should be accessible to rural practitioners through locating them in rural regional centres and, where appropriate, making use of distance education methods including modern information technology.

4.2 Generally rural continuing medical education programs should be developed by rural doctors for rural doctors.

4.3 Development of appropriate university postgraduate diplomas and degrees available via distance education so as to allow more remote rural doctors to pursue higher university studies without leaving their towns or practices.

5. **Appropriate academic positions, professional development and financial support for rural doctor-teachers to encourage rural health research and education.**

5.1 Rural Medical Education and Research Centres should be established in rural areas with the aim of co-ordinating undergraduate education, postgraduate vocational training, and continuing medical education for rural practitioners. Such Centres greatly facilitate implementation of all

World Organisation of Family Doctors

previous recommendations. An important consequence of establishing Rural Medical Education and Research Centres is development of reciprocal links between country hospitals/practices and medical schools/teaching hospitals.

6.   **Medical schools should take responsibility to educate appropriately skilled doctors to meet the needs of their general geographic region including underserved areas and should play a key role in providing regional support for health professionals and accessible tertiary heath care.**

7.   **Development of appropriate needs based and culturally sensitive rural health care resources with local community involvement, regional cooperation and government support.**

    7.1   Provide appropriate funding to develop and maintain hospital and other health services and referral resources to meet the needs of people in rural and remote communities.

    7.2   Establish rural community health centres with facilities and support for doctors and other health professionals.

8.   **Improved professional and personal/family conditions in rural practice to promote retention of rural doctors. Strategies include:**

    8.1   Locum relief schemes should be established to permit release of rural family physicians to undertake continuing education as well as recreation and other forms of leave.

    8.2   Targeted financial support for rural practice such as:

        8.2.1   Funding models that provide security and flexibility for the doctor to and recognise the physician as a community resource.

        8.2.2   Additional payments to rural practitioners in recognition of the higher level of clinical responsibility, services provided and on call demands.

        8.2.3   Specific incentive payments for practicing in isolated/underserved areas

        8.2.4   Financial assistance to maintain the economic viability of at least two doctors working together in a rural location.

        8.2.5   Funding for travel and other costs for the doctor to attend continuing medical education.

    8.3   Specific programs to meet the needs of rural doctors' spouses and families such as:

        8.3.1   Spouse and family support networks.

        8.3.2   Financial assistance with accommodation for the doctor and family.

        8.3.3   Financial assistance to facilitate education of the doctor's family.

8.3.4   Funding to permit travel by the doctor and family for recreation and other forms of leave and to visit family members undertaking secondary or tertiary education.

8.3.5   Assistance in developing employment opportunities for the doctor's spouse.

9.   **Development and implementation of national rural health strategies with central government support.   This requires:**

9.1   Cooperative involvement of communities, doctors and other health care professionals, hospitals, medical schools, professional organisations, and governments at all levels. Establishment of national rural health research and education organisations can facilitate this process.

World Organisation of Family Doctors

References

This Wonca Policy is based on experiences in many countries around the world. The following list of references highlights key issues:

1.   Australian Health Ministers Conference. **National Rural Health Strategy.** Australian Government Publishing Service, Canberra, 1994.

2.   Rural Undergraduate Steering Committee. Rural Doctors: **Reforming undergraduate medical education for rural practice.** Australian Commonwealth Department of Human Services and Health. Australian Government Publishing Service, Canberra, 1994.

3.   Rural medicine design project. **Training curriculum surgery, anaesthesia and obstetrics for rural general practice.** Faculty of Rural Medicine, Royal Australian College of General Practitioners, Sydney. 1992.

4.   Association of American Medical Colleges. **Rural Health : A challenge for medical education. Proceedings of 1990 invitational symposium.** Academic Medicine 65: Supplement 1-126. 1990.

5.   Littlemeyer M, Martin D. **Academic Initiatives to address physician supply in rural areas in the United States : A compendium.** Association of American Medical Colleges, Washington, 1991.

6.   American Academy of Family Physicians. **Rural Family Practice: You can make a difference.** American Academy of Family Physicians, Kansas City. 1989.

7.   Canadian Medical Association. **Report of the advisory panel on the provision of medical services in underserviced regions.** Canadian Medical Association, Ottawa. 1992.

8.   Blackwood R, McNab J. **A portrait of rural family practice: Problems and Priorities.** College of Family Physicians of Canada, Toronto. 1991.

9.   Stiratanaban A and Sangprasert B. **The Rural Area Project (RAP) in Thailand: curriculum development.** Medical Education 17:374-377, 1983.

10.   Carter R G. **The relation between personal characteristics of physicians and practice location in Manitoba.** CMAJ 136:366-368, 1987.

11.   Asuzu M C. **The influence of undergraduate clinical training on the attitude of medical students to rural medical practice in Nigeria.** African Journal of Medicine & Medical Sciences 18:245-250, 1989.

12.   Poulose K P and Natarajan P K. **Re-orientation of medical education in India past, present and future.** Indian Journal of Public Health. 33:55-58, 1989.

Policy on Training for Rural Practice

13. Hickner J M. **Training for rural practice in Australia 1990.** Medical Journal of Australia 154:111-118, 1991.

14. Rosenblatt R A, Whitcomb M E, Cullen T J, Lishner D M and Hart L G. **Which medical schools produce rural physicians?** JAMA 268:1559-1565, 1992.

15. Strasser R P. **Attitudes of Victorian rural general practitioners to country practice and training.** Australian Family Physician 21(7). 808-812, 1992.

16. Umland B, Waterman R, Wiese W, Duban S, Mennin S and Kaufman A. **Learning from a rural physician program in China.** Academic Medicine 67:307-309, 1992.

17. Magnus J H and Tollan A. **Rural doctor recruitment: does medical education in rural districts recruit doctors to rural areas?** Medical Education 25:250-253, 1993.

18. Gray J D, Steeves L C and Blackburn J W. **The Dalhousie University experience of training residents in many small communities.** Academic Medicine 69(10):847-851, 1994.

An extensive list of published articles on education for rural practice has been collected, collated and annotated by Dr James Rourke. This publication "Education for rural practice: Goals and opportunities: An annotated bibliography", is available at cost through the Australian Rural Health Research Institute Moe, Victoria 3825 Australia.

CHAPTER 12

The importance of being different

Ruth Wilson

NOMINATED CLASSIC PAPER

Ian McWhinney. The importance of being different. *British Journal of General Practice*, 1996; 46: 433–36.

This article, published in 1996, came at a time when family medicine (at least in Canada) was at a low ebb. Medical student interest in becoming a family doctor was low, and working conditions were poor. Family doctors felt demoralised and weren't sure if they were valued by patients or policy-makers. Ian McWhinney's four simple but elegant themes gave us a language and philosophy to explain to ourselves, and to others, the difference and the necessity of our discipline to modern medicine.

In the words of Ian McWhinney, 'It is the only discipline to define itself in terms of relationships, especially the doctor–patient relationship'.

This simple claim is extraordinarily helpful to us in defining just who we are as family physicians. The medical student is often asked, 'What are you going to specialise in?' The student aiming for a career in family medicine may say, after some foot-shuffling, 'Oh, I'm just going to be a GP' or perhaps 'I'm specialising in family medicine'. To be able to respond that one is part of a discipline, which has at its heart being a personal physician, is both true and immediately understandable to the public.

This article's three other points are elegant elaborations on the aphorism credited to Hippocrates, 'It is more important to know what sort of person has a disease than to know what sort of disease a person has.' William Osler, a fellow Canadian, proclaimed: 'The good physician treats the disease; the great physician treats the patient who has the disease.'

By claiming the relationship between the doctor and the patient as being at the heart of family medicine, Ian McWhinney places family doctors firmly in the heritage of patient-centred holistic healers. But he goes beyond this, to make the bold claim that we are unique in defining ourselves by this noble tradition.

ABOUT THE AUTHOR OF THIS PAPER

Ian Renwick McWhinney OC (1926– 2012) was born in Burnley, England, the son of a general practitioner. Following his medical training at Cambridge University, he joined his father in general practice in Stratford-upon-Avon for 13 years. Recruited by the University of Western Ontario to London in Ontario, Canada, in 1968, he became the first Professor of Family Medicine in Canada. He remained at what is now called Western University for the rest of his career. He is acknowledged as the 'father of family medicine' for his work in establishing family medicine as an academic discipline. His insightful writings, his compassionate disposition, and his passion for the importance of family medicine have made him renowned worldwide. His *Textbook of Family Medicine* is now its third edition. Ian was married to Betty, and they were the parents of two children.

ABOUT THE NOMINATOR OF THIS PAPER

Ruth Wilson has served as president of the College of Family Physicians of Canada and as the North American Regional President of the World Organization of Family Doctors (WONCA). Her practice as a family physician included 11 years in remote communities in Canada, and 26 years in Kingston, Ontario, where she currently includes obstetrics in her practice. In 2015 she was made a Member of the Order of Canada for her contributions to improving primary care and for her leadership in family medicine.

> 'Keep a diary, or some notes. The first few years of practice one is caught up in mastering the technical aspects of the discipline. You may forget what you don't write down, and recalling the stories of individuals you meet over the years will be a source of pleasure, perhaps of research (as in the example of William Pickles), and a testament to your vocation.'

> *Professor Ruth Wilson C.M., Canada*

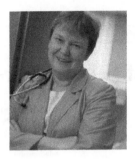

Attribution:

We attribute the original publication of *The importance of being different* to *British Journal of General Practice*. With thanks to Moira Davies and the Royal College of General Practitioners.

WILLIAM PICKLES LECTURE 1996

The importance of being different

IAN R McWHINNEY

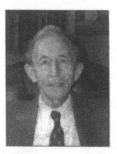

IT is an honour to give the William Pickles Lecture, and it is especially pleasing to give it in this part of Scotland, so near the birthplace of James Mackenzie. Mackenzie and Pickles were two of the most distinguished scientists general practice has produced. Mackenzie did his original research in Burnley on the western edge of the Pennines; Pickles did his in Aysgarth, on the eastern edge, only 35 miles away. Pickles must have known Burnley well, for he married a Burnley woman. There is no indication that the two men ever met. Even so, Pickles was profoundly influenced by Mackenzie's work. It was his reading in 1926 of Mackenzie's *Principles of Diagnosis and Treatment in Heart Conditions* that inspired Pickles to begin his research into the epidemiology of infectious diseases.

Both Mackenzie and Pickles used key features of general practice as foundations of their research method. Mackenzie's observations on the natural history of heart disease depended on his caring for the same patients over many years. Pickles' observations on the spread of infections used his knowledge of person-to-person contacts in his rural practice. Then, as now, our discipline's greatest contributions to medicine sprang from the things that made it different.

In an article based on interviews with all 12 academic general practitioners (GPs) and a sample of full-time GPs in Scotland in 1975, Reid[1] described the academic GPs' sense of alienation from the academic mainstream, and from their colleagues in full-time practice. They felt 'marginal' in the medical school. Academic general practice has made considerable progress since then, yet we still, I believe, do not fit comfortably into the academic milieu. To gain acceptance, it is said, general practice must become less pragmatic, more theoretical and more productive in quantitative research. My own view is that general practice is marginal because it differs in fundamental ways from the academic mainstream and that our value to medicine lies in the differences. Eventually, I think, the academic mainstream will become more like us than *vice versa*. I will describe four ways in which general practice is different, most of which are shared with other primary care disciplines.

I R McWhinney, MD, FRCGP, FCFP(C), FRCP, professor emeritus, Centre for Studies in Family Medicine, The University of Western Ontario, London, Ontario, Canada. The text is based on the 1996 William Pickles Lecture, which was delivered at the Spring Meeting of the Royal College of General Practitioners in Aberdeen on 14 April 1996.
Submitted: 5 March 1996; accepted: 15 March 1996.

© *British Journal of General Practice*, 1996, **46**, 433-436.

1. It is the only discipline to define itself in terms of relationships, especially the doctor–patient relationship

Other fields define themselves in terms of content: diseases, organ systems or technologies. Clinicians in other fields form relationships with patients, but in general practice, the relationship is usually *prior* to content. We know people before we know what their illnesses will be. It is, of course, possible to define a content of general practice, based on the common conditions presenting to GPs at a particular time and place. But, strictly speaking, the content for a particular doctor is whatever conditions her patients happen to have. Other relationships also define our work. By caring for members of a family, the family doctor may become part of the complex of family relationships, and many of us share with our patients the same community and habitat.

Defining our field in these terms has consequences, both positive and negative. Not to be tied to a particular technology or set of diseases is liberating. It gives general practice a quality of unexpectedness and a flexibility in adapting to change. On the other hand, it is poorly understood in a society that seems to place less and less value on relationships. One major consequence is that we cannot be comfortable with the mechanical metaphor which dominates medicine, or with the mind/body dualism derived from it. Another is that the value we place on relationships influences our valuation of knowledge. Those who value relationships tend to know the world by experience rather than by what Charles Taylor[2] calls 'instrumental' and 'disengaged' reason. Experience engages our feelings as well as our intellect. The emotions play a very significant part in general practice, and as I will maintain, are seriously neglected in medicine as a whole.

2. General practitioners tend to think in terms of individual patients rather than generalized abstractions

When the conversation is about a disease, we are likely to say: 'That reminds me of Mrs X.' We have difficulty thinking about diseases as separate from the people who 'have' them. Reid[1] observed of the full-time GPs she interviewed that some 'could not talk about general practice except in terms of their specific patients'. This trait, I believe, arises from the intimacy of the doctor–patient relationship in general practice. The closer we are to a person, the more we are aware of their individual particulars, and the more difficult it is to think of them as members of a class. 'We instinctively recoil,' wrote William James, 'from seeing an object to which our emotions and affections are committed, handled by the intellect as any other object is handled. The first thing the intellect does with an object is to class it along with something else. But any object that is infinitely important to us and awakens our devotion feels to us as if it must be *sui generis* and unique.'[3]

In classifying, we distance ourselves from experience. In Umberto Eco's novel *The Name of the Rose*,[4] Brother William explains to Adso how he identified the abbot's horse as they climbed the hill to the monastery: 'If you see something from a distance, and you do not understand what it is, you will be content with defining it as an animal, even if you do not know whether it is a horse or an ass. And when it is still closer you will be able to say it is a horse, even if you do not yet know its name. Only when you are at the proper distance will you see that it is Brucellus, the abbot's horse, and that will be full knowledge, the learning of the singular.'*

I R McWhinney   William Pickles Lecture 1996

The closer we are, the fuller our knowledge of particulars. The greater the distance, the greater the degree of abstraction. Medicine has gained great predictive power by distancing itself enough from individual patients to see the abstraction (the disease) rather than the individual. This is now what we refer to as the diagnosis, although in former times physicians spoke of diagnosing a patient, not a disease. If we look closely, every patient is different in some way. It is in the care of patients that knowledge of particulars becomes crucial. Care is about attention to detail. 'Caring is not about categories,' wrote Arthur Frank,[5] reflecting on his own illness. 'A large acquaintance with particulars,' said William James,[3] 'often makes us wiser than the possession of abstract formulas, however deep.'

Of course, we need the abstractions too, especially for making causal inferences and applying powerful technologies. The ideal is an integration of the two kinds of knowledge: an ability to see the universal in the particular. There are penalties for dwelling too much in one or the other. For physicians who dwell too much in the particulars, there is a risk of missing the forest for the trees. For those who dwell too much in abstractions, the risk is detachment from the patient's experience and a lack of feeling for his or her suffering. Abstraction produces accounts of experience that, stripped of their affective colouring, are far removed from the realities of life.

These two kinds of knowledge are illuminated by Alfred Korzybski's[6] vivid metaphor of the map and the territory. We can get to know a territory by studying the map, which is made by abstracting certain features and ignoring others. The map helps us to find our way, but knowing the territory from the map is not the same as knowing it by dwelling in it. A native knows his territory by feeling part of it. His knowledge is visceral, much of it tacit and difficult to articulate, as with the peasant farmer who knows that a new scheme will not work on his land, but cannot give his reasons to the expert. We cannot experience the beauty or the terror of a landscape by reading the map. Of course, one can get passionate about maps. There is a thrill in making a good diagnosis (finding our place on the map), and there can be beauty in a radiograph. But this is not the same as a feeling for the patient's experience of illness — and patients are very quick to sense the difference. If we are to be healers as well as technicians, we have at some point to set aside our maps and walk hand-in-hand with our patients through the territory.

In the modern university, abstraction and disengaged reason reign supreme. Knowledge has been separated from experience, thinking from feeling. The educational challenge we face is correcting, in Margaret Donaldson's[7] words, 'the imbalance between intellectual and emotional development'. In medicine, the standard diagnostic method is an outstanding example of the imbalance. The physician is required to categorize the illness, but not to attend to the patient's feelings or understand his experience. Stephen Toulmin[8] contrasts the modern paradigm of knowledge with the one which dominated the learned world of the Renaissance, when scholars were 'as concerned with circumstantial questions of practice in medicine, law or morals, as with any timeless, universal matters of philosophical theory.' With the coming of the Enlightenment, this was replaced by a paradigm which removed knowledge from its context: *'abstract axioms were in, concrete diversity was out, general principles were in, particular cases were out.'* I suspect that some of our discomfort in the medical school is due to our different valuation of knowledge.

*Excerpt from *The Name of the Rose* by Umberto Eco, © 1980 by Gruppo Editoriale Fabbri-Bonpiani, Sonzogno, Etas S.p.A., English translation ©1983 by Harcourt Brace & Company and Martin Secker & Warburg Ltd., reprinted by permission of Harcourt Brace & Company and Martin Secker & Warburg Ltd.

3. General practice is based on an organismic rather than a mechanistic metaphor of biology

The metaphors we use in medicine are often very revealing about the way we think. The metaphor of the human body as a machine speaks volumes about the modern idea of healing. Even though the body has some machine-like features, everything we do for the health of the body depends on the healing powers of nature. Living organisms have properties possessed by no machine: growth, regeneration, healing, learning, self-organization and self-transcendence. At its most successful, medicine works in supporting these natural processes. Surgeons drain abscesses, set fractures, repair wounds, relieve obstructions. Immunization strengthens the organism's defences. The most effective drugs are those which support natural defences and maintain balance in the *milieu interieur*. The traditional regimens of balanced nutrition, rest, sound sleep, exercise, relief of pain and anxiety, and personal support are all measures which support the organism's healing powers.

What does it mean to think organismically? An organism is a particular, that is 'it occupies a region of space, persists through time, has boundaries and has an environment.'[9] The point about particulars is that their behaviour cannot be explained or predicted solely by applying the general laws of science. Whether or not the law will apply to a particular will depend on its history and its context or environment. There is an inherent uncertainty about all particular applications of general scientific principles. The more complex the particular, the greater the uncertainty, and a sick patient is a very complex organism. To think organismically is to 'think complexity' and to accept uncertainty. Generalizations must be framed in terms such as: 'given this context, the following will for the most part apply.' Of all the clinical disciplines, general practice operates at the highest level of complexity.

Organismic thinking is multilevel and non-linear. Organisms maintain themselves in a state of dynamic equilibrium by a reciprocal or circular flow of information at all levels, and between organism and environment. Through these multilevel channels, change in any part can reverberate through the whole organism and to its surroundings. The necessity of constant information flow can be seen in the destabilizing effects on humans of sensory deprivation. Information is carried in the form of symbols conveying messages that are decoded at the appropriate level of the organism. At lower levels, information is carried by hormones and neurotransmitters. At the level of the whole organism, it is carried by stimuli reaching the special senses, among which are the words and other symbols by which meaning is expressed in human relationships. This provides the background for our accumulating knowledge of the effect of relationships on health and disease.

The transition from mechanistic to organismic thinking requires a radical change in our notion of disease causation. Medicine has been dominated by a doctrine of specific aetiology: a cause for each disease. We have learned to think of a causal agent as a force acting in linear fashion on a passive object, as when a moving billiard ball hits a stationary one. In self-organizing systems such as organisms, causation is non-linear. The multiple feedback loops between organism and environment, and between all levels of the organism, require us to think in causal networks, not straight lines. Moreover, the organism is not a passive object. The 'specific cause' of an illness may only be the trigger which releases a process that is already a potential of the organism. The causes which maintain an illness and inhibit healing may be different from the causes which initiated it, and these may include the organism's own maladaptive behaviour. Therapeutic measures may act not on a causal agent, but on the body's defences, as appears to be the case with the therapeutic benefits of human relationships. In a complex system, cause and effect are not usually close to each other in time and space, and since organic processes are maintained or changed by multiple influences, it is difficult to predict the consequences of an intervention.[10] It is true that we can still isolate one link in the causal network as our point of intervention, as when we prescribe an antibiotic, but even in these instances we should be aware of the whole context in which we are operating, and of the reciprocal effects of our intervention. The complexity of the illnesses we encounter in general practice make it natural for us to think in this way. Does isolation from social supports cause depression, or does depression cause the isolation? Did this life event cause the depression or was it only the trigger, releasing a depression in a susceptible individual? In human science, we can establish relationships between events, but it is often difficult to establish cause. Does this imply therapeutic impotence? No, but it does require a change from simplistic causal thinking to thinking about how change can be facilitated in complex systems.

With the transition from mechanistic to organismic thinking, either/or questions become meaningless, especially those which take the form 'Is disease X psychogenic or organic?' A recent editorial in the *New England Journal of Medicine* said: 'Migraine is a neurobiologic, not a psychogenic disorder.'[11] Why can it not be both?

In their capacity for self-organization, learning and self-transcendence, organisms behave in a way that is 'mindful'. This is not simply a mind 'in the brain', but one which is immanent in the whole body. Every level of the organism — from the molecular upwards — has a capacity for autonomous activity and for integrating its activity with the whole. Each level can transmit and receive coded messages that convey meaning. The immune system, for long thought to be isolated, is connected reciprocally with the neuroendocrine systems through neural networks and circulating neurotransmitters. The immune system can learn from experience and can distinguish 'self' from 'not self'. A large body of evidence indicates that emotions can influence immune function, thus providing a physiological link between life experience and the course and outcome of illness.[12] As John Cassell[13] predicted, relationships act at this intermediate level of host resistance, not as causal agents for specific diseases. Social isolation, for example, increases mortality from virtually all causes of death. The notion of a separate group of psychosomatic diseases is therefore obsolete. In any disease, social factors can be part of the causal web and human relationships can be part of the healing process.

The immanent mind knows the world through bodily feelings. The separation of thinking from feeling, and the relegation of emotion to a limited role, is being rendered untenable by cognitive science. Psychologists from Freud to Piaget have shown that thinking and feeling do not occur in isolation: emotion is necessary for cognition, especially for giving meaning to our experience. Neuroscience now tells us that the connection is embodied in the structure and function of the brain.[14] Experiences that are significant to us are laid down as memory in our neural circuits, with the affective colouring which imbues them with meanings for us. The events of our lives are woven into a personal narrative which not only gives us our sense of self, but enables us to interpret and give personal meaning to each new experience.[15] The 'body as machine' is replaced by a new metaphor — the embodied mind[16] — and our new language speaks of the mind–body, not the mind *and* the body. Our understanding comes from bodily experience of the world interpreted always in terms of our personal story. This approach takes very seriously the knowledge derived from experience.

When applied to medicine, it makes patients' experiences of illness an important aspect of medical knowledge. This is the domain of qualitative research — a natural field of inquiry for general practice.

I believe we are living through the final breakdown of the dualistic world view — a situation with profound implications for us, as we turn to the fourth difference.

4. General practice is the only major field which transcends the dualistic division between mind and body

This division runs through medicine like a geological fault. Most clinical disciplines lie on one side or the other: internal medicine, surgery and paediatrics on one side; psychiatry, child psychiatry and psychogeriatrics on the other. Separate taxonomies of disease lie on either side: textbooks of medicine and surgery on one, the *Diagnostic and Statistical Manual of Mental Disorders* on the other. We divide therapies into the physical and the psychological. In clinical practice, internists and surgeons do not normally explore the emotions, psychiatrists do not examine the body. Since general practice defines itself in terms of relationships, it cannot divide in this way.

Without this artificial barrier, the relationship between patient and doctor can develop through many encounters for all kinds of illness. In examining and attending to the body, we are also attending to the mind. Mental states are expressed in posture, movement and muscle tone, and examining the body can trigger the expression of feeling. Body therapies can heal the mind; mental therapies can heal the body. Psychotherapy need not be separate from therapy for the body: indeed, it is doubtful whether in general practice we should call it 'psychotherapy'. For most of us, I suspect, it is a question of listening, supporting, reassuring, encouraging the expression of feelings and the reinterpretation of perceptions we call cognitive therapy. This is something we do for all patients, not only for those with 'psychiatric' illness. The more we learn about the placebo effect, the more it appears to be the healing power of the doctor–patient relationship through symbolic acts and rituals.[17] Since the effect is strengthened by each new experience of the relationship, it has a special importance for us in general practice. In the course of time, the relationship with the doctor can become part of the patient's own narrative. I began by saying that general practice has no technology to call its own. I will now modify this and say that our therapeutic tool is ourselves in the healing relationship — the drug 'doctor' as Balint called it.[18]

One of the legacies of dualism is the clinical method we have inherited from the nineteenth century, a method which leaves it to psychiatrists to attend to the emotions. It is not surprising, therefore, that moves to reform our clinical method have come from general practice. The essence of the patient-centred method[19] is that the doctor attends to feelings, emotions and moods, as well as categorizing the patient's illness. What does it mean to attend to a patient's feelings, emotions and moods? Understanding the emotions is person to person, and we cannot attend to another person's emotions without attending to our own. The key skill is attentive listening. To listen to a person with total, undivided attention is one of the greatest gifts we can bestow.[20] It is listening not only with our ears, but with all our faculties, especially with an open heart. We cannot do this if our eyes are on our 'map' or if we are thinking what to say next, or if we are consumed by our own negative emotions. If we can achieve this state of openness, we find that our responses to the patient spring naturally from some inner source. Needleman[21] describes this attentive state as 'non-egoistic, impersonal love', a love we call charity (to the Greeks *agape*). It is not an emotion in

I R McWhinney   William Pickles Lecture 1996

the usual sense and does not depend on affection. The Good Samaritan did what was needful for the man he rescued, then went on his way. As physicians we can do likewise, whatever our discipline. But for general practitioners, there is an additional dimension — the long-term relationship with patients, in the course of which affections grow. Of the four loves — affection, friendship, eros and charity — C. S. Lewis[22] called affection the humblest and most widely diffused. When combined with charity, the warmth of affection must surely be a healing force, but it comes with a price, for the relationship between doctor and patient is subject to the same stresses and weaknesses as other human relationships. So we see both love and hate, trust and mistrust, betrayal and forgiveness, irretrievable breakdown and survival of the relationship in spite of difficulties. Unacknowledged negative emotions, such as fear, helplessness, anxiety, anger and guilt, may be acted out by the doctor in avoidance, indifference, rejection and even cruelty. The doctor's own need for affection may be stronger than his ability to give it. It is the egoistic emotions, so destructive of human relationships, that prevent us from responding to suffering with our authentic feelings. The priest and the Levite 'passed by on the other side', no doubt giving themselves very good reasons.

We can only attend to a patient's feelings and emotions if we know our own, but self-knowledge is neglected in medical education, perhaps because the path to this knowledge is so long and hard. Egoistic emotions often come disguised as virtues and we all have a great capacity for self-deception. But there are pathways to this knowledge and medical education could find a place for them. Could medicine become a self-reflective discipline? The idea may seem preposterous. Yet I think it must, if we are to be healers as well as competent technologists. By living in a world of abstractions and neglecting our own emotional development, we have erected an invisible barrier between ourselves and our patients. We protect ourselves by growing a hard shell which makes openness difficult, and our patients interpret this as cold indifference or rejection. A contemporary novelist has referred to our profession's 'stunted emotions'.[23] Even psychiatry is not a model of self-reflectiveness. As Bettelheim[24] and Needleman[21] have noted, psychiatry has directed its attention more to *other people's* emotions. Rather than turn our attention inwards, we are driven by our culture to put our faith in new abstractions such as systems theory, not seeing that, however useful they may be as 'maps', they can come between us and our patients.

The four differences I have described are all of a piece. Giving primacy to long-term relationships directs our attention to the particulars of illness; and the complexity of illness in the context of relationships makes it difficult for us to think in mechanistic and dualistic terms. But we have hardly begun to see the advantages of our position. Transcending the 'fault line' should make general practice the ideal therapeutic setting for the many disorders which, like chronic pain, do not fit neatly on one side or the other. The more we learn about the effect of supportive relationships on cancer and other chronic diseases, the more redundant the fault line becomes.[25,26] To realize our potential, however, we have other work to do. Thinking in the way I have described may be natural for us, but it is still difficult, for we are all, to some extent, prisoners of an unreformed clinical method and the language of linear causation and mind/body dualism. The fault line runs through the affect-denying clinical method which dominates the modern medical school. Not until this is reformed will emotions and relationships have the place in medicine they deserve. Finally, to become self-reflective, medicine will have to go through a huge cultural change. In these changes, general practice is already some distance along the way. The importance of being different is that we can lead the way.

References

1. Reid M. Marginal man: the identity dilemma of the academic general practitioner. *Symbolic Interaction* 1982; **5:** 325-342.
2. Taylor C. *The malaise of modernity*. Concord, Ontario: Anansi Press, 1991.
3. James W. *The varieties of religious experience: a study in human nature*. New York, NY: New American Library, 1958.
4. Eco U. *The name of the rose*. New York, NY: Warner Books, 1984.
5. Frank A. *At the will of the body: reflections on illness*. Boston, MA: Houghton Mifflin, 1992.
6. Korzybski A. *Science and sanity: an introduction to non-Aristotelian systems and general semantics*, 4th edn. Lake Bille, CT: International Non-Aristotelian Library Publishing Co., 1958.
7. Donaldson M. *Human minds: an exploration*. London: Penguin Books, 1992.
8. Toulmin S. *Cosmopolis: the hidden agenda of modernity*. Chicago, IL: University of Chicago Press, 1990.
9. Gorovitz S, MacIntyre A. Toward a theory of medical fallibility. *J Med Philosophy* 1976; **1:** 51-71.
10. Briggs J, Peat DF. *Turbulent mirror: an illustrated guide to chaos theory and the science of wholeness*. New York, NY: Harper & Row, 1989.
11. Olesen J. Understanding the biological basis of migraine. *N Engl J Med* 1994; **331:** 1713-1714.
12. Ader R, Felten SC, Cohen N (eds). *Psychoneuroimmunology*. New York, NY: Academic Press, 1991.
13. Cassel J. The contribution of the social environment to host resistance. *Am J Epidemiol* 1976; **104:** 107-123.
14. Damasio AR. *Descartes' error: emotion, reason, and the human brain*. New York, NY: Putnam, 1994.
15. Bruner JS. *Acts of meaning*. Boston, MA: Harvard University Press, 1990.
16. Varela FJ, Thompson E, Rosch E. *The embodied mind: cognitive science and human experience*. Cambridge, MA: MIT Press, 1993.
17. Peck C, Coleman G. Implications of placebo theory for clinical research and practice. *Theor Med* 1991; **12:** 247-270.
18. Balint M. *The doctor, his patient, and the illness*. London: Pitman Medical, 1964.
19. Stewart M, Brown JB, Weston WW, *et al. Patient-centered medicine: transforming the clinical method*. Thousand Oaks, CA: Sage Publications, 1995.
20. Remen RN. Wholeness. In: Moyers B (ed.). *Healing and the mind*. New York, NY: Doubleday, 1993.
21. Needleman J. *The way of the physician*. London: Penguin Books, 1992.
22. Lewis CS. *The four loves*. Glasgow: Fount Paperbacks, 1982.
23. Price R. *A whole new life: an illness and a healing*. New York, NY: Atheneum, 1994.
24. Bettelheim B. *Freud and man's soul*. New York, NY: Random House, 1994.
25. Fawzy FI, Fawzy NW, Hyun CS. Short-term psychiatric intervention for patients with malignant melanoma: effects on psychological state, coping, and the immune system. In: Lewis CE, O'Sullivan C, Barraclough J (eds). *The psychoimmunology of cancer*. Oxford: Oxford University Press, 1994.
26. Spiegel D, Bloom J, Yalom ID. Effect of psychosocial treatment on survival of patients with metastatic breast cancer. *Lancet* 1989; **ii:** 888-891.

Acknowledgements
I thank Sudi Devanesen, Tom Freeman, Brian Hennen, Betty McWhinney, Paul Rainsberry, Walter Rosser and Wayne Weston for their helpful comments; also Bette Cunningham for preparing the manuscript.

Address for correspondence
Ian R McWhinney, Professor Emeritus, Department of Family Medicine, Kresge Building, The University of Western Ontario, London, Ontario, Canada N6A 5C1.

CHAPTER 13

Family doctors and evidence-based medicine

Lubna Al-Ansary

NOMINATED CLASSIC PAPER

Alastair McColl, Helen Smith, Peter White, Jenny Field. General practitioners' perceptions of the route to evidence based medicine: a questionnaire survey. *British Medical Journal*, 1998; 316: 361–65.

This landmark study, conducted in the south of England, was the first to assess the different aspects of putting evidence into practice by general practitioners (GPs). The objectives were to determine the attitude of GPs towards evidence-based medicine (EBM), and their related educational needs. The participants generally welcomed EBM, and agreed that it improves patient care, but they had a low level of awareness of secondary sources of evidence and, even if aware, many did not use them. The major perceived barrier to practising EBM was lack of personal time. These findings have been consistent in all repeats of this study regardless of the specialty, health professional group or the country in which surveys have been conducted.

This paper concluded that promoting and improving access to summaries of evidence, rather than teaching all GPs literature searching and critical appraisal, should be the way of encouraging evidence-based general practice. GPs who are skilled in accessing and interpreting evidence can be encouraged to develop local evidence-based guidelines and advice. These conclusions have paved the way for reshaping the future of evidence-based practice in family medicine as well as other general specialties.

The following decades have witnessed the development and evolution of many of the iconic secondary sources of evidence such as Clinical Evidence/Best Practice, DynaMed and UpToDate, and the Cochrane Library and Database of Systematic Reviews, which have become important sources of trusted evidence.

The medical profession recognised that developing and implementing evidence-based guidance, based on systematic reviews, would be the way to put evidence into practice, thereby improving quality of care and saving cost. This paradigm shift was manifested by national organisations such as the National Health and Medical Research Council (Australia), National Institute for Health and Care Excellence (NICE) and the Scottish Intercollegiate Guidelines Network (SIGN) (United Kingdom), the National Guideline Clearinghouse and the Institute of Medicine standards for developing trustworthy guidelines (United States of America), and The Guidelines International Network (G-I-N). Safe and effective patient care can be fostered by facilitating networking about health professionals, promoting excellence in clinical care, and helping international organisations and individuals to create high-quality clinical practice guidelines.

ABOUT THE AUTHORS OF THIS PAPER

This research team was based at the University of Southampton, which was responsible for the Wessex Primary Care Research Network, a network of hundreds of general practices in the South of England involved in large-scale clinical trials led by staff of the academic department of Primary Medical Care. Helen Smith, at the time a senior lecturer in primary care, led the Wessex Research Network before being appointed to the first chair of general practice at the new Brighton and Sussex Medical School. Alastair McColl was a lecturer in public health medicine, Jenny Field was a senior lecturer in primary care, and Peter White was a GP based at the Nightingale Surgery in nearby Romsey.

The Wessex Research Network was established in 1993 as a tripartite initiative between the Department of Primary Medical Care, University of Southampton, the Wessex Faculty of the Royal College of General Practitioners, and the research and development directorate of the former Wessex Regional Health Authority. At the time of this research, the research network comprised 483 practices. Primary Care Research Networks in the United Kingdom, linked to academic departments, were established to bring together healthcare professionals interested in primary care research, and to promote research awareness and high-quality research by practitioners, and involvement in collaborative research projects.

ABOUT THE NOMINATOR OF THIS PAPER

Professor Lubna A. Al-Ansary is a family doctor and Professor and Consultant with the Department of Family and Community Medicine at King Saud University in

Riyadh in Saudi Arabia, where she holds the Sheikh Abdullah Bahamdan Research Chair for Evidence-Based Health Care and Knowledge Translation.

Lubna is an international leader in evidence-based medicine in family medicine, and serves as a member of the board of trustees of the Guidelines International Network (G-I-N). She has the distinction of being a member of the Health Committee of the Al-Shura (Consultative) Council, a legislative body of 150 members appointed to advise the King on issues that are important to Saudi Arabia.

> 'One of the key sets of skills that you need to acquire in order to provide proficient patient-centred care is to base your decisions on valid and relevant information. In other words, you need to learn the skills of evidence-based healthcare. At this period of time, you are blessed to be able to enjoy the fruits of more than two decades of work to promote and support evidence-based practice. This is an opportunity and you should make the most out of it.'

Professor Lubna A. Al-Ansary, Saudi Arabia

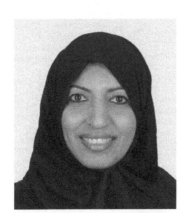

Attribution:

We attribute the original publication of *General practitioners' perceptions of the route to evidence based medicine: a questionnaire survey* to *British Medical Journal*. With thanks to Editor in Chief, Fiona Godlee, and Laura Lacey.

Information in practice

General practitioners' perceptions of the route to evidence based medicine: a questionnaire survey

Alastair McColl, Helen Smith, Peter White, Jenny Field

Abstract

Objectives: To determine the attitude of general practitioners towards evidence based medicine and their related educational needs.
Design: A questionnaire study of general practitioners.
Setting: General practice in the former Wessex region, England.
Subjects: Randomly selected sample of 25% of all general practitioners (452), of whom 302 replied.
Main outcome measures: Respondents' attitude towards evidence based medicine, ability to access and interpret evidence, perceived barriers to practising evidence based medicine, and best method of moving from opinion based to evidence based medicine.
Results: Respondents mainly welcomed evidence based medicine and agreed that its practice improves patient care. They had a low level of awareness of extracting journals, review publications, and databases (only 40% knew of the *Cochrane Database of Systematic Reviews*), and, even if aware, many did not use them. In their surgeries 20% had access to bibliographic databases and 17% to the world wide web. Most had some understanding of the technical terms used. The major perceived barrier to practising evidence based medicine was lack of personal time. Respondents thought the most appropriate way to move towards evidence based general practice was by using evidence based guidelines or proposals developed by colleagues.
Conclusion: Promoting and improving access to summaries of evidence, rather than teaching all general practitioners literature searching and critical appraisal, would be the more appropriate method of encouraging evidence based general practice. General practitioners who are skilled in accessing and interpreting evidence should be encouraged to develop local evidence based guidelines and advice.

Introduction

Evidence based medicine is being promoted in general practice as throughout the NHS. General practitioners can attend workshops on how to practice and teach it, research networks promote its use, the Cochrane Library has an increasing number of systematic reviews relevant to general practice, and the journal *Evidence-Based Medicine* regularly contains summaries

of general practice topics. Books on evidence based medicine present common general practice questions, show how to critically appraise papers, and to evaluate different sorts of evidence. Critical appraisal is now part of the MRCGP exam. Recent papers have highlighted the need for evidence based general practice,[1][2] the role of evidence based guidelines in the management of conditions common to general practice,[3-5] and the estimated proportion of interventions in general practice that are based on evidence.[6] One paper has described the problems that may arise in general practice from overreliance on evidence based medicine.[7] These included the potential lack of applicability of the biomedical perspective and the role of opinion in tailoring evidence to a patient's context and preferences.

In the United Kingdom, however, very little is known about general practitioners' attitudes towards evidence based medicine, the extent of their skills to access and interpret evidence, the barriers to moving from opinion based to evidence based practice, and the additional support necessary to incorporate evidence based medicine into everyday general practice. The objectives of this study were to determine the attitude of general practitioners towards evidence based medicine and their related educational needs. Postgraduate tutors, health authorities, and the Wessex Primary Care Research Network (WReN) required this information to inform local strategies aimed at encouraging general practitioners to implement evidence based medicine. Early approaches used in Wessex included workshops on critical appraisal and evidence based medicine and training in performing literature search as part of courses on research methods. After initial local enthusiasm, however, it had become harder to recruit general practitioners to such training events.

To fulfil the objectives of the study we set out to identify general practitioners'
- Attitude towards evidence based medicine
- Awareness and perceived usefulness of relevant extracting journals, review publications, and databases
- Ability to access relevant databases and the world wide web
- Understanding of technical terms used in evidence based medicine
- Views on the perceived major barriers to practising evidence based medicine
- Views on how best to move from opinion based to evidence based medicine.

Wessex Primary Care Research Network, Primary Medical Care, University of Southampton, Aldermoor Health Centre, Southampton SO16 5ST
Alastair McColl, *lecturer in public health medicine*
Helen Smith, *senior lecturer in primary care*

Nightingale Surgery, Great Well Drive, Romsey, Hampshire SO51 7QN
Peter White, *general practitioner tutor*

Primary Medical Care, University of Southampton
Jenny Field, *senior lecturer in primary care*

Correspondence to:
Dr Alastair McColl

BMJ 1998;316:361–5

Survey questionnaire appears on our website

Information in practice

Subject and methods

In April 1997 we sent a questionnaire to 452 general practitioner principals in the former Wessex region in south England. These represented 25% of all Wessex general practitioner principals obtained from a national database,[8] who were randomly selected by means of random numbers generated by Microsoft Excel with supervision from a statistician.

The covering letter for the questionnaire included a definition of evidence based medicine as the "conscientious, explicit and judicious use of current best evidence in making decisions about the care of individual patients. Its practice means integrating individual clinical expertise with the best available external clinical evidence from systematic research."[9]

The questionnaire consisted of

* Visual analogue scales to determine the general practitioners' attitudes towards evidence based medicine
* Closed questions to assess their awareness of and perceived usefulness of extracting journals, review publications, and databases relevant to evidence based medicine; their ability to access Medline or other bibliographic databases and the world wide web; their

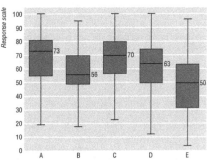

Attitudes of 293 general practitioners towards evidence based medicine: (A) attitude towards current promotion of evidence based medicine (100=extremely welcoming, 0=extremely unwelcoming); (B) perceived attitude of colleagues towards evidence based medicine (100=extremely welcoming, 0=extremely unwelcoming); (C) practising evidence based medicine improved patient care (100=strongly agree, 0=strongly disagree); (D) perceived usefulness of evidence based medicine in day to day management of patients (100=extremely useful, 0=totally useless); (E) estimated percentage of respondent's clinical practice that is evidence based. Box plots show maximum and minimum values, median, and first and third quartiles

Table 1 Characteristics of 302 respondents* and 148 non-respondents to postal questionnaire of general practitioners in former Wessex region. Values are numbers (percentages) of subjects unless stated otherwise

	Respondents	Non-respondents	P value of difference
Personal characteristics			
Men	210/301 (70)	103/141 (73)†	0.48
MRCGP	183/298 (61)	35/148 (24)	<0.0001
Full time principals	242/300 (81)	Unavailable	
Practice characteristics			
WReN member‡	41/302 (14)	5/148 (3)	<0.05
Undergraduate teaching practice	185/297 (62)	81/148 (55)	0.13
Postgraduate training practice	154/299 (52)	Unavailable	
Practice size less than 5000	61/299 (20)	Unavailable	
Mean No of full time equivalent partners	4.7	Unavailable	
Fundholding practice	165/298 (55)	Unavailable	
Setting:			
Rural	56/300 (19)	Unavailable	
Urban	129/300 (43)	Unavailable	
Mixed	115/300 (38)	Unavailable	

*Some respondents did not answer all the questions.
†We were unable to determine the sex of some of the non-respondents.
‡Wessex Primary Care Research Network.

Table 2 Awareness of 302 general practitioners* of extracting journals, review publications, and databases relevant to evidence based medicine and their usefulness. Values are numbers (percentages) of subjects who ticked each response

Publication	Unaware	Aware but not used	Read	Used to help in clinical decision making
Bandolier (published in Oxford)	141/294 (48)	49/294 (17)	55/294 (19)	49/294 (17)
Evidence-Based Medicine (BMJ publishing group)	83/287 (29)	132/287 (46)	52/287 (18)	20/287 (7)
Effective Health Care Bulletins (Universities of Leeds and York)	115/287 (40)	48/287 (17)	81/287 (28)	43/287 (15)
Cochrane Database of Systematic Reviews (part of *Cochrane Library*)	169/284 (60)	89/284 (31)	15/284 (5)	11/284 (4)
Database of Abstracts of Reviews of Effectiveness (part of *Cochrane Library*)	231/283 (82)	43/283 (15)	7/283 (2)	2/283 (1)
Evidence-Based Purchasing (South and West R&D)	232/283 (82)	36/283 (13)	12/283 (4)	3/283 (1)

*Some respondents did not answer all the questions.

understanding of technical terms; and their views on how best to move from opinion based practice to evidence based medicine

* A free text section to determine their views on the major barriers to practising evidence based medicine in general practice. These brief statements were coded and grouped by AMcC. (For details of the questionnaire, see copy included in this article on the *BMJ* website www.bmj.com).

We sent reminders to non-respondents in June and July 1997, and data on non-respondents were collected by AMcC from teaching and research networks and the 1997 *Medical Directory*.[10]

We entered the data into a spreadsheet. We initially identified 38 categories, but these were grouped into broader categories during the analysis. We analysed data from the visual analogue scales using SPSS for Windows 6.1.2 and analysed the other data using Microsoft Excel 5.0. We compared differences between respondents and non-respondents using the χ^2 test.

Results

Of the 452 questionnaires we sent out, two were returned because the general practitioners had retired. We received 302 replies (67%) to the remaining 450 questionnaires. Table 1 compares the characteristics of the respondents and non-respondents.

Attitudes towards evidence based medicine—The figure shows the responding general practitioners' attitudes towards evidence based medicine. Most were welcoming towards the current promotion of evidence based medicine (A), although colleagues were perceived to be less welcoming (B), and most agreed that practising evidence based medicine improved patient care (C) and that research findings were useful in the day to day management of patients (D). The median value for the estimated percentage of the respondents' clinical practice that was evidence based was 50% (E).

Awareness and perceived usefulness of relevant information sources—Table 2 shows that the doctors had a low level of awareness of extracting journals, review publications, and databases relevant to evidence based medicine. Only 40% of respondents were aware of the *Cochrane Database of Systematic Reviews*, 52% of *Bandolier*, and 60% of *Effective Health Care Bulletins*.

Access to relevant databases and the world wide web—Only 20% (41/220) of respondents had access to Medline or other bibliographic databases at their surgery while 76% (173/227) had access at their local library and 21% (45/219) at their home. They also lacked access to the world wide web: only 17% (40/236) had access at their surgery, 41% (73/178) at their local library, and 29% (71/247) at their home. In the previous year 51% (102/201) had used Medline or another database for literature searching or had asked someone to do a search on their behalf, and 12 had searched on more than 10 occasions. Of these 102 doctors, 28 reported having had some training in literature searching, while a total of 16% (47/297) had received formal training in search strategies. At least 11 of those trained had not made a literature search in the previous year. Those trained in searching were more likely to have access to Medline or another database in their home (30% (14/47) v 11% (27/250)) and in their surgery (32% (15/47) v 12% (29/250)).

Understanding of technical terms used in evidence based medicine—Most of the respondents had some understanding of the technical terms used in evidence based medicine, and a third felt able to explain to others the meaning of some of these terms (table 3). However, only 15% (44/290) understood publication bias and could explain it to others. A considerable proportion who did not understand the terms expressed a desire to understand (9-48%). In total 39% (115/297) had received formal training in critical appraisal.

Views on major barriers to practising evidence based medicine—The main perceived barrier to practising evidence based medicine in general practice was a lack of personal time (table 4).

Views on how best to move from opinion based to evidence based medicine—Most of the respondents (57%) thought that the most appropriate way to move from opinion based practice to evidence based medicine was "using evidence based guidelines or protocols developed by colleagues for use by others," while 37% thought it should be by "seeking and applying evidence based summaries" and only 5% by "identifying and appraising the primary literature or systematic reviews" (table 5).

Discussion

Methodological issues

A response rate of 67% is a considerable achievement as response rates to questionnaire surveys among general practitioners are dropping.[11] Respondents were more likely to be members of the Royal College of General Practitioners and the Wessex Primary Care Research Network. Other questionnaire studies have suggested that members of the royal college are more innovative[12] and more "enthusiastic" to participate in quality assessment[13] than non-members. The difference between the respondents' attitude and their perception of their colleagues' attitudes could be explained by a

Table 3 Understanding of 302 general practitioners* of technical terms used in evidence based medicine. Values are numbers (percentages) of subjects who ticked each response

Term	It would not be helpful for me to understand	Don't understand but would like to	Some understanding	Understand and could explain to others
Relative risk	7/291 (2)	31/291 (11)	157/291 (54)	96/291 (33)
Absolute risk	7/291 (2)	40/291 (14)	153/291 (53)	91/291 (31)
Systematic review	8/288 (3)	55/288 (19)	160/288 (56)	65/288 (23)
Odds ratio	27/289 (9)	138/289 (48)	92/289 (32)	31/289 (11)
Meta-analysis	12/291 (4)	63/291 (22)	120/291 (41)	96/291 (33)
Clinical effectiveness	5/290 (2)	27/290 (9)	165/290 (57)	93/290 (32)
Number needed to treat	6/288 (2)	54/288 (19)	126/288 (44)	102/288 (35)
Confidence interval	17/290 (6)	90/290 (31)	124/290 (43)	59/290 (20)
Heterogeneity	20/289 (7)	124/289 (43)	116/289 (40)	29/289 (10)
Publication bias	21/290 (7)	88/290 (30)	133/290 (46)	44/290 (15)

*Some respondents did not answer all the questions.

more positive attitude of respondents towards evidence based medicine than non-respondents.

Our subjects were general practitioners rather than primary healthcare teams. Our narrow focus was partly due to the availability of an adequate sampling frame, but we are sending a similar questionnaire to practice nurses to widen our understanding of evidence based health care in primary care.

Interpretation of findings

Attitudes towards evidence based medicine—Although most of the respondents agreed that practising evidence based medicine improved patient care, the median value for the estimated percentage of their clinical practice that was evidence based was 50%. However, this was a self reported question, and it had limitations. This estimate was considerably less than one from a retrospective review of case notes, which concluded that over 80% of interventions in general

Table 4 Perceived major barriers to practising evidence based medicine in general practice reported by 242 general practitioners*

Perceived barrier	No of responses
Lack of personal time	171
Context of primary care:	62
Personal and organisational inertia	35
Morale in general practice	6
Lack of investment by health authorities and trusts	4
Difficulties in involving whole practice	5
No financial gain in using evidence based medicine	8
Closed lists	4
The evidence itself:	59
Lack of hard evidence	20
Evidence not related to context of primary care	16
Too much evidence	9
Availability and access to information	14
Attitudes of patients:	44
Patients' expectations	23
Patients demanding ineffective treatment	11
The need for lengthy discussions with patients	6
An ignorant media	4
General practitioners themselves:	35
Attitudes of colleagues	29
Lack of critical appraisal skills	2
Evidence based medicine seen as threat	4
Others	3

*Only 80% of the 302 respondents answered these questions. Respondents gave more than one answer

Information in practice

Table 5 Views of 302 general practitioners* on ways of moving from opinion based practice to evidence based general practice. Values are numbers (percentages)

Method of moving towards evidence based medicine	Method currently using	Method of interest for future use	Most appropriate method
a) Learning the skills of evidence based medicine	84/297 (28)	101/296 (34)	15/281 (5)
b) Seeking and applying evidence based summaries	215/297 (72)	229/296 (77)	105/281 (37)
c) Using evidence based practice guidelines or protocols	249/297 (84)	230/296 (78)	161/281 (57)
Doctors currently using method (a)—Learning the skills of evidence based medicine			
a) Learning the skills of evidence based medicine	—	62/84 (74)	12/84 (14)
b) Seeking and applying evidence based summaries	67/84 (80)	64/84 (76)	28/84 (33)
c) Using evidence based practice guidelines or protocols	69/84 (82)	64/84 (76)	39/84 (46)
Doctors currently using method (b)—Seeking and applying evidence based summaries			
a) Learning the skills of evidence based medicine	67/215 (31)	82/215 (38)	11/215 (5)
b) Seeking and applying evidence based summaries	—	191/215 (89)	96/215 (45)
c) Using evidence based practice guidelines or protocols	174/215 (81)	170/215 (79)	96/215 (45)
Doctors currently using method (c)—Using evidence based practice guidelines or protocols			
a) Learning the skills of evidence based medicine	69/249 (28)	82/249 (33)	8/249 (3)
b) Seeking and applying evidence based summaries	174/249 (70)	194/249 (78)	80/249 (32)
c) Using evidence based practice guidelines or protocols	—	200/249 (80)	146/249 (59)

*Some respondents did not answer all the questions. In the questionnaire, method (a) was described as "by learning the skills of evidence-based medicine i.e. to identify and appraise the primary literature or systematic reviews oneself"; method (b) was "by seeking and applying evidence-based summaries, which give the clinical 'bottom line.' Such summaries may be obtained from abstracting journals"; and method (c) was "by using evidence based practice guidelines or protocols developed by colleagues for use by others." Respondents were allowed more than one response when asked what methods they were currently using and would be interested in using in the future but only one response when asked which of these methods they thought was most appropriate in general practice.

practice were evidence based.[6] The methods used were criticised, as the quality of evidence was not reviewed and non-experimental evidence was included.[14 15] The case notes may not have been representative of typical consultations, as only recorded consultations with a primary diagnosis and intervention were used and in general practice patients rarely enter the consulting room with a discrete, one dimensional problem.[15 16] Other reviews have suggested that evidence based medicine is less relevant to general practice than other specialties because it mainly addresses the biomedical perspective of diagnosis from a doctor centred paradigm[7] and does not integrate quantitative and qualitative research, epidemiology, and psychology and the skills of public health and family medicine.[17]

Awareness of relevant information sources—Respondents showed a low level of awareness of extracting journals, review publications, and databases relevant to evidence based medicine. Attempts have been made to find out who uses the Cochrane Database[18] and whether obstetricians and gynaecologists were aware of and used it,[19] but there have been no such studies of general practitioners. The practice of evidence based medicine involves integrating individual clinical expertise with the best available external clinical evidence from systematic research.[9] Much of this clinical evidence in primary care has already been identified, critically appraised, and packaged in extracting journals and databases.[2]

Health authorities in Wessex send *Effective Health Care Bulletins* to every general practice, and *Bandolier* and *Evidence-Based Purchasing* are available to general practitioners on request without charge. Respondents may not have been aware of the formal title of some of these publications despite having read them and so we may have underestimated awareness. Of the general practitioners who were aware of these sources, 13-46% did not use them. Further studies with interviews are needed to understand why this is so. Without current best evidence, medical practice risks becoming out of date, to the detriment of patients.[9]

Access to relevant databases and the world wide web—Less than a fifth of the respondents had access to a relevant database or world wide web in their surgeries. Although almost all general practices have computers, access to the internet cannot be available on machines that hold patient data. Sackett suggested that, to improve efficiency, evidence must travel to general practitioners' surgeries as they can spend twice as long travelling to a medical library as reading in it.[20] The respondents thought that 75% of their local libraries had access to Medline or other relevant databases and that only 42% had access to the world wide web. In reality all 12 libraries had access to Medline, and 10 had access to the world wide web (J Stephenson, personal communication). The resource implications of advertising and improving access to evidence, at local libraries and in doctors' surgeries, should be considered. Primary care research networks may have a role in this, as shown by Starnet in the South Thames region.[21]

Understanding of technical terms—Our respondents showed a partial understanding of the technical terms used in evidence based medicine. Interpretation of evidence is a key element in practising evidence based medicine, and this partial understanding could hinder interpretation and make cascading of evidence to other members of the primary care team more difficult.

Views on major barriers to practising evidence based medicine—The barriers described in this study are more pragmatic than some of those identified in other papers.[7 17] Lack of personal time was the main perceived barrier. There are ways of increasing the time available for practising evidence based medicine.[2 20] This time could be spent more efficiently by changing the emphasis of postgraduate education away from lectures and toward training in accessing and interpreting evidence and then spending time putting these skills into practice. Two general practitioners in a Southampton pilot project receive postgraduate education payments for preparing summaries of evidence based medicine for their practices. Dawes suggested that a general practitioner who spent an hour a week searching and reading would make huge strides in implementing evidence.[2]

A considerable proportion of respondents perceived personal and organisational inertia and the attitudes of colleagues as a major barrier. Tensions between doctors in general practices may lead to difficulties in investing in technology to access evidence and in failures to agree practice policies on clinical management that are evidence based. However, the attitudes of patients were also seen as a barrier.

Views on how best to move to evidence based medicine—The focus of workshops on critical appraisal and evidence based medicine in Wessex has been on training healthcare workers to identify and appraise primary literature or systematic reviews. However, few respondents thought that this was the most appropriate way to move from opinion based to evidence based medicine. Most thought that the best way was by using evidence based guidelines or protocols developed by colleagues for use by others. Only 14% of those currently identifying and appraising primary literature or systematic reviews thought this was the best method.

Conclusions

Postgraduate tutors, health authorities, and primary care research networks are attempting to encourage general practitioners to implement evidence based general practice. They should refocus their efforts on promoting and improving access to summaries of evidence. They should also encourage local general practitioners working in localities or commissioning groups, who are themselves skilled in accessing and interpreting evidence, to develop local evidence based guidelines and advice. This may be a more effective approach to harness the interest and welcoming attitude of general practitioners towards evidence based medicine than trying to teach all general practitioners skills in search and critical appraisal.

We thank the Wessex general practitioners who took part in this survey.

Contributors: HS developed the original idea and questionnaire. AMcC, HS, PW, and JF refined the questionnaire and jointly wrote the paper. Chris Spencer-Jones, Paul Roderick, and Ruairidh Milne gave advice on the questionnaire. AMcC coordinated the distribution and follow up of the questionnaire, coded the free text sections, and performed the data analysis. Wendy Davis coded the rest of the questionnaire and provided administrative support. Mark Mullee advised on the random sampling. AMcC is guarantor for the paper.

Funding: The Wessex Primary Care Research Network is funded by the South and West Research and Development Directorate. The Southampton GP Tutor Educational Fund paid for the coding and entry of data.

Conflict of interest: None.

Key messages

- Despite considerable variation in 302 general practitioners' attitudes to the promotion of evidence based medicine, most were welcoming and agreed that it improved patient care
- There was a low level of awareness of extracting journals, review publications, and databases relevant to evidence based medicine, and the major perceived barrier to its practice was lack of personal time
- In their surgery only 20% of general practitioners had access to Medline or other bibliographic databases and 17% had access to the world wide web
- Most had some understanding of the technical terms used in evidence based medicine, but less than a third felt able to explain to others the meaning of these terms
- Respondents thought that the best way to move from opinion based practice towards evidence based medicine was by using evidence based guidelines or protocols developed by colleagues

1   Risdale L. Evidence-based learning for general practice. *Br J Gen Pract* 1996;46:503-4.
2   Dawes M. On the need for evidence-based general and family practice. *Evidence-Based Med* 1996;1:68-9.
3   Baker R, Carney TA, Cobbe S, Farmer A, Feder G, Fox KAA, et al. North of England evidence based guidelines development project: summary version of evidence based guideline for the primary care management of stable angina. *BMJ* 1996;312:827-32.
4   North of England Asthma Guideline Development Group. North of England evidence based guidelines development project: summary version of evidence based guideline for the primary care management of asthma in adults. *BMJ* 1996;312:762-6.
5   Eccles M, Clapp Z, Grimshaw J, Adams PC, Higgins B, Purves I, et al. North of England evidence based guidelines development project: methods of guideline development. *BMJ* 1996;312:760-2.
6   Gill P, Dowell AC, Neal RD, Smith N, Heywood P, Wilson AE. Evidence based general practice: a retrospective study of interventions in one training practice. *BMJ* 1996;312:819-21.
7   Jacobson LD, Edwards AGK, Granier SK, Butler CC. Evidence based medicine and general practice. *Br J Gen Pract* 1997;47:449-52.
8   Information Management Group. *Organisations codes file*. Leeds: NHS Executive, 1997.
9   Sackett DL, Rosenberg WMC, Gray JAM, Haynes RB, Richardson WS. Evidence based medicine: What it is and what it isn't. It's about integrating individual clinical expertise and the best external evidence. *BMJ* 1996;312:71-2.
10 *The Medical Directory, 1997*. London: Financial Times Healthcare, 1997.
11 McAvoy BR, Kaner EFS. General practice surveys: a questionnaire too far? *BMJ* 1996;313:732-3.
12 Bosanquet N. Quality of care in general practice—lessons from the past. *J R Coll Gen Pract* 1989;39:88-90.
13 Fraser RC, Gosling JT. Information systems for general practitioners for quality assessment: I. Responses of the doctors. *BMJ* 1985;291:1473-6.
14 Chikwe J. Evidence based general practice: findings of study should prompt debate. *BMJ* 1996;313:114-5.
15 Meakin R, Lloyd M, Ward M. Evidence based general practice: studies using sophisticated methods are needed. *BMJ* 1996;313:114.
16 Greenhalgh T. "Is my practice evidence-based?" *BMJ* 1996;313:957-8.
17 MacAuley D. The integration of evidence based medicine and personal care in family practice. *Ir J Med Sci* 1996;165:289-91.
18 Hyde C. Who uses the Cochrane pregnancy and childbirth database? *BMJ* 1995;310:1140-1.
19 Paterson-Brown S, Wyatt JC, Fisk NM. Are clinicians interested in up to date reviews of effective care? *BMJ* 1993;307:1464.
20 Sackett DL. ...so little time, and.... *Evidence-Based Med* 1997;2:39.
21 Pickering A. *Evidence-based health care—a resource pack*. London: Kings College School of Medicine and Dentistry, 1997.

(Accepted 28 November 1997)

CHAPTER 14

The contribution of family medicine research to improving global healthcare

Waris Qidwai

NOMINATED CLASSIC PAPER

Chris van Weel, Walter W. Rosser. Improving health care globally: a critical review of the necessity of family medicine research and recommendations to build research capacity. *Annals of Family Medicine*, 2004; 2(Suppl. 2): S5–S16.

This paper is a pioneering manuscript about the need for capacity building in primary care research. It was based on an historic invitational conference, held in 2003 in Kingston in Canada. For the first time researchers from 34 countries from across the globe participated in a primary care research capacity building conference that examined primary care research from a global perspective. The linkage of primary care research with improvements in global healthcare makes this paper and its recommendations of immense practical value. The paper outlines nine evidence-based, consensus recommendations for capacity building. There is particular emphasis on primary care research in developing countries and on the ethical aspects of research. It highlights the status of primary care research as it existed globally in 2003. It was through this historic paper that policy-makers were sensitised to the need for capacity building in primary care research. This paper offers insight into how primary care researchers, even today, can examine and realign primary care research strategies to improve healthcare globally. This paper will continue to be relevant to primary care researchers from across the globe, as it offers a basis for continuing future capacity building in primary care research.

ABOUT THE AUTHORS OF THIS PAPER

Chris van Weel is a family doctor and primary care researcher from the Netherlands. He was Professor of General Practice and Head of the Department of Primary and Community Care at Radboud University in Nijmegen in the Netherlands from 1985 to 2012. He was president of the World Organization of Family Doctors (WONCA) from 2007 to 2010. He has special research interests in chronic diseases in family practice, and the development of academic practice-based research networks.

Walter Rosser is a family doctor and an academic leader in Canada, having served as Head of Family Medicine at McMaster University, the University of Toronto, and Queen's University in Kingston. He has worked throughout his career to develop and influence policy and guidelines that affect the environment in which family doctors practise, to make that environment more conducive to research, and to promote the application of research evidence into clinical practice. He has promoted practice-based research networks, which he sees as the 'laboratories' in which primary care research is conducted.

ABOUT THE NOMINATOR OF THIS PAPER

Professor Waris Qidwai is Chairman of the Department of Family Medicine at Aga Khan University in Karachi in Pakistan. He has been the chair of the working party on research of the World Organization of Family Doctors (WONCA). He has played an important role in the promotion of family medicine and primary care research in his country, region and around the world.

> 'Family medicine is an emerging medical specialty in many parts of the world, and is considered mandatory for the success of healthcare delivery, resulting in better healthcare at a lower cost. It is through working together that we will be able to ensure that family medicine gets its due recognition in medical practice in every country of the world.'

Professor Waris Qidwai, Pakistan

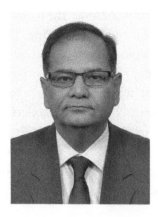

Attribution:

We attribute the original publication of *Improving health care globally: a critical review of the necessity of family medicine research and recommendations to build research capacity* to *Annals of Family Medicine*. With thanks to Kurt Stange, Joshua Freeman, Stephanie Hanaway, Mindy Cleary and Doug Henley at the American Academy of Family Physicians, and to all participants at the Kingston Conference.

Improving Health Care Globally: A Critical Review of the Necessity of Family Medicine Research and Recommendations to Build Research Capacity

Chris van Weel, MD, PhD, FRCGP[1]

Walter W. Rosser, MD, CCFP, FCFP, MRCGP(UK)[2]

[1] Department of Family Medicine, University Medical Centre Nijmegen, Nijmegen, The Netherlands

[2] Department of Family Medicine, Queens University, Kingston, Ontario, Canada

ABSTRACT

An invitational conference led by the World Organization of Family Doctors (Wonca) involving selected delegates from 34 countries was held in Kingston, Ontario, Canada, March 8 to12, 2003. The conference theme was "Improving Health Globally: The Necessity of Family Medicine Research." Guiding conference discussions was the value that to improve health care worldwide, strong, evidence-based primary care is indispensable. Eight papers reviewed before the meeting formed the basic material from which the conference developed 9 recommendations. Wonca, as an international body of family medicine, was regarded as particularly suited to pursue these conference recommendations:

1. Research achievements in family medicine should be displayed to policy makers, health (insurance) authorities, and academic leaders in a systematic way.
2. In all countries, sentinel practice systems should be developed to provide surveillance reports on illness and diseases that have the greatest impact on the population's health and wellness in the community.
3. A clearinghouse should be organized to provide a central repository of knowledge about family medicine research expertise, training, and mentoring.
4. National research institutes and university departments of family medicine with a research mission should be developed.
5. Practice-based research networks should be developed around the world.
6. Family medicine research journals, conferences, and Web sites should be strengthened to disseminate research findings internationally, and their use coordinated. Improved representation of family medicine research journals in databases, such as Index Medicus, should be pursued.
7. Funding of international collaborative research in family medicine should be facilitated.
8. International ethical guidelines, with an international ethical review process, should be developed in particular for participatory (action) research, where researchers work in partnership with communities.
9. When implementing these recommendations, the specific needs and implications for developing countries should be addressed.

The Wonca executive committee has reviewed these recommendations and the supporting rationale for each. They plan to follow the recommendations, but to do so will require the support and cooperation of many individuals, organizations, and national governments around the world.

Ann Fam Med 2004;2(Suppl 2):S5-S16. DOI: 10.1370/afm.194.

Conflict of interest: none reported

CORRESPONDING AUTHOR

Chris van Weel, MD, PhD, FRCGP
Department of Family Medicine
University Medical Centre Nijmegen
229-HAG, PO Box 9101
6500 HB Nijmegen, The Netherlands
C.vanWeel@HAG.umcn.nl

INTRODUCTION

The aim of medicine everywhere is to provide safe, effective, efficient, timely, patient-centered, and equitable care.[1] To pursue this aim, strengthening primary care—the point of first contact with the health care system for most people—is important. Most people receive formal medical care in primary care,[2,3] and it is in that setting most episodes of illness are treated. Family medicine is a key discipline of primary care, and in many countries family physicians are the only physicians directly accessible to the public.[4] Clinical decisions made on first encounters often determine whether health care resources are appropriately used.[2,5-7] Strengthening the knowledge base in primary care will contribute to better medical care for all.

Against this background an invitational conference was organized by the World Organization of Family Doctors (Wonca) to explore ways to improve the status of family medicine research, expand the evidence base of family physicians, and contribute to better health care worldwide. This article summarizes the conference discussions and presents recommendations proposed by the 74 conference attendees from 34 countries.

Although key components of primary care, family medicine and primary care are not identical concepts. Family physicians in different countries work with other primary care professionals in a variety of arrangements. Because of the international divergence in primary care structure, we wish to clarify that the target discipline of this paper is family medicine. Throughout the document family medicine and family physician (FP) are used and should be interpreted as the European, Australian, and New Zealand "general practice" and "general practitioner."

METHODS: THE CONFERENCE PROCESSES

The international conference organized by Wonca, in Kingston, Ontario, Canada, from March 8 to 11, 2003, provided the material for this article. Participants were leaders in primary care research in their countries. The meeting was initiated, organized, and chaired by the authors. Before the meeting every participant was asked to read 8 papers that had been written and peer reviewed by 4 reviewers especially for the conference.[8-15] Each paper addressed different aspects of family medicine research. After the opening keynote address,[16] the author of each paper had 10 minutes to comment on suggestions provided through the peer-review process. These comments were followed by a further 10 minutes of comments about the paper made by an individual from outside family medicine research.[17] Papers were modified after the meeting on the basis of the peer review and feedback from conference participants and the guest editor for this supplement.

Conference participants then convened into 8 small groups for an extended discussion of the issues raised by each paper. Each group included representatives from both developed and developing countries, as well as those from outside the family medicine research arena. Feedback from the small groups was provided to the assembled conference. This feedback highlighted the most important points in each paper, identified gaps in content, and provided 1 or 2 recommendations. From this process several issues were identified for more discussion. The program plan allowed time for additional discussions by small groups, with reports back to the full assembly. Designated reporters for each group recorded all small-group proceedings.

The oral and written proceedings from 48 small-group sessions and the large-group discussions were reviewed and consolidated by the authors into this article. The findings are grouped in relation to the main conclusions and recommendations formulated during the conference. Vignettes provided in the text were developed from 2 sources. Some were chosen from two 1-hour sessions in which participants from 11 countries had 10 minutes to present a unique development. The other source was ideas emerging from group discussions during the conference. Vignettes were chosen for their ability to serve as models that are transferable to other settings.

During the large-group sessions all recommendations were reviewed and consolidated into the final 9 that were viewed by the assembly as best contributing to further development of family medicine research internationally. The need for concerted actions on these recommendations was stressed, and the conference identified the key role of Wonca in implementation. For clarity in this article, the recommendations have been formulated as generic statements. Draft versions of this report were sent to conference participants for their comments on two occasions, and all comments received have been considered for incorporation into the paper.

RESULTS

Research in Family Medicine Improves Patient Care and Health

FPs provide their services in direct contact with the communities where patients live and work: the ecology of health care[3] (see Green, Figure 1[9(p24)]). FPs work at the interface between community and the health care system. They treat most health problems in their own clinical setting, and coordinate with other sectors of the health care system for the management of an important minority of health problems. Family medicine research helps sustain the proper functioning of health care systems and guarantees access to health care on the basis of individuals' needs in a framework of equity of access for all persons. Substantial research from family medicine supports these statements,[6,18] but health care funders, planners, publishers, and others often have poor under-

---

Vignette 1. Clinical Uncertainty

Clinical uncertainty is an inherent aspect of first-contact medical care and should be distinguished from insecurity of individual practitioners. FPs have developed the methods to deal with clinical uncertainty that are based on the scientific concept of increasing the pretest likelihood of a disease. By watchful waiting, 40% of undifferentiated problems encountered by FPs will resolve without ever meeting the criteria of a specific diagnosis. The remaining 60% of problems will develop signs and symptoms that will increase the pretest likelihood of a specific diagnosis. The strategy of watchful waiting, which is unacceptable in most secondary and tertiary care practice, saves unknown but large expenditures in health care investigations that would otherwise be wasted.[18,21]

---

standing of the current contribution of family medicine research and of its potential to improve health. To improve the profile and understanding of family medicine research in the medical research community, family medicine research must be more widely disseminated.

Recommendation 1

Wonca should develop a strategy to display research achievements in family medicine to policy makers, health funders, and academic leaders.

Problem Solving in Family Medicine

In family medicine problem solving has often been characterized as coping with the clinical uncertainty arising from the breadth of the clinical field.[3] Forty percent of all new undifferentiated health problems never evolve into a condition that meets the criteria for a diagnosis according to the International Classification of Primary Care (ICPC)[19] or the International Classification of Diseases (ICD-10); yet, in the remaining 60% of these problems, there is the possibility of every disease known to man.[18,20] The way clinical uncertainty implicit in the early signs and symptoms of disease is managed determines the efficiency and effectiveness of patient care and the appropriate use of primary and secondary care diagnostic and therapeutic facilities (Vignette 1). The more common the health condition, however, the less it is studied,[22] and available studies from selected populations and tertiary care centers are difficult to translate to family medicine.[23] For these reasons only, rigorous research of common health problems in the community, derived from the clinical context of family medicine, will

appropriately support FPs in their management of clinical uncertainty[20,24] and increase the precision of their problem solving. Family medicine research will promote understanding of the origins and natural history of disease and will identify factors that enable health, as well as determinants of seeking and receiving health care.

Research to improve FP problem solving must include the broader context of patient care,[25] the biopsychosocial reality of patients and their families with their values and expectations, and the socioeconomic and cultural determinants of health. Including the patients' context requires a mixture of methods and approaches in family medicine research. The application of different paradigms is also an expression of the complexity of family medicine research.

Transfer and Implementation

The transfer and implementation of new knowledge and skills gained from research in family medicine are essential to achieve the full potential of benefits to be gained for health in any community. There is a need to assess and value new knowledge in relation to the study population from which it was derived, and to determine whether the results can be generalized to other patient populations. It is important to appraise critically the potential risks and benefits of any innovation for patients in each family medicine setting.[21] The concepts of evidence-based medicine provide one framework to assess the value of new innovations for each community[21,26-28] (Vignette 2). There is a further need to better understand current practices and to analyze how to transfer best practices effectively to change the delivery of health care in the community, while considering each patient's personal context. Participation in practice-

---

Vignette 2. Research and Clinical Decision Making in Family Practice

Finding out where research fails in its support for clinical decision making is challenging for researchers. The Dutch College of General Practitioners has developed evidence-based guidelines for family physicians for the most common health problems in primary care. Seventy-six practice guidelines are published in Dutch, 7 in English[27] (Web site: http: //nhg.artsennet.nl?s=4512). These guidelines summarize available evidence; at the same time, they single out where no research is available to support family physicians in their key decisions.

In a critical analysis of the first 70 guidelines, more than 800 important diagnostic and therapeutic decision areas were found to be insufficiently supported by scientific evidence.[29] This information is fed back to primary care researchers to focus their support on the greatest needs of practitioners.

The Dutch college has organized a fund for research of common disorders in family medicine. This fund, which was first available in 2002, is integrated into the research program of the national medical and health research organization,[30] and its research programming is tuned to the identified priorities. In the last 2 years, 16 studies have been published on a wide variety of common subjects, such as infectious conjunctivitis, impetigo, complaints in the mouth, and therapy for emotional problems in family practice, among others. The results of these studies have been already published in Dutch and English medical journals.[31,32]

---

based research greatly facilitates the transfer of research findings into regular practice routines.[33-35]

Developing Appropriate Health Policy

The development of appropriate health policy to support community-oriented care for patients requires insight into the functioning and integration of health care services, their accessibility for all who need care, and ultimately their sustainability in communities and countries.[36] Policy will be improved through a better understanding of the implications for secondary and tertiary care of preventive, diagnostic, and therapeutic interventions in family medicine. Maynard has argued that what is best (but expensive) for individuals can restrict care for others and may not be the best for populations.[37] A comprehensive assessment of their community's health can help FPs choose the most effective interventions to improve individual patients' health within the prevailing circumstances. As providing anticipatory (preventive) care is an integral part of family medicine, more family medicine research should also address the benefits and risks of preventive care and health promotion—assessing the outcomes of both for a long period.[38] For instance, long-term assessment has recently cast doubts about previously celebrated protective effects of hormone replacement therapy (HRT) on heart disease.[39] Earlier involvement of FPs in these investigations might have exposed the harms of prolonged HRT therapy that are only now being uncovered.[40]

Long-term monitoring of health outcomes[38,41] in the community is likely best achieved through development of sentinel practices or practice-based research networks (PBRNs) (Vignette 3). Development PBRNs in countries with underdeveloped primary care delivery systems should assist in capacity building.[34,35,43] In developing countries, the promotion of very simple recording systems in networks can have a dramatic effect on detecting sources of serious illness in the community (contaminated water supply); by removing these sources, we improve the health status of the community.[44,45] Simple recording systems can also powerfully inform priority setting in developing countries and encourage more efficient use of limited resources.

Domain of Family Medicine Research

Research in family medicine should be driven by questions, problems, and challenges that are derived from FPs' practices and that respect the complexity of the health problems FPs encounter. Implicit in this idea is the need to bring to family medicine research a variety of medical and behavioral disciplines. This apparent overlap with other disciplines may have contributed to confusion in defining the family medicine research domain. Family medicine research is any study that addresses questions of

---

Vignette 3. Practice-Based Research Networks

In an effort to support the development of practice-based research networks (PBRNs) around the world, the International Federation of Primary Care Research Networks (IFPCRN) organizes PBRNs from developed and developing countries that function in a variety of health care systems. The objective of IFPCRN is to stimulate the formation of PBRNs, to offer peer support and provide a forum to meet and exchange information, and to stimulate joint research. It meets during scientific primary care conferences (Wonca, North American Primary Care Research Group [NAPCRG]) and through e-mail. Membership is open to everyone either involved in or in the process of setting-up a PBRN.[42]

---

importance to FPs with the objective to improve the care of patients. It is essential to focus research on the priorities of family medicine. Effective family medicine research requires a culture in the discipline of family medicine that is more supportive of the value of research.

Additional Benefits of Research

The benefits of family medicine research also include the effects it can have on the profession. By increasing professional confidence and promoting intellectual growth and richness, the morale of the profession will be improved. A number of countries are experiencing low morale among FPs and a decline in interest of medical students to enter family medicine as a career.[46] Development of research networks and programs in community practice will combat dissatisfaction and improve the intellectual stimulation for FPs overcoming concerns about the sustainability of the primary health care base in several countries.[47] For the discipline of family medicine, research can enhance institutional and academic status, increase the visibility of the benefits of family medicine for health care, and lead to improved professional standards. Development of family medicine research will promote standardization of terminology and diagnostic and therapeutic procedures, which in turn can enhance cooperation nationally and internationally.[19,48-50]

Recommendation 2

Wonca should seek the development in all its member countries of sentinel practices to provide surveillance reports on illness and diseases that have the greatest impact on patients' health and wellness in the community.

Recommendation 3

Wonca should organize a clearinghouse for the world's research expertise, training, and mentoring.

Building Research Capacity

Building research capacity and introducing a research culture are essential to realize the potential of family medicine research. The conference provided a rich variety of ideas, proposals, and recommendations to these ends. The discussion identified 3 general objectives for capacity building that will raise the quality of research while they make family medicine research more visible.[51-56]

Three General Objectives for Capacity Building
There are 3 general objectives for research capacity building in family medicine:

1. Organizing a tight and enduring link between clinical practice and a research environment (changing the climate to supporting inquiry in the discipline)

2. Establishing an improved working relationship between family medicine researchers and the wider scientific community

3. Providing research training and a career path for family medicine researchers

Essential to research capacity building is access to a research infrastructure for researchers to meet for critical reviews of their proposals and findings, presentation of their projects, and dissemination of their results.[57] An impressive number of proposals emerging from this discussion were experience-based (Vignettes 4-8). Three models integrated various aspects of capacity building and will be described in more depth: PBRNs, mentoring programs, and participatory research.

Link Community-Based Physicians With a Research Environment
Developing a strong and enduring link between community-based FPs and a research environment will only occur with improvements in the interface between practice and research. Achieving this objective will require increased involvement of practicing FPs on all levels: as research leaders, participants, contributors, and users.[10,13] A valuable first step is in turning passive users of research information into actively involved users. Action research or participatory research that involves communities in conducting and owning the research results is an effective method to involve FPs more directly in the research needs of their community.[63] Critical appraisal of research information requires knowledge that incorporates the principles of evidence-based medicine. Direct feedback about one's own clinical performance promotes the professional use of research. Other research capacity-building strategies include the involvement of FPs on scientific panels of foundations and funding agencies, reviewing papers for (primary care) journals, and participation in audit

Vignette 4. The Scottish School of Primary Care

Capacity building for primary care research is illustrated by the Scottish School of Primary Care, founded in 2000 to build capacity for primary care research, create a culture in which research is valued and rewarded, and provide a research infrastructure to improve patient care.[51-53] It directs its activities in particular at research and development in the National Health Service.

As a virtual institute, this school without walls has created a critical mass of practitioners and researchers by promoting research skills and methodological expertise, interpersonal programs, and organizational programs. It is open for everyone with a primary care research interest in Scotland and promotes interprofessional projects in particular. It coordinates funding for research collaborations (obtaining $2 million for 4 programs) and coordinates the Scottish MSc.

It persuaded every health board in Scotland to pool their small sums of money into a single 3-year program of research worth $1.2 million and ensured a forefront position in the current postgenomic Biobank project. Major collaborative studies undertaken are (1) an investigation into the delay between the initial symptoms of breast and bowel cancer in rural and deprived communities in 3 regions of Scotland, and (2) a randomized controlled trial of steroids and antiviral medications in Bell's palsy. The school was modeled after the Netherlands school of primary care research.

Vignette 5. The Netherlands School of Primary Care Research CaRe

The Netherlands School of Primary Care Research (CaRe) is a center of research in primary care.[56] It is also a virtual institute to promote medical doctor and doctoral (MD/PhD) programs for primary care (family medicine, health science, epidemiology, ethics, medical informatics, nursing). It was founded in 1995 by the universities of Maastricht, Nijmegen, and Vrije Universiteit, Amsterdam, and the Netherlands Institute of Health Care Research (NIVEL). It is recognized by the Royal Netherlands Academy of Sciences as a research center of excellence. The research program focuses on (1) promotion and health education, (2) determinants of long-term outcome of illness, (3) effectiveness of diagnostic and therapeutic interventions, and (4) quality of care, and (5) international aspects of primary care. Three practice-based research networks are linked to the research program.

The core of the school's mission is PhD training. Since 1995, more than 20 PhD theses have been completed. The combined registrar and PhD training is a particular feature of training to enhance retention of research trained practitioners into clinical practice.

Vignette 6. Encourage Primary Care Research and Retain Researchers

The Brisbane Initiative pursues excellence in primary care research through international cooperation in advanced research training.[58,59] The initiative comes from a number of established research groups in Europe, Australia, and North America. Specifically the initiative is directed at recruiting the most talented researchers in primary care and retaining them for a senior research career. As well as courses for advanced research skills, opportunities for exchange visits, fellowships, and research collaborations are promoted. Of particular concern is the need for primary care researchers to continue their involvement in patient care, resulting in shorter leaves than most academics demand.

Vignette 7. Estonia, Trinidad and Tobago, and the Caribbean

Family medicine has been growing in Estonia and in Trinidad and Tobago. In Estonia after the Russian occupation ended in the early 1990s, there was a strong desire to move away from a Russian polyclinic system of primary health care delivery. Margus Lember and some other academic and physician leaders in the country developed a 750-hour curriculum to retrain the physicians from the former system into a family medicine personal care model to deliver health care. By 2000 more than 1,000 Estonian physicians completed the program and are practicing in a new model of health care delivery. There are now 2 residency training programs, so new graduates have access to training in family medicine.[60]

A native of Trinidad and Tobago, Rohan Mahiraj spent 2 years in Toronto obtaining a master's degree in community health (family medicine). He then returned to Trinidad and Tobago and developed a fellowship program for the University of West Indies. Thirty-five physicians who were practicing in the community have taken the program of weekly sessions distributed over 2 years and passed a rigorous examination to obtain their fellowship. It is hoped that the external funding for the program will continue to allow another 2 classes of up to 20 to complete the program and that the government will make the program an integral part of the educational system. A similar program functions in Jamaica, and a small residency program has been functioning in Barbados for more than 20 years. These 3 programs plan to cooperate using distance learning courses.

Vignette 8. Regional Research Development

To encourage researchers and research development on a regional basis, the European General Practice Research Network (EGPRN)[61] has since the 1970s organized a platform for aspiring family medicine researchers to meet and interact. Currently each year the network organizes stand-alone research meetings and sessions in the Wonca European regional conference. The emphasis was initially on mentoring individuals, which has resulted in a tight international network of experienced researchers. Increasingly this network also focuses on the development of a research culture in family medicine and on international research collaboration.[57,62] The result has been research development on local, national, and regional levels.

provides an excellent model for setting an initial level of funding for primary care research.[55] The establishment of research funds specifically directed at research in family medicine will substantially stimulate new studies. An example is provided by the positive experience of the Dutch College of General Practitioners fund for common morbidity in family practice.[30-32] The initiative based its program on established needs of family medicine for research evidence.[27,29,64] (Vignette 2). Research assessment tools of the medical research council of the Netherlands are used in reviewing projects funded by this program. This model improves the relationship between family medicine researchers and the medical research establishment and builds the credibility of family medicine research. Research funders will be rewarded by improvement in the health status of their communities. The reward for universities and research institutes will also be in establishing closer links with the communities that they serve.[64-67] The Australian government has committed $50 million dollars to establishing a primary health care research infrastructure.[67] This investment supports the founding of the new Australian Primary Health Care Research Institute, funds family medicine research in university departments of family medicine and rural health, finances fellowships and a scholarship program, and pays for grant-based research projects in primary care (Vignette 9).

Recommendation 4

Wonca should stimulate the development of national research institutes and university departments of family medicine with a research mission.

Research Training and Career Paths

Providing research training and career paths for FP researchers should be fostered. In most regions courses for education in basic research skills are available. To sustain benefits from the skills of those receiving research training, the tension between research development and demands from clinical work and teaching must be addressed.[54] Family medicine faces similar tensions between clinical and research demand to most other clinical specialties.[68] Partnering in research with other specialties would foster research in all clinical domains. Universities with their departments of family medicine are in an

projects. The role of data collectors should be regarded as a helpful first step to becoming an active participant as researcher. Equally important, though, is the role of validating the research question and methods for FPs and reviewing the implications of research findings. PBRNs and practices that consider research interests in the selection of their staff and providers should be supported.

National medical colleges, university departments of family medicine, and family medicine research institutes provide the focal points for capacity-building activities, and their establishment in every country should be promoted. These organizations and institutions can promote effective transfer of research knowledge into practice by producing guidelines, organizing conferences for practitioners and researchers, and supporting researchers with special-interest group forums, journal clubs, and family medicine research journals.

The British example of allocating a percentage of the national health care budget to research in proportion to the spending in the primary healthy care sector

Vignette 9. Structuring Primary Care Research

The Australian Primary Health Care Research Evaluation Development (PHCRED) had been structuring primary care research in a comprehensive way. The PHCRED[67] strategy was developed by the Commonwealth Department of Health and Aging in consultation with General Practice Partnership Advisory Council. The strategy supports several elements that will provide support to general practice and primary health care research community. The aim is to develop both research capacity and the fields of knowledge that support the evidence base for general practice and primary health care services. The elements of the strategy include (1) a primary health care research institute, (2) a research priority-setting process, (3) a research capacity-building fund for university departments of general practice and rural health, (4) project grants in the area of primary health care, and (5) a primary health care fellowship and scholarship program for 2002 scholars. The amount of funding was $50 million for 5 years from 2001 to 2005.

excellent position to lead the way by building partnerships with other researchers in biomedicine, health, and social sciences.[13] In a number of countries, however, universities are conspicuously lacking in primary care development.

All academic FPs require protected time for research, and candidates for such positions should demonstrate that they can use this time. To achieve this goal, there is a need for research-training programs (including supported fellowships, masters' degrees, and doctorates) in family medicine research. Although there are a number of these programs in different countries, including some distance learning programs, there still needs to be an international clearinghouse so that potential researchers can easily review all available training opportunities. A number of centers of excellence[51,56,58,59] can serve as a role model for other sites that might be considering similar development (Vignettes 4, 5, and 6). Promoting the benefits and domain of family medicine research should begin in undergraduate education programs, where students should be encouraged to develop their

own research projects and to assist FP researchers on funded studies. Residency and registrar training programs should include instruction in critical appraisal of the literature, a focus on accessing and using research evidence in practice, and participating in research projects of their own. Combined residency and research-training programs need to be developed to prepare clinical scientists for a research career. Such programs are currently available in the Netherlands[69] and Canada.[70] These programs extend the length of vocational training but lead to a dual clinical and research qualification. Researchers in family medicine also need a career track and protected research time.[51,56]

Independent research institutes can present a valuable alternative to universities, as illustrated by the experiences in Italy (Vignette 10). This model works by stimulating universities and institutes to extend their mission into the community and to focus on health problems that have the greatest impact on the population.[64,65] The prevailing research culture is thereby changed, with an expansion of family medicine research opportunities.[12,13]

PBRNs and Research Capacity Building

PBRNs contribute to research capacity building by (1) collecting empirical data from family medicine, (2) connecting FPs to researchers and focusing research on important questions from practice, (3) disseminating research results in practice, and (4) stimulating research interest among FPs.

PBRNs have developed in a number of countries.[34,35,42,66,72-77] These networks are sometimes also referred to as primary care research networks. The key element of PBRNs is the bond between practice and research, and for that reason, that they are practice based is essential and therefore is used here. PBRN practices can consist of all (medical and paramedical) professionals who practice in primary care. The

Vignette 10. Linking Family Medicine Research to Biomedical Research: The Italian Example

Successfully linking family practice research to the biomedical research infrastructure, where no university network is available, the Centro Studie e Recerche Medicina Generale (CseRMeG) in Italy brings together family physicians to improve primary care through research and development. A feature of primary care research in Italy is the absence of university involvement. The network has established a working relation with the Institute Mario Negri—a private research institute—for methodological support and cooperation. The result has been a number of studies, of which the Primary Prevention Project on the effectiveness of low-dose aspirin and vitamin E on cardiovascular events in high-risk patients is the best known.[65] This trial stands as a landmark randomized controlled trial in primary care. In addition, the network has published a textbook of family medicine.[71]

Vignette 11. Uncovering Common Primary Care Health Problems in Developing Countries

In an effort to uncover the hidden burden of illness in primary care, the South African sentinel practices network (SASPAN)[75] organized a network of family practices to identify and study the most common health problems. This solution addresses a major problem of primary care in developing countries by providing empirical data on the major health problems in and challenges for family practice. The network covers the most deprived areas, and its practices are faced with substantial mismatch between the demands of their practice population and the limited available resources. Among its main findings are studies of population need. Its work is currently supporting primary care by using their available resources more effectively and efficiently for patients with human immunodeficiency virus infection and acquired immunodeficiency syndrome.

potential for research capacity building makes PBRNs a powerful generic tool, the development of which must be encouraged in every country (Vignette 3, 11).

PBRN principles have been practiced for decades in a number of groups. In particular, in the United Kingdom and the Netherlands there is a tradition of more than 20 years of practice-directed research, resulting in high-quality data collection.[78] This accomplishment is undoubtedly related to the central position of general practice in the health care system of these countries; patients are listed with the same practice and physician for decades, making the denominator of epidemiological data straightforward. These registration strategies not only help FPs build a longitudinal overview of patients' episodes of illness and medical care but also encourage research that applies this information to defined populations. Even where patients can directly access specialists without referral, examples of developing research networks and databases exist,[34,35,72,75,77,79] illustrating the generic nature of PBRNs. A recent German initiative illustrates benefits from links between primary and secondary care and specific specialties.[80]

Analysis of empirical data directly derived from patient care is a critical step in the development of a family medicine research culture.[76,77,79] The strength of PBRNs is their grounding in practice, with a strong value of ownership by participating FPs[34,66] and a bottom-up approach to answering research questions that are derived from practice. Once the research questions are answered, the results can be implemented in the networks, where the practitioners have a sense of ownership of the findings. A concern about a bottom-up research network is the potential for lack of rigor and too much free-floating research. Many countries deal with this potential problem by linking PBRNs to university departments that provide supervision and methodological support for studies.[41,66,74] PBRNs are also a way for universities and research institutes to broaden their research activities into the community and into primary care.

Among the most important contributions of PBRNs may be in the longitudinal collection and monitoring of morbidity data. Information about care collected during a short period is of limited relevance—and occasionally misleading.[38] Longitudinal research with long-term follow-up of patients' health status can make a major contribution to better understanding of illness and disease. To achieve this goal in a PBRN, it is necessary to obtain long-term commitment from practices to continue to provide high-quality and consist data for many years. This outcome has been achieved in The Netherlands, resulting in databases that can be used as an index to recruit and select patients for research on the basis of their lifetime characteristics.[41,74,78,81]

Recommendation 5

Wonca should organize an expert group to provide advice for the development of PBRNs around the world.

Mentoring

Mentoring is an essential capacity-building tool in all research programs at local, national, and international levels. Formal mentoring processes include masters' degrees, medical doctor (MD), and doctoral (PhD) programs and courses. Mentors need not be based in the same institution or even, for that matter, in the same country as those they are mentoring. Mentoring by an experienced researcher of an FP interested in research in an underdeveloped country can be a powerful way to build family medicine research capacity.[82] Capacity building in underdeveloped countries may also occur with external support partnerships with overseas family medicine university departments (Vignettes 7, 12, and 13). These partnerships should be on equal terms and could include student and faculty exchanges between departments.

Two mentoring approaches can be distinguished: (1) mentorship for interested individual FP researchers, and (2) mentorship between organizations, institutions and countries. There is overlap among these two approaches, and the first may lead into the second.

Two examples of mentoring individual FPs to foster research skills are (1) the 5-weekend research programs in Canada,[83,84] and (2) the activities of the European General Practice Research Network[13,57,61,62] (Vignette 8). These examples stimulate FPs with a research question arising from their practice to participate in partnership with a (university-based) researcher. Mentoring can increase research knowledge and understanding in the discipline in a relatively short period.

An example of programmatic mentoring is the Bosnia-Herzegovina project (Vignette 13), to which many more experiences in eastern[84-86] and southern Europe,[87-89] Latin America (Vignette 12), and Africa[90] can be added. By training future leaders through mentorship, optimal conditions are created to transfer research expertise from one region or country to another. Mentorship might also go beyond research to include support of education. Mentoring should be based on partnerships among universities, research institutes, and national colleges.

In the dissemination of research, conferences, journals, and Web sites play a key role. Primary care output is in danger of losing its visibility when research methods and cross-disciplinary partnerships disperse the family medicine profile of the work. The good working relationships of family medicine with many other disciplines makes loss of visibility a real danger. A Web site linkage from an international foundation family medicine Web site should be pursued. Indexing family medicine journals in a database also provides a powerful method to focus research output, but unfortunately the profile of family medicine journals in the most prestigious database, Index Medicus, is insufficient.

Recommendation 6

Wonca should promote research journals, conferences, and Web sites for the international dissemination of research findings and coordinate their display. A wider representation of family medicine research journals in databases like Index Medicus should be pursued

Recommendation 7

Wonca should facilitate funding of international collaborative research.

Participatory Research

In addition to PBRNs and mentoring, participatory research[63,91,92] has become an established method to answer questions arising from communities. Through engaging in participatory research FPs can both use their position in the communities in which they practice and strengthen their understanding of those communities. Participatory research has in particular established its value in the introduction of (primary) health care in deprived communities by improving social and economic conditions, and effecting equity in care. Reducing distrust of an agenda of research and of care that is perceived as coming from outside—and being imposed upon—the community is the key value of participatory research and results in partnerships between family medicine researchers and the community under study. Participatory research is the process of producing new knowledge by "systematic inquiry, with the collaboration of those affected by the issue being studied, for the purposes of education and taking action or effecting social change."[91] The 3 primary features of participatory research are collaboration, mutual education, and action that is relevant to the community based on the research results. Participatory research encourages partnerships between researcher and community with the goal of incorporating both researcher and community expertise throughout the research process. Participatory research also promotes community capacity building and sustainability beyond research funding. A goal is that research subjects should own the research process, develop skills, and use research results

---

Vignette 12. Brazil: International Partnerships and Mentoring

In 1985 Brazil, a country with the fourth largest land mass in the world and 175 million people, moved from a military dictatorship to a democracy. Between 1987 and 1990 a new constitution was developed guaranteeing every Brazilian basic health care. In 1993 the Programe Sauda Familiale program was initiated to address the health care needs of more than two thirds of the population who had little or no access to primary health care. The federal government began building 40,000 health clinics, sharing the operating costs with municipalities. As the clinics were built, there were no physicians, nurses, or dentists with any training in primary health care. None of the 92 medical schools had a department of family medicine, and no graduates had any experience in delivery of primary health care.

A delegation from the City of Curitiba visited North America to find a university willing to provide education for the health care providers in 92 clinics the city had established by 1995. The Department of Family and Community Medicine at the University of Toronto developed a 10-month program delivered in 5 sessions of 3 days over 1 year. The first 18 participants promised to teach the program to others after they completed the program. The program was based on the 4 principles of Canadian family medicine and also used adult education principles. After the first session, 7 teams of 2 persons each began delivering the program to colleagues. More teachers were identified in the second round. After 7 years there are more than 5,000 graduates of the program in 9 states. There are 4 residency programs in family medicine, and state and national associations have been formed. There is evidence for improving health status in the countries population.[44] Interest in research in primary care has been increasing among those who have graduated from the program, with a growth in paper presentations at society meetings.

Vignette 13. Bosnia-Herzegovina Family Medicine Development

The Queen's University–Bosnia-Herzegovina Family Medicine Development Project began in 1995 when the war was still active in Sarajevo. The Queen's University School of Rehabilitation started a program in 1995 to provide community-based physical rehabilitation to war victims. The health care system was in disarray, with most medical facilities shattered and the education system in chaos. Dr Geoff Hodgetts from Queen's Department of Family Medicine, saw an opportunity to assist the Ministry of Health and Medical Faculties to rebuild medicine in a family medicine model, a major change from the Russian polyclinic system of the former Yugoslavia. During the past 7 years, 4 Bosnian medical faculties have developed departments of family medicine, overseeing 6 family medicine residency programs in more than 20 family medicine teaching centers. There are now more than 175 physicians who have graduated from the 3-year residency program, and many hundreds of nurses and other physicians have received training in primary care. The medical culture has undergone fundamental changes including the legal, political, and cultural aspects of health care. This model will be sustainable into the new future of Bosnia. Twenty-eight papers using research and evidence-based methods were presented by graduates from the program at the Wonca Europe meeting in Slovenia. This event provides evidence of the research capacity building potential of international partnerships.

---

to improve their quality of life and plan for future health needs. Results of participatory research have local applicability and are transferable to other communities.[63]

Given the critical relation between researchers and a community (as much as with individuals under study), the potential benefits and harms for involved communities should be appraised in ethical reviews of studies. The conference identified a problem with ethical review guidelines that are insufficiently focused on the position of communities in study designs.

Recommendation 8

Wonca should organize international ethical review guidelines in particular of participatory (action) research, where researchers work in partnership with communities. These guidelines should address the protection of the community as well as the individual.

Research in Developing Countries

Research in developing countries was reviewed extensively by the assembly, addressing the concern that developing countries had specific needs requiring extra attention. Often the capacity-building strategies that work elsewhere can be used for developing countries, and examples have been provided in the sections discussing PBRNs and mentoring. Mentorship from more developed countries provides powerful opportunities to have substantial effects from the investment of limited resources. Mentoring should be directed at the needs of the developing country rather than driven by the priorities of (commercial) mentors with insufficient ethical review.

Strategies for promoting family medicine research in developing countries should take account of the fact that FPs are often overwhelmed by clinical demands in chaotic systems. There are a number of examples where PBRNs have had a great impact on improving health in developing countries by applying simple recording methods (Vignettes 11, 12). On a larger scale, their epidemiologic analyses could dramatically improve the countries response to community needs.[44,45,75] Focusing on PBRNs and mentoring the well-developed principles of community-oriented primary care in these environments have the potential to contribute to lasting and sustainable improvements in health and wellness.[93-95] Even small amounts of money—for example 1% or 2% of the national budget for health—could, under these circumstances, effect enormous improvement in the health of a country's population.

Recommendation 9

In all recommendations made to support family medicine research, Wonca should address the specific needs and implications for developing countries.

CONCLUSIONS AND RECOMMENDATIONS

It was concluded that through family medicine research the effectiveness and efficiency of health care in all countries could be improved. Strengthening family medicine research is essential to enhance the role of FPs in health care systems, to improve the optimal functioning of health care systems, and to improve the health of populations.

Analysis of the conference discussion identified strengths in family medicine research from around the world and found further resources to support its devel-opment. Mentoring aspiring researchers or research organizations is increasingly driven by international organizations and provides a practical strategy for building research capacity. PBRNs are providing more information on health problems and their solutions in communities. The development of PBRNs can be supported by international collaboration.

In several European countries FPs are playing leadership roles in the biomedical research community, providing encouraging signs that FPs have broken out of their isolation from the research community. There is a need, however, to be more articulate about the achievements of family medicine research and the potential this research holds for improved medical care and improved health.

Mentoring FP researchers and PBRNs promotes a bottom-up research agenda based on evidence gaps experienced in practice. At the same time, the link of family medicine research and researchers with university departments and research institutes is important to enhance rigorous studies methods. A multidisciplinary approach is essential to combine the paradigm of illness and disease with the paradigm of whole patients and their vulnerability or resilience to illness and health-related behavior.[20,96,97] This is the context of family medicine and the complex environment that family medicine research should be able to address.

No country can reasonably expect to improve their health care system without strong primary care. Because of their central service and leadership role in primary care, FPs worldwide must enter into research and development of their research-based discipline. If implemented, the above recommendations will substantially strengthen family medicine research around the world and enhance the care FPs render. Strengthening family medicine research will result in not a few but millions of people benefiting.

To read or post commentaries in response to this article, see it online at http://www.annfamed.org/cgi/content/full/2/suppl_2/S5.

Key words: Family practice; general practice; research development; capacity building, world health

A version of this paper was presented at the Wonca Research Conference, Kingston, Ontario, Canada, March 8-11, 2003.

References

1. Institute of Medicine. Committee on Quality of Health Care in America. *Crossing the Quality Chasm. A New Health System for the 21st Century.* Washington, DC: National Academies Press; 2001.

2. Starfield B. Is primary care essential? *Lancet.* 1994; 344:129-133.

3. Green LA, Fryer, GE, Yawn, BP, Lanier D, Dovey, SM. The ecology of medical care revisited. *N Engl J Med.* 2001; 344:2021-2025.

4. van Weel, C. International research and the discipline of family medicine. *Eur J Gen Pract.* 1999; 5:110-115.

5. Wonca Europe. The European definition of general practice/family medicine. Wonca Europe 2002. Available at: http://www.globalfamilydoctor.com/publications/Euro_Def.pdf. Accessed March 10, 2004.

6. Donaldson M, Yordy K, Vanselow N, eds. *Defining Primary Care: An Interim Report*. Washington, DC: Institute of Medicine; 1994.

7. Rosser WW, Dovey S, Green LA, Phillips R, Fryer E. The evolving role of the family physician in Canada. *Can Med Association J* (Submitted).

8. De Maeseneer JM, De Sutter A. Why research in family medicine? *Ann Fam Med.* 2004;2:(Suppl 2):S17-S22.

9. Green LA. The research domain of family medicine. *Ann Fam Med.* 2004;2(Suppl 2):S23-S29.

10. Del Mar C, Askew D. Building family medicine research capacity. *Ann Fam Med.* 2004;2(Suppl 2):S35-S40.

11. Hutchinson A, Becker L. Styles and methods of family medicine: their impact on the research agenda. *Ann Fam Med.* 2004;2(Suppl 2): S41-S44.

12. Lam CLK. The 21st century: the age of family medicine research? *Ann Fam Med.* 2004;2(Suppl 2):S50-S54.

13. Svab I. Changing research culture. *Ann Fam Med.* 2004;2(Suppl 2): S30-S34.

14. Bentzen N. Family medicine research: implications for Wonca. *Ann Fam Med.* 2004;2(Suppl 2):S45-S49.

15. Sparks B., Gupta S. Research in family medicine in developing countries. *Ann Fam Med.* 2004;2(Suppl 2):S55-S59.

16. Herbert CP. Future of research in family medicine: where to from here? *Ann Fam Med.* 2004;2(Suppl 2):S60-S64.

17. Anonymous. Is primary-care research a lost cause? *Lancet.* 2003; 361:977.

18. Starfield B. Primary Care: *Balancing Health Needs, Services And Technology*. New York, NY: Oxford University Press; 1998.

19. Wonca International Classification Committee. *International Classification of Primary Care, ICPC-2*. 2nd ed. Oxford: Oxford Press, 1998.

20. McWhinney IR. *A Textbook of Family Medicine*. 2nd ed. New York, NY: Oxford University Press; 1997.

21. Rosser WW, Shafir MS. *Evidence-Based Family Medicine*. Hamilton, Decker Inc. 1998.

22. De Melker RA. Diseases: the more common the less studied. *Fam Pract.* 1995;12:84-87.

23. Rosser WW. Applying evidence from randomized controlled trials in general practice. *Lancet.* 1999;353: 661-663.

24. Okkes IM, Oskam SK, Lamberts H. The probability of specific diagnoses for patients presenting with common symptoms to Dutch family physicians. *J Fam Pract.* 2002;51:31-36.

25. van Weel C. Examination of context of medicine. *Lancet.* 2001;357: 733-734.

26. Cochrane collaboration Web site. Available at: http://www.cochrane. org. Accessed March 10, 2004.

27. Dutch College of Family Physicians. Available at: http://nhg.artsennet.nl/content/resources/AMGATE_6059_104_TICH_L748610903/AMGATE_6059_104_TICH_R119952487066081 Accessed March 9, 2004.

28. Guideline Advisory Committee of the Ontario Medical Association/Ministry of Health and Long Term Care of Ontario Web site. Available at: http://www.gacguidelines.ca/. Accessed March 9, 2004.

29. Dutch College of General Practitioners (NHG) Overview of under-researched areas in family medicine. Available at: http://nhg.artsennet.nl/content/resources/AMGATE_6059_104_TICH_L866838437/AMGATE_6059_104_TICH_R1196231005919511 also: Tasche M, Oosterberg E, Kolnaar B, Rosmalen K. Inventarisatie van lacunes in huisartsgeneeskundige kennis. HuisartsWet. 2001;44:91-95. Accessed March 9, 2004.

30. ZonMW research fund 'common morbidity in general practice'. Available at: http://zonmw.collexis.net/default.asp?key=prog. Accessed March 10, 2004.

31. Deconnick S, Boeke AJP, van der Waal I, et al. Incidence and management of oral conditions in general practice. *Br J Gen Pract.* 2003;53:130-133.

32. Koning S, van Suijlekom LWA, Nouwen JL, et al. Fusidic acid cream in the treatment of impetigo in general practice: double blind randomised placebo controlled trial. *Br Med J.* 2002;324:203-206.

33. van Weel C, Gouma DJ, Lamberts SWJ. De bijdrage van klinisch wetenschappelijk onderzoek aan een betere patientenzorg [English abstract]. *Ned Tijdschr Geneesk.* 2003:147:229-233.

34. Nutting PA, Beasley JW, Werner JJ. Asking and answering questions in practice: practice based research networks build the science base of family practice. *JAMA.* 1999; 281:686-688.

35. Green LA, Dovey SM. Practice-based primary care research networks. They work and are ready for full development and support. *BMJ.* 2001;322:567-568.

36. Nutting PA, ed. *Community-Oriented Primary Care: From Principle to Practice.* Washington, DC: US Department of Health and Human Service; 1987.

37. Maynard A. Evidence-based medicine: an incomplete method for informing treatment choices. *Lancet.* 1997;349:126-128.

38. Pincus T. Analyzing long-term outcomes of clinical care without randomized comtrolled clinical trials: the consecutive patient questionnaire database. *J Mind-Body Health.* 1997;13:3-32.

39. Writing Group for the Women's Health Initiative Investigators. Risks and benefits of estrogen plus progesterone in healthy postmenopausal women: principle results from the Women's Health Initiative randomized trial. *JAMA.* 2002;288:321-333.

40. Lagro-Janssen ALM, Rosser WW, van Weel C. Breast cancer and hormone replacement Therapy: up to general practice to collect the pieces. *Lancet.* 2003;362:414-415.

41. de Grauw W, van de Lisdonk EH, van den Hoogen HJM, van Weel C. Cardiovascular morbidity and mortality of type 2 diabetes patients. *Diabetic Med.* 1995;12:117-122.

42. International Federation of Primary Care Research Networks. Available at: http://groups.msn.com/IFPCRN. Accessed March 09, 2004.

43. Lionis C, Trell E. Health needs assessment in general practice: the Cetan approach. *Eur J Gen Pract.* 1999;5:75-77.

44. Sant'Ana AM, Rosser W, Talbot Y. Five years of health care in Sao Jose. *Fam Pract.* 2002;19:410-415.

45. Isaakidis P, Swingler GH, Piennaar EE, Volmink NJ, Ioannina JPA. Relations between burden of disease and randomized evidence in sub-Sahara Africa: survey of research. *Br Med J.* 202;324:702-705.

46. Del Mar CB, Freeman GK, van Weel C. Only a GP: is the solution to the general practice crisis intellectual? *Med J Aust.* 2003;179: 26-29.

47. Rosser W. The decline of family medicine as a career choice. *CMAJ.* 2002;166:1419-1420.

48. Okkes, IM, Jamoulle, M., Lamberts, H., Bentzen, N. ICPC-2-E, the electronic version of ICPC-2. Differences with the printed version and the consequences. *Fam Pract.* 2000;17:101-106.

49. Bentzen N, ed. An international glossary for general practice/family medicine. *Fam Pract.* 1995;12: 341-369.

50. Bentzen N, ed. Wonca Dictionary of General/Family Practice. Copenhagen: *Maanedsskrift for Praktisk Laegegering*, 2003. Available at: http://www.globalfamilydoctor.com. Accessed March 11, 2004.

51. Scottish School of Primary Care. Available at: http://www.sspc.uk.com. Accessed March 09, 2004.

52. Sullivan FM, Lewison G, Clarkson J. What Scottish primary care researchers are doing to recover their standing in the UK. *Health Bull (Edinb).* 2002;60:1-4.

53. Wyke S, Bond C, Morrison J, Ryan K, Sullivan F, for the Office Primary Care Implementation Committee. Research priorities in primary care. A report from the CSO's primary care implementation committee. *Health Bull (Edinb).* 2000 58:426-433.

54. North American Primary Care Research Group Committee on Building Research Capacity and the American Family Medicine Organizations Research Subcommittee. What does it mean to build research capacity? *Fam Med* 2002;34:678-684.

55. Mant D. *Research and Development in Primary Care. National Working Group Report.* Bristol, NHS Executive South and West; 1997.

56. The Netherlands School of Primary Care Research (CaRe). Available at: http://www.researchschoolcare.nl. Accessed March 9, 2004.

57. Lionis C, Stoffers HEJH, Hummers–Pradier E, Griffiths F, Rotar-Pavlic D, Rethans JJ. Setting priorities and identifying barriers for general practice research in Europe. Results from an EGPRN meeting. EGPRN report 2003. Email address EGPRN: hanny.prick@hag.unimaas.nl. Accessed March 10, 2004.

58. van Weel C. The Brisbane Initiative: International Advanced Education for Primary Care Research. The Brisbane Initiative: pursuing advanced research training and the establishment of a future research leadership for primary care. 2003. Available at: http://www.globalfamilydoctor.com .Accessed March 09, 2004.

59. Kochen MM. Excellence in primary care research: which requirements are needed? *Eur J Gen Pract.* 2003;9:39-40.

60. Kalda R, Maaroos HI, Lember M. Motivation and satisfaction among Estonian family doctors working in different settings. *Eur J Gen Pract.* 2000;6:9-15.

61. The European General Practitioners Research Network (EGPRN). Available at: http://www.egprw.org. Accessed March 09, 2004.

62. Royen P van, Griffith F, Lionis C, Rethans JJ, Sandholzer H, Gali F. A research strategy for EGPRW. *Eur J Gen Pract.* 2000;6:69-71.

63. Mccauly AC, Gibson N, Freeman W, et al. Participatory research maximises community and lay involvement. *Br Med J.* 1999;319:774-778.

64. Interfaculty Council of Departments of General Practice: Report results academic practices network 1992-1997 (Interfacing Overleg Huisartsgeneeskunde: Rapportage Academisch Werkveld Huisartsgeneeskunde 1992-1997). Nijmegen: Department of General Practice, University of Nijmegen, 1998.

65. Collaborative group of the Primary Prevention Project (PPP). Low-dose aspirin and vitamin E in people at cardiovascular risk. *Lancet.* 2001;357:89-95.

66. van Weel C, Smith H, Beasley JW. Family practice research networks. Experience from three countries. *J Fam Pract.* 2000;49:938-943.

67. Australian Gouvernment Department of Health and Ageing's Primary Health Care Research, Evaluation Development Strategy. Available at: http://www.phcris.org.au/resources/phcred/PHC_RED_framemet.html. Accessed March 09, 2004.

68. Anonymous. Researcher, clinician or teacher? *Lancet.* 2001;357: 1543.

69. The Netherlands Organisation of Scientific Research and Zon/MW, programme 'Clinician-researcher'. Available at http://www.zonmw.nl/index.asp?a = 32111&rs = 3789&rp = 1. Accessed March 11, 2004.

70. Queens University FP/MSc researcher residency program. Queens University Department of Family Medicine, Kingston, Ontario, Canada. July 2003. Available at: http://www.queensu.ca/fmed/resprojects.htm. Accessed March 09, 2004.

71. Caimi V, Tombesi M, eds. *Medicina Generale.* Turin, Unione Tipografico-Editrice Torinese; 2003.

72. Gunn J. Should Australia develop primary care research networks? *Med J Aust.* 2002;177:63-66.

73. Smith HD, Dunleavey J. Wessex primary care research network: a report on two years progress. *Southampton Health Journal.* 1996;3: 43-47.

74. Metsemakers JF, Hoppener P, Knottnerus JA, Kocken RJ, Limonard CB. Computerized health information in The Netherlands: a registration network of family practices. *Br J Gen Pract.* 1992;42:102-6. Registratie Netwerk Huisartsen (RNH) Available at: http://www.hag.unimaas.nl/RNH. Accessed March 09, 2004).

75. Pather MK. *SASPREN – South African Sentinel Practitioner Research Network Family Practitioner Primary Health Care Surveillance Project. Report for 2000/2001.* Stellenbosch Department of Family Medicine and Primary Care: University of Stellenbosch; 2002.

76. Culpepper L, Froom J. The International Primary Care network: purpose, methods and policies. *Fam Med.* 1988;20:197-201.

77. Green LA, Wood M, Becker L, et al. The Ambulatory sentinel Practice Network: purpose, methods and policies. *J Fam Pract.* 1984;18:275-280.

78. van Weel, C. Validating long term morbidity recording. *J Epidemiol Commun Health.* 1995;49(Suppl 1):29-32.

79. De Maeseneer JM. Huisartsgeneeskunde: een Verkenning [dissertation, English summary]. Belgium: University of Ghent; 1989.

80. Bundesministerium für Bildung und Forschung, networks of competence. Available at: http://www.kompetenznetze.de/index.php?sprache = 2. Accessed March 10, 2004.

81. Lamberts H, Brouwer HJ, Mohrs J. *Reason for Encounter, Episode and Process-oriented Standard Output From the Transition Project.* Amsterdam Department of General Practice/Family Medicine: University of Amsterdam; 1991.

82. Costello A, Zumla A. Moving to research partnerships in developing countries. *BMJ.* 2000;321:827-829.

83. Talbot Y, Batty H, Rosser W. Five weekend national family medicine fellowship: program for faculty development. *Can Fam Phys.* 1997;43: 2151-2157.

84. Department of Family Medicine, Queens University Kingston Ontario /Ontario College of Family Physicians. Five weekend research program: Available at: http://www.queensu.ca/fmed/CSPC-OCFP.htm. Accessed March 12, 2004.

85. Evans PR. Medicine in Europe: the changing scene in general practice in Europe. *Br Med J* 1994:308:645-648.

86. Svab I, Yaphe Y, Correia de Sousa J, Passerine G. An international course for faculty development in family medicine: the Slovenian model. *Med Educ.* 1999;33: 80-81.

87. Kounalakis D, Lionis C, Okkes I, Lamberts H. Developing an appropriate EPR system for the Greek primary care setting. *J Med Sys.* 2003;27:239-246.

88. Koutis A, Isacsson A, Lionis C, Lindholm L, Svenninger K, Fioretos M. Differences in the diagnosis panorama in primary health care in Dalby, Sweden and Spili, Crete. *Scand J Soc Med.* 1993;21:51-58.

89. Lionis C, Koutis A, Antonakis N, Isacsson A, Lindhol L, Fioretos M. Mortality rates in a cardiovascular 'low risk' population in rural Crete. *Fam Pract.* 1993;10:300-304.

90. De Maeseneer J. Optimisation of the vocational training in family medicine in South-Africa: a contribution to the realisation of health for all [Vlir - Own Initiatives. EI - SEL2003-14]. Ghent, Department of Family Medicine and Primary Health Care, 2003. Available at: http://allserv.rug.ac.be/ ~ apeleman/huisartsgeneeskunde Folder/huisartsgeneeskunde/NewFiles/hoofdmenu/hoofdmenu.htm. Accessed March 09, 2004.

91. Green LW, George MA, Daniel M, et al. *Study of Participatory Research in Health Promotion.* Ottawa: Royal Society of Canada; 1994.

92. Phillips WR, Grams GD. Involving patients in a primary care research meeting worked well. *BMJ.* 2003; 326:1329.

93. Iliffe S, Lenihan P, Wallace P, Drennan V, Blanchard M, Harris A. Applying community-oriented primary care methods in British general practice: a case study. *Br J Gen Pract.* 2002:52:646-651.

94. Nutting PA, Wood M, Conner EM. Community oriented primary care in the United States. A status report. *JAMA.* 1985;253:1763-1766.

95. Kark SL, Kark E. An alternative strategy in community health care: community-oriented primary health care. *Isr J Med Sci.* 1983;19:707-713.

96. McWhinney IR. Being a general practitioner: what it means. *Eur J Gen Pract.* 2000;6:135-139.

97. Huygen FJA. *Family Medicine: The Medical Life History Of Families.* New York, NY: Brunner Maze;1982.

CHAPTER 15

Family medicine development in Eastern Europe

Bohumil Seifert

NOMINATED CLASSIC PAPER

Igor Švab, Danica Rotar Pavlič, Smiljka Radić, Paula Vainiomäki. General practice east of Eden: an overview of general practice in Eastern Europe. *Croatian Medical Journal*, 2004; 45(5): 537–42.

The countries of Central and Eastern Europe (CEE) experienced dramatic changes at the end of the 20th century, including changes in primary healthcare. Primary care had been strongly influenced by a specialist polyclinic system, called the Semashko system, and had subsided into international isolation. In the 1990s primary care had a chance to recover its appropriate role and position within the healthcare system.

This was a great time for those of us in CEE, despite the fact that our journey back to Europe was difficult. General practice was in a very poor state. Its recognition among other medical specialties was low, its image was bad, and it had difficulty attracting doctors. General practice was seen as a second-choice discipline. General practitioners in CEE had few international contacts and very limited international experience.

But we were enthusiastic. In the 1990s we suddenly faced many new perspectives and possibilities. We could travel and meet foreign colleagues, participate in courses and conferences, join WONCA networks, and engage in research and quality projects. We learned, absorbed and adopted ideas, knowledge and skills. Finally we decided also to meet the challenge of working together internationally.

I was lucky to belong to a generation of enthusiastic general practitioners from CEE, many of whom later became global WONCA and network leaders, including Igor Švab, Janko Kersnik and Matea Bulc from Slovenia, Mladenka Vrcić-Keglević from Croatia, Adam Windak from Poland, and Václav Beneš from the Czech Republic.

There are a few articles in scientific journals reporting and reflecting on these exciting developments and this Guest Editorial, written by Professor Igor Švab and colleagues, is one of the most significant. This paper is about the lessons that were learnt in the CEE region, showing the growth of general practice in all its European diversity. There are many aspects and issues highlighted in the paper, which remain high on the agenda of general practice in Europe, including the need for further development of the academic discipline of general practice, the recruitment of the next generation of family physicians, and the mutual benefits of collaboration. One of the key messages from this paper is about the past, current and future role of WONCA Europe – the European Society of General Practice/Family Medicine, serving as a platform for learning and for sharing successes and challenges, and functioning as a forum where communication between general practitioners and other parties can be fostered.

ABOUT THE LEAD AUTHOR OF THIS PAPER

Igor Švab graduated from the Ljubljana medical faculty in Slovenia in 1981. From 1983 to 1991, he worked as a rural GP. In 1991, he moved to the National Institute of Public Health in Ljubljana to help run the vocational training scheme for general practitioners in Slovenia. During this time, he started his PhD studies on multivariate analysis of the reasons for referral from general practice. Igor continues to work in part-time general practice, as well as being Professor of Family Medicine in the Department of Family Medicine at the Ljubljana University School of Medicine.

For many years, Igor has contributed to the development of general practice in an outstanding way, both nationally and internationally. He served as President of WONCA Europe from 2004 to 2010. His major contributions to WONCA have been in his role as an ambassador for family medicine and WONCA in the countries of CEE. He has been involved in many family medicine development projects, especially in the development of family medicine in Estonia, Turkey, Montenegro and Macedonia. In 2010, in recognition of his many contributions to European general practice, Igor was awarded Fellowship of WONCA, the global organisation's highest honour, following nomination by the Royal College of General Practitioners and the Dutch College of General Practitioners.

ABOUT THE NOMINATOR OF THIS PAPER

Associate Professor Bohumil Seifert is an academic general practitioner and head of the Department of General Practice at the Charles University in Prague in the Czech

Republic. He has been a Czech representative on WONCA's European and World Councils and on several international family doctor networks. He chaired the Host Organizing Committee of WONCA's World Conference, in Prague, in June 2013.

> 'One of the things I realised during my medical training was that no other discipline was wide-ranging enough to satisfy my need for a comprehensive approach to human beings. You would probably find all other medical specialities fascinating but you would always be missing something.'

Associate Professor Bohumil Seifert, Czech Republic

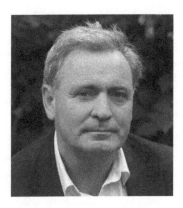

Attribution:

We attribute the original publication of *General practice east of Eden: an overview of general practice in Eastern Europe* to *Croatian Medical Journal*. With thanks to Editor in Chief, Professor Srećko Gajović.

CROATIAN MEDICAL JOURNAL

CMJ

45(5):537-542,2004

GUEST EDITORIAL

General Practice East of Eden: an Overview of General Practice in Eastern Europe

Igor Švab[1], Danica Rotar Pavlič[1], Smiljka Radić[2], Paula Vainiomäki[3]

[1]Department of Family Medicine, Ljubljana University School of Medicine, Ljubljana, Slovenia; [2]Primary Health Center Zemun, Zemun, Serbia and Montenegro; [3]Task Force on Communicable Disease Control in the Baltic Sea Region STAKES, Helsinki; and General Practice, University Hospital, Turku, Finland

Aim. To review the status of family medicine in Eastern European countries, specifically the position of the discipline within the health care system, its academic status, and expected trends in the development of the discipline.

Methods. We used available data in the literature and information gathered from personal contacts with members of European Society of General Practice/Family Medicine (ESGP/FM) expert groups, European Academy of Teachers in General Practice (EURACT), and European General Practice Research Network (EGPRN). Personal interviews with key informants from countries that do not have members in these organizations were used. We also performed a Medline search using terms "primary health care" and "family medicine".

Results. It was difficult to get standardized information about the issues addressed. In some countries, contact persons and articles were impossible to find. Because of that, information from some countries is lacking (e.g. Belarus, Ukraine, the Kavkaz states and Central Asian republics). The information from the 14 countries showed that family medicine was formally widely recognized as a specific discipline. In 13 of them, there were some programs of vocational training. In 10 countries, academic recognition has resulted in rapid development in the past two decades, especially after 1989, but in Bulgaria and Moldova we found no evidence of family medicine departments.

Conclusion. The position of general practice in most Central and Eastern European countries is formally adequate, but a lot of effort will still be needed to achieve the desired level of its recognition and quality.

Key words: delivery of health care; Europe, Eastern; family practice; health policy; primary health care; Turkey

Europe is characterized by diversity in all areas of society. One of the areas of diversity is the way health care is delivered. There is a powerful movement towards integration in the European Union (EU) and the countries which want to join it. The process is pushing the systems closer in many areas, including health care. But the countries that do not belong to the European Union lack this kind of overall trend towards integration. On the other hand, these countries comprise a bigger population and land area than EU member nations, especially if Europe is defined according to the World Health Organization (WHO) criteria (1,2).

Family medicine has for a very long time been recognized as the key element of a good health care system. This importance is stressed in many declarations, policy papers, and research articles. The countries of Central and Eastern Europe have made significant changes to their health care systems in the last twenty years and have invariably declared family medicine a cornerstone of their new policies. The question remains whether family medicine in these countries has been able to meet the challenges put forward by policymakers and was provided with sufficient resources to meet these challenges. This phenomenon occurred in many countries, but especially in Russia. There are many declarations concerning the importance of family medicine, yet the actual results indicate that family medicine is largely ignored (3-5). Anecdotal information about the actual position of family medicine in these countries gives rise to speculations about large differences.

Family medicine is largely influenced by the context in which it is practiced (6). The issues that are of great relevance to a British general practitioner are not at all relevant to a physician working in Bosnia and Herzegovina. Although the principles are the same, the issues may be tremendously different (7). Countries that want to change their health care systems by raising the importance of primary health care need to take into consideration the actual situation in the country and its potential to carry out the necessary tasks.

The European Society of General Practice/Family Medicine (ESGP/FM) clearly identified the area of Central and Eastern Europe as a priority for the development of the discipline. Although the society represents the biggest and strongest region within the world organization, all of the European countries are

Švab et al: General Practice in Eastern Europe   Croat Med J 2004;45:537-542

still not members, and some of the members are in great need of support. As part of this strategy, the ESGP/FM executive board has deliberately located its meetings in countries of Central and Eastern Europe (e.g. Sarajevo, Belgrade, Ankara) in order to support the development of the discipline in these countries and to gain clearer information about the actual position of general practice.

Three sets of issues invariably come under consideration when the position of family medicine is discussed:

1) the position of the discipline within the health care system (whether family medicine is officially recognized as a separate discipline with distinct training and a professional society);

2) the academic status of the discipline (the position of family medicine within the universities); and

3) what the existing plans are for the development of family medicine in the future.

The impression from informal contacts is that many very interesting activities are going on in these countries and some of them are of a clear benefit to the development of the discipline. Yet such informal information is hardly adequate to assess the situation of family medicine in a country in order to make policy decisions. Other sources of information would be useful, but there is a lack of good quality comparable data and good quality published papers in this area.

In order to get a clearer picture of the position of family medicine in the countries of Central and Eastern Europe and to create a basis for a clearer policy in this exciting region, an attempt was made to provide an overview of the situation in these countries by focusing on these three issues. This overview is based on the information from resource persons within the society and readily available published information.

Methods

In order to gather the information, we first approached resource persons from two European network organizations that represent their country in either the European Academy of Teachers in General Practice (EURACT) or the European General Practice Research Network (EGPRN). This approach was used for Estonia, Lithuania, Poland, Czech Republic, Romania, Slovakia, and Turkey. The second source of information was used for countries that have no representatives in the European network organizations of general practice (Latvia, Russia, Moldova). In these cases an expert who is running family medicine development programs in these countries (PV) was used as a resource person and co-author of this article. The third source of information were field visits and contacts with local family physicians and representatives of family medicine organizations. This approach was used for Slovenia, Croatia, Bosnia and Herzegovina, Serbia and Montenegro, and Turkey. A semi-structured interview was conducted with each of them, addressing all three issues. In addition, respondents were asked to provide written information about the most relevant issues in family medicine in the countries they were interviewed about.

As a validation, supplemental information about the situation in the countries was sought from other sources. Most of this additional information was obtained by a Medline search of literature describing the development of family medicine in these countries. In the search, the following descriptors and their combinations were used: Primary Health Care; Family Practice; Europe, Eastern; Baltic States; Bosnia-Herzegovina; Croatia; Czech Republic; Estonia; Latvia; Lithuania; Moldova; Poland; Romania; Russia; Slovenia; Slovakia; Turkey; and Yugoslavia. Additional in-

formation about these issues was also sought by a simple general Internet search using the same descriptors. The analysis yielded 18 articles when combining the term "family medicine" with the name of a specific country and 57 articles when combining the term "primary health care" with the name of the country. In cases of Czech Republic, Latvia, Lithuania, Moldova, and Slovakia, no articles were found.

Results

Position of Discipline within Health Care System

The position of family medicine in these countries is strongly influenced by the health care systems that have existed in the past (Table 1). Two main systems can be identified, whose legacy has influenced the position of the discipline. Countries that were part of the former USSR (Russia, Estonia, Latvia, Lithuania, Belarus, Moldova, Ukraine, Georgia, Armenia, Azerbaijan, Kazakhstan, Turkmenistan, Uzbekistan, Tajikistan, and Kyrgyzstan) and its satellites (Poland, Czech Republic, Slovakia, Hungary, Bulgaria, and Romania) have had the Shemasko system of health care, based on a system of specialist policlinics. Family medicine was often not officially recognized or promoted, because it was believed that good quality health care could only be delivered by specialists. In addition, basic medical education led to a specialist level degree, and no real generalists existed. In contrast, the countries of former Yugoslavia have had a firmly established position of family medicine, which was (at least formally) considered to be a specialty equal to others. The Yugoslav system also included vocational training for general practice, which was introduced in 1961, although it was not obligatory. The other important reason for the much better position of the discipline within the health care system was the Andrija Štampar School of Public Health, which was a center of expertise and training in this area and the collaborative center for the WHO in primary care (8).

The other factor that has strongly influenced the current position of family medicine was the motivation of policymakers to make changes in society that would demonstrate the shift away from the old systems. In the countries that had a Shemashko system of health care, this motivation was especially strong, as in Estonia (9) and to a lesser extent, Latvia and Lithuania (10). In these countries, most of general practice service was performed by therapists, who are doctors, working in primary care, not specifically educated to be general practitioners. They mostly do not take care of women and children or perform surgical procedures. This practically meant that their main work was largely administrative. The introduction of a new health care system, based on family medicine, was recognized as a priority of health care policymakers and has received strong support from the government, enabling the retraining of therapists into family physicians.

Other countries have been more careful in introducing changes, shifting from the old policlinic system to a new one much more gradually. Some countries made formal changes to their health care system in the past, but have started to introduce change recently (e.g. Bulgaria), while in others there is no indi-

Švab et al: General Practice in Eastern Europe

Croat Med J 2004;45:537-542

Table 1. Overview of information about the development of family medicine in selected countries. Countries are listed in alphabetic order according to 3 areas of interest: position of family medicine within the health care system, academic status of the discipline, and future trends*

Country	Position within the system	Academic status	Trends and comments
Bulgaria	FM officially recognized ESGP/FM member vocational training exists	no departments	slow development
Bosnia and Herzegovina	FM officially recognized ESGP/FM member vocational training exists	departments exist	external support ending
Croatia	FM officially recognized ESGP/FM member vocational training reestablished after a period of stagnation	departments exist	leading country in FM development in former Yugoslavia
Czech Republic	FM officially recognized ESGP/FM member vocational training exists	departments exist	
Estonia	FM officially recognized ESGP/FM member vocational training exists	departments exist	successful cooperation with Finland
Latvia	FM officially recognized ESGP/FM member vocational training exists	no department	some academic development
Lithuania	FM officially recognized ESGP/FM member vocational training exists	department exists	retraining in progress
Moldova	FM not yet recognized not a member of ESGP/FM no vocational training	no departments	no real development
Poland	FM officially recognized ESGP/FM member vocational training exists	departments exist	many EU-funded programs
Romania	FM officially recognized ESGP/FM member vocational training exists	departments exist	cooperation with The Netherlands
Russia	FM officially recognized not a member of ESGP/FM program of vocational training exists	departments exist	implementation of vocational training not yet properly organized, many programs, great need
Serbia and Montenegro	FM officially recognized applied for membership of ESGP/FM vocational training exist	departments exist	period of a long isolation
Slovenia	FM officially recognized ESGP/FM member vocational training exists	departments exist	
Turkey	FM officially recognized ESGP/FM member vocational training exists	departments exist	

*Abbreviations: FM – Family medicine; ESGP/FM – European Society of General Practice/Family Medicine.

cation that the situation is likely to change in the near future (e.g. Moldova). In Russia, the concept of family medicine was introduced in 1992 by a federal order. Due to problems in its implementation, a new law was passed in 2002 to ratify an official position for family medicine among the medical disciplines and also to define responsibilities of family doctors and nurses in addition to the equipment needed. The big drop-out rate from the profession (according to estimates, only 20-30% of trained and retrained family doctors practice their profession, often because of poor salary) and not enough family doctors' posts are impeding implementation.

Enthusiasm for change also varied greatly among the countries of former Yugoslavia. Some, like Slovenia, have opted for a slow transition from a previous health care system to a new one, and have introduced changes gradually, without abandoning the system of existing health centers. On the other hand, others have experienced dramatic changes. Bosnia and Herzegovina has been faced with the destruction of the entire health care system and has experimented with various models, based on foreign help. The most successful aid program in this country was based on the premise that family medicine has to be introduced from scratch, and that the previous system is of no use. Serbia and Montenegro, however, have not implemented any changes in the system, and have started to consider the possibility only recently.

Turkey has a health care system which does not resemble the ones mentioned above. Currently, primary health care is largely provided by therapists on the primary level, but family medicine as a specialty is recognized and there are plans for its implementation on a larger scale.

Teamwork is one of the important characteristics of family doctors' work, and nurses are supposed to be important team members. The position of nurses and the availability of family and public health nurses' services differ considerably among these countries. In Russia, nurses have not been officially considered as health professionals and understandably this makes team work difficult. The new federal order, issued in 2002, will probably change the situa-

Švab et al: General Practice in Eastern Europe   Croat Med J 2004;45:537-542

tion for the better. In Baltic countries, the conditions for family doctors' nurses are variable: in Estonia, the family doctor is responsible for providing nurses services within his/her office region. In Latvia, authorities supervise and pay for nurses' services in the rural areas, but not in the cities. The situation in former Yugoslavia was very different, since nurses were always considered as an integral part of the family medicine team, and were hired and paid by the health centers, just like doctors.

Academic Status of Discipline

The key indicator of the academic status of the discipline is its position within the university. The Shemashko system did not recognize family medicine as an academic discipline; therefore no departments of family medicine existed. The transition of systems in the 1990's was marked by a rapid growth of departments of family medicine. Quite often the heads of departments were not family physicians by training, but rather other clinical specialists who had fulfilled the academic criteria for the position. Again, the Baltic States, especially Estonia, were very successful in establishing the position of family medicine within the university. Successes in establishing departments of family medicine were also reported in Lithuania, Poland (11), Romania (12), Hungary, Czech Republic, and Slovakia. Their role and position seems variable. Some are independent, with a strong contribution to the university (e.g. Tartu, Krakow), while some still struggle for proper recognition. On the other hand, there are still countries (e.g. Moldova) that have no departments or teaching of family medicine at the university level. In northwest Russia, there are several recently established departments of family medicine at the university level. Undergraduate level teaching will be provided mainly through optional courses, but postgraduate training has a more formal position within the federally defined curricula (13,14).

The countries of former Yugoslavia, on the other hand, have traditionally had departments of general practice, mainly due to the Andrija Štampar School of Public Health, which was the center of academic development in this region. The department of general practice in Zagreb has existed since 1974 and was involved in undergraduate and postgraduate education. Departments in Rijeka, Osijek, and Split have also been founded in Croatia. General practice was also taught in Belgrade on the postgraduate level. The isolation of Serbia was one of the reasons why the academic development in this country was halted and now faces serious problems due to lack of young experts. The department in Ljubljana, Slovenia, was established in 1995 and has become a major player in the development of the discipline. In Bosnia and Herzegovina, the departments were created as a part of the development of family medicine programs after the war (15).

Reports from Turkey indicate very strong development of the academic position of family medicine, with departments being rapidly established throughout the country (16).

Future Trends

The expected overall trends in family medicine development are positive. All the respondents were positive about the future position of the discipline and its academic development, which seems rather rapid. Nevertheless, some threats were also identified. One of the main threats in the development of family medicine is the political will of policymakers to continue current development programs. Political instability in some of the countries, leading to changes in government policies is also an important issue. Bosnia and Herzegovina, which has relied heavily on support from external sources, is faced with the problem of developing the discipline further while the externally funded projects are ending and the agencies that have supported the development of family medicine are moving to other places. Rapid changes are anticipated in Serbia and Montenegro which are now being introduced to international cooperation after a rather long period of isolation.

The assessment of the challenges facing family medicine in Lithuania seems applicable to the whole region: 1) to make all graduate family doctors practice as family doctors, 2) to regard prevention as more important than problem solving, 3) to make family doctors provide the full scope of services, and 4) to create incentives to deliver high quality and comprehensive services using team approach.

Discussion

As in any survey, the validity of our information is of key importance. Because of the nature of our information gathering, bias by informants could be problematic. We have tried to minimize this risk. We have been very careful in trying to select the appropriate informants and decided that the EURACT council members who represent family medicine teachers from every country should have the best insight into the academic position of family medicine in these countries. Although in most cases we had only one informant, we tried to validate the information and to support it with information from other sources: e.g. the Internet and published articles. A Medline search proved a good method of validating information, especially for Estonia, Poland, Croatia, and Bosnia and Herzegovina. However, we were not successful in obtaining informants from some countries of interest (e.g. Belarus, Ukraine, the Kavkaz states, and the Central Asian republics). This clearly limits the scope of this paper, but a comprehensive overview of the situation was never our aim.

We have managed to identify some important and relevant dilemmas.

Relation to Heritage

Primary health care is provided in every health care system, still it differs in the way in which it is provided. The functions of family medicine can be, ideally, performed by well trained family physicians or, in a less favorable situation, by other therapists that do not have adequate knowledge of the discipline and gain some of this knowledge intuitively by working in practice. It seems interesting that our informants often

Švab et al: General Practice in Eastern Europe   Croat Med J 2004;45:537-542

expressed the view that family medicine did not previously exist in the countries that have been successful in its radical introduction. It seems that the role of former district therapists did not fulfill even the basic requirements of family medicine and that they are now very aware of progress made in recent years. The need to start from the beginning and to reject everything that existed before the reform was most often mentioned in relation to existing therapists, especially in the countries of the post-Shemashko systems. Powerful motivation to give up the Shemashko system has also had less beneficial by-products, e.g. many preventive services were withdrawn for a long time. Nursing as a profession also partly disappeared, and efforts have been put into re-establishing the system. This was probably an indication that the system was not providing adequate results and services.   Still there are problems in implementing the family doctor-based health care e.g. in providing adequate posts and resources for family doctors (Moldova, Russia).

The relation to heritage is more complex in the countries of former Yugoslavia (17-19). Although the health care systems at the beginning were almost the same, the approach to change was different. Some have kept the system unchanged, some have made modifications, while the others have totally abandoned it. This probably reflects the quality that the previous system has achieved in the various countries. A similar dilemma is seen in Turkey, where academic family physicians have problems in establishing dialogue with existing therapists, who have a genuine need to further develop their discipline but do not have enough formal training. Cooperation of both groups of therapists would generally be recommended, since it could create a synergy. But, on the other hand, it can also be a cause of problems and may put a stop to the further development of family medicine, and result in the duplication of general practice societies and their unnecessary competition.

In former Yugoslavia, a further dilemma exists, which relates to the former specialization of general practice. Since almost all of the countries have decided to start a new specialty of family medicine, three groups of general practitioners now exist: untrained general practitioners, trained "specialists in general practice" and new "specialists in family medicine." In some countries, family medicine is recognized as a continuum of the previous specialty of general practice (Slovenia), whereas in others (e.g. Bosnia and Herzegovina), it is considered as being completely different and the relation is less clear.

Reliance on Own Sources or External Support?

There are two aspects of this dilemma. The first is how much of general practice development should be left to foreign experts and how much needs to be done locally. There are many good examples of bilateral cooperation: Finland and Estonia, The Netherlands and Romania, Canada and Bosnia and Herzegovina. Foreign experts in most of these cases bring with them the latest expertise in the field of family medicine, but often lack experience and insight into the local situation, which may create problems in implementing suggested solutions in the local setting. One key measure of success of such an approach is whether the changes suggested by the program will be sustainable after the program is over. Sustainability and relevance to the local situation should be strongly emphasized in program planning, performing and also in the phasing-out situation.

The other aspect of this problem relates to the academic position of the discipline. Almost all countries have identified the need for the academic development of the discipline, although the approaches have differed. Some countries have staffed departments with clinical specialists who have fulfilled academic criteria in order to speed up the process of academic development. If the new chairs are able to incorporate the principles of family medicine in teaching and research, this approach is useful. But the danger of introducing a clinical specialist who fails to teach the principles of the discipline, but instead transfers their specialty clinical teaching to yet another department, seems real.

One critical issue is the recruitment of the younger generation of family physicians. In many retraining programs, especially in Russia, professionals near retirement have been the main group interested in retraining to become family doctors. To sustain the family medicine movement, incentives have to be created, especially directed towards the younger generation.

In conclusion, our survey showed that family medicine was almost universally recognized as a specific discipline. Some countries have shown great improvement in the development of the discipline over the last two decades, especially after 1989. Strategies for achieving this position have differed and were full of difficulties. Even if one can be positive about the achievements of the past, the current position of family medicine differs among the countries. Whereas in some countries, family medicine has been clearly established and has a strong academic position, equal to the position in the EU (Estonia, Slovenia, and Croatia), in many countries family medicine is still in its infancy and will need support. This is an important challenge for international organizations of family medicine. The benefits of collaboration are mutual. The role of the European society of family medicine in this respect is to foster communication between general practitioners in the field and the policymakers and to serve as a forum where these successes and challenges can be discussed and learned from.

Acknowledgements

The authors greatly acknowledge the help in obtaining the information about the situation to the following respondents: European Academy of Teachers in Family Medicine council members – Okay Basak, Ivanka Bogrova, Margus Lember, Iuliana Popa, Mladenka Vrcić Keglević, Adam Windak, and Egle Žebiene; European General Practice Research Network members – Heidi Ingrid Maaroos and Hakan Yaman.

References

1 Saltman RB, Figueras J, Sakellarides C, editors. Critical challenges for health care reform in Europe. Buckingham (UK): Open University Press; 1998.

2 Saltman RB, Figueras J, editors. European health care reform: analysis of current strategies. Copenhagen: Regional Office for Europe, World Health Organisation; 1997.

3 Barker LR. Recent trans-European initiatives in general practice. Arch Fam Med. 1999;8:379-81.

4 Boelen C, Haq C, Hunt V, Rivo M, Shahady E. Improving health systems: the contribution of family medicine; a guidebook. Singapore: WONCA (World Academy of Family Doctors), Bestprint publications; 2002.

5 Boerma WG, Fleming DM. The role of general practice in primary health care. Geneva: World Health Organization; 1998.

6 Boerma WG. Profiles of general practice in Europe. An international study of variation in the tasks of general practitioners. Utrecht, The Netherlands: NIVEL; 2003.

7 Allen J, Gay B, Crebolder H, Heyrman J, Svab I, Ram P. The European definitions of the key features of the discipline of general practice: the role of the GP and core competencies. Br J Gen Pract. 2002;52:526-7.

8 Borovečki A, Belicza B, Orešković S. 75th anniversary of Andrija Stampar School of Public Health – what can we learn from our past for the future? Croat Med J. 2002;43:371-3.

9 Lember M. A policy of introducing a new contract and funding system of general practice in Estonia. Int J Health Plann Manage. 2002;17:41-53.

10 Lovkyte L, Reamy J, Padaiga Z. Physicians resources in Lithuania: change comes slowly. Croat Med J. 2003; 44:207-13

11 Okkes IM, Polderman GO, Fryer GE, Yamada T, Bujak M, Oskam SK, et al. The role of family practice in different health care systems: a comparison of reasons for encounter, diagnoses, and interventions in primary care

populations in the Netherlands, Japan, Poland, and the United States. J Fam Pract. 2002;51:72-3.

12 Van Es JC. Dutch-Romanian connection on family medicine. Lancet. 2001;357:1713.

13 Toon PD. Reforming the Russian health service. BMJ. 1998;317:741-2.

14 Ministry of Health of the Russian Federation. Order No 350. On improving the out-patient care to the population of Russian Federation. November 20, 2002.

15 Godwin M, Hodgetts G, Bardon E, Seguin R, Packer D, Geddes J. Primary care in Bosnia and Herzegovina. Health care and health status in general practice ambulatory care centers. Can Fam Physician. 2001;47:289-97.

16 Ersoy F, Sarp N. Restructuring the primary health care services and changing profile of family physicians in Turkey. Fam Pract. 1998;15:576-8.

17 Hebrang A. Reorganization of the Croatian health care system. Croat Med J. 1994;35:130-6.

18 Hrabač B, Ljubić B, Bagarić I. Basic package of health entitlements and solidarity in the Federation of Bosnia and Herzegovina. Croat Med J. 2000;41:287-93.

19 Hebrang A, Henigsberg N, Erdeljic V, Foro S, Turek S, Zlatar M. Privatization of the Croatian health care system: effect on indicators of health care accessibility in general medicine [in Croatian]. Lijec Vjesn. 2002;124: 239-43.

Correspondence to:
Igor Švab
Department of Family Medicine
Ljubljana University School of Medicine
Poljanski nasip 58
1000 Ljubljana, Slovenia
igor.svab@mf.uni-lj.si

CHAPTER 16

New perspectives on evidence-based medicine

Trisha Greenhalgh

NOMINATED CLASSIC PAPER

John Gabbay, Andrée le May. Evidence based guidelines or collectively constructed 'mindlines?' Ethnographic study of knowledge management in primary care. *British Medical Journal*, 2004; 329: 1013.

In early 2004, Tony Delamothe, Deputy Editor of the *British Medical Journal* (BMJ), asked me to referee this paper, which he was 'pretty sure' he was going to reject. But after reading it, I could not have been more at odds with Tony's initial inclination. I thought this was the most important paper I'd ever been sent to referee by the BMJ.

Why? Because, at multiple levels (philosophical, theoretical, methodological, empirical), this paper confronted the prevailing wisdom on evidence-based guidelines. Philosophically and theoretically, it challenged two key assumptions: that research-based knowledge could be unproblematically captured and codified in written guidelines, and that clinical practice was, more or less, a rational exercise in applying this abstracted knowledge. Rather, suggested Gabbay and le May, research knowledge, as applied to clinical practice in particular situations ('knowledge-in-practice-in-context'), was both individually embodied and socially shared; a defining feature was its fluidity and continuing contestation within a community of practitioners over time.

Methodologically, the paper rejected evidence-based medicine's hierarchy of evidence (which would privilege randomised trials of guideline-on versus guideline-off with a goal of reaching normative conclusions about what *should* happen) in favour of a naturalistic (ethnographic) design that carefully studied what actually *did* happen in clinical medicine.

Empirically, this study found that 'practitioners did not go through the steps that are traditionally associated with the linear-rational model of evidence based health care – not once in the whole time we were observing them'. Rather, good clinicians embodied key aspects of guidelines; they applied them intuitively and engaged with them critically and collectively – in rather the same way as good parents engage critically and collectively with parenting handbooks.

This paper has been widely cited and has inspired a genre of critical research into evidence-based practice.

ABOUT THE AUTHORS OF THIS PAPER

John Gabbay and Andrée le May, who work as equal partners, are professors emeriti at the University of Southampton in the United Kingdom. Each has devoted their career to the interface of research, practice, education and management; together they now research how knowledge enters clinical practice, policy and learning. Having qualified in medicine, John worked at Cambridge University on the historical and social origins of medical knowledge before he entered public health. In the 1980s in Oxford and London he became interested in health services organisation, involving himself in the development and evaluation of clinical audit. Until 2004 he directed the Wessex Institute for Health Research and Development, and the National Coordinating Centre for Health Technology Assessment in the United Kingdom.

Andrée graduated from Chelsea College and Charing Cross Hospital with a degree in nursing and registration as a general nurse. Before starting her first lecturing post at Surrey University in 1990, she held a variety of community nursing posts, and a Department of Health Doctoral Studentship for studies on touch and older people. However, it was working as an 'R&D specialist nurse' in London that irretrievably immersed her in trying to help practitioners use best evidence in everyday practice.

ABOUT THE NOMINATOR OF THIS PAPER

Trisha Greenhalgh is Professor of Primary Care Health Sciences at the University of Oxford. She studied Medical, Social and Political Sciences at the University of Cambridge and Clinical Medicine at Oxford before training as an academic general practitioner. She leads a programme of research at the interface between the social sciences and medicine.

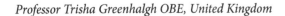

'Family comes first.'

Professor Trisha Greenhalgh OBE, United Kingdom

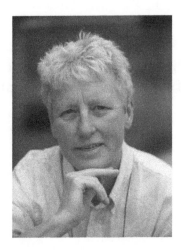

Attribution:

We attribute the original publication of *Evidence based guidelines or collectively constructed 'mindlines?'* to *British Medical Journal*.

With thanks to Editor in Chief, Fiona Godlee, and Laura Lacey.

Primary care

Evidence based guidelines or collectively constructed "mindlines?" Ethnographic study of knowledge management in primary care

John Gabbay, Andrée le May

Abstract

Objective To explore in depth how primary care clinicians (general practitioners and practice nurses) derive their individual and collective healthcare decisions.

Design Ethnographic study using standard methods (non-participant observation, semistructured interviews, and documentary review) over two years to collect data, which were analysed thematically.

Setting Two general practices, one in the south of England and the other in the north of England.

Participants Nine doctors, three nurses, one phlebotomist, and associated medical staff in one practice provided the initial data; the emerging model was checked for transferability with general practitioners in the second practice.

Results Clinicians rarely accessed and used explicit evidence from research or other sources directly, but relied on "mindlines"—collectively reinforced, internalised, tacit guidelines. These were informed by brief reading but mainly by their own and their colleagues' experience, their interactions with each other and with opinion leaders, patients, and pharmaceutical representatives, and other sources of largely tacit knowledge. Mediated by organisational demands and constraints, mindlines were iteratively negotiated with a variety of key actors, often through a range of informal interactions in fluid "communities of practice," resulting in socially constructed "knowledge in practice."

Conclusions These findings highlight the potential advantage of exploiting existing formal and informal networking as a key to conveying evidence to clinicians.

Introduction

The promotion of evidence based health care over the past decade has resulted in several dilemmas. Firstly, the proponents of evidence based health care advocate importing explicit knowledge from the world of research and incorporating it into practice,[1-3] whereas the parallel vogue for knowledge management in the industrial sector has emphasised methods to elicit and promulgate practitioners' tacit knowledge or "knowledge in practice."[4-8] Secondly, many clinicians are concerned that the evidence based healthcare movement may, in its understandable enthusiasm to reduce idiosyncratic, suboptimal practice, undervalue the importance of tacit clinical knowledge in practice by naively promoting prescriptive guidelines that encourage "cookbook" practice. Thirdly, the overwhelming influence of local context on attempts to change clinical practice has presented almost insuperable challenges to the search for simple generalised techniques for implementing research evidence.[9-12]

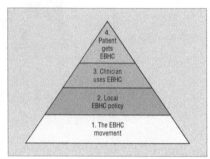

Fig 1   Four levels of evidence based health care

Fourthly, the evidence from psychologists about the role of shortcuts such as "scripts," "heuristics," and "rules of thumb" in clinical decision making,[13-15] which itself tends to play down the social and organisational context, has been generally forgotten in the over-rationalist model implicit in evidence based health care.

Successful implementation of research evidence will require a deeper understanding of the processes of collective "sense making" by which knowledge, both explicit and tacit and from whatever sources, is negotiated, constructed, and internalised in routine practice. Raw research information can be transformed into knowledge in practice at many levels, so it is helpful to consider evidence based health care separately as (1) a social movement with clear values and conventions[16]; (2) a local context in which evidence based policies are agreed; (3) an individual clinician using the accepted evidence based approach; and (4) patients receiving evidence based treatment (fig 1).

Although each of these different levels can operate independently (for instance, a patient might serendipitously receive an evidence based treatment when none of the other levels of evidence based health care is in place), they tend to be closely related. Yet much of the work on the implementation of research evidence conflates them or ignores their inter-relationships.

We set out to illuminate some of the reasons behind the inherent tensions described above. Our research aimed to study explicitly the ways in which primary care practitioners—general practitioners (GPs) and practice nurses—use evidence in their day to day decisions about the management of patients, both at an individual level (levels 3 and 4) and in their collective discussions about best practice (level 2), and how these interact. We were interested to understand the social and organisational

Primary care

processes by which evidence, information, and knowledge—tacit or explicit—become transformed into knowledge in practice.

Methods

Ethnography underpinned the data collection, analysis, and interpretation phases of our study.[17-19] We purposively selected and gained access to two highly regarded general practices. "Lawndale," where we did our main ethnography, is a rural teaching practice in the south of England; the practice population is relatively elderly and middle class. The other practice, "Urbchester" is a contrasting, university based, inner city practice in the north of England, which treats a high proportion of unemployed and immigrant patients as well as students. We used Urbchester to expand and check out our findings from Lawndale.

In Lawndale we studied all of the practitioners (nine doctors, including one GP trainee; three nurses; and a phlebotomist) and associated administrative staff intermittently over two years. We analysed their use of information and knowledge in clinician-patient interactions in the general practitioners' surgeries and nurses' clinics and in practice meetings. We collected data through non-participant observation and semistructured formal and informal interviews, supplemented where appropriate by documentary review of guidelines or practice protocols. Typically, we would briefly discuss a clinical encounter to explore why the clinician believed he or she had acted in a particular way. The observations and informal interviews were detailed in fieldwork notes; four of the formal interviews were tape recorded and transcribed.

We also used unstructured non-participant observation to study a range of other clinician-clinician and clinician-support staff interactions in Lawndale practice meetings in which practice policy was reflected on and formulated. Three of these meeting were recorded and transcribed, we documented the others by using written fieldwork notes, as our piloting suggested that verbatim transcription was not a cost effective method for our purposes. Our complete dataset (box 1) therefore included individual clinical and general policy making encounters, with an auditable trail of fieldwork notes and thematic analyses.

The principal analysis focused on our records of the observations and interviews. We analysed these thematically by noting and coding each piece of information in the fieldwork notes and interview transcripts and allocating these to emerging themes (this was done independently by JG for GP focused data and by AIM for nurse focused data); both researchers then discussed and iteratively reviewed these as the themes developed. This process involved transferring each relevant statement in the field notes and interview transcripts on to around 500 hundred "Post-it" notes and clustering these into emerging themes (box 2). Our analysis was informed by several theoretical frameworks rather than being a simple grounded theory approach. We were, for example, mindful of the role of social and organisational context in the construction and use of knowledge,[8-12] of collective sense making,[20] and of the role of communities of practice in knowledge management.[21-23] However, we were not testing any hypothesis or preconceived models. During this process, we noted incidents atypical of the emerging model, which we used to further develop the analysis.

From such preliminary analysis we derived a theoretical model of the ways in which evidence and information became built into clinical or policy decisions. We used data collected from our observations and interviews in the Urbchester practice (three GP surgeries and one routine partners' meeting; three semistructured informal one to one interviews; and several short

discussions with the GPs) to confirm the model's transferability. We then "tested" the credibility of this emerging model with the research participants in Lawndale and subsequently also at seminar presentations with other practitioners from a range of sectors, which helped us to refine the model.[24]

Results and discussion

Use of guidelines

We found that the individual practitioners did not go through the steps that are traditionally associated with the linear-rational model of evidence based health care[1-3]—not once in the whole time we were observing them. Neither while we observed them did they read the many clinical guidelines available to them in paper form or electronically, except to point to one of the laminated guidelines on the wall in order to explain something to a patient or to us. They told us that they would look through guidelines at their leisure, either in preparation for a practice meeting at which they were expected to bring the practice policy for a given clinical condition up to date or more informally to ensure that their own practice was generally up to standard. For example, one partner told us that when a new guideline arrived in the post he would leaf through it—as long as it looked authoritative and well produced—to reassure himself that there was nothing major that needed changing in his practice. If there was, he would discuss it with colleagues before deciding how to handle the discrepancy. The nurses told us that they would turn to guidelines when faced with an unfamiliar problem, and that once they were familiar with the procedure—for nurse triage of presenting patients, for example—they would rarely if ever look at the guideline again. Although the practice's sophisticated

---

Box 1: Summary of data sources from Lawndale

Observations and informal interviews
10 GP surgeries
6 sets of home visits by GPs
4 nurse led surgeries
1 interview and half day observation with practice manager
Practice meetings:
  1 lunchtime executive meeting
  3 routine partners' meetings
  1 continuing professional development meeting
  1 meeting of administrative staff
  1 awayday of all practice staff
  1 awayday of partners and practice manager
  1 practice meeting on coronary heart disease audit
Multiple informal coffee room gatherings and one to one and informal group discussions
10 "quality practice award" meetings of practice staff (all the quality practice award meetings over one year, of which three were recorded and transcribed)
1 quality practice award nurse team meeting
1 meeting of GP representatives from all local practices to discuss primary care trust-wide coronary heart disease audit
7 "new GP contract" meetings of practice staff
1 "new GP contract" meeting of GPs only

Formal interviews
3 interviews with GPs
1 group interview with clinic staff (practice nurses and phlebotomist)

Documentary sources
Practice guidelines, manuals, and protocols
One partner's "fellowship by assessment" portfolio
"Quality practice award" submission drafts

computer system allowed easy direct access to several accepted expert systems, and more generally to the internet, GPs very rarely used them. Their own average estimates were usually that they might use such facilities less than once every week; even then it would probably be only to download information to give to patients. Indeed, we never saw them use such systems to solve a clinical problem in real time.

Networks

Rather than directly accessing new knowledge in the literature or from the internet and other written sources, the practitioners nearly always took shortcuts to acquiring what they thought would be the best evidence base from sources that they trusted. These sources included the popular doctors' and nurses' magazines mailed free of charge to practices in the United Kingdom. Most importantly, however, the shortcut to the best up to date practice was—for the GPs—via their professional networks among other doctors. The nurses had far fewer opportunities for such external networking and relied more on localised links between themselves, the practice doctors, and the community nurses linked to the surgery.

Box 2: From data to interpretation: example of process of analysis

During a conversation about the way in which the partners learn from each other, a Lawndale GP had told JG that they tended to use "anecdotes with a purpose." This comment was noted on a Post-it sticker, together with the date and field book reference. We placed the sticker on the whiteboard among a growing cluster of around 30 similar notes in a section labelled "Meetings." Other items there included "I'm generally OK about it if a partner later disagrees with my diagnosis or my actions," which had been noted six months earlier in a chat about the extent to which GPs discussed their cases; another item, from five months earlier, noted that the senior partner had smilingly admitted that his "younger partners would gently point out" where his practice was not up to date. We felt that these data seemed to relate to another note about how the practice's policy on statins had developed from the practitioners' individual decisions, which they had shared through informal chats, eventually leading to a formal meeting in which one partner led an audit on use of statins; this, they said, had been followed by argument and discussion and someone agreeing to read up some detail and report back. So perhaps the relevant heading was not only "Meetings," we decided, but broader than that: so we added the label "Each other."

Near to this cluster was a note of an ironic joke—made in the coffee room when a local consultant was visiting—about how GPs "always keep up with the all research literature [ha ha]." We recalled, on returning to the field notes, how avidly the partners capitalised on the consultant's visit to find out about the latest developments in his field and to ask him—both through the coffee room chat and at a lunchtime seminar—about some recent difficult cases. Was this not, we asked ourselves, an example of the importance of "Meetings," rather an "Each other?" Or was it "Education/CPD?" We also linked it to a nearby cluster called "Opinion leaders" and then realised that although many opinion leaders were external to the practice, some were internal, as in the example of statins policy development. This was amply confirmed when we later saw how partners took leading roles—for example, on asthma or diabetes—at formal practice meetings. It became clear as this train of analysis developed that once the group had entrusted themselves to the expertise of an external or internal opinion leader, they would not then question the evidence source. Moreover, they often vaguely referred to those same "meetings with each other" when we asked them to reflect on the reasons for decisions about individual patients. So was this indicative of collective mindline development?

Networking was vital in order to know which colleagues to trust. A great deal of the social interaction and professional comings and goings between doctors, nurses, and other practice staff (and beyond) could be seen as a way of checking out who or what were the most authoritative and trustworthy sources and ascertaining what "they say." However, our participants rarely if ever questioned whether "they" (that is, authoritative sources) practised the linear-rational process traditionally linked to evidence based health care (fig 1, levels 1 and 2), or even the extent to which the views that they conveyed were rooted in explicit research evidence (level 3). This was simply assumed on the basis of trust in "their" expertise. In contrast, the views relayed to practitioners by pharmaceutical representatives, and to a lesser extent the centre of the NHS, were regarded with considerable scepticism, although that did not necessarily mean that they were without influence, as the practitioners themselves admitted. The local primary care trust pharmaceutical adviser had, however, earned the respect of the practitioners and was a highly trusted source.

"Mindlines"

In short, we found that clinicians rarely accessed, appraised, and used explicit evidence directly from research or other formal sources; rare exceptions were where they might consult such sources after dealing with a case that had particularly challenged them. Instead, they relied on what we have called "mindlines," collectively reinforced, internalised tacit guidelines, which were informed by brief reading, but mainly by their interactions with each other and with opinion leaders, patients, and pharmaceutical representatives and by other sources of largely tacit knowledge that built on their early training and their own and their colleagues' experience. The clinicians, in general, would refine their mindlines by acquiring tacit knowledge from trusted sources, mainly their colleagues, in ways that were mediated by the organisational features of the practice, such as the nature and frequency of meetings, the practice ethos, and its financial and structural features, including the computer system.

When describing what we call mindlines, clinicians told us, for example, that they were grown from experience and from people who are trusted; they were "stored in my head" but could be shared and tested and then internalised through discussion, while leaving room for individual flexibility. Once compiled, each individual practitioner's mindlines were adjusted by checking them out against what was learnt from brief reading or from discussions with colleagues, either within or outside the practice. The mindline might well be modified when applied to an individual patient after discussion and negotiation during the consultation; at this stage patients' ideas of what is the appropriate evidence about their particular case (their own personal history, what their family has experienced, what they have read in the media, and so on) could influence the application or even the continuing development of the mindline. Further adjustment might subsequently happen during swapping stories with colleagues or in audit or "critical incident meetings." In those rare challenging cases in which practitioners felt they did not have a ready mindline, they would later read up or ask around so that they could develop one for the future.

Mindlines were therefore iteratively negotiated with a variety of key actors, often through a range of informal interactions in fluid communities of practice, interactions with and experience of patients, and practice meetings. The result was day to day practice based on socially constituted knowledge (fig 2).

We observed the same pattern of knowledge management in the "quality practice award" and other practice meetings. When

Primary care

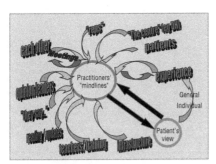

Fig 2   Construction of mindlines

formulating a practice protocol for the management of a given condition, clinicians relied on one of the partners with a special interest in that field to produce a summary of current best practice (box 3). These discussions sometimes resulted in modification of the computerised protocols that were available to prompt clinical actions, but which were not often actually needed as they had already been internalised through the discussions.

Conclusions and implications

Transferability of the model
Our ethnography was based largely on one practice and checked in a contrasting practice; further similar work will be needed to determine the transferability of our findings to other centres. Although the sample consisted of hundreds of interactions and events carried out by more than 15 practitioners, these were all within just two practices, which each had particular organisational cultures. We know of other practices, for example, where

---

Box 3: Developing protocols

We ascertained from interviewing the doctor developing the practice protocol for heart failure that she did so largely by accessing local hospital guidelines produced by a team led by a respected local cardiologist, who she assumed had "drawn upon all the evidence." She supplemented this by reading two sets of published guidelines and synthesising these sources with her own current practice. When she presented the suggested protocol to the practice team, they robustly debated it on the basis of

• Its practicability

• The other clinicians' experience of patients in their own practice

• The acceptability of variations between their own routines

• The ways in which the practice team and computer system could assist or hinder the execution and recording of the new protocol

• The level at which the new protocol might improve remuneration as well as provide high quality care

• Comparisons with other well regarded practices (either local or on the internet)

Although some partners had assumed that she had used the national service framework for coronary heart disease, they were not surprised or concerned to discover that she had not. The scientific basis of the suggestions was rarely questioned during the meeting; rather, it was taken for granted that they were sound, as they were based on trusted sources within and outside the practice

---

partners make more use of online information in their day to day practice and practices where very little communication occurs between the clinicians and no recognisable "community of practice" exists. To test our model it would be necessary to explore how knowledge is put into practice in such different organisational structures and cultures. Nevertheless, the two practices used were acknowledged to be among the best in their localities; our results therefore strongly suggest that it is unrealistic to expect even the best clinicians to rely on the full process of evidence based health care promulgated by its advocates (fig 1, level 1).

Knowledge in practice
We need to recognise that—just as the literature on knowledge management describes in other fields[4 7 25]—clinicians usually work not with explicit codified knowledge (such as guidelines) but with "knowledge in practice." We found that our sample instinctively did this by constantly comparing their own and each others' tacit and explicit knowledge as they formulated their mindlines. In doing so, they omitted any explicit checks of the quality of the evidence base, but relied instead on their "communities of practice."[21 22 26] This was a social process that entailed a range of largely local "actor networks" (human, paper, and electronic) as sources of evidence.[27 28] Thus, to return to the dilemmas that we listed in our introduction, mindlines, because they encapsulate tacit and explicit knowledge sources, are a buffer against rigid cookbook adherence to codified knowledge; and because they emerge from practitioners' communities of practice and actor networks, they may be the key to designing generalised techniques for implementing research that capitalise on, rather than try to factor out, the power of local context.

We believe that mindlines are more complex than the "heuristics" and "rules of thumb" described elsewhere.[14 15] Although similar to the concept of "scripts,"[15] in so far as they are learnt, internalised sequences of thought and behaviour that people find it almost impossible to articulate, mindlines seem to be more reliant on professional interactions. They are more flexible than scripts, more like internalised guidelines—hence our new term. Even so, mindlines may seem to be a dangerous shortcut when compared with the formal model of evidence based health care. However, their use is unsurprising, as there is every reason to suppose that it is knowledge in practice that is needed for practising a knowledge based profession, and practitioners do not have the time (nor usually the skills) to rigorously review and combine all the key sources of tacit and explicit knowledge themselves. Thus the real skill of the practitioner might be expected to be that of learning reliably from the knowledge of trusted sources either individually or through working in a community of practice.

Implications
If this is the case, we need to make sure that the knowledge of the key opinion leaders, from medical or nursing school onwards, is based on research and experiential evidence and wherever appropriate follows the evidence based healthcare model. Training in critical appraisal of research might therefore be most usefully targeted at those who are likely to be the opinion leaders to whom most practitioners turn for their knowledge.[29 30] Moreover, the teaching of evidence based health care might also include explanation of the role of communities of practice, the strengths and weaknesses of taking such shortcuts, and each practitioner's potential role in helping to shore up and strengthen the evidence base of the mindlines of their colleagues.

If our findings are correct, practitioners have a collective professional responsibility to ensure that mindlines are based on

What is already known on this topic

Considerable work has been done to elucidate the factors that help to get research into clinical practice

A large knowledge management literature from other sectors indicates that tacit rather than explicit research based knowledge underpins much professional work

Very little detailed observation of the ways in which clinicians derive and use their knowledge in practice, either collectively or individually, has been reported

What this study adds

Primary care clinicians work in "communities of practice," combining information from a wide range of sources into "mindlines" (internalised, collectively reinforced tacit guidelines), which they use to inform their practice

This has important implications for the dissemination and use of clinical research findings

research evidence wherever possible. In order to do this, the potential of networking as part of continuing professional development must be recognised and fostered, and appropriate information must be targeted, through a variety of routes, to the relevant individuals. This also has important implications for the dissemination of new clinical research findings by using not the sources of knowledge that researchers and the government think practitioners should use but the actual sources that they do use.

We thank Dale Webb, who carried out some of the formal interviews. Above all we thank the staff of "Lawndale" for their forbearance in allowing us to "hang around" over all this time and learn so much from them about the day to day practice of primary care. Thanks also to the "Urbchester" GPs for the very fruitful time spent there.

Contributors: Both authors jointly conceived and designed the study, did the fieldwork, and wrote the paper. They are joint guarantors.

Funding: Grant from former Department of Health South East Regional Office R&D Directorate.

Competing interests: None declared.

1   Muir Gray J. *Evidence-based healthcare: how to make health policy and management decisions.* Edinburgh: Churchill Livingstone, 1998.
2   Haines A, Donald A, eds. *Getting research into practice.* London: BMJ Books, 1998.
3   Trinder L, Reynolds S, eds. *Evidence-based practice: a critical appraisal.* Oxford: Blackwell Science, 2000.
4   Davenport TK, Prusak L. *Working knowledge: how organisations manage what they know.* Boston: Harvard Business Press, 1998.
5   Polanyi M. *Personal knowledge: towards a post-critical philosophy.* London: Routledge and Kegan Paul, 1958.
6   Polanyi M. *The tacit dimension.* London: Routledge and Kegan Paul, 1967.
7   Nonaka I, Takeuchi H. *The knowledge creating company: how Japanese companies create the dynamics of innovation.* Oxford: Oxford University Press, 1995.
8   Lave J. The values of quantification. In: Law J, ed. *Power, action and belief: a new sociology of knowledge?* (Sociological Review Monograph 32.) London: Routledge and Kegan Paul, 1986.
9   Dopson S, Fitzgerald L, Ferlie E, Gabbay J, Locock L. No magic targets! Changing clinical practice to become more evidence based. *Health Care Manag Rev* 2002;27:35-47.
10 Le May A, Mulhall A, Alexander C. Bridging the research practice gap: exploring the research cultures of practitioners and managers. *J Adv Nurs* 1998;28:428-37.
11 Fitzgerald L, Ferlie E, Wood M, Hawkins C. Interlocking interactions, the diffusion of innovations in health care. *Hum Relat* 2002;55:1429-49.
12 Ferlie E, Fitzgerald L, Wood M. Getting evidence into clinical practice: an organisational behaviour perspective. *J Health Serv Res Policy* 2000;5:96-102.
13 Hamm RM. Medical decision scripts: combining cognitive scripts and judgement strategies to account fully for medical decision making. In: Hardman D, Macchi L, eds. *Thinking: psychological perspectives on reasoning, judgement and decision making.* London and New York: John Wiley and Sons, 2003:315-45.
14 Andre M, Borgquist L, Foldevi M, Molstad S. Asking for 'rules of thumb': a way to discover tacit knowledge in general practice. *Fam Pract* 2002;19:617-22.
15 Andre M, Borgquist L, Molstad S. Use of rules of thumb in the consultation in general practice—an act of balance between the individual and the general perspective. *Fam Pract* 2003;20:514-9.
16 Pope CJ. Resisting evidence: the study of evidence-based medicine as a contemporary social movement. *Health: An Interdisciplinary Journal for the Social Study of Health, Illness and Medicine* 2003;7:267-82.
17 Eriksen TH. *Small places, large issues: an introduction to social and cultural anthropology.* London: Pluto Press, 2001.
18 Agar MH. *The professional stranger.* San Diego: Academic Press, 1996.
19 Spradley JP. *The ethnographic interview.* Florida: Harcourt Brace Jovanovich, 1979.
20 Weick K. *Sensemaking in organizations.* Thousand Oaks, CA: Sage Publications, 1995.
21 Wenger E. *Communities of practice: learning, meaning and identity.* New York: Cambridge University Press, 1998.
22 Brown JS, Duguid P. Organisational learning and communities of practice: towards a unified view of working, learning, and innovation. *Organisational Science* 1991;2:40-57.
23 Gabbay J, le May A, Jefferson H, Webb D, Lovelock R, Powell J, et al. A case study of knowledge management in multi-agency consumer-informed "communities of practice": implications for evidence-based policy development in health and social services. *Health: An interdisciplinary Journal for the Social Study of Health, Illness and Medicine* 2003;7:283-310.
24 Lincoln Y, Guba R. *Naturalistic inquiry.* Beverly Hills: Sage, 1985.
25 Choo CW. *The knowing organization: how organizations use information to construct meaning, create knowledge and make decisions.* New York and Oxford: Oxford University Press, 1998.
26 Brown JS, Duguid P. *The social life of information.* Boston: Harvard Business School Press, 2000.
27 Latour B. *Science in action: how to follow scientists and engineers through society.* Boston: Harvard University Press, 1988.
28 Callon M. Some elements of a sociology of translation: domestication of the scallops and the fishermen of St Brieuc Bay. In: Law J, ed. *Power, action and belief: a new sociology of knowledge?* (Sociological Review Monograph 32.) London: Routledge and Kegan Paul, 1986.
29 Coleman JS, Katz E, Menzel H. *Medical innovation, a diffusion study.* Indianapolis: Dobbs Merrill, 1966.
30 Locock L, Dopson S, Chambers D, Gabbay J. Understanding the role of opinion leaders in improving clinical effectiveness. *Soc Sci Med* 2001;53:745-57.

(Accepted 7 September 2004)

bmj.com 2004;329:1013

Wessex Institute for Health Research and Development, Community Clinical Sciences, University of Southampton, Southampton SO16 7PX
John Gabbay *professor of public health*

School of Nursing and Midwifery, University of Southampton
Andrée le May *reader in nursing*
Correspondence to: J Gabbay j.gabbay@soton.ac.uk

CHAPTER 17

The contribution of primary care to health systems and health

Shannon Barkley

NOMINATED CLASSIC PAPER

Barbara Starfield, Leiyu Shi, James Macinko. Contribution of primary care to health systems and health. *Milbank Quarterly*, 2005; 83: 457–502.

This landmark review presents decades of evidence from international sources that uniformly demonstrate the undeniable benefits of health systems founded on high-quality primary care. Increased primary care, whether measured by (1) supply of primary care physicians (family and general practitioners, general internists, and general paediatricians) per population, (2) people who report a primary care physician as their regular source of healthcare, or (3) the receipt of high-quality primary care, results in lower mortality, better health outcomes, and better perceptions of health status, distributed more equitably and compensating for disparities caused by social determinants of health, all at lower cost. In short, primary care gets us where we want to be.

What's more, countries that reinforce the foundational role of primary healthcare with supportive policies improve the quality of primary care. Relevant policies identified in this review include the equitable distribution of health resources according to health needs, a high proportion of primary care physicians to other specialists, financial coverage through publically accountable means, low co-payments for health services, and the higher relative earnings of primary care physicians compared to other specialists.

This review is a manifesto for physicians and policy-makers who seek to improve the health of all people, particularly populations who suffer the consequences of social deprivation. It offers validation and purpose to primary care providers – in reality one of the health system's greatest assets – who are, too often, overworked and undervalued, and also provides clear organising principles for policy-makers seeking to improve the health outcomes that matter most and respond to the needs and expectations of people.

Recognising that the benefits of primary care are amplified when care is higher quality, this paper presents a clear call for study of performance measurement and improvement of primary care systems globally, focused on the factors that most influence outcomes.

ABOUT THE LEAD AUTHOR OF THIS PAPER

Barbara Starfield (1932–2011) was an accomplished physician, health systems researcher and champion of the need for strong primary care systems worldwide. She earned her medical degree from State University of New York, where she graduated magna cum laude in 1959. Barbara then completed her internship and residency in paediatrics at the Harriet Lane Home at the Johns Hopkins Hospital. She earned her master of public health degree at Johns Hopkins School of Hygiene and Public Health in 1962. As a professor at Hopkins, she went on to lead the Division of Health Policy in the Department of Health Policy and Management, and was founding director of the Primary Care Policy Center. Her work led to the development of important tools for assessing morbidity burden and service delivery performance, including the Adjusted Clinical Groups System, the Primary Care Assessment Tools (PCAT) and the Child Health and Illness Profile (CHIP). She served on many government and professional committees, including the National Committee on Vital and Health Statistics. She was also a member of the Institute of Medicine. She was the co-founder and first President of the International Society for Equity in Health.

ABOUT THE NOMINATOR OF THIS PAPER

Dr Shannon Barkley is the technical lead on Primary Health Care at the World Health Organization. As a family doctor, she has been involved with the development of effective primary healthcare among underserved communities internationally through clinical practice, family medicine education, research, performance assessment and improvement and service delivery policy.

> 'Life's harshest realities affect our patients, our priorities may differ from those who organise our health systems, and change can be slow. Despite the challenges, our position as family doctors remains one of privilege: we

see humanity at its most human. Realise your potential to positively affect patients, colleagues, health systems and society.'

Dr Shannon Barkley, United States of America

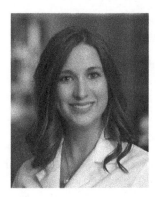

Attribution:

We attribute the original publication of *Contribution of primary care to health systems and health* to *Milbank Quarterly*, published by Wiley. With thanks to Paulette Goldweber and Emma Willcox at Wiley.

Contribution of Primary Care to Health Systems and Health

BARBARA STARFIELD, LEIYU SHI, and JAMES MACINKO

Johns Hopkins University; New York University

Evidence of the health-promoting influence of primary care has been accumulating ever since researchers have been able to distinguish primary care from other aspects of the health services delivery system. This evidence shows that primary care helps prevent illness and death, regardless of whether the care is characterized by supply of primary care physicians, a relationship with a source of primary care, or the receipt of important features of primary care. The evidence also shows that primary care (in contrast to specialty care) is associated with a more equitable distribution of health in populations, a finding that holds in both cross-national and within-national studies. The means by which primary care improves health have been identified, thus suggesting ways to improve overall health and reduce differences in health across major population subgroups.

Key Words: Primary care, health outcomes, population health.

THE TERM *PRIMARY CARE* IS THOUGHT TO DATE BACK TO ABOUT 1920, when the Dawson Report was released in the United Kingdom. That report, an official "white paper," mentioned "primary health care centres," intended to become the hub of regionalized services in that country. Although primary care came to be the cornerstone of the health services system in the United Kingdom as well as in many other countries, no comparable focus developed in the United States. Indeed, the formation of one after another specialty board

Address correspondence to: Barbara Starfield, Department of Health Policy and Management, Johns Hopkins Bloomberg School of Public Health, 624 N. Broadway, Room 406, Baltimore, MD 21205 (email: bstarfie@jhsph.edu).

The Milbank Quarterly, Vol. 83, No. 3, 2005 (pp. 457–502)
© 2005 Milbank Memorial Fund. Published by Blackwell Publishing.

in the early decades of the 20th century signaled the increasing specialization of the U.S. physician workforce (Stevens 1971). The GI Bill of Rights, which supported the further training of physicians returning from service in World War II, helped increase the specialization of many who had been general practitioners (generalists) before the war. At that time, general practitioners were physicians who lacked additional training after graduation from medical school, apart from a short clinical internship.

Concerned that the survival of generalist physicians would be threatened by the disproportionate increase in the supply of specialists in the United States—to the detriment of generalist practice—family physicians, working with international colleagues, established standards for credentialing the new "specialty" of family practice. Thus, in the 1960s and 1970s, longer postgraduate training became part of generalist physicians' preparation for practice. This recognition of a "specialty" of primary care, which, in the United States, covered general internal medicine as well as general pediatrics, resulted in two reports from the Institute of Medicine (IOM) (Donaldson et al. 1996; IOM 1978). These reports defined primary care as "the provision of integrated, accessible health care services by clinicians who are accountable for addressing a large majority of personal health care needs, developing a sustained partnership with patients, and practicing in the context of family and community." This definition is consistent with at least two international reports (WONCA 1991; World Health Organization 1978) and has been used to measure the four main features of primary care services: first-contact access for each new need; long-term person- (not disease) focused care; comprehensive care for most health needs; and coordinated care when it must be sought elsewhere. Primary care is assessed as "good" according to how well these four features are fulfilled. For some purposes, an orientation toward family and community is included as well (Starfield 1998).

Despite the greater recognition of the importance of primary care to health services systems (World Health Organization 1978, 2003), professionals have recently called for increasing even further the supply of specialist physicians in the United States (Cooper et al. 2002). Compared with other industrialized nations, the United States already has a surplus of specialists, but not of primary care physicians. On the basis of the studies reviewed in this article, we believe that health of the U.S. population will improve if this maldistribution is corrected. Specifically, a greater emphasis on primary care can be expected to lower the costs

Contribution of Primary Care to Health Systems and Health   459

of care, improve health through access to more appropriate services, and reduce the inequities in the population's health.

We first review the evidence concerning the relationship between primary care and health, using three different measures of primary care. The effect of health policy on primary care and health can also be determined by between-country comparisons, which we summarize next. We then consider the impact of primary care in reducing disparities in health across population groups. After a section on cost considerations, we discuss why primary care would be expected to have a beneficial effect on health. We then look at the analyses' limitations and discuss the likely nature of primary care in the future in accordance with the policy implications of this evidence.

Reviewing the Evidence

We used research on the effects of primary care on health from studies of the supply of primary care physicians, studies of people who identified a primary care physician as their regular source of care, and studies linking the receipt of high-quality primary care services with health status. These three lines of evidence represent a progressively stronger demonstration that primary care improves health by showing, first, that health is better in areas with more primary care physicians; second, that people who receive care from primary care physicians are healthier; and, third, that the characteristics of primary care are associated with better health. We used three systematic literature reviews of primary care (Atun 2004; Engstrom, Foldevi, and Borgquist 2001; Health Council of the Netherlands 2004), supplemented by our own compilation of articles in major national and international general medical journals. We concentrated on publications written in English and mainly on studies from the United States (which accounted for most of them). We did, however, include studies from other countries if they addressed primary care, as measured by at least one of the three types of studies. A study's inclusion or exclusion did not depend on its findings. Rather, the only criterion for inclusion was a clear conceptualization of primary care, systematic data collection and analysis, and comparison populations. Several studies in the systematic literature reviews, although uniformly favorable to primary care, did not meet these criteria and therefore were excluded.

460   *B. Starfield, L. Shi, and J. Macinko*

Primary Care and Health

Health Outcomes and the Supply of Primary Care Physicians

As a group, these studies covered a variety of health outcomes: total and cause-specific mortality, low birth weight, and self-reported health. They examined the relationship between the supply of primary care physicians and health at different levels of geographic aggregation (state, county, metropolitan, and nonmetropolitan regions); controlled for various population characteristics (such as income, education, and racial distribution); and used several different analytic approaches (standard regressions, path analyses) in individual years (cross-sectional) as well as over time (longitudinal).

The number of primary care physicians per 10,000 population is the measure of "supply." Primary care physicians include family and general practitioners, general internists, and general pediatricians. These three types of physicians constitute the primary care physician workforce and have been shown to provide the highest levels of primary care characteristics in their practices (Weiner and Starfield 1983).

Studies in the early 1990s (Shi 1992, 1994) showed that those U.S. states with higher ratios of primary care physicians to population had better health outcomes, including lower rates of all causes of mortality: mortality from heart disease, cancer, or stroke; infant mortality; low birth weight; and poor self-reported health, even after controlling for sociodemographic measures (percentages of elderly, urban, and minority; education; income; unemployment; pollution) and lifestyle factors (seatbelt use, obesity, and smoking). Vogel and Ackerman (1998) subsequently showed that the supply of primary care physicians was associated with an increase in life span and with reduced low birth-weight rates.

Other studies added sophistication to these early studies by examining the relationship between primary care and health after considering other potentially confounding characteristics. One of these confounders was income inequality, or the extent to which income is concentrated in certain social groups rather than being equitably distributed. In 1999, Shi and colleagues reported that both primary care and income inequality had a strong and significant influence on life expectancy, total mortality, stroke mortality, and postneonatal mortality at the state level. They also found smoking rates to be related to these outcomes, but the effect

Contribution of Primary Care to Health Systems and Health   461

of the primary care physician supply persisted after they controlled for smoking (Shi et al. 1999). A later study confirmed these findings, this time using self-assessed health as the health outcome (Shi and Starfield 2000). These relationships remained significant after controlling for age, sex, race/ethnicity, education, paid work (employment and type of employment), hourly wage, family income, health insurance, physical health (SF-12), and smoking.

Additional studies examined the influence of the supply of primary care physicians at the state level while also taking into account the supply of specialist physicians. These analyses found, in the same year as well as in time-lagged (between 1985 and 1995) analyses, that the supply of primary care physicians was significantly associated with lower all-cause mortality, whereas a greater supply of specialty physicians was associated with higher mortality. When the supply of primary care physicians was disaggregated into family physicians, general internists, and pediatricians, only the supply of family physicians showed a significant relationship to lower mortality (Shi et al. 2003a).

Mortality attributed to cerebrovascular stroke also was found to be influenced by the supply of primary care physicians. Using 11 years of state-level data and adjusting for income inequality, educational level, unemployment, racial/ethnic composition, and percentage of urban residents, the supply of primary care physicians remained significantly associated with reduced mortality and even wiped out the adverse effect of income inequality (Shi et al. 2003b).

Consistent with these findings for total and cause-specific mortality, the reduction in low birth weight at the state level was significantly associated with the supply of primary care physicians in the concurrent year as well as after one-, three-, and five-year lag periods (Shi et al. 2004). A greater supply of primary care physicians was associated with lower infant mortality as well and persisted after controlling for various socioeconomic characteristics and income inequality.

County-level analyses confirmed the positive influence of an adequate supply of primary care physicians by showing that all-cause mortality, heart disease mortality, and cancer mortality were lower where the supply of primary care physicians was greater. When urban areas (counties including a city with at least 50,000 people) and nonurban areas were examined separately (Shi et al. 2005b), nonurban counties with a greater number of primary care physicians experienced 2 percent lower all-cause mortality, 4 percent lower heart disease mortality, and 3 percent lower

462   *B. Starfield, L. Shi, and J. Macinko*

cancer mortality than did nonurban counties with a smaller number of primary care physicians. In urban areas, however, the relationship appeared more complex, possibly resulting from the lesser degree of income inequality and the greater racial differences in urban areas. A study of premature mortality (mortality before age 75) in U.S. metropolitan, urban, and rural areas found inconsistent relationships to the supply of primary care physicians, possibly owing to a statistical instability in the way in which the supply of physicians was categorized, which was inappropriate for areas with great variability in both the supply and the population size (Mansfield et al. 1999).

Analyses conducted in counties in the state of Florida used cervical cancer mortality as the health outcome. Controlling for a variety of county-level characteristics (percentage of whites, low educational level, median household income, percentage of married females, and urban/nonurban), each one per 10,000 population increase in the supply of family physicians was associated with a decrease in mortality of 0.65 per 100,000 population. That is, a one-third increase in the supply of family physicians was associated with a 20 percent lower mortality rate from cervical cancer. The positive effect of primary care was also found in the significant relationship between reduced mortality and the supply of general internists, but not the supply of obstetrician-gynecologists (Campbell et al. 2003).

The relationship between primary care physician supply and better health is not limited to studies in the United States. In England, the standardized mortality ratio for all-cause mortality at 15 to 64 years of age is lower in areas with a greater supply of general practitioners. (In England, pediatricians and internists are not considered, and do not function as, primary care physicians.) Each additional general practitioner per 10,000 population (a 15 to 20 percent increase) is associated with about a 6 percent decrease in mortality (Gulliford 2002). A later study (Gulliford et al. 2004) found that the ratio of general practitioners to population was significantly associated with lower all-cause mortality, acute myocardial infarction mortality, avoidable mortality, acute hospital admissions (both chronic and acute), and teenage pregnancies, but the statistical significance disappeared after controlling for socioeconomic deprivation and for partnership size, which the authors interpreted as suggesting that the structural characteristics of primary care practices may have had a greater impact on health outcomes than did the mere presence of primary care physicians.

Contribution of Primary Care to Health Systems and Health 463

The supply of general practitioners also has high salience for in-hospital mortality; that is, it is more closely associated with lower in-hospital standardized mortality than is the total number of physicians per 100 hospital beds (Jarman et al. 1999).

In summary, the studies consistently show a relationship between more or better primary care and most of the health outcomes studied. Primary care was associated with improved health outcomes, regardless of the year (1980–1995), after variable lag periods between the assessment of primary care and of health outcomes, level of analysis (state, county, or local area), or type of outcome as measured by all-cause mortality, heart disease mortality, stroke mortality, infant mortality, low birth weight, life expectancy, and self-rated health. All but a few studies found this effect for cancer mortality. The magnitude of improvement associated with an increase of one primary care physician per 10,000 population (a 12.6 percent increase over the current average supply) averaged 5.3 percent. The results of these studies suggest that as many as 127,617 deaths per year in the United States could be averted through such an increase in the number of primary care physicians (Macinko, Starfield, and Shi 2005).

Patients' Relationship to Primary Care Facilities and Providers

Because a greater number of primary care physicians does not necessarily mean that all people in the area have greater access to or receipt of primary care services, analyses considering people's relationships to or experiences with a primary care practitioner are helpful to determining the association between primary care and health outcome. Thus the second line of evidence for the positive impact of primary care on health comes from comparing the health of people who do or do not have a primary care physician as their regular source of care.

A nationally representative survey showed that adult U.S. respondents who reported having a primary care physician rather than a specialist as their regular source of care had lower subsequent five-year mortality rates after controlling for initial differences in health status, demographic characteristics, health insurance status, health perceptions, reported diagnoses, and smoking status (Franks and Fiscella 1998). That is, people who identify a primary care physician as their usual source of

464   *B. Starfield, L. Shi, and J. Macinko*

care are healthier, regardless of their initial health or various demographic characteristics.

U.S. populations served by community health centers, which are required to emphasize primary care as a condition for federal funding, are healthier than populations with comparable levels of social deprivation receiving care in other types of physicians' offices or clinics (O'Malley et al. 2005). People receiving care in community health centers receive more of the indicated preventive services than does the general population (Agency for Healthcare Research and Quality 2004). A comparison of rural patients receiving care in these community health centers with patients receiving care in other types of facilities showed that despite being sicker, they are significantly more likely to have received a Pap smear in the previous three years and to have been vaccinated against pneumococcal infection and less likely to have low-birth-weight babies (Regan et al. 2003).

In some health systems, both in the United States and abroad, people normally go to their primary care physician before seeking care elsewhere (such as from another type of physician). Spain passed a law in the mid-1980s that strengthened primary care by reorganizing services to better achieve the main features of primary care, which led to the establishment of a national program of primary health care centers. The impact of this reform on health was evaluated after ten years by examining mortality rates for some major causes of death (Villalbi et al. 1999). Death rates associated with hypertension and stroke fell most in those areas in which the reform was first implemented. There even were fewer deaths from lung cancer in those areas with primary care reform than in other areas. Health outcomes that would not be expected to be influenced by primary care, for example, perinatal mortality, did not differ across the areas.

Outcomes of care after surgery in Canada also were shown to be better when care was sought from a primary care physician who then referred children to specialists for recurrent tonsillitis or otitis media, compared with self-referral to a specialist (Roos 1979). The referred children had fewer postoperative complications, fewer respiratory episodes following surgery, and fewer episodes of otitis media after surgery, thus implying that specialist interventions were more appropriate when patients were referred from primary care.

Finally, we note that Cuba and Costa Rica, which reformed their health systems to provide people with a source of primary care, now have much lower infant mortality rates than do other countries in Latin America. In

Cuba, infant mortality rates now are on a par with those in the United States (PAHO 2005; Riveron Corteguera 2000; Waitzkin et al. 1997).

The findings from studies of the impact of actually receiving care from a primary care source consistently show benefits for a variety of health and health-related outcomes.

How Well the Characteristics of Primary Care Are Achieved

As we noted earlier, until recently primary care could be assessed only by determining the type of physician who provided it: family physicians, general internists, and general pediatricians in the United States; and family physicians or general practitioners in most other industrialized countries. The intensive examination of criteria for the designation of "primary care" in the most recent half century encouraged the development of tools to assess the adequacy of those health delivery characteristics that together define the practice of primary care. This development then enabled us to examine the extent to which the receipt of better primary care is associated with better health.

Using these new methods, several studies have demonstrated a positive association between the adequacy of the features of primary care and the provision of preventive services. A cross-sectional study using a representative sample of 2,889 patients in Ohio evaluated the aforementioned four attributes of primary care for their relationship to the delivery of preventive services. After controlling for the patients' age, race, health, and insurance in the hierarchical linear regression model (HLM), each of the measured primary care attributes was significantly associated with patients' being up to date on screening, immunization, and health habit–counseling services (Flocke, Stange, and Zyzanski 1998). According to another study, adolescents with the same regular source of care for preventive and illness care (one indication that the source is focused on providing primary care) were much more likely to receive the indicated preventive care and less likely to seek care in emergency rooms (Ryan et al. 2001).

The positive impact of primary care also was shown by comparing the self-assessed health of those who received better primary care (as assessed by the health delivery characteristics of primary care) with those who reported less adequate primary care. Among those who reported better

466   *B. Starfield, L. Shi, and J. Macinko*

primary care, more than 5 percent fewer people reported poor health and 6 percent fewer reported depression than did people experiencing less adequate primary care. Considering only those who reported the *best* primary care experiences, 8 percent fewer reported poor health, and more than 10 percent fewer reported feeling depressed, compared with those who received less adequate primary care (Shi et al. 2002).

Studies in two different areas of Brazil confirmed the relationship between the adequacy of primary care delivery characteristics and self-reported health. In a study in Petropolis, Macinko, Almeida, and Sa (2005) showed that patients who had better primary care experiences were more likely to report better health, even after adjusting for other salient characteristics such as their age, whether or not they had a chronic illness or a recent illness, household wealth, educational level, and the type of facility in which they received their care. Using parents' reports of their children's primary care, Erno Harzheim and colleagues confirmed these findings in a study conducted in Porto Alegre (Harzheim 2005, personal communication).

International Comparisons

International comparisons extended our examination of the impact of primary care according to the achievement of its characteristics. Studies of the characteristics of different health systems were particularly useful because they enabled us to assess the impact of various policy characteristics on the practice and outcomes of primary care. Three studies, one using data from the mid-1980s and two from a decade later, demonstrated not only that countries with stronger primary care generally had a healthier population but also that certain aspects of policy were important to establishing strong primary care practice.

The first study examined the association of primary care with health outcomes through an international comparison conducted in 11 industrialized countries (Starfield 1991, 1994). Each country's primary care was rated according to the four main characteristics of primary care practice: first-contact care, person-focused care over time, comprehensive care, and coordinated care, as well as family orientation and community orientation. Policy characteristics were the attempts to distribute health services resources equitably (according to the extent of health needs in different areas of the country); universal or near-universal financial coverage guaranteed by a publicly accountable body (government or government-regulated insurance carriers); low or no copayments for health services; percentage of physicians who were not primary care physicians; and professional earnings of primary care physicians relative to those of other specialists. (Operational definitions of these indicators and the method of scoring them are described in Starfield 1998.) The first important finding is that the score for the practice characteristics was highly correlated with the score for the policy characteristics. That is, the adequate delivery of primary care services was associated with supportive governmental policies. The second finding is that those countries with low primary care scores as a group had poorer health outcomes, most notably for indicators in early childhood, particularly low birth weight and postneonatal mortality.

A more recent comparison, with 13 countries and an expanded set of indicators of both primary care policy characteristics and health outcomes, also showed better health outcomes for the primary care–oriented countries even after controlling for income inequality and smoking rates, most significantly for postneonatal mortality ($r = .74$, $p < .001$) and rates of low birth weight ($r = .38$, $p < .001$). Countries with weak primary care also performed less well on most major aspects of health, including mental health, such as years of potential life lost because of suicide (Starfield and Shi 2002). The positive impact of primary care orientation on low birth-weight rates may reflect a beneficial effect of primary care on mothers' health *before* pregnancy (Davey Smith and Lynch 2004; Starfield and Shi 2002). The characteristics of primary care practice present in countries with high primary care scores and absent in countries with low primary care scores were the degree of comprehensiveness of primary care (i.e., the extent to which primary care practitioners provided a broader range of services rather than making referrals to specialists for those services) and a family orientation (the degree to which services were provided to all family members by the same practitioner). The most consistent policy characteristics were the government's attempts to distribute resources equitably, universal financial coverage that was either under the aegis of the government or regulated by the government, and low or no patient cost sharing for primary care services (Starfield and Shi 2002). The latter two were studied and confirmed by Or (2001).

The positive contributions of primary care to health also were found in a much more extensive time-series analysis of 18 industrialized

468   *B. Starfield, L. Shi, and J. Macinko*

countries, including the United States (Macinko, Starfield, and Shi 2003). The stronger the country's primary care orientation (as measured by the same scoring system as in the earlier international comparison) was, the lower the rates were of all-cause mortality, all-cause premature mortality, and cause-specific premature mortality from asthma and bronchitis, emphysema and pneumonia, cardiovascular disease, and heart disease. This relationship held even after controlling for various system characteristics (GDP per capita, total physicians per 1,000 population, percentage of elderly people) and population characteristics, including the average number of ambulatory care visits, per capita income, alcohol consumption, and tobacco consumption. The analyses estimated that increasing a country's primary care score by five points (on a 20-point scale) would be expected to reduce premature deaths from asthma and bronchitis by as much as 6.5 percent and that the reduction in premature mortality for heart disease could be as high as 15 percent.

Data from this study were analyzed as well to ascertain the robustness of primary care scores over time. The average primary care score increased by nearly one point from the 1970s to the 1990s. Countries that performed well in the 1970s remained high performers in each succeeding decade. When countries were divided into high and low performers (above or below the mean for each decade), no country crossed the threshold from low to high or from high to low, but the score of some countries changed. One country's score fell over time; Germany lowered access to ambulatory care services by imposing higher copayments, thus lowering its overall primary care score (OECD 2001). In general, policy changes over time paralleled improvements in primary care practice. For example, in the late 1980s and early 1990s, Spain strengthened its primary care by moving to a tax-based financing system, improving its geographic allocation of funds, and increasing the supply of family physicians as well as developing primary health care centers that improved integration, family orientation, coordination of care, and health promotion services (Larizgoitia and Starfield 1997). The United States' score rose slightly over time, almost entirely resulting from the greater participation of Americans in health maintenance organizations (HMOs), which tend, on average, to use a higher percentage of primary care practitioners (Weiner 2004) and have (at least among the not-for-profit HMOs) a tradition of community involvement (Stevens and Shi 2003).

Primary Care and Disparities
in Health Outcomes

Both the World Health Organization and many countries (including the United States) have recognized the existence of marked disparities (inequities) in health across population subgroups and have identified reductions (and, for the United States, even elimination) of these as a priority (Sachs and McArthur 2005; U.S. Department of Health and Human Services 2000). In reviewing the impact of primary care on reductions in disparities in health, we looked at studies of physician supply, studies of the association with a primary care physician, and studies of the receipt of services that fulfilled the criteria for primary care delivery.

Higher ratios of primary care physicians to population are associated with relatively greater effects on various aspects of health in more socially deprived areas (as measured by high levels of income inequality). Areas with abundant primary care resources and high income inequality have a 17 percent *lower* postneonatal mortality rate (compared with the population mean), whereas the postneonatal mortality rate in areas of high income inequality and few primary care resources was 7 percent *higher*. For stroke mortality, the comparable figures were 2 percent *lower* mortality where the primary care resources were abundant and 1 percent *higher* where the primary care resources were scarce (calculated from data in Shi et al. 1999). These findings are even more striking in the case of self-reported health. Income inequality and primary care were significantly associated with self-rated health, but the supply of primary care physicians significantly reduced the effects of income inequality on self-reported health status (Shi and Starfield 2000). People in high-income-inequality areas were 33 percent more likely to report fair or poor health if the primary care resources were few (calculated from data in Shi and Starfield 2000).

As in state-level analyses, the adverse impact of income inequality on all-cause mortality, heart disease mortality, and cancer mortality was considerably diminished where the number of primary care physicians in county-level analyses was high (Shi et al. 2005a).

The supply of primary care physicians in the U.S. states has a larger positive impact on low birth weight and infant mortality in areas with high social inequality than it does in areas with less social inequality (Shi et al. 2004).

470   *B. Starfield, L. Shi, and J. Macinko*

Eleven years of state-level data found the supply of primary care physicians to be significantly related to lower all-cause mortality rates in both African American and white populations, after controlling for income inequality and socioeconomic characteristics (metropolitan area, percentage of unemployed, and educational levels). In these state-level analyses, the supply of primary care physicians had a greater positive impact on mortality among African Americans than among whites. The inclusions of both the supply of primary care physicians and sociodemographic characteristics eliminated the negative impact of income inequality. The association between a greater supply of primary care physicians and lower total mortality was found to be four times greater in the African American population than in the white majority population, indicating a reduction in racial disparities in mortality in the U.S. states (Shi et al. 2005c). But when exploring further the relationship between the supply of primary care physicians and health outcomes in African American and white populations in metropolitan areas of the United States, both the supply of primary care and income inequality were significantly associated with total mortality rates in the white population, whereas only income inequality maintained its significant relationships in African American populations (Shi and Starfield 2001). The authors interpreted this finding as suggesting that in many urban areas, a great supply of primary care physicians does not ensure certain population subgroups' access to primary care; they may receive their care in places such as hospital clinics and emergency rooms, which do not emphasize primary care.

The equity-related effect of having a good primary care source also was found in the study that examined the degree of primary care–oriented services that people received. Good primary care experiences were associated with reductions in the adverse effects of income inequality on health, with fewer differences in self-rated health between higher and lower income-inequality areas where primary care experiences were stronger (Shi et al. 2002). Although similar in the direction of effect, the relationship to "feeling depressed" was not statistically significant.

In county-level analyses that stratified urban areas by race, the supply of primary care physicians had a strong and significant influence on white mortality in both low- and high-income-inequality areas, but only a weak association with African American mortality in low-income-inequality areas and no significant association in high-income-inequality areas (Shi et al. 2005b).

Thus, the U.S. studies showed that an adequate supply of primary care physicians reduced disparities in health across racial and socioeconomic groups. Multivariate analyses controlling for individual, community, and state-level characteristics provided strong evidence for the association of primary care with fewer disparities in several aspects of health.

These conclusions are buttressed by a study comparing the type of place where care is received. Disparities in low-birth-weight percentages between the majority white and African American infants are fewer in infants of mothers receiving care in primary care–oriented community health centers, compared with the population as a whole. In both white and African American populations in both urban and rural areas in the United States, the rates of low birth weight were lower, in both absolute numbers and ratios of rates, where the source of care was a community health center (Politzer et al. 2001).

A study of civil servants in the United Kingdom, where access to primary care physicians is universal, found that socioeconomic differences in coronary heart disease mortality were *not* a result of differences in cardiac care (Britton et al. 2004). Another exploration of the effect of primary care found that blacks in London did not have greater rates of diabetes-related lower-extremity amputation than whites did (Leggetter et al. 2002), whereas blacks in the United States had rates two to three times higher than that in the white population. In the United Kingdom, the rates were lower in black men than in the white population, a difference wholly accounted for by lower rates of smoking, neuropathy, and peripheral vascular disease. The findings persisted even after controlling for socioeconomic differences, thus confirming other findings (van Doorslaer, Koolman, and Jones 2004) that a health system oriented toward primary care services (such as in the United Kingdom) reduced the disparities in health care so prominent in the United States (Agency for Healthcare Research and Quality 2004).

Primary care programs aimed at improving health in deprived populations in less developed countries succeeded in narrowing the gaps in health between socially deprived and more socially advantaged populations. A matched case-control study in Mexico (Reyes et al. 1997) found that some aspects of primary care delivery had an important independent effect on reducing the odds of children dying in socially deprived areas. These processes included adequate referral mechanisms, continuity of care (being seen by the same provider at each visit), and being attended

472   *B. Starfield, L. Shi, and J. Macinko*

in a public facility designed to provide primary care. A study in Bolivia (Perry et al. 1998) found that a community-based approach to planning primary health care services in socially deprived areas lowered the mortality of children under age five compared with adjacent similar areas or the country as a whole.

The Costa Rican primary care reforms, which were instituted first in the most socially deprived areas, illustrate the importance of primary care in reducing health disparities. These reforms included transferring the responsibility for providing health care from the Ministry of Health to the Costa Rican Social Security Fund (CCSS), expanding the number of primary care facilities—particularly in underserved areas—and reorganizing primary care into "integrated primary care teams" or EBAIS (equipos básicos de atención integral en salud), which consist of teams of health professionals assigned to a geographic region covering about 1,000 households (Rosero-Bixby 2004b). By 1985, Costa Rica's life expectancy reached 74 years, and infant mortality rates fell from 60 per 1,000 live births in 1970 to 19 per 1,000 live births, levels comparable to those in more developed countries. The improvements in primary health care were estimated to have reduced infant mortality by between 40 percent and 75 percent, depending on the particular study (Haines and Avery 1982; Klijzing and Taylor 1982; Rosero-Bixby 1986). For every five additional years after primary health care (PHC) reform, child mortality fell by 13 percent, and adult mortality fell by 4 percent. The study's quasi-experimental nature provided evidence of the power of PHC policies and provision of services to improve health, above and beyond improvements in social and economic indicators (which the longitudinal analyses controlled for) (Rosero-Bixby 2004a).

Studies in other developing countries show the considerable potential of primary care to reduce the large disparities associated with socioeconomic deprivation. In seven African countries, the wealthiest 20 percent of the population receives well over three times as much financial benefit from overall government spending as does the poorest 20 percent of the population (40 percent versus 12 percent). For primary care services, the ratio of rich to poor in the distribution of government expenditures was notably lower (23 percent to the top group versus 15 percent to the lowest group) (Castro-Leal et al. 2000), leading one international expert to conclude that "from an equity perspective, the move toward primary care represents a clear step in the right direction" (Gwatkin 2001, 720). An analysis of preventable deaths in children concluded that in the 42 countries accounting for 90 percent of child deaths worldwide, 63 percent could have been prevented by the full implementation of primary care. The primary care interventions included integrated care addressing the very common problems of diarrhea, pneumonia, measles, malaria, HIV/AIDS, preterm delivery, neonatal tetanus, and neonatal sepsis (Jones et al. 2003).

Except in metropolitan areas, where a greater supply of primary care physicians alone may not be associated with reductions in disparities between African Americans and whites, the findings of fewer disparities by primary care were consistent across all types of studies and were particularly marked in studies examining the actual receipt of primary care services.

Costs of Care

In addition to its relationship to better health outcomes, the supply of primary care physicians was associated with lower total costs of health services. Areas with higher ratios of primary care physicians to population had much lower total health care costs than did other areas, possibly partly because of better preventive care and lower hospitalization rates. This was demonstrated to be the case for the total U.S. adult population (Franks and Fiscella 1998), as well as among U.S. elderly living in metropolitan areas (Mark et al. 1996; Welch et al. 1993). Baicker and Chandra's (2004) analysis showed a linear decrease in Medicare spending along with an increase in the supply of primary care physicians, as well as better quality of care (as measured by 24 indicators concerning the treatment of six common medical conditions). In contrast, the supply of specialists was associated with more spending and poorer care.

Care for illnesses common in the population, for example, community-acquired pneumonia, was more expensive if provided by specialists than if provided by generalists, with no difference in outcomes (Rosser 1996; Whittle et al. 1998).

Consistent with the findings within countries, international comparisons of primary care showed that those countries with weaker primary care had significantly higher costs ($r = .61, p < .001$) (Starfield and Shi 2002).

474   *B. Starfield, L. Shi, and J. Macinko*

Rationale for the Benefits of Primary Care for Health

Six mechanisms, alone and in combination, may account for the beneficial impact of primary care on population health. They are (1) greater access to needed services, (2) better quality of care, (3) a greater focus on prevention, (4) early management of health problems, (5) the cumulative effect of the main primary care delivery characteristics, and (6) the role of primary care in reducing unnecessary and potentially harmful specialist care.

1. *Primary care increases access to health services for relatively deprived population groups.* Primary care, as the point of first contact with health services, facilitates entry to the rest of the health system. With the exception of the United States, most industrialized countries have achieved universal and equitable access to primary health services, some of them directly provided and others through the assurance of financial coverage for visits (van Doorslaer, Koolman, and Jones 2004). In the United States, however, socially deprived population subgroups are more likely than more advantaged people to lack a regular source of care. The evidence is striking with regard to family income, for which there are marked gradients in having a regular source of care, hovering around 80 percent for the poor and near-poor to nearly 90 percent for those in the middle income range, approaching 95 percent for those with high incomes, and increasing over time from 1999 to 2001 for mainly those with high incomes (Agency for Healthcare Research and Quality 2004).

   The principal benefit of health insurance in the United States is facilitating access to primary care (Lillie-Blanton and Hoffman 2005; Starfield and Shi 2004). Socially deprived population groups that do not have health insurance are less likely to have a source of primary care and thus have less access to the entire health system. Over the past several decades, attempts to improve access have been mainly the expansion of eligibility for reimbursement by public funds through Medicare, Medicaid, and related programs like the State Child Health Insurance Program. Some, but not all, of these efforts have been accompanied by incentives or even mandated enrollment with a regular source of care, and disparities in identification with a regular source of care have been reduced. However, differences in the receipt of good primary care services persist (Seid, Stevens, and Varni 2003; Shi 1999; Stevens and Shi 2002; Taira et al. 1997). Shi's national study of adults (1999) demonstrated not only differences in the likelihood of having a regular source but also (and more marked) differences in the type of that regular source, with minorities more likely to report a place rather than a person as their regular source of care; to have a specialist (other than a primary care physician) if they reported a physician as their source of care; and to experience longer delays in obtaining needed services after controlling for having a regular source of care. The same was found for children (Newacheck, Hughes, and Stoddard 1996). Other studies show that minority children are more likely to use an emergency room as their source of care (Weitzman, Byrd, and Auinger 1999). After controlling for having a regular source of care, there were few if any differences in reporting difficulty in obtaining needed services.

Analyses reported by Weinick and Krauss (2000) and Lieu, Newacheck, and McManus (1993) confirmed the finding of fewer or no difficulties in access to care when the source is a primary care source. Once they do have access to adequate primary care services, deprived minority groups often report better experiences with their care than the majority white population does, particularly when the studies were conducted in organized health care settings that, by design, eliminated many of the access barriers to primary care services (Morales et al. 2001; Murray-Garcia et al. 2000; Taira et al. 1997).

In sum, one of the main functions of a primary care source is reducing or eliminating difficulty with access to needed health services.

2. *The contribution of primary care to the quality of clinical care.* Studies designed by specialists to compare the quality of care of specialty and generalist practices often find that specialists are better at adhering to guidelines. For example, adhering to guidelines for asthma management was better in practices of specialists dealing with asthma (Bartter and Pratter 1996), and gastroenterologists used antibiotic therapy for *helicobacter pylori* earlier than

B. Starfield, L. Shi, and J. Macinko

generalists did (unless the generalists were in a group practice with gastroenterologists) (Hirth, Fendrick, and Chernew 1996). Most studies comparing generalists and specialists concluded that the condition-specific quality of care provided by specialists was better when the condition was in the specialist's area of special interest, using indicators of quality of care such as the performance of disease-specific preventive procedures, the performance of indicated laboratory tests for monitoring disease status, and the prescription of relevant medications (Harrold, Field, and Gurwitz 1999).

The findings concerning the superior quality of care by specialists were not, however, confirmed by other studies. In demonstrating the effectiveness of primary care for diabetes, general practitioner (GP) diabetic clinics in the United Kingdom were found to do as well as hospital specialists in monitoring for diabetic complications (Parnell, Zalin, and Clarke 1993). In addition, in systems in which the GPs were given additional educational support and had an organized system for recall, GPs' care of diabetic patients was better than that of specialists in hospitals. In such situations, patients of GPs had lower mortality rates and better glycemic control than did patients treated by specialists (Griffin and Kinmonth 1998). Rates of complications, readmission to the hospital, and length of convalescence were the same after early discharge from the hospital after minor surgery, regardless of whether the care was provided by the hospital's outpatient department or general practitioners (Kaag, Wijkel, and de Jong 1996). Moreover, the few studies planned and executed by generalists (Donohoe 1998; Grumbach et al. 1999) concluded that the quality of care was the same or that primary care was better. These differences suggest differences in the conceptualization of appropriate "outcomes" by the two types of physicians, with specialists more concerned with specific disease-related measures and adherence to guidelines for these diseases and primary care physicians more targeted to multiple aspects of health, that is, "generic" health. Assessing generic outcomes, or quality of care *other* than for the particular conditions under study, is important because comorbidity is common and causes more visits to both generalists and specialists than do most specific conditions (Starfield et al. 2003; Starfield et al. 2005a). If the interest is in patients' health (rather than disease processes or outcomes) as the proper focus of health services, primary care provides superior care, especially for conditions commonly seen in primary care, by focusing not primarily on the condition but on the condition in the context of the patient's other health problems or concerns.

In short, primary care physicians do at least as well as specialists in caring for specific common diseases, and they do better overall when the measures of quality are generic. For less common conditions, the care provided by primary care physicians with appropriate backup from specialists may be the best; for rare conditions, appropriate specialist care is undoubtedly important, as primary care physicians would not see such conditions frequently enough to maintain competence in managing them.

3. *The impact of primary care on prevention.* The evidence strongly shows that it is in primary care that preventive interventions are best when they are not related to any one disease or organ system. Examples of these "generic" (i.e., not limited to a particular disease or type of disease) measures are breast-feeding, not smoking, using seat belts, using smoke detectors, being physically active, and eating a healthy diet. Those U.S. states with higher ratios of primary care physicians to population have lower smoking rates, less obesity, and higher seatbelt use than do states with lower ratios of primary care physicians to population (Shi 1994; Shi and Starfield 2000). Good primary care, as determined by peoples' ratings of its main characteristics, is positively associated with smoking cessation and influenza immunization, as shown in an ongoing 60-community study in the United States (Saver 2002). The likelihood of disadvantaged children's making any preventive visits is much greater when their source of care is a good primary care practitioner (Gadomski, Jenkins, and Nichols 1998).

To the extent that many preventive activities stress the early detection of specific diseases (secondary prevention), the quality of primary care (compared with specialty care) would not necessarily be expected to be better. However, the evidence suggests otherwise for common conditions that are in the purview of primary care. A greater supply of family physicians (although not necessarily internists) is associated with an earlier detection of breast cancer, colon cancer, cervical cancer, and melanoma (Campbell et al. 2003; Ferrante et al. 2000; Roetzheim et al. 1999, 2000). Ferrante and

478   *B. Starfield, L. Shi, and J. Macinko*

colleagues (2000) found that each tenth-percentile increase in the supply of primary care physicians was associated with a statistically significant 4 percent increase in the odds of a diagnosis in an early (rather than late) stage. Most mammograms (87 percent) are ordered by primary care physicians (Schappert 1994); moreover, a physician's advice to have mammograms enhances their receipt (Breen and Kessler 1994; Campbell et al. 2003; Fox, Siu, and Stein 1994; NCI Breast Cancer Screening Consortium 1990; Roetzheim et al. 1999, 2000). Another study of differences between primary care physicians and specialists caring for patients with hypertension, non-insulin-dependent diabetes, recent myocardial infarction, or depression showed that the only preventive care procedures better performed by specialists were checks for foot ulcers and infection status in endocrinologists' diabetic patients (Greenfield et al. 1992). Moreover, approaches to prevention in primary care practice were more generic and resulted in more improvement in patients' health status than was the case in specialty-oriented practices (Bertakis et al. 1998). When the data were from the general community rather than from practices, having a good primary care source was the major determinant of receiving even disease-focused preventive care, consisting of blood pressure screening, clinical breast exams, mammograms, and Pap smears (Bindman et al. 1996).

4. *The impact of primary care on the early management of health problems.* Another indication of the benefit of primary care is its demonstrated impact on managing health problems before they are serious enough to require hospitalization or emergency services. Several studies support this conclusion.

Shea and colleagues (1992) examined the relationship between having a primary care physician as the source of care and hospitalization for reasons that should be preventable by good primary care. Men with hypertension who were admitted to the hospital from the emergency room in a large metropolitan area were divided into two groups. One group was composed of those who were admitted for a preventable complication of hypertension; the other group was admitted for a condition unrelated to hypertension. The study found that those admitted for the preventable complication were four times more likely to lack a primary care provider than were those admitted for a condition unrelated to hypertension, even after considering other factors such as absence of health insurance, level of compliance with antihypertensive regimens, and alcohol or drug use–related problems, thus indicating that those men with a primary care provider were relatively better protected against hospitalization for a preventable complication of a common medical problem.

In the United Kingdom, each 15 to 20 percent increase in GP supply per 10,000 population was significantly associated with a decrease in hospital admission rates of about 14 per 100,000 for acute illnesses and about 11 per 100,000 for chronic illnesses, even after controlling for the degree of social deprivation in the area in which people live, their social class, ethnicity, and limiting long-term illness (Gulliford 2002).

In the United States, rates of hospitalization for conditions that should be preventable by exposure to good primary care (ambulatory care–sensitive conditions, or ACSC) are strongly associated with socioeconomic deprivation, at least in part because socially disadvantaged populations are less likely to have a good source of primary care (Agency for Healthcare Research and Quality 2004; Hansell 1991; Stevens and Shi 2002). In contrast, in Spain, the rates of hospitalization for these conditions were *not* associated with socioeconomic characteristics, indicating that the Spanish health system's primary care orientation reduced the hospitalization rates for these conditions despite social disadvantage (Casanova, Colomer, and Starfield 1996; Casanova and Starfield 1995).

In a large multispecialty comparison of hospitalization rates, Greenfield and colleagues found that the rates of hospitalization were 100 percent higher when, compared with family physicians, the ongoing care was provided by cardiologists and 50 percent higher when it was provided by endocrinologists (Greenfield et al. 1992).

The literature is consistent in showing that lower rates of hospitalization for ACSC are strongly associated with the receipt of primary care. Geographic areas with more family and general practitioners have lower hospitalization rates for these types of conditions, including diabetes mellitus, hypertension, and pneumonia (Parchman and Culler 1994). Children receiving their care from a primary care source that fulfills the criteria for its main

B. Starfield, L. Shi, and J. Macinko

characteristics have lower hospitalization rates for these conditions as well as lower hospitalization rates overall. These findings are associated with the greater receipt of preventive care from primary care providers (Gadomski, Jenkins, and Nichols 1998). Rates of hospital admissions of children are lower in those U.S. communities in which primary care physicians are more involved in caring for children both before and during hospitalization (Perrin et al. 1996). Adolescents with the same regular source of care for preventive and illness care are less likely to seek care in emergency rooms (Ryan et al. 2001). An analysis of national Medicare data showed that the elderly in the United States who are in fair or poor health are more likely to experience a potentially preventable hospitalization if they live in a county designated as a primary care shortage area (Parchman and Culler 1999).

Only two studies failed to find a positive impact for the supply of primary care physicians and hospitalizations for conditions sensitive to primary care management. Each of the studies was conducted in only one state, New York or North Carolina (Ricketts et al. 2001; Schreiber and Zielinski 1997). In both studies, socioeconomic characteristics were more salient, and so it is possible that in some places, the availability of more primary care physicians did not necessarily mean that deprived populations had access to them. A later study in one of those states (New York) showed that the ratio of primary care physicians to population was one of the more salient factors associated with lower levels of hospitalizations for ACSC (Friedman and Basu 2001).

5. *The accumulated contribution of primary care characteristics to more appropriate care.* As noted in regard to quality of care, the beneficial effects of primary care on mortality and morbidity can be attributed, at least in part, to the focus of primary care on the person rather than on the management of particular diseases. Care focuses on the person when practitioners attend to overall aspects of the patient's health rather than to the care of his or her specific diseases; it focuses on achieving better outcomes for health in all its aspects rather than on the procedures directed at improving the processes or outcomes of care for particular conditions. Other aspects of health services delivery that are characteristic of primary care also have been associated with better health outcomes. Although an extensive review of the positive contribution of each

of these characteristics is outside the scope of this review (which concerns primary care as an entity within health service systems) and has been covered elsewhere (Starfield 1998), a brief summary of these contributions explains why primary care as a whole might have positive effects.

We noted earlier that an important element of primary care is its role as the first contact for patients when a problem develops. In a seminal article entitled "Gatekeeping Revisited—Protecting Patients from Overtreatment," Franks, Clancy, and Nutting (1992) made the case for seeing a primary care physician before seeking care from another type of physician. Having a relationship with a primary care practitioner who can serve as an initial point of contact is strongly and statistically significantly associated with less use of specialists and emergency rooms (Hurley, Freund, and Taylor 1989; Martin et al. 1989). *Continuity* of care, which implies that individuals use their primary source of care over time for most of their health care needs, is associated with greater satisfaction, better compliance, and lower hospitalization and emergency room use (Freeman and Hjortdahl 1997; Mainous and Gill 1998; Rosenblatt et al. 2000; Weiss and Blustein 1996). Previous knowledge of a patient, which reflects good continuity of care, increases the doctor's odds of recognizing psychosocial problems influencing the patient's health (Gulbrandsen, Hjortdahl, and Fugelli 1997). Both continuity and first-contact attributes of primary care ensure greater efficiency of services in the time saved in the consultation, less use of laboratory tests, and fewer health care expenditures (Forrest and Starfield 1996, 1998; Hjortdahl and Borchgrevink 1991; Raddish, Horn, and Sharkey 1999; Roos, Carriere, and Friesen 1998). Very short-term relationships with physicians are associated with poor outcomes. For example, veterans with a chronic disease who did not have a previous relationship with a primary care physician were randomized to receive an intervention of increased follow-up by a newly assigned nurse and a primary care physician after they were discharged from the hospital. Rehospitalization rates six months later were higher in this intervention group (Weinberger, Oddone, and Henderson 1996), thus indicating that relationships over time are an important component of primary care. (The study did not assess rehospitalization rates for veterans who already had a primary care provider,

B. Starfield, L. Shi, and J. Macinko

and it may be that the assignment of such a provider to people without an existing relationship led to the discovery of new conditions not previously recognized and requiring hospitalization.) At least two years of a relationship (and as many as five) are generally required for patients and practitioners to get to know each other well enough to provide optimal person-focused care (Starfield 1998, 175). A freely chosen primary care practitioner provides better assurance of a good relationship than does assigning a practitioner (Starfield 1998, 151). The evidence is strong regarding the benefits of an ongoing relationship with a particular provider rather than with a particular place or no place at all. People with no source of primary care are more likely to be hospitalized, to delay seeking needed and timely preventive care, to receive care in emergency departments, and to have higher subsequent mortality and higher health care costs, and they are less likely to see a physician in the presence of symptoms. People with just a place (such as a particular hospital clinic) are somewhat better off than those without a regular source of care, in that they are more likely to keep their appointments, have fewer hospitalizations and lower costs, and receive generally better preventive care. In addition, people who report a particular doctor as their regular source of care receive more appropriate preventive care, are more likely to have their problems recognized, have fewer diagnostic tests and fewer prescriptions, have fewer hospitalizations and visits to emergency departments, and are more likely to have more accurate diagnoses and lower costs of care than are either people having a particular place or people having no place at all as their regular source of care (Starfield 1998, chap. 8).

The benefits of the other two main attributes of good primary care (comprehensiveness and coordination) are less well documented, but the existing evidence was summarized by Starfield (1998, chaps. 10 and 11).

6. *The role of primary care in reducing unnecessary or inappropriate specialty care.* Nearly all studies of specialist services concluded that there is either no effect or an adverse effect on major health outcomes from increasing the supply of specialists in the United States, which already has a much greater supply of such physicians than do other industrialized countries (Starfield et al. 2005b). This

evidence addresses a wide variety of population health outcomes, including all-cause (total) mortality; heart and cerebrovascular disease mortality; cancer mortality; postneonatal, neonatal, and total infant mortality; and low birth weight; as well as the early detection of various cancers, including cervical cancer, colorectal cancers, breast cancer, and melanoma (the evidence was reviewed by Starfield et al. 2005b). The evidence is also consistent that first contact with a primary care physician (before seeking care from a specialist) is associated with more appropriate, more effective, and less costly care (Starfield 1998, chap. 7).

Other countries, most notably the United Kingdom and the Netherlands, have led the way with primary care innovations to reduce the inappropriate use of specialist services. These include making better use of information systems and video communications as well as consulting with specialists in primary care settings.

The adverse effects of seeking care directly from nonprimary care specialists have a strong theoretical basis. Since these specialists are trained in the hospital, the patients seen by specialists are not representative of the way in which patients present symptoms in community settings, because the latter have a much lower prior probability of serious illness requiring the services of a specialist. The properties of diagnostic tests (sensitivity, specificity, predictive power of a positive test) are much different in populations with a high prevalence of serious illness than they are in community settings and thus much different in specialty care than in primary care settings. The result is that specialists practicing in the community overestimate the likelihood of illness in the patients they see, with the consequently inappropriate use of diagnostic and therapeutic modalities, both of which raise the likelihood of adverse effects (Franks, Clancy, and Nutting 1992; Hashem, Chi, and Friedman 2003; Sox 1996). Compared with other Anglophone countries, people in the United States experience more adverse effects and medical errors (Schoen et al. 2004). This, combined with evidence concerning the adverse effects of greater supplies of specialists and estimates of the likelihood of adverse effects of medical care, may at least partly explain the United States' low ranking on health status relative to that of similarly industrialized countries.

Potential Limitations of Interpretations of Effectiveness of Primary Care

Despite the consistency of the findings from various types of studies, areas, and populations and the theoretical rationale for benefit of primary care on population health, it is possible that the results may be overinterpreted. Those countries and areas in which primary care is strongest (however measured) may be areas in which other social interventions (such as income supports and welfare policies that influence health) also are strongest. So far, the effort to identify the social policies that have a great influence on health has not been successful (Graham and Kelly 2004).

Moreover, the mere presence of primary care physicians may not reflect the availability of primary care services to certain population groups. At least two of the reviewed analyses in urban counties showed that the supply of primary care physicians is less closely related to the health of urban African Americans than it is for urban whites or for African Americans in rural areas. This is likely due to the poorer distribution of primary care physicians in more deprived urban areas, with the consequently greater need to seek care in such places as hospital outpatient units and emergency rooms. Supporting this hypothesis are two lines of evidence. First, African Americans are more likely than whites to report having their regular source of care in a facility (such as a hospital) and to report a specialist as their regular source of care (Shi 1999). That is, primary care physicians in urban areas tend to locate in more socially advantaged areas (Weiner et al. 1982). As a result, hospital clinics with predominantly hospital-based physicians not trained to provide the important features of primary care become the "default" regular source of care. Second, even in the presence of adequate primary care resources, African Americans may be less likely than other racial and ethnic groups to use primary care when other resources (such as hospital clinics) are available; this has been demonstrated to be the case for the medical care of inner-city infants (Hoffmann, Broyles, and Tyson 1997). State-level analyses are not as susceptible to this type of possible error because primary care is more evenly distributed than is specialty care (Shi and Starfield 2001).

If the supply of primary care physicians is less closely associated with health outcomes in urban African Americans than in whites because of difficulties in access to them, the demonstrated association between supply and health outcomes may actually underestimate the potential impact

Contribution of Primary Care to Health Systems and Health   485

of primary care services, particularly for deprived populations. Moreover, the studies that use alternative measures of primary care, including relationships with a primary care physician and studies considering the adequacy of primary care health services delivery characteristics, all confirm the conclusion that care meeting the criteria for primary care is associated with the better health of those populations receiving it, with a greater impact in more deprived populations.

Primary Care in the Future

What issues remain to be addressed in primary care to improve its contribution to the health of populations and equity in distribution of health? A pervasive U.S. focus on "access" to health services rather than on the type of health services has detracted from the need to ensure that services are provided in the most appropriate places. The existing national data health interview surveys combine various safety net providers into one group so that people receiving their care from hospital outpatient clinics are not distinguishable from those receiving care from primary care–oriented clinics. Combining primary care–focused community health centers with hospital emergency and outpatient departments as "safety net providers" masks the high positive contributions to the health of the former with the lesser primary care focus of the latter. Apart from the Community Health Center program of the federal Health Resources and Services Administration and the commitment of certain not-for-profit health care organizations to strong primary care (Weiner 2004), little or nothing has been done to ensure that other "regular sources of care" fulfill the criteria for good primary care. In most other industrialized countries, primary care physicians are clearly distinguished from other physicians, and where people receive care is easily identified as primary care or specialty care. Greater appreciation that it is primary care that plays a major role in ensuring access to appropriate health services should provide the rationale for better distinguishing primary care from specialty care in data on the use of health services in the United States.

At the very least, primary care must be recognized as a distinct aspect of a health services system. There now are well-validated methods (e.g., see Shi, Starfield, and Xu 2001; Starfield et al. 1998) to assess both the presence and the characteristics of primary care, and all sources of data on use of health services should include at least a few of these

486   *B. Starfield, L. Shi, and J. Macinko*

measures. Understanding people's primary care experiences (rather than or in addition to their satisfaction), including the extent to which they receive the range of services appropriate to their needs and have the care they receive elsewhere coordinated and integrated, are important to evaluating the adequacy of health services.

In contrast to the situation in primary care, for which intensive conceptual and methodologic study over the past several decades has clarified its most important aspects, professional specialty groups in the United States have made little if any attempt to define the practice of "specialism" or the circumstances that should lead to seeking care from specialists. Referrals to specialists apparently have three functions: short-term consultation for diagnosis or management, referral for long-term management of specific illnesses, and recurrent consultation for periodic management. A study of referrals from 80 office-based family practices showed that by far the most referrals for common conditions (over 50 percent of all referrals to most types of specialists) were expected to be for a short term (less than 12 months) and that for more than 50 percent, they were for consultation only (no direct intervention) (Starfield et al. 2002). Very little is known, however, about the relative frequency of these functions from the viewpoint of specialty practice. One report (Hewlett et al. 2005) indicated that about 75 percent of visits to a pulmonary specialty clinic were just for "checkups," even though the patients' primary care physicians, once they had access to the specialists' reports, could just as easily perform this function and report the findings to the specialists. Such an approach to reducing the number of visits to specialists could lower the demand for a greater supply of specialists; it at least deserves to be tested. There is an urgent need for information about the indications for specialty care and about the impact on outcomes of excessive use of specialists.

Major challenges to primary care practice concern (1) recognizing and managing comorbidity, (2) preventing the adverse effects of medical interventions, (3) maintaining a high quality of the important characteristics of primary care practice, and (4) improving equity in health services and in the health of populations (Starfield 2001).

1. Historically, principles of delivery of medical care have been based on preventing and managing specific diseases. In the current climate of evidence-based medicine, guidelines for the management of diseases are proliferating and increasingly used. The

development of guidelines is generally based on evidence from the literature that certain modes of management achieve better outcomes than others do. The "gold standard" for evidence is the randomized controlled clinical trial, which generally excludes, as a requirement for participation in the trial, individuals with co-morbid conditions. Comorbidity (the simultaneous presence of apparently unrelated conditions) is common in the population and is not randomly distributed. Although comorbidity becomes more common with age, it is in the young that comorbidity occurs much more frequently than expected by the chance occurrence of two or more conditions (van den Akker et al. 1998). (That is, the frequency of illness is much greater in the old than in the young, so there is much greater likelihood that two unrelated illnesses will be found together. In the young, illness is much less common, so that it is statistically much less likely that two or more will be found together, although in fact this is the case.) Data systems should be developed that provide a much better basis for examining the distribution and nature of comorbidity in primary care; ascertainment of the impact of baseline risks on comorbidity; likelihood of responsiveness to treatment in the presence of comorbidity; and susceptibility to adverse effects of medical interventions. Moreover, the applicability to primary care of guidelines developed from randomized controlled clinical trials may be more limited than is generally thought, even apart from the issue of comorbidity (Kravitz, Duan, and Braslow 2004; Rothwell 2005), particularly when considering the issue of disease-specific versus overall clinical end points (Fleming 2005).

2. Primary care practitioners are in the best position to detect the occurrence of potentially adverse effects of medical interventions, particularly those stemming from drug reactions and interactions. In systems of care oriented to primary care (including some HMOs in the United States), the primary care practitioner is, by far, the most commonly seen physician, for patients with *all* degrees of comorbidity and for both single common conditions and comorbid conditions. Only when individual conditions are uncommon are specialists the type of physician most frequently seen, and only for that condition (*not* for comorbid conditions) (Starfield et al. 2003; Starfield et al. 2005a). Thus, primary care physicians are more likely to see the adverse events that result from their own

488   *B. Starfield, L. Shi, and J. Macinko*

care as well as the care of others whom the patient may see. The challenge for primary care is to establish systems to code unexpected symptoms or signs and to create information systems that could serve as early warnings of the occurrence of adverse events in persons previously subjected to particular types of interventions. It is possible that the International Classification of Primary Care (ICPC) (Lamberts, Wood, and Hofmans-Okkes 1993), which provides a straightforward classification of problems encountered in primary care while maintaining comparability with the better known International Classification of Diseases (originally developed to code causes of death), could serve as the basis for recording and classifying these symptoms and signs in the United States, as it is already being used in several other countries.

3. Improvement in clinical quality and in performance with respect to the main features of primary care practice is a challenge for primary care practice. Although each of these features is known to confer benefits on health, the remaining issues require consideration.

   • To what extent can teams of practitioners provide first-contact care without interfering with the benefits of continuing interpersonal relationships between particular practitioners and patients?

   • Ongoing person-focused care means that care should be focused on the person rather than on the disease. Can teams of practitioners fulfill this function?

   • Comprehensiveness means that all problems in the population should be cared for in primary care (with short-term referral as needed), except those that are too unusual (generally a frequency of less than one or two per thousand in the population served) for the primary care practitioner or team to treat competently. How can data systems provide the information needed to decide when problems are best met in primary care, when they can be best dealt with in primary care with appropriate specialty backup, and when patients need to be seen by a specialist?

   • Coordination of care means that the primary care practice must integrate all aspects of care when patients must be seen elsewhere. Because 13 to 20 percent (depending on various assumptions) of an average practice population requires a referral each year, this burden is considerable. Very few health systems, even those that rate high on primary care, achieve high coordination of care, at least as measured by transfer of information from primary care physicians to specialists and vice versa. Systems to facilitate coordinating efforts are urgently needed. Lessons might be gleaned from the experiences of some health systems. For example, and despite the design limitations (Talbot-Smith et al. 2004) of the study comparing the Kaiser-Permanente health care plan in the United States with the National Health Service in the United Kingdom (Feachem, Sekhri, and White 2002), the lower hospitalization rates and lower resource use in the United States may well be a result of a system specifically designed to enhance coordination between primary care physicians and specialists.

4. The achievement of equity in health services and health is an imperative everywhere. Primary care is inherently a more equitable level of care than other levels of care. It is less costly (hence sparing resources that could be devoted to providing better services to more disadvantaged populations), and through its key features, it narrows disparities in health between more and less socially deprived population groups. The extent to which primary care in fact does result in more equity depends on the availability of information about the needs in the various areas in which primary care practices are located. Better information systems, at both the area and practice levels, would enhance the already-strong benefits of primary care to the health of individuals, population subgroups, and populations (National Committee for Vital and Health Statistics 2001).

The Relevance of Policy

The relatively poor performance of the United States on major health indicators, despite per capita health care expenditures that are much higher than those of any other country, is a pressing concern for policymakers, the business community (which has, historically, paid for much of the health insurance in the country), and, ultimately, taxpayers. Efforts to improve the system to achieve better health at lower cost are rapidly becoming imperative. Primary care offers an effective and efficient approach to achieve that goal. Evidence of the benefits of a health

490   *B. Starfield, L. Shi, and J. Macinko*

system with a strong primary care base is abundant and consistent. These benefits are not limited to one or only a few aspects of health but, rather, extend to the major causes of death and disorders as well as to reducing disparities in health across major population subgroups, including racial and ethnic minorities as well as socially deprived adults and children.

Federally qualified community health centers (CHCs) currently serve more than 3,600 urban and rural communities, which are typically low-income inner-city or resource-poor rural communities. But they serve only one-quarter of all people living below the poverty level, one in seven people living under 200 percent of poverty level, and one of eight uninsured Americans (Proser, Shin, and Hawkins 2005). Expansion of the CHC network well beyond the current supply is one appropriate strategy.

Other policy strategies would strengthen primary care on a broader level (Starfield and Simpson 1993). These include (but are not limited to) changes in the method of reimbursing primary care physicians and, particularly, better reimbursement rates for primary care services for both common conditions and for the important primary care delivery characteristics. Establishing a more rational basis for referrals and improving the coordination between primary care and specialist physicians would make primary care practice more challenging and intellectually rewarding. States could encourage a better distribution of physicians (both primary care and specialists) by tailoring their licensing policies to health needs in different areas or by providing financial incentives for practicing in underserved areas, as is done in some other countries. Incentives for training primary care practitioners could be improved by reorienting federal support for graduate medical education toward training primary care physicians. Similarly, loan forgiveness for primary care practitioners could be expanded. Reducing the amount of paperwork needed to file claims and encouraging the creation of electronic medical records would greatly reduce the tedium of record keeping in practice and, at the same time, make time to improve the self-monitoring of the quality of care. Bonus payments for team practice could enhance the comprehensiveness of primary care. Special recognition of best primary care practices could enhance public recognition of the importance of primary care and its characteristics. Finally, offering more funds for research on primary care, including the support of collaborative practice-based networks (Lanier 2005; Wasserman, Slora, and Bocian 2003), would help meet the intellectual challenges of expanding our knowledge base for the practice of both primary care and specialty care.

Contribution of Primary Care to Health Systems and Health 491

References

Agency for Healthcare Research and Quality. 2004. *2004 National Healthcare Disparities Report.* AHRQ Publication no. 05-0014. Rockville, Md.

Atun, R. 2004. *What Are the Advantages and Disadvantages of Restructuring a Health Care System to Be More Focused on Primary Care Services?* London: Health Evidence Network.

Baicker, K., and A. Chandra. 2004. Medicare Spending, the Physician Workforce, and Beneficiaries' Quality of Care. *Health Affairs* W4:184–97 (http://content.healthaffairs.org/cgi/reprint/hlthaff.w4.184v1.pdf).

Bartter, T., and M.R. Pratter. 1996. Asthma: Better Outcome at Lower Cost? The Role of the Expert in the Care System. *Chest* 110:1589–96.

Bertakis, K.D., E.J. Callahan, L.J. Helms, R. Azari, J.A. Robbins, and J. Miller. 1998. Physician Practice Styles and Patient Outcomes: Differences between Family Practice and General Internal Medicine. *Medical Care* 36:879–91.

Bindman, A.B., K. Grumbach, D. Osmond, K. Vranizan, and A.L. Stewart. 1996. Primary Care and Receipt of Preventive Services. *Journal of General Internal Medicine* 11:269–76.

Breen, N., and L. Kessler. 1994. Changes in the Use of Screening Mammography: Evidence from the 1987 and 1990 National Health Interview Surveys. *American Journal of Public Health* 84:62–7.

Britton, A., M. Shipley, M. Marmot, and H. Hemingway. 2004. Does Access to Cardiac Investigation and Treatment Contribute to Social and Ethnic Differences in Coronary Heart Disease? Whitehall II Prospective Cohort Study. *British Medical Journal* 329:318–23.

Campbell, R.J., A.M. Ramirez, K. Perez, and R.G. Roetzheim. 2003. Cervical Cancer Rates and the Supply of Primary Care Physicians in Florida. *Family Medicine* 35:60–64.

Casanova, C., C. Colomer, and B. Starfield. 1996. Pediatric Hospitalization Due to Ambulatory Care-Sensitive Conditions in Valencia (Spain). *International Journal for Quality in Health Care* 8:51–9.

Casanova, C., and B. Starfield. 1995. Hospitalizations of Children and Access to Primary Care: A Cross-National Comparison. *International Journal of Health Services* 25:283–94.

Castro-Leal, F., J. Dayton, L. Demery, and K. Mehra. 2000. Public Spending on Health Care in Africa: Do the Poor Benefit? *Bulletin of the World Health Organization* 78:66–74.

Cooper, R.A., T.E. Getzen, H.J. McKee, and P. Laud. 2002. Economic and Demographic Trends Signal an Impending Physician Shortage. *Health Affairs* 21:140–54.

492   *B. Starfield, L. Shi, and J. Macinko*

Davey Smith, G., and J. Lynch. 2004. Commentary: Social Capital, Social Epidemiology and Disease Aetiology. *International Journal of Epidemiology* 33:691–700.

Donaldson, M.S., K.D. Yordy, K.N. Lohr, and N.A. Vanselow. 1996. *Primary Care: America's Health in a New Era*. Washington, D.C.: National Academy Press.

Donohoe, M.T. 1998. Comparing Generalist and Specialty Care: Discrepancies, Deficiencies, and Excesses. *Archives of Internal Medicine* 158:1596–1608.

Engstrom, S., M. Foldevi, and L. Borgquist. 2001. Is General Practice Effective? A Systematic Literature Review. *Scandinavian Journal of Primary Health Care* 19:131–44.

Feachem, R.G., N.K. Sekhri, and K.L. White. 2002. Getting More for Their Dollar: A Comparison of the NHS with California's Kaiser Permanente. *British Medical Journal* 324:135–41.

Ferrante, J.M., E.C. Gonzalez, N. Pal, and R.G. Roetzheim. 2000. Effects of Physician Supply on Early Detection of Breast Cancer. *Journal of the American Board of Family Practice* 13:408–14.

Fleming, T.R. 2005. Surrogate Endpoints and FDA's Accelerated Approval Process. *Health Affairs* 24:67–78.

Flocke, S.A., K.C. Stange, and S.J. Zyzanski. 1998. The Association of Attributes of Primary Care with the Delivery of Clinical Preventive Services. *Medical Care* 36:AS21–30.

Forrest, C.B., and B. Starfield. 1996. The Effect of First-Contact Care with Primary Care Clinicians on Ambulatory Health Care Expenditures. *Journal of Family Practice* 43:40–48.

Forrest, C.B., and B. Starfield. 1998. Entry into Primary Care and Continuity: The Effects of Access. *American Journal of Public Health* 88:1330–36.

Fox, S.A., A.L. Siu, and J.A. Stein. 1994. The Importance of Physician Communication on Breast Cancer Screening of Older Women. *Archives of Internal Medicine* 154:2058–68.

Franks, P., C.M. Clancy, and P.A. Nutting. 1992. Gatekeeping Revisited—Protecting Patients from Overtreatment. *New England Journal of Medicine* 327:424–9.

Franks, P., and K. Fiscella. 1998. Primary Care Physicians and Specialists as Personal Physicians. Health Care Expenditures and Mortality Experience. *Journal of Family Practice* 47:105–9.

Freeman, G., and P. Hjortdahl. 1997. What Future for Continuity of Care in General Practice? *British Medical Journal* 314:1870–73.

Friedman, B., and J. Basu. 2001. Health Insurance, Primary Care, and Preventable Hospitalization of Children in a Large State. *American Journal of Managed Care* 7:473–81.

Gadomski, A., P. Jenkins, and M. Nichols. 1998. Impact of a Medicaid Primary Care Provider and Preventive Care on Pediatric Hospitalization. *Pediatrics* 101:E1 (http://www.pediatrics.org/cgi/content/full/101/3/e1).

Graham, H., and M.P. Kelly. 2004. *Health Inequalities: Concepts, Frameworks, and Policy*. London: National Health Service/Health Development Agency. Available at http://www.publichealth.nice.org.uk/page.aspx?o=502453 (accessed April 5, 2005).

Greenfield, S., E.C. Nelson, M. Zubkoff, W. Manning, W. Rogers, R.L. Kravitz, A. Keller, A.R. Tarlov, and J.E. Ware Jr. 1992. Variations in Resource Utilization among Medical Specialties and Systems of Care. Results from the Medical Outcomes Study. *Journal of the American Medical Association* 267:1624–30.

Griffin, S., and A. Kinmonth. 1998. *Diabetes Care: The Effectiveness of Systems for Routine Surveillance for People with Diabetes*. Cochrane Library.

Grumbach, K., J.V. Selby, J.A. Schmittdiel, and C.P. Quesenberry Jr. 1999. Quality of Primary Care Practice in a Large HMO according to Physician Specialty. *Health Services Research* 34:485–502.

Gulbrandsen, P., P. Hjortdahl, and P. Fugelli. 1997. General Practitioners' Knowledge of Their Patients' Psychosocial Problems: Multipractice Questionnaire Survey. *British Medical Journal* 314:1014–8.

Gulliford, M.C. 2002. Availability of Primary Care Doctors and Population Health in England: Is There an Association? *Journal of Public Health Medicine* 24:252–4.

Gulliford, M.C., R.H. Jack, G. Adams, and O.C. Ukoumunne. 2004. Availability and Structure of Primary Medical Care Services and Population Health and Health Care Indicators in England. *BMC Health Services Research* 4:12.

Gwatkin, D.R. 2001. The Need for Equity-Oriented Health Sector Reforms. *International Journal of Epidemiology* 30:720–23.

Haines, M., and R. Avery. 1982. Differential Infant and Child Mortality in Costa Rica. *Population Studies* 36:31–43.

Hansell, M.J. 1991. Sociodemographic Factors and the Quality of Prenatal Care. *American Journal of Public Health* 81:1023–8.

Harrold, L.R., T.S. Field, and J.H. Gurwitz. 1999. Knowledge, Patterns of Care, and Outcomes of Care for Generalists and Specialists. *Journal of General Internal Medicine* 14:499–511.

Hashem, A., M.T. Chi, and C.P. Friedman. 2003. Medical Errors as a Result of Specialization. *Journal of Biomedical Informatics* 36:61–9.

Health Council of the Netherlands. 2004. *European Primary Care*. Publication no. 2004/20E. The Hague.

494   *B. Starfield, L. Shi, and J. Macinko*

Hewlett, S., J. Kirwan, J. Pollock, K. Mitchell, M. Hehir, P.S. Blair, D. Memel, and M.G. Perry. 2005. Patient Initiated Outpatient Follow up in Rheumatoid Arthritis: Six Year Randomised Controlled Trial. *British Medical Journal* 330:171–5.

Hirth, R.A., A.M. Fendrick, and M.E. Chernew. 1996. Specialist and Generalist Physicians' Adoption of Antibiotic Therapy to Eradicate *Helicobacter pylori* Infection. *Medical Care* 34:1199–1204.

Hjortdahl, P., and C.F. Borchgrevink. 1991. Continuity of Care: Influence of General Practitioners' Knowledge about Their Patients on Use of Resources in Consultations. *British Medical Journal* 303:1181–4.

Hoffmann, C., R.S. Broyles, and J.E. Tyson. 1997. Emergency Room Visits Despite the Availability of Primary Care: A Study of High Risk Inner City Infants. *American Journal of Medical Science* 313:99–103.

Hurley, R.E., D.A. Freund, and D.E. Taylor. 1989. Emergency Room Use and Primary Care Case Management: Evidence from Four Medicaid Demonstration Programs. *American Journal of Public Health* 79:843–6.

Institute of Medicine (IOM). 1978. *A Manpower Policy for Primary Health Care.* IOM Publication 78-02. Washington, D.C.: National Academy of Sciences.

Jarman, B., S. Gault, B. Alves, A. Hider, S. Dolan, A. Cook, B. Hurwitz, and L.I. Iezzoni. 1999. Explaining Differences in English Hospital Death Rates Using Routinely Collected Data. *British Medical Journal* 318:1515–20.

Jones, G., R.W. Steketee, R.E. Black, Z.A. Bhutta, and S.S. Morris. 2003. How Many Child Deaths Can We Prevent This Year? *Lancet* 362:65–71.

Kaag, M.E., D. Wijkel, and D. de Jong. 1996. Primary Health Care Replacing Hospital Care—The Effect on Quality of Care. *International Journal for Quality in Health Care* 8:367–73.

Klijzing, F., and H. Taylor. 1982. The Decline of Infant Mortality in Costa Rica, 1950–73: Modernization or Technological Diffusion? *Malaysian Journal of Tropical Geography* 5:22–9.

Kravitz, R.L., N. Duan, and J. Braslow. 2004. Evidence-Based Medicine, Heterogeneity of Treatment Effects, and the Trouble with Averages. *Milbank Quarterly* 82:661–87.

Lamberts, H., M. Wood, and I. Hofmans-Okkes. 1993. *The International Classification of Primary Care in the European Community.* Oxford: Oxford University Press.

Lanier, D. 2005. Primary Care Practice-Based Research Comes of Age in the United States. *Annals of Family Medicine* 3:S2–4.

Larizgoitia, I., and B. Starfield. 1997. Reform of Primary Health Care: The Case of Spain. *Health Policy* 41:121–37.

Leggetter, S., N. Chaturvedi, J.H. Fuller, and M.E. Edmonds. 2002. Ethnicity and Risk of Diabetes-Related Lower Extremity Amputation: A Population-Based, Case-Control Study of African Caribbeans and Europeans in the United Kingdom. *Archives of Internal Medicine* 162:73–8.

Lieu, T.A., P.W. Newacheck, and M.A. McManus. 1993. Race, Ethnicity, and Access to Ambulatory Care among U.S. Adolescents. *American Journal of Public Health* 83:960–5.

Lillie-Blanton, M., and C. Hoffman. 2005. The Role of Health Insurance Coverage in Reducing Racial/Ethnic Disparities in Health Care. *Health Affairs* 24:398–408.

Macinko, J., C. Almeida, and P. Sa. 2005. Evaluating Primary Care Services in Brazil: A Rapid Appraisal Methodology. Unpublished manuscript.

Macinko, J., B. Starfield, and L. Shi. 2003. The Contribution of Primary Care Systems to Health Outcomes within Organization for Economic Cooperation and Development (OECD) Countries, 1970–1998. *Health Services Research* 38:831–65.

Macinko, J., B. Starfield, and L. Shi. 2005. Quantifying the Health Benefits of Primary Care Physician Supply in the United States. Unpublished manuscript.

Mainous, A.G. III, and J.M. Gill. 1998. The Importance of Continuity of Care in the Likelihood of Future Hospitalization: Is Site of Care Equivalent to a Primary Clinician? *American Journal of Public Health* 88:1539–41.

Mansfield, C.J., J.L. Wilson, E.J. Kobrinski, and J. Mitchell. 1999. Premature Mortality in the United States: The Roles of Geographic Area, Socioeconomic Status, Household Type, and Availability of Medical Care. *American Journal of Public Health* 89:893–8.

Mark, D.H., M.S. Gottlieb, B.B. Zellner, V.K. Chetty, and J.E. Midtling. 1996. Medicare Costs in Urban Areas and the Supply of Primary Care Physicians. *Journal of Family Practice* 43:33–9.

Martin, D.P., P. Diehr, K.F. Price, and W.C. Richardson. 1989. Effect of a Gatekeeper Plan on Health Services Use and Charges: A Randomized Trial. *American Journal of Public Health* 79:1628–32.

Morales, L.S., M.N. Elliott, R. Weech-Maldonado, K.L. Spritzer, and R.D. Hays. 2001. Differences in CAHPS Adult Survey Reports and Ratings by Race and Ethnicity: An Analysis of the National CAHPS Benchmarking Data 1.0. *Health Services Research* 36:595–617.

Murray-Garcia, J.L., J.V. Selby, J. Schmittdiel, K. Grumbach, and C.P. Quesenberry Jr. 2000. Racial and Ethnic Differences in a Patient

496   *B. Starfield, L. Shi, and J. Macinko*

Survey: Patients' Values, Ratings, and Reports Regarding Physician Primary Care Performance in a Large Health Maintenance Organization. *Medical Care* 38:300–10.

National Committee for Vital and Health Statistics. 2001. *Information for Health: A Strategy for Building the National Health Information Infrastructure.* Washington, D.C.: U.S. Department of Health and Human Services.

NCI Breast Cancer Screening Consortium. 1990. Screening Mammography: A Missed Clinical Opportunity? *Journal of the American Medical Association* 264:54–8.

Newacheck, P.W., D.C. Hughes, and J.J. Stoddard. 1996. Children's Access to Primary Care: Differences by Race, Income, and Insurance Status. *Pediatrics* 97:26–32.

O'Malley, A.S., C.B. Forrest, R.M. Politzer, J.T. Wulu, and L. Shi. 2005. Health Center Trends, 1994–2001: What Do They Portend for the Federal Growth Initiative? *Health Affairs* 24:465–72.

Or, Z. 2001. *Exploring the Effects of Health Care on Mortality across OECD Countries.* Labour Market and Social Policy Occasional Papers no. 46. Paris: Organization for Economic Cooperation and Development.

Organization for Economic Cooperation and Development (OECD). 2001. *Health Data 2001: A Comparative Analysis of 30 Countries.* Paris.

Pan American Health Organization (PAHO). 2005. *Regional Core Health Data.* Washington, D.C. Available at http://www.paho.org/English/SHA/coredata/tabulator/newTabulator.htm (accessed June 8, 2005).

Parchman, M.L., and S.D. Culler. 1994. Primary Care Physicians and Avoidable Hospitalizations. *Journal of Family Practice* 39:123–8.

Parchman, M.L., and S.D. Culler. 1999. Preventable Hospitalizations in Primary Care Shortage Areas. An Analysis of Vulnerable Medicare Beneficiaries. *Archives of Family Medicine* 8:487–91.

Parnell, S.J., A.M. Zalin, and C.W. Clarke. 1993. Care of Diabetic Patients in Hospital Clinics and General Practice Clinics: A Study in Dudley. *British Journal of General Practice* 43:65–9; erratum 1993; 43 (369):163.

Perrin, J.M., P. Greenspan, S.R. Bloom, D. Finkelstein, S. Yazdgerdi, J.M. Leventhal, L. Rodewald, P. Szilagyi, and C.J. Homer. 1996. Primary Care Involvement among Hospitalized Children. *Archives of Pediatric and Adolescent Medicine* 150:479–86.

Perry, H., N. Robison, D. Chavez, O. Taja, C. Hilari, D. Shanklin, and J. Wyon. 1998. The Census-Based, Impact-Oriented Approach: Its Effectiveness in Promoting Child Health in Bolivia. *Health Policy and Planning* 13:140–51.

Contribution of Primary Care to Health Systems and Health   497

Politzer, R.M., J. Yoon, L. Shi, R.G. Hughes, J. Regan, and M.H. Gaston. 2001. Inequality in America: The Contribution of Health Centers in Reducing and Eliminating Disparities in Access to Care. *Medical Care Research and Review* 58:234–48.

Proser, M., P. Shin, and D. Hawkins. 2005. *A Nation's Health at Risk III: Growing Uninsured, Budget Cutbacks Challenge President's Initiative to Put a Health Center in Every Poor County.* Washington, D.C.: National Association of Community Health Centers and George Washington University.

Raddish, M., S.D. Horn, and P.D. Sharkey. 1999. Continuity of Care: Is It Cost Effective? *American Journal of Managed Care* 5:727–34.

Regan, J., A.H. Schempf, J. Yoon, and R.M. Politzer. 2003. The Role of Federally Funded Health Centers in Serving the Rural Population. *Journal of Rural Health* 19:117–24.

Reyes, H., R. Perez-Cuevas, J. Salmeron, P. Tome, H. Guiscafre, and G. Gutierrez. 1997. Infant Mortality Due to Acute Respiratory Infections: The Influence of Primary Care Processes. *Health Policy and Planning* 12:214–23.

Ricketts, T.C., R. Randolph, H.A. Howard, D. Pathman, and T. Carey. 2001. Hospitalization Rates as Indicators of Access to Primary Care. *Health and Place* 7:27–38.

Riveron Corteguera, R. 2000. Estrategias para reducir la mortalidad infantil. Cuba 1995–1999. *Revista Cubana de Pediatria* 72:147–64.

Roetzheim, R.G., N. Pal, E.C. Gonzalez, J.M. Ferrante, D.J. Van Durme, J.Z. Ayanian, and J.P. Krischer. 1999. The Effects of Physician Supply on the Early Detection of Colorectal Cancer. *Journal of Family Practice* 48:850–58.

Roetzheim, R.G., N. Pal, D.J. Van Durme, D. Wathington, J.M. Ferrante, E.C. Gonzalez, and J.P. Krischer. 2000. Increasing Supplies of Dermatologists and Family Physicians Are Associated with Earlier Stage of Melanoma Detection. *Journal of the American Academy of Dermatology* 43:211–8.

Roos, N.P. 1979. Who Should Do the Surgery? Tonsillectomy-Adenoidectomy in One Canadian Province. *Inquiry* 16:73–83.

Roos, N.P., K.C. Carriere, and D. Friesen. 1998. Factors Influencing the Frequency of Visits by Hypertensive Patients to Primary Care Physicians in Winnipeg. *Canadian Medical Association Journal* 159:777–83.

Rosenblatt, R.A., G.E. Wright, L.M. Baldwin, L. Chan, P. Clitherow, F.M. Chen, and L.G. Hart. 2000. The Effect of the Doctor-Patient Relationship on Emergency Department Use among the Elderly. *American Journal of Public Health* 90:97–102.

Rosero-Bixby, L. 1986. Infant Mortality in Costa Rica: Explaining the Recent Decline. *Studies in Family Planning* 17:57–65.

498   *B. Starfield, L. Shi, and J. Macinko*

Rosero-Bixby, L. 2004a. Evaluación del impacto de la reforma del sector de la salud en Costa Rica mediante un estudio cuasiexperimental. *Revista Panamamericana de Salud Publica* 15:94–103.

Rosero-Bixby, L. 2004b. Spatial Access to Health Care in Costa Rica and Its Equity: A GIS-Based Study. *Social Science and Medicine* 58:1271–84.

Rosser, W.W. 1996. Approach to Diagnosis by Primary Care Clinicians and Specialists: Is There a Difference? *Journal of Family Practice* 42:139–44.

Rothwell, P.M. 2005. Treating Individuals 2. Subgroup Analysis in Randomised Controlled Trials: Importance, Indications, and Interpretation. *Lancet* 365:176–86.

Ryan, S., A. Riley, M. Kang, and B. Starfield. 2001. The Effects of Regular Source of Care and Health Need on Medical Care Use among Rural Adolescents. *Archives of Pediatric and Adolescent Medicine* 155:184–90.

Sachs, J.D., and J.W. McArthur. 2005. The Millennium Project: A Plan for Meeting the Millennium Development Goals. *Lancet* 365:347–53.

Saver, B. 2002. Financing and Organization Findings Brief. *Academy for Research and Health Care Policy* 5:1–2.

Schappert, S.M. 1994. National Ambulatory Medical Care Survey 1991. *Vital and Health Statistics* 13:1–110.

Schoen, C., R. Osborn, P.T. Huynh, M. Doty, K. Davis, K. Zapert, and J. Peugh. 2004. Primary Care and Health System Performance: Adults' Experiences in Five Countries. *Health Affairs* W4:487–503.

Schreiber, S., and T. Zielinski. 1997. The Meaning of Ambulatory Care Sensitive Admissions: Urban and Rural Perspectives. *Journal of Rural Health* 13:276–84.

Seid, M., G.D. Stevens, and J.W. Varni. 2003. Parents' Perceptions of Pediatric Primary Care Quality: Effects of Race/Ethnicity, Language, and Access. *Health Services Research* 38:1009–31.

Shea, S., D. Misra, M.H. Ehrlich, L. Field, and C.K. Francis. 1992. Predisposing Factors for Severe, Uncontrolled Hypertension in an Inner-City Minority Population. *New England Journal of Medicine* 327:776–81.

Shi, L. 1992. The Relationship between Primary Care and Life Chances. *Journal of Health Care for the Poor and Underserved* 3:321–35.

Shi, L. 1994. Primary Care, Specialty Care, and Life Chances. *International Journal of Health Services* 24:431–58.

Shi, L. 1999. Experience of Primary Care by Racial and Ethnic Groups in the United States. *Medical Care* 37:1068–77.

Contribution of Primary Care to Health Systems and Health   499

Shi, L., J. Macinko, B. Starfield, R. Politzer, J. Wulu, and J. Xu. 2005a. Primary Care, Social Inequalities, and All-Cause, Heart Disease, and Cancer Mortality in U.S. Counties, 1990. *American Journal of Public Health* 95:674–80.

Shi, L., J. Macinko, B. Starfield, R. Politzer, J. Wulu, and J. Xu. 2005b. Primary Care, Social Inequalities, and All-Cause, Heart Disease, and Cancer Mortality in U.S. Counties: A Comparison of Urban and Rural Areas. *Public Health* 119:699–710.

Shi, L., J. Macinko, B. Starfield, R. Politzer, and J. Xu. 2005c. Primary Care, Race, and Mortality in U.S. States. *Social Science and Medicine* 61:65–75.

Shi, L., J. Macinko, B. Starfield, J. Wulu, J. Regan, and R. Politzer. 2003a. The Relationship between Primary Care, Income Inequality, and Mortality in the United States, 1980–1995. *Journal of the American Board of Family Practice* 16:412–22.

Shi, L., J. Macinko, B. Starfield, J. Xu, and R. Politzer. 2003b. Primary Care, Income Inequality, and Stroke Mortality in the United States. A Longitudinal Analysis, 1985–1995. *Stroke* 34:1958–64.

Shi, L., J. Macinko, B. Starfield, J. Xu, J. Regan, R. Politzer, and J. Wulu. 2004. Primary Care, Infant Mortality, and Low Birth Weight in the States of the USA. *Journal of Epidemiology and Community Health* 58:374–80.

Shi, L., and B. Starfield. 2000. Primary Care, Income Inequality, and Self-Rated Health in the United States: A Mixed-Level Analysis. *International Journal of Health Services* 30:541–55.

Shi, L., and B. Starfield. 2001. The Effect of Primary Care Physician Supply and Income Inequality on Mortality among Blacks and Whites in U.S. Metropolitan Areas. *American Journal of Public Health* 91:1246–50.

Shi, L., B. Starfield, B.P. Kennedy, and I. Kawachi. 1999. Income Inequality, Primary Care, and Health Indicators. *Journal of Family Practice* 48:275–84.

Shi, L., B. Starfield, R. Politzer, and J. Regan. 2002. Primary Care, Self-Rated Health, and Reductions in Social Disparities in Health. *Health Services Research* 37:529–50.

Shi, L., B. Starfield, and J. Xu. 2001. Validating the Adult Primary Care Assessment Tool. *Journal of Family Practice* 50:161W–175W (http://jfponline.com/content/2001/02/jfp_0201_01610.asp).

Sox, H.C. 1996. Decision-Making: A Comparison of Referral Practice and Primary Care. *Journal of Family Practice* 42:155–60.

Starfield, B. 1991. Primary Care and Health. A Cross-National Comparison. *Journal of the American Medical Association* 266:2268–71.

Starfield, B. 1994. Is Primary Care Essential? *Lancet* 344:1129–33.

500   *B. Starfield, L. Shi, and J. Macinko*

Starfield, B. 1998. *Primary Care: Balancing Health Needs, Services, and Technology*. New York: Oxford University Press.

Starfield, B. 2001. New Paradigms for Quality in Primary Care. *British Journal of General Practice* 51:303–9.

Starfield, B., C. Cassady, J. Nanda, C.B. Forrest, and R. Berk. 1998. Consumer Experiences and Provider Perceptions of the Quality of Primary Care: Implications for Managed Care. *Journal of Family Practice* 46:216–26.

Starfield, B., C.B. Forrest, P.A. Nutting, and S. von Schrader. 2002. Variability in Physician Referral Decisions. *Journal of the American Board of Family Practice* 15:473–80.

Starfield, B., K.W. Lemke, T. Bernhardt, S.S. Foldes, C.B. Forrest, and J.P. Weiner. 2003. Comorbidity: Implications for the Importance of Primary Care in "Case" Management. *Annals of Family Medicine* 1:8–14.

Starfield, B., K.W. Lemke, R. Herbert, W.D. Pavlovich, and G. Anderson. 2005a. Comorbidity and the Use of Primary Care and Specialist Care in the Elderly. *Annals of Family Medicine*, in press.

Starfield, B., and L. Shi. 2002. Policy Relevant Determinants of Health: An International Perspective. *Health Policy* 60:201–18.

Starfield, B., and L. Shi. 2004. The Medical Home, Access to Care, and Insurance: A Review of Evidence. *Pediatrics* 113:1493–8.

Starfield, B., L. Shi, A. Grover, and J. Macinko. 2005b. The Role of Evidence in Physician Workforce Policy. *Health Affairs* W5:97–107 (http://content.healthaffairs.org/cgi/reprint/hlthaff.w5.97v1).

Starfield, B., and L. Simpson. 1993. Primary Care as Part of U.S. Health Services Reform. *Journal of the American Medical Association* 269:3136–9.

Stevens, G.D., and L. Shi. 2002. Racial and Ethnic Disparities in the Quality of Primary Care for Children. *Journal of Family Practice* 51:573.

Stevens, G.D., and L. Shi. 2003. Racial and Ethnic Disparities in the Primary Care Experiences of Children: A Review of the Literature. *Medical Care Research and Review* 60:3–30.

Stevens, R. 1971. *American Medicine and the Public Interest*. New Haven, Conn.: Yale University Press.

Taira, D.A., D.G. Safran, T.B. Seto, W.H. Rogers, M. Kosinski, J.E. Ware, N. Lieberman, and A.R. Tarlov. 1997. Asian-American Patient Ratings of Physician Primary Care Performance. *Journal of General Internal Medicine* 12:237–42.

Talbot-Smith, A., S. Gnani, A.M. Pollock, and D.P. Gray. 2004. Questioning the Claims from Kaiser. *British Journal of General Practice* 54:415–21.

U.S. Department of Health and Human Services. 2000. *Healthy People 2010*. 2nd ed., with *Understanding and Improving Health and Objectives for Improving Health*. Washington, D.C.: U.S. Government Printing Office.

van den Akker, M., F. Buntinx, J.F. Metsemakers, S. Roos, and J.A. Knottnerus. 1998. Multimorbidity in General Practice: Prevalence, Incidence, and Determinants of Co-occurring Chronic and Recurrent Diseases. *Journal of Clinical Epidemiology* 51:367–75.

van Doorslaer, E., X. Koolman, and A.M. Jones. 2004. Explaining Income-Related Inequalities in Doctor Utilisation in Europe. *Health Economics* 13:629–47.

Villalbi, J.R., A. Guarga, M.I. Pasarin, M. Gil, C. Borrell, M. Ferran, and E. Cirera. 1999. An Evaluation of the Impact of Primary Care Reform on Health. *Atención Primaria* 24:468–74.

Vogel, R.L., and R.J. Ackermann. 1998. Is Primary Care Physician Supply Correlated with Health Outcomes? *International Journal of Health Services* 28:183–96.

Waitzkin, H., K. Wald, R. Kee, R. Danielson, and L. Robinson. 1997. Primary Care in Cuba: Low- and High-Technology Developments Pertinent to Family Medicine. *Journal of Family Practice* 45:250–58.

Wasserman, R., E. Slora, and A. Bocian. 2003. Current Status of Pediatric Practice-Based Research Networks. *Current Problems in Pediatric and Adolescent Health Care* 33:115–23.

Weinberger, M., E.Z. Oddone, and W.G. Henderson. 1996. Does Increased Access to Primary Care Reduce Hospital Readmissions? Veterans Affairs Cooperative Study Group on Primary Care and Hospital Readmission. *New England Journal of Medicine* 334:1441–7.

Weiner, J.P. 2004. Prepaid Group Practice Staffing and U.S. Physician Supply: Lessons for Workforce Policy. *Health Affairs* (suppl.) Web Exclusives: W4–59.

Weiner, J.P., L.E. Kassel, T.D. Baker, and B.H. Lane. 1982. Baltimore City Primary Care Study: The Role of the Office-Based Physician. *Maryland State Medical Journal* 31:48–52.

Weiner, J.P., and B. Starfield. 1983. Measurement of the Primary Care Roles of Office-Based Physicians. *American Journal of Public Health* 73:666–71.

Weinick, R.M., and N.A. Krauss. 2000. Racial/Ethnic Differences in Children's Access to Care. *American Journal of Public Health* 90: 1771–4.

Weiss, L.J., and J. Blustein. 1996. Faithful Patients: The Effect of Long-Term Physician-Patient Relationships on the Costs and Use of Health Care by Older Americans. *American Journal of Public Health* 86:1742–7.

502   *B. Starfield, L. Shi, and J. Macinko*

Weitzman, M., R.S. Byrd, and P. Auinger. 1999. Black and White Middle Class Children Who Have Private Health Insurance in the United States. *Pediatrics* 104:151–7.

Welch, W.P., M.E. Miller, H.G. Welch, E.S. Fisher, and J.E. Wennberg. 1993. Geographic Variation in Expenditures for Physicians' Services in the United States. *New England Journal of Medicine* 328:621–7.

Whittle, J., C.J. Lin, J.R. Lave, M.J. Fine, K.M. Delaney, D.Z. Joyce, W.W. Young, and W.N. Kapoor. 1998. Relationship of Provider Characteristics to Outcomes, Process, and Costs of Care for Community-Acquired Pneumonia. *Medical Care* 36:977–87.

World Health Organization. 1978. *Declaration of Alma-Ata: International Conference on Primary Health Care, Alma-Ata, USSR, 6–12 September 1978.* Geneva. Available at http://www.who.int/hpr/NPH/docs/declaration_almaata.pdf (accessed December 30, 2004).

World Health Organization. 2003. *A Global Review of Primary Health Care: Emerging Messages.* Geneva.

World Organization of National Colleges, Academies and Academic Association of General Practitioners/Family Physicians (WONCA). 1991. *The Role of the General Practitioner/Family Physician in Health Care Systems.* Victoria.

Acknowledgments: This work was funded in part by the Bureau of Health Professions, U.S. Department of Health and Human Services. The authors gratefully acknowledge the advice of Dr. Neil Holtzman in writing this article.

CHAPTER 18

The development of family medicine in Latin America

Maria Inez Padula Anderson

NOMINATED CLASSIC PAPER

Julio Ceitlin. La medicina familiar en América Latina (Family medicine in Latin America). *Revista de Atención Primária*, 2006; 38: 469–70 (published in Spanish).

'The future of family medicine in Latin America is a story we start writing every day.' These words form the conclusion of Julio Ceitlin's paper on family medicine in Latin America. This paper provides an update of family medicine in 12 countries of the region, and includes reflections and comparative analysis, providing a vision about the continuing development of our specialty across Latin America.

Julio pointed out two phenomena of the 20th century that had strongly influenced the organisation of healthcare delivery and, therefore, the organisation of primary care. Firstly, the reform of the health systems in many countries, driven by the influence of international agencies, such as the World Bank. Secondly, the concept of managed care, influenced by globalisation, that has brought forward ideas such as 'health services as a commodity', and the role of 'family doctor as a barrier keeper to limit the access of patients to secondary or tertiary levels, in order to lower costs'.

But unlike many high-income countries, where economic crises affecting health systems have occurred after the large-scale development of family medicine, Julio reminds us that in most Latin American countries these crises occurred before family medicine had been fully developed.

Julio also highlights some valuable achievements and calls for attention to the strategic sequence used in many countries in the region to develop family medicine. This has seen the creation of primary care services with the characteristics of family medicine (care model), then organisation of postgraduate educational programmes within these services to train family doctors (teaching model), followed by the establishment of professional associations of specialist family doctors (professional model). He also highlights the inclusion of family medicine into the undergraduate medical school at universities (university model).

Julio writes, 'The fate of family medicine depends on the existence of well-trained family physicians; their number and distribution will define the degree of population coverage. All this depends on clear political decisions. However, to achieve satisfactory levels of development does not ensure the permanence of the model, as evidenced by the crisis in family medicine and primary care in some developed countries.'

He adds, 'Primary Care, like any other social process, presents ups and downs due to internal crises or attacks of ideological forces or socioeconomic movements, as happens today with globalisation, neo-liberalism or with multinational or supranational entrepreneurship interventions into the delivery of health care. Those responsible for the development [of family medicine] need to be the family doctors themselves, the society they belong to, and the people, their patients.'

ABOUT THE AUTHOR OF THIS PAPER

Julio Ceitlin was the Founder and Chairman of the Department of Family Medicine at the University of Buenos Aires Medical School in Argentina. He was born in Lithuania, in 1923, and his family moved to Argentina when he was one year old. He was the first president of the Iberoamericana Confederation of Family Medicine and is considered one of the founders of family medicine in Latin America. He established the first Family Medicine residency programme in Argentina in 1984, led the creation of the Argentine Association of Family Medicine, and introduced family medicine into the medical curriculum at his university. Julio became Program Director of the Pan-American Federation of Associations of Medical Schools (PAFAMS) in 1971, and through this role directed the Community Medicine Program, an international programme involving seven Latin American countries.

At the time of publication, Julio was 93 years old, still very active, in good health and continuing to work to ensure the future of family medicine. Julio remains a strong influence, not only for family doctors in Latin America, but for family doctors all around the world.

ABOUT THE NOMINATOR OF THIS PAPER

Professor Maria Inez Padula Anderson is a Brazilian family doctor, primary care researcher and medical educator. Following her graduation from the School of

Medicine at the Rio de Janeiro State University, and postgraduate training in family and community medicine, and a PhD in public health, Inez was appointed Professor of Family and Community Medicine at the Rio de Janeiro State University, and has been coordinator of the family medicine residency programme, and head of the Department of Family Medicine. She was president of the Brazilian Society of Family and Community Medicine from 2002 to 2006, and regional president of the World Organization of Family Doctors (WONCA) Iberoamericana Confederation of Family Medicine (CIMF) from 2013 to 2016.

'I had the opportunity of meeting Julio Ceitlin, for the first time, two years ago, in Argentina. At 92 years of age, he remained firm and secure in his conviction that family medicine is the medical specialty that people will need most during their lives. Julio Ceitlin, with his commitment to the importance of being faithful and persistent, and to making a difference for all people, provides an example we should all follow.'

Professor Maria Inez Padula Anderson, Brazil

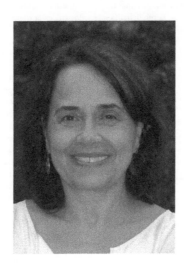

Attribution:

We attribute the original publication of *La medicina familiar en América Latina* to *Revista de Atención Primária*, the journal of the Spanish Society of Family and Community Medicine (SEMFYC), published by Elsevier España S.L. With thanks to Dr Julio Ceitlin for permission to reproduce this article, to Dr Josep Basora, SEMFYC President, and to Dr Juanjo Mascort Roca.

SERIES

Localizador web
Artículo 177.424

LA MEDICINA FAMILIAR EN AMÉRICA LATINA

Coordinador de la serie: Julio Ceitlin

La medicina familiar en América Latina. Presentación

Julio Ceitlin

Introducción

Por haber participado activamente en los pasos iniciales de la especialidad, fue para mí una gran satisfacción recibir la invitación del Dr. Amando Martín Zurro para coordinar una serie de artículos sobre la medicina familiar en América Latina. Esta serie presenta una puesta al día de la medicina familiar en 12 países de la región. La metodología para su preparación fue la siguiente: invitamos a médicos de familia que ocupan posiciones de liderazgo a escribir un artículo sobre su respectivo país; se preparó un esquema común al que todos debían ceñirse que incluía, además de los datos, una reflexión sobre el futuro de la medicina familiar en su propio país. La primera versión de cada trabajo fue editada y devuelta al autor para una segunda revisión

y se solicitaron aclaraciones sobre aspectos que no estaban claros; una vez editada, se volvió a enviar esta segunda versión a los autores para su aprobación y la versión final, enviada para su publicación. El grupo de artículos y/o informes de los 12 países me permitió elaborar algunas reflexiones, hacer un análisis comparativo y esbozar algunas conclusiones, lo que se presenta a continuación. La realización periódica de esfuerzos de este tipo nos permite tener una visión analítica y también de conjunto sobre el desarrollo de nuestra especialidad.

América Latina es un conjunto de países en desarrollo en los cuales la medicina familiar tuvo una evolución interesante. Aunque el comienzo fue muy parecido en los diferentes países latinoamericanos, la realidad actual ofrece un panorama muy disímil.

Centro de Estudios en Medicina Familiar Ian McWhinney. Centro Privado de Medicina Familiar afiliado a la USC. Buenos Aires. Argentina.

Introducción. Se presenta una serie de artículos sobre la medicina familiar en 12 países de América Latina, escritos por médicos de familia que ocupan posiciones de liderazgo en sus respectivos ámbitos. Como coordinador de la serie, ofrezco a continuación una visión de las características más salientes del conjunto. Lo escrito aquí no agota el análisis porque los trabajos tienen un contenido muy rico que servirá para otras conclusiones.
La medicina familiar y el seguro social. La medicina familiar comenzó como servicio al público en los sistemas de salud de la seguridad social en 5 países: Bolivia, El Salvador, México, Panamá y Venezuela. Se agregaron luego los seguros sociales de Colombia y Argentina.
La medicina familiar y los ministerios de Salud. La medicina familiar se desarrolló preponderantemente en los ministerios de salud en 2 países: Cuba y Uruguay, dadas las características de sus sistemas de salud, pero también se organizaron programas en los Ministerios de Salud de Bolivia, El Salvador, México y Paraguay.
Posgrados y universidad. Los posgrados (residencias) que entrenan a los médicos de familia tienen carácter universitario en 5 países: Bolivia, Colombia, México, Uruguay y Venezuela.
Pregrado y medicina familiar. Se enseña medicina familiar en el currículo de pregrado en escuelas de medicina de 9 países: Argentina, Bolivia, Colombia, Cuba, México, Panamá, Paraguay, Uruguay y Venezuela.
Futuro de la especialidad según los autores: ¿qué hacer? *a*) Redefinir el perfil del médico de familia, volver a las fuentes e incorporar nuevas ideas; *b*) más financiación para residencias; *c*) conversión de médicos generales; *d*) difundir los conceptos de la medicina familiar, y *e*) insertar la medicina familiar en la reforma de los servicios de salud
Dificultades o problemas. *a*) Faltan políticas nacionales para utilizar a los médicos familiares; *b*) no hay oferta de trabajo para médicos de familia; *c*) oposición de otras especialidades; *d*) en uno de los países el gobierno introduce, por motivos ideológicos, una competencia con la medicina familiar local (que lleva 20 años de desarrollo exitoso) con el apoyo y la financiación de la medicina general integral.
Visión. Sólo en 2 casos se expresa optimismo franco: en uno es sólo subjetivo y en el otro está basado en datos objetivos.
Médicos familiares y población. Finalmente, se presenta un análisis cuantitativo del número de médicos de familia formados hasta el presente en relación con la población del respectivo país.

Palabras clave: Medicina familiar. América Latina. Desarrollo.

Un poco de historia

Los primeros programas de medicina familiar se desarrollaron en México en la década de los setenta. Este país tiene el honor de haber organizado el primero de los programas de medicina familiar de América Latina, en el Instituto Mexicano de los Seguros Sociales (IMSS); una vez creado el servicio para el público, el IMSS tuvo la necesidad de organizar su propio programa educativo para formar el recurso humano que necesitaba en esta especialidad. El programa logró rápidamente el reconocimiento de la Universidad Nacional Autónoma de México (UNAM), que en 1975 crea el departamento de medicina familiar, primero en ese país y en la región, que recientemente celebró sus 30 años de existencia.

En esa misma década se establecen también servicios de medicina familiar en Panamá y Bolivia, acompañados de los respectivos programas formativos; cabe destacar que Bolivia tenía entonces un convenio de cooperación con el seguro social mexicano que le prestó su ayuda para este propósito.

Después de los primeros tanteos, el desarrollo más pujante en la región comienza a partir de la creación del Centro Internacional para la Medicina Familiar (CIMF) en 1981. Unos pocos datos sobre lo realizado en la década de los años ochenta dan una idea de la magnitud del proceso: en ese período se crearon residencias de medicina familiar en 13 países de América Latina, se fundaron sociedades nacionales de medicina familiar, se organizaron reuniones in-

SERIES | Ceitlin J.
La medicina familiar en América Latina. Presentación

ternacionales de las incipientes sociedades y se realizaron otras reuniones con autoridades de salud; además, se concretaron actividades de intercambio de residentes y docentes. Al comenzar la década de los ochenta había medicina familiar en 3 países (México, Panamá y Bolivia) con un total de 21 programas (denominamos «Programa de medicina familiar» a una organización que ofrece servicios de atención primaria atendido por médicos de la especialidad y que además tiene un programa educativo de posgrado, del tipo residencia médica, en el que se forman médicos de familia). Diez años después, en 1990, los países con medicina familiar eran 18: Argentina, Bolivia, Brasil, Colombia, Costa Rica, Cuba, Chile, República Dominicana, Ecuador, Jamaica, México, Nicaragua, Panamá, Paraguay, Perú, Puerto Rico, Uruguay y Venezuela, y reunían un total de 160 programas.

«Este éxito puede ser atribuido a la confluencia de varios factores, como la promoción de la atención primaria de salud por las organizaciones internacionales como OMS, OPS; la mayor conciencia de los gobiernos latinoamericanos sobre la necesidad de desarrollar sistemas eficientes y coste-efectivos que ofrecieran buenos servicios de salud a sus poblaciones; la influencia de líderes que habían tomado el estandarte de la medicina familiar como factor de calidad y excelencia de la atención primaria, entre los que pueden mencionarse a José Narro en México, Pedro Iturbe en Venezuela, Tomas Owens en Panamá, Cosme Ordóñez en Cuba y Julio Ceitlin en Argentina... El desarrollo de la especialidad en Canadá y Estados Unidos sirvió como estímulo adicional a este proceso[1].»

Vinculada desde hace 5 siglos a la cultura hispánica, no es de extrañar que, tras la entrada de España al movimiento de medicina familiar, se produjeran influencias recíprocas con América Latina, principalmente a través del CIMF, donde el grupo español desempeñó un importante papel.

La última década del siglo XX trajo de la mano 2 fenómenos de enorme influencia sobre los sistemas de salud y, por ende, sobre la atención primaria: la reforma de los sistemas de salud, impulsada por los organismos internacionales y el concepto de medicina gerenciada o gestionada *(managed care)*, todo esto en un marco signado por la globalización. Para entender mejor este fenómeno es importante destacar que, en esa década, el liderazgo internacional del movimiento de reforma lo tuvieron los entes financieros, Banco Mundial, BID, por encima de los organismos específicos de salud, OMS, OPS. Así, se pusieron en boga conceptos tales como «los servicios de salud como mercancía» y se impulsó el de la función del «médico de familia como barrera o portero» del sistema de salud *(gatekeeper)*, cuya misión es limitar el acceso de los pacientes a niveles más complejos del sistema, con el objeto de bajar costes. Nada más injusto, porque ese concepto nunca fue sostenido por los fundadores de la medicina familiar, quienes concebían al médico de familia como facilitador, coordina-

dor, orientador y cuidador de sus pacientes aun en los niveles más complejos del sistema.

En la década de los noventa, la atención primaria de salud de América Latina no sólo recibió la influencia de los cambios demográficos y epidemiológicos que ya venían haciendo lo suyo, sino también los embates de los conceptos procedentes de la globalización. Aunque el desarrollo de la atención primaria de la salud no tuvo oposición oficial, en la práctica careció de apoyo real por falta de claras decisiones políticas; ningún gobierno de América Latina dictó una resolución parecida al Real Decreto de 1978 (en España) disponiendo que: «El médico de familia constituye la figura fundamental del sistema sanitario y tiene como misión realizar una atención médica integrada y completa a los miembros de la comunidad».

A diferencia de lo ocurrido en los países desarrollados, en los cuales la crisis se produjo con posterioridad a un gran desarrollo de la atención primaria/medicina familiar, en la mayoría de los países de América Latina la atención primaria presenta una crisis desde fines de la década de los noventa, aun antes de haberse desarrollado plenamente.

Algunos eventos habidos en esa década constituyen verdaderos «contramovimientos»:

1. En noviembre de 1994 se realizó la Conferencia sobre Medicina Familiar en la Reforma de los Servicios de Salud de las Américas organizado por WONCA/OMS, en London, Ontario, Canadá. El documento aprobado tiene un título sugerente: «Hacer que la práctica médica sea más relevante a las necesidades de salud de la comunidad».

2. En septiembre de 1996, con el auspicio del gobierno Argentino, OPS, CIMF y WONCA, tuvo lugar en Buenos Aires una conferencia regional de líderes y expertos de las Américas, sobre «La medicina familiar en la reforma de los servicios de salud». Fue la continuación y tuvo similar orientación a la Conferencia de Ontario. Allí se aprobó la Declaración de Buenos Aires, cuyas recomendaciones más importantes siguen vigentes:

– Las escuelas y facultades de medicina deben implementar procesos de inserción de la medicina familiar dentro de los planes curriculares del pregrado, que permitan al alumno un contacto temprano, gradual y continuo con los principios universales y las modalidades de práctica de esta disciplina.

– Con base en sus características particulares, cada país debe desarrollar modelos integrales de atención a la salud, que permitan utilizar de manera óptima los principios y las ventajas de la práctica de la medicina familiar, convirtiéndola en la vía de entrada a los servicios de salud.

Ya en este siglo, la Resolución de los Ministros de Salud de las Américas aprobada en septiembre del año 2005 constituye un reconocimiento franco del deficiente estado de la atención primaria de salud en esta región:

– Solicitar a los Estados miembros que:

1. Hagan esfuerzos para que el desarrollo de la atención primaria cuente con los recursos necesarios que aseguren su contribución a la reducción de las desigualdades en salud.

2. Renueven su compromiso con el fortalecimiento a largo plazo de las capacidades en lo que respecta a los recursos humanos requeridos para la atención primaria de salud.

3. Reconozcan el potencial de la atención primaria de salud para llevar a cabo una reorientación de los servicios con criterio de promoción de la salud.

4. Promuevan el mantenimiento y el fortalecimiento de los sistemas de información y vigilancia en la atención primaria de salud.

5. Respalden la participación activa de las comunidades locales en la atención primaria de salud.

Como se ve, un cuarto de siglo no había sido suficiente para alcanzar las metas originales planteadas en Alma Ata y, según algunos autores, la situación había empeorado por lo menos en cuanto a accesibilidad y equidad en la utilización de los servicios de salud.

A pesar de todo, algunos logros

Aunque el panorama general de la atención primaria y la medicina familiar en América Latina es carencial e insatisfactorio, pueden mencionarse algunas realizaciones valiosas: el logro de estatus universitario para la disciplina, los programas de conversión de médicos generales, la creación de una entidad para impulsar la investigación en medicina familiar, y la difusión de los principios e instrumentos de la medicina familiar entre otros especialistas.

Si repasamos la secuencia estratégica utilizada en la región para desarrollar la medicina familiar se observa lo siguiente: primero, la creación de servicios de atención primaria con características de medicina familiar (modelo asistencial); a continuación, organización en esos servicios de programas educativos de posgrado para entrenar a médicos de familia (modelo docente); a medida que se formaban los médicos de familia, constitución de las asociaciones profesionales respectivas (modelo profesional) e incorporación como docentes a los programas educativos de los que habían salido. Bastante más tarde se produce la inclusión de la disciplina en la Universidad, en el currículum de grado, en posgrado o en ambos (modelo universitario).

En el año 2000, el Grupo de Panamá, un grupo interuniversitario, cuyo propósito era promover la medicina familiar académica en América Latina, realizó una encuesta sobre la enseñanza de la medicina familiar en las facultades de medicina de México, Argentina, Panamá y Colombia. Los resultados fueron los siguientes: de las 65 escuelas que contestaron la encuesta, 40 respondieron afirmativamente; de éstas, en 22 escuelas se enseña en el currículo de grado, en 11, tanto en grado como en postgrado y en 7 escuelas, solamente en posgrado. En cuanto a la estructura académica que soporta la enseñanza, 10 son departamentos, 13 cátedras, 5 cursos y 5 con otro formato. En el 80% de las escuelas que tenían medicina familiar en el currículo de grado (33), la materia era obligatoria[1]. Al comparar la situación con la de Estados Unidos y Canadá en ese mismo año (en Estados Unidos el 93% de las escuelas de medicina tiene departamentos académicos y en Canadá, todas las escuelas los tienen), observamos que todavía estamos lejos. La importancia del estatus académico universitario se relaciona con el prestigio de la especialidad y de quienes la practican, así como con la difusión y la influencia interprofesional.

Número de médicos de familia

Es casi obvia la importancia de lo cuantitativo en la generación de cambios cualitativos. De ahí que el número de especialistas en medicina familiar, en relación con la población de cuya atención primaria son responsables, tiene singular importancia. La experiencia internacional permite calcular aproximadamente el número de médicos de familia necesarios para una ciudad, región o país.

Si aceptamos que el médico familiar está directamente relacionado a la calidad de los servicios de atención primaria y, por lo tanto, su número constituye un factor fundamental para asegurar una cobertura adecuada de servicios de atención primaria de alta calidad, los datos de los 12 países de América Latina que comprende esta serie y que están incluidos en la tabla 1 son los siguientes: población total del país, total de médicos de familia del país según los respectivos reportes, cantidad de población por cada médico de familia, número ideal de médicos de familia calculado a razón de 2.000 habitantes por médico, diferencia entre el número ideal y el real.

TABLA 1	Número de médicos de familia en los países de América Latina				
	País	Población total (en millones de habitantes)	Total MF	N.º habitantes/ MF	N.º ideal MF	Diferencia
1	Cuba	11,2	33.000	339	5.600	+27400
2	México	103,4	37.000	2.800	51.700	−14.700
3	Venezuela	24,3	1.700	4.300	12.150	−10.450
4	Argentina	38,7	2.500	15.480	19.350	−16.850
5	Paraguay	6,3	400	15.750	3.150	−2.750
6	Bolivia	8,4	400	21.000	4.200	−3.800
7	Uruguay	3,4	130	26.153	1.700	−1.570
8	Panamá	2,9	40	72.500	1.450	−1.410
9	El Salvador	6,7	52	130.000	3.350	−3.300
10	Ecuador	13,4	50	268.000	6.700	−6.650
11	Colombia	41,0	150	273.000	20.500	−20.350
12	Perú	28,0	62	451.600	14.000	−13.940

MF: médicos de familia.

SERIES | Ceitlin J.
La medicina familiar en América Latina. Presentación

El caso de Cuba es singular porque tiene la mayor proporción de médicos de familia por habitantes (1/339) debido a un sistema centralizado y a una política de firme apoyo a la atención primaria de calidad encabezada por médicos de familia. Este exceso de médicos familiares de acuerdo con los parámetros internacionales es utilizado para misiones de colaboración internacional en otros países.

La situación de los demás países estudiados es la siguiente:

1. México: en poco más de 30 años ha llegado a una proporción equilibrada (1/2.800).
2. Venezuela: en poco más de 20 años alcanzó una proporción cercana a lo razonable (1/4.300).
3. En la franja de 10.000-20.000 agrupamos a 2 países: Argentina (1/15.480) y Paraguay (1/15.750).
4. En la franja entre 20.000 y 30.0000 se encuentran Bolivia (1/21.000) y Uruguay (1/26.000).
5. Panamá, con la proporción de 1/72.000, presenta insuficiencias mayores.
6. En el último grupo de los estudiados, Ecuador, Colombia y Perú, los países tienen que proporciones que son ampliamente insuficientes (1/268.000; 1/273.000 y 1/450.000, respectivamente) a pesar de tener un tiempo de desarrollo similar.

El destino de la medicina familiar y, a nuestro entender, el de la atención primaria de buena calidad depende de la existencia de médicos de familia bien formados; su número y su distribución definirán la mayor o menor cobertura poblacional. Todo esto depende de decisiones políticas claras, como las que ha habido en los casos de México o Cuba, y España, para citar un ejemplo extracontinental. Sin embargo, alcanzar grados de desarrollo satisfactorio no asegura la permanencia del modelo, como lo demuestran las crisis de la medicina familiar y la atención primaria en el Reino Unido, España, Estados Unidos y Canadá. La atención primaria, como cualquier otro proceso social, presenta vaivenes por crisis internas o por embates de fuerzas ideológicas o movimientos socioeconómicos, como sucede en la actualidad con la globalización, el neoliberalismo o la intervención del empresariado multinacional o supranacional en el campo de la salud, según lo expresado claramente por Iona Heath[2].

El futuro de la medicina familiar en América Latina es una historia que empezamos a escribir cada día. Elementos principales de ese desarrollo son: decisiones políticas de salud, inserción universitaria, difusión del rol de los médicos de familia en el sistema y la sociedad, exposición de otros especialistas a los principios e instrumentos de la medicina familiar, reconversión de médicos que trabajan en atención primaria a médicos de familia, y fomento de la investigación en atención primaria/medicina familiar con formación de investigadores en este campo.

Los responsables a partir de ahora son los médicos familiares, las sociedades que los agrupan y el público, sus pacientes.

Bibliografía

1. Knox L, Ceitlin J, Hahn RH. Slow Progress: predoctoral education in family practice in four Latin American countries. Fam Med. 2003;35:591-5.
2. Ceitlin J. APS: desde Alma Ata hasta hoy: luces y sombras vistas desde Buenos Aires. Conferencia presentada en el I Congreso Extremeño de Atención Primaria, celebrado el 5 de mayo de 2006.

CHAPTER 19

The importance of research in family medicine

Felicity Goodyear-Smith

NOMINATED CLASSIC PAPER

Paul Little, Michael Moore, Greg Warner, Joan Dunleavy, Ian Williamson. Longer term outcomes from a randomised trial of prescribing strategies in otitis media. *British Journal of General Practice*, 2006; 56(524): 176–82.

Although Cochrane reviews indicate minimal or no benefit from antibiotics for acute otitis media in children, as well as for other upper respiratory tract infections including sore throat and the common cold, antibiotics continue to be used for these conditions, and they are often prescribed in family medicine clinics. Overprescribing of antibiotics for self-limiting conditions is an international problem. A previous randomised controlled trial study, by Paul Little and his research team, demonstrated that the strategy of delayed, compared with immediate, prescribing is effective in reducing unnecessary antibiotic use in children over six months old with acute otitis media. While immediate prescribing of antibiotics reduced the duration of the illness, this benefit occurred mainly after the first 24 hours, when symptoms were already resolving, and needs to be weighed against the risk of side-effects, and the danger of developing antibiotic resistance. Prescribing on the basis of patients' belief in, and expectation for, antibiotics is likely to increase pressure on doctors to prescribe, and hence increase antibiotic use.

This paper reports on a follow-up study which found that a 'wait and see' approach was acceptable to most parents and resulted in a 76% reduction in the use of antibiotics. One-year follow-up reported in this study found that the delayed prescribing strategy did not significantly increase reported episodes of earache.

This paper is important because it addresses a commonplace condition, and offers a pragmatic, cost-effective intervention that not only reduces antibiotic use, but also enhances communication between patients and their general practitioner (GP), and facilitates parents' ability to self-manage in the future.

This paper also exemplifies the importance and nature of family medicine research, which focuses on people rather than conditions, and places interventions within their social contexts. Addressing people's attitudes, beliefs, expectations and values, and providing care within a person's family and social context, are as important as focusing on biomedical components of disease.

ABOUT THE LEAD AUTHOR OF THIS PAPER

Professor Paul Little is Professor of Primary Care Research in the Faculty of Medicine at the University of Southampton in England. He has had a distinguished career in conducting rigorous family medicine research, with a focus on studies where the findings directly lead to improvements in clinical practice.

Paul was the first GP to be awarded a Wellcome health services research training fellowship, for research on health promotion, and the first GP to be awarded a Medical Research Council Clinician Scientist Fellowship, for research on common self-limiting illness.

Paul's two main areas of research interest are health promotion and the management of common self-limiting illnesses. These topics link evidence about effectiveness with the effect of management of patient beliefs and behaviour, which enables better understanding of the importance of the patient-centred approach to the consultation. His current major areas of research are in enabling behaviour change both for health professionals and in empowering patients.

ABOUT THE NOMINATOR OF THIS PAPER

Professor Felicity Goodyear-Smith is a general practitioner and is currently academic head of the Department of General Practice & Primary Health Care at the University of Auckland in New Zealand. She is the founding editor-in-chief of the *Journal of Primary Health Care*, and chair of the World Organization of Family Doctors (WONCA) Working Party on Research from 2016.

> 'Family medicine involves the care of people and their families over time. Best practice involves the application of empirical evidence in the context of people's lives, taking into account a complex array of factors such as attitudes, beliefs, values, social and legal issues and resource constraints to facilitate collaborative decision making.'

Professor Felicity Goodyear-Smith, New Zealand

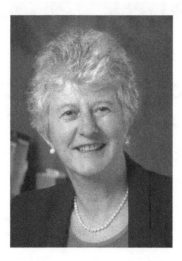

Attribution:

We attribute the original publication of *Longer term outcomes from a randomised trial of prescribing strategies in otitis media* to *British Journal of General Practice*. With thanks to Professor Roger Jones and Moira Davies.

Longer term outcomes from a randomised trial of prescribing strategies in otitis media

Paul Little, Michael Moore, Greg Warner, Joan Dunleavy and Ian Williamson

ABSTRACT

Background
There are limited data about the longer-term outcomes in acute otitis media (AOM) when comparing the realistic alternatives of immediate prescription of antibiotics and a 'wait and see' or delayed prescribing policy.

Aim
The aim was to assess the medium and longer term outcomes of two prescribing strategies for otitis media.

Design of study
Follow-up of a randomised controlled trial cohort.

Setting
Primary care.

Method
Three-hundred and fifteen children aged 6 months to 10 years presenting with AOM were randomised to immediate antibiotics, or antibiotics delayed at the parents discretion 72 hours if the child still had significant otalgia or fever, or was not improving. Episodes of earache since study entry were documented, and a poor score (of 9 or more — the top 20%) on a reliable six-item functional rating scale (Cronbach's α = 0.75).

Results
The delayed prescribing strategy did not significantly increase reported episodes of earache in the 3 months since randomisation (odds ratio [OR] = 0.89; 95% confidence interval [CI] = 0.48 to 1.65) or over 1 year (OR = 1.03; 95% CI = 0.60 to 1.78) nor of poor scores on the function scale at 3 months (OR = 1.16; 95% CI = 0.61 to 2.22) or 1 year (OR = 1.12; 95% CI = 0.57 to 2.19), and controlling for subsequent antibiotic use after the randomised episode did not alter these estimates. The number of prior episodes of AOM documented in the doctor's notes predicted episodes of earache reported (0, 1, ≥2 episodes, respectively; OR = 1, 2.42, 2.61; χ^2 for trend 8.04; P<0.01). There was weaker evidence that prior episodes also predicted poor function at 1 year (OR = 1, 1.86, 2.28; χ^2 for trend 5.49; P = 0.019). For children with recurrent AOM (two or more previous episodes documented in the doctor's notes, n = 43) there was possible evidence of fewer episodes of earache in the 3 months since study entry in the immediate antibiotic group (10% compared to 39% in the delayed group, χ^2 4.8, P = 0.029), but no effect from randomisation to 1 year.

Conclusions
For most children, delayed prescribing is not likely to have adverse longer-term consequences. Children with recurrent AOM are more likely to have poorer outcomes. Secondary analysis should be treated with caution and requires confirmation, but suggests that treating such children with antibiotics immediately may not alter longer-term outcomes.

Keywords
antibiotics; otitis media; prescribing strategies; randomised controlled trial.

INTRODUCTION

Otitis media is one of the most common acute respiratory conditions managed in primary care, yet treatment is controversial.[1-3] Evidence from systematic reviews suggests marginal benefit from antibiotics for most children:[4] an estimated 18 children have to be treated for one child to benefit from symptom resolution during the next week. Prescribing for all children is also likely to encourage attendance in future episodes, increase pressure on doctors to prescribe, increase antibiotic use,[5-6] and increase antibiotic resistance.[3,9] A large Dutch cohort documented that waiting for 72 hours before symptomatic treatment is safe: the only child to develop mastoiditis was not given antibiotics after 72 hours despite remaining unwell.[10]

Although most children are likely to obtain marginal benefit from immediate antibiotics in the short term, there are several unanswered issues: is there likely to be benefit in the longer term — particularly for outcomes important to parents — what factors predict adverse outcome, and whether 'at risk' subgroups are likely to benefit from treatment. We have reported the short-term results of a trial which compared the 'wait and see approach' with immediate antibiotics,[11] and demonstrated that for most children there was marginal short-term benefit

P Little, MD, MRCP, FRCGP, professor of primary care research; M Moore, BMed Sci, MSc, MRCP, FRCGP, senior lecturer; C Gould, BSc, research assistant; J Dunleavy, BEd(Hons), research coordinator; I Williamson, MD, MRCGP, FRCS, senior lecturer, Community Clinical Sciences (Primary Medical Care Group), University of Southampton, Aldermoor Health Centre, Southampton. G Warner, MA(Camb), MRCGP, DCH, DRCOGGP, Nightingale Surgery, Romsey, Hampshire.

Address for correspondence
Dr Paul Little, Community Clinical Sciences (Primary Medical Care Group), University of Southampton, Aldermoor Health Centre, Aldermoor Close, Southampton SO15 6ST. E-mail: p.little@soton.ac.uk

Submitted: 23 June 2003; **Editor's response:** 23 September 2003; **final acceptance:** 29 July 2005.

©*British Journal of General Practice* 2006; **56:** 176–182.

of immediate antibiotics with no significant difference in pain or distress scores — since what benefit there was from antibiotics mainly occurred after the first 24–48 hours when symptoms are milder.[12] We now report the predictors of poor medium- and longer-term outcome from this trial cohort.

METHOD

This study was approved by several local research ethics committees. The methods[12] and referencing of the discussion about the pragmatic diagnostic criteria we used have previously been reported in full elsewhere.[1,12-17] Children were eligible if they were aged 6 months to 10 years, attending their doctor with acute otalgia and otoscopic evidence of acute inflammation, and using the same photographic examples of each physical sign to guide physicians as in a previous trial.[13,17] Where children were too young to specifically document otalgia from the history (under 3 years old), then otoscopic evidence only was a sufficient entry criteria. The study design and trial flow are shown in Figure 1.

Intervention

After written consent, patients were randomised when the doctor opened a sealed numbered opaque envelope containing a standardised advice sheet[5,6,12] for one of two groups:

1. Immediate antibiotics: amoxicillin according to *British National Formulary* guidelines, and the same dosaging regime as the previous largest blinded trial from primary care[13] (or erythromycin if allergic to penicillin);
2. Delayed antibiotics: as in (1), but patients were asked to wait for 72 hours after seeing the doctor before considering using the prescription. Parents were advised to use antibiotics if their child had significant otalgia or fever after 72 hours, or if discharge lasted for 10 days or more.

How this fits in

There is very limited data from previous randomised trials about longer-term outcomes in acute otitis media from either prescribing immediately or delayed prescribing. The delayed prescribing strategy did not significantly increase the risk of earache or poor function at 3 months or 1 year. Secondary analysis provides some weaker evidence that children with previous recurrent otitis media were at risk of poorer outcomes in the longer term. However the data from this study suggest that prescribing antibiotics is not likely to modify this.

Outcome measurement and other documentation

Prior episodes. Blind to randomisation group, a researcher extracted information about attendance with prior episodes of otitis media from the medical notes.

Questionnaire. A questionnaire was sent at 3 months and then at 1 year after study entry to parents, with second and third mailing to non-responders asking about earache and functioning. The emphasis was to measure outcomes likely to be important to parents:

- Earache: the questionnaire asked parents whether there had been any further episodes of earache since study entry. We have previously shown evidence of the validity of parental rating of pain/earache.[12] We report earache since study entry at both 3 months (that is, from randomisation to 3 months), and also 1 year (that is, from randomisation to 1 year);
- Child functioning: the questionnaire also contained seven questions that parents scored about their child's language and social functioning: mishearing what is said; speech difficult to understand; shouts; has poor pronunciation; difficulty learning to read; poor concentration; and, is a daydreamer. These questions were a subset of questions from a previous study which provided 14 descriptions of how hearing impairment with chronic secretory otitis media presents:[18] the seven questions used were shown in a sample of 140 school children to have good inter-rater reliability between parents and teachers — and were thus more likely to be clinically useful. Each question was scored on a 3-point Likert scale (0 = does not apply, 1 = sometimes applies, and 2 = definitely applies). Factor analysis of the seven questions in this cohort showed a one-factor solution explaining 90% of the variance with all items loading strongly onto the factor (loading 0.50 or more) except difficulty reading. Thus, in our analysis we used the six-item function scale based on a simple sum of the six questions (that is, all questions except difficulty reading): this scale has a Cronbachs's α value of 0.75 — in the optimal range,[19] suggesting that it is reliable. Clearly the rating scale is not appropriate for children with little or no language (such as those under 2 years of age), but this trial cohort had very few very young children: by the 1-year follow-up only 3.5% were aged under 2 years, 10.5% under 3 years, and 24% under 4 years. A cut-off of 9 on the score represents a group of children performing poorly (the worst 20%), where their parents felt, on average, all items sometimes applied and at least three out of six items definitely applied.

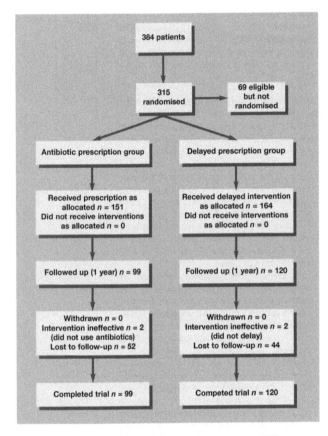

Figure 1. Study design and trial flow diagram.

significant in univariate analysis at the 5% level were entered by forward selection, starting with the most significant first, and retained if they remained significant at the 5% level. Variables that predicted poor outcome were then used to identify clinical subgroups, and the estimated effect of antibiotic in those subgroups was assessed by the χ^2 test for dichotomous outcomes. To assess the effect of intervention for continuous outcomes we used the *t* test. Our primary analyses were the randomised comparisons, and the assessment of the role of prior episodes of otitis media in predicting subsequent episodes of otalgia. Our secondary analyses were the assessment of risk factors for poor function, and the assessment of benefit of antibiotics in the higher-risk subgroups. Secondary analyses should be treated with caution in view of the danger of type I error.

RESULTS
At 3 months and 1 year, responses were received from 223 (71%) and 219 (70%) participants, respectively. There was no difference in the characteristics of responders compared with non-responders in those receiving immediate antibiotics (47% and 51%, respectively; $P = 0.55$), vomiting (18% and 22%; $P = 0.54$) prior episodes of otitis media (46% and 48%; $P = 0.94$), discharge (26% and 26%; $P = 0.91$), aged 3 years and under (42% and 36%; $P = 0.34$) and with a bulging drum (46% and 49%; $P = 0.58$). There was good agreement between reported collection of antibiotic prescriptions and actual collection, and good differentiation between antibiotic and delayed groups in the number who took an antibiotic prescription.[12]

The effect of prescribing strategies
The delayed prescribing strategy did not significantly increase risk of earache at 3 months (OR = 0.89; 95% confidence interval [CI] = 0.48 to 1.65) or 1 year (OR = 1.03; 95% CI = 0.60 to 1.78), or poor scores on the function scale at 3 months (OR = 1.37; 95% CI = 0.72 to 2.60) or 1 year (OR = 1.16; 95% CI = 0.61 to 2.23). Controlling for subsequent antibiotic use (that is, after the randomised episode) did not significantly alter the estimates for any of the above outcomes (OR = 0.85, 0.80, 1.43, 1.16, respectively). To check that the negative result for the function score could not be explained by the particular cut-off, we also assessed the function score as a continuous variable: the delayed prescribing strategy made very little difference at 3 months ($\beta = 0.14$; 95% CI = -0.68 to 0.39; $P = 0.60$) or 1 year ($\beta = -0.05$; 95% CI = -0.49 to 0.58; $P = 0.87$).

Sample size (for 80% power and 95% confidence using the Epi Info sample size program)
The original sample size calculation was based on short-term outcomes:[12] to detect a 15% difference in the number of children better by 72 hours after seeing their doctor required 233 children, or 291 children in total, allowing for up to 20% loss to follow-up. We recruited 315 children: we estimated that this sample size allowing for up to 30% non-response to follow-up questionnaires, would allow detection of risk factors for adverse outcomes with an odds ratio (OR) of 2.5 (that is, a significant risk factor) — assuming adverse outcomes occur in 50% of children (earache reported at 3 months or 1 year), and assuming the prevalence of risk factors varies from 20–65%.

Analysis
We assessed the effect of intervention and predictors of poor outcome using logistic regression for dichotomous outcomes. Variables

Table 1. Predictors of episodes of earache reported after 3 months.

	Had earache n (%)	Did not have earache n (%)	Crude OR (95% CI)	Adjusted OR (95% CI)[a]	LR χ^2 (P-value)
Symptoms and signs:					
High temperature	11 (21)	23 (14)	1.66 (0.75 to 3.68)	1.62 (0.71 to 3.71)	1.25 (0.26)
Vomiting	8 (16)	32 (19)	0.78 (0.34 to 1.83)	0.63 (0.26 to 1.52)	1.13 (0.29)
Ear discharge	20 (39)	35 (21)	2.43 (1.24 to 4.78)	2.57 (1.29 to 5.13)	7.04 (0.004)
Bulging drum	30 (58)	71 (42)	1.86 (0.99 to 3.50)	2.18 (1.13 to 4.20)	5.50 (0.019)
Past history — prior episodes of otitis media:					
0	78 (53)	26 (54)	1	1	0.52 (0.77)
1	37 (25)	11 (23)	0.89 (0.40 to 2.00)	0.80 (0.34 to 1.84)	
2	32 (22)	11 (23)	1.03 (0.46 to 2.33)	0.75 (0.30 to 1.85)	
Family/social factors — child care:					
Playgroup	13 (29)	29 (22)	1	1	0.43 (0.81)
Nursery	4 (9)	19 (14)	0.47 (0.13 to 1.66)	0.65 (0.17 to 2.45)	
School	28 (62)	86 (64)	0.73 (0.33 to 1.59)	0.83 (0.36 to 1.92)	

OR = odds ratio. LR = likelihood ratio. [a]Adjusted for significant predictors of outcome. Other variable assessed in models and shown not to predict outcome: asthma, eczema, exposure to smoke in the home, educational status of parents, history of breast feeding, past and current use of dummy, sibling having had otitis media.

Predictors of poor outcome

Predictors of poor outcome are shown in Tables 1–4. Prior episodes of otitis media documented in the doctor's notes predicted episodes of earache reported since study entry after 1 year, and the secondary outcomes (weaker evidence) of parental rating of function at both 3 months and 1 year. Other factors that possibly predict poor outcome were bulging drum and ear discharge in the index episode, which predicted episodes of earache in the 3 months since study entry.

Does treatment with antibiotics in subgroups with poor outcome predict response?

This was a secondary subgroup analysis and as such should be treated with caution. In children with recurrent otitis media (≥ 2 previous episodes) ($n = 43$), there was weaker evidence and fewer episodes of

Table 2. Predictors of episodes of earache reported after 1 year.

	Had earache n (%)	Did not have earache n (%)	Crude OR (95% CI)	Adjusted OR (95% CI)[a]	LR χ^2 (P-value)
Symptoms and signs:					
High temperature	18 (21)	18 (13)	1.73 (0.84 to 3.55)	1.88 (0.85 to 4.17)	2.40 (0.12)
Vomiting	19 (24)	26 (20)	1.28 (0.66 to 2.50)	1.45 (0.72 to 2.92)	1.09 (0.30)
Ear discharge	27 (34)	32 (24)	1.61 (0.87 to 2.96)	1.40 (0.72 to 2.69)	0.98 (0.32)
Bulging drum	42 (50)	63 (47)	1.13 (0.65 to 1.95)	1.01 (0.56 to 1.83)	0.00 (0.98)
Past history — prior episodes of otitis media:					
0	28 (37)	73 (60)	1	1	8.04 (0.005) (test for trend)
1	26 (35)	28 (23)	2.42 (1.22 to 4.82)	2.42 (1.22 to 4.82)	
2	21 (28)	21 (17)	2.61 (1.24 to 5.49)	2.61 (1.24 to 5.49)	
Family/social factors — child care:					
Playgroup	14 (25)	19 (21)	1	1	1.52 (0.47)
Nursery	7 (12)	15 (15)	0.68 (0.22 to 2.12)	0.46 (0.13 to 1.62)	
School	36 (63)	58 (64)	0.84 (0.38 to 1.89)	0.79 (0.33 to 1.90)	

OR = odds ratio. LR = likelihood ratio. [a]Adjusted for significant predictors of outcome. Other variable assessed in models and shown not to predict outcome: asthma, eczema, exposure to smoke in the home, educational status of parents, history of breast feeding, past and current use of dummy, sibling having had otitis media.

Table 3. Predictors of poor score (9 or more) on function scale after 3 months.

	Had poor function n (%)	Did not have poor function n (%)	Crude OR (95% CI)	Adjusted OR (95% CI)[a]	LR χ^2 (P-value)
Symptoms and signs:					
High temperature	8 (16)	26 (15)	1.12 (0.47 to 2.65)	0.96 (0.36 to 2.59)	0.01 (0.94)
Vomiting	13 (27)	27 (16)	1.93 (0.90 to 4.10)	1.96 (0.88 to 4.40)	2.58 (0.11)
Ear discharge	18 (37)	38 (22)	2.03 (1.03 to 4.03)	1.96 (0.94 to 4.11)	3.12 (0.077)
Bulging drum	22 (46)	80 (46)	0.99 (0.52 to 1.89)	0.99 (0.49 to 1.97)	0.0 (0.97)
Past history — prior episodes of otitis media:					
0	17 (40)	88 (58)	1	1	4.95 (0.026) (test for trend)
1	12 (28)	36 (24)	1.73 (0.75 to 3.98)	1.73 (0.75 to 3.98)	
2	14 (33)	29 (19)	2.50 (1.10 to 5.69)	2.50 (1.10 to 5.69)	
Family/social factors — child care:					
Playgroup	9 (21)	34 (25)	1	1	4.79 (0.091)
Nursery	2 (5)	21 (15)	0.36 (0.07 to 1.83)	0.31 (0.06 to 1.65)	
School	31 (74)	84 (60)	1.39 (0.60 to 3.24)	1.36 (0.54 to 3.38)	

OR = odds ratio. LR = likelihood ratio. [a]Adjusted for significant predictors of outcome. Other variable assessed in models and shown not to predict outcome: asthma, eczema, exposure to smoke in the home, educational status of parents, history of breast feeding, past and current use of dummy, sibling having had otitis media.

earache were reported in the 3 months since study entry (immediate antibiotics 10%; delayed 39%; χ^2 4.8; $P = 0.029$). There was a similar effect for poor functioning at 3 months (20% compared to 44%; χ^2 2.69; $P = 0.10$). However, in the same group of children, immediate treatment with antibiotics did not predict outcome for parental rating of poor functioning at 1 year (30% and 32%) or episodes of earache reported since study entry at 1 year (47% and 52%).

DISCUSSION
Summary of main findings
This randomised controlled trial of antibiotic prescribing strategies for acute otitis media in typical primary care settings suggests that delayed prescribing does not result in adverse medium- to longer-term outcomes. Children with recurrent episodes are likely to have poorer outcome, and secondary analysis of this subgroup — which should

Table 4. Predictors of poor score (9 or more) on function scale after 1 year.

	Had poor function n (%)	Did not have poor function n (%)	Crude OR (95% CI)	Adjusted OR (95% CI)[a]	LR χ^2 (P-value)
Symptoms and signs:					
High temperature	9 (19)	28 (16)	1.24 (0.54–2.86)	1.53 (0.64–3.66)	0.89 (0.35)
Vomiting	12 (26)	35 (21)	1.35 (0.63–2.88)	1.28 (0.59–2.78)	0.38 (0.54)
Ear discharge	18 (39)	42 (25)	1.94 (0.98–3.86)	1.62 (0.79–3.32)	1.67 (0.20)
Bulging drum	23 (50)	83 (47)	1.11 (0.58–2.12)	1.03 (0.52–2.02)	0.01 (0.94)
Past history — prior episodes of otitis media:					
0	17 (37)	87 (57)	1	1	4.56 (0.033) (test for trend)
1	16 (35)	38 (25)	2.15 (0.99–4.71)	2.15 (0.99–4.71)	
2	13 (28)	29 (19)	2.29 (0.99–5.29)	2.29 (0.99–5.29)	
Family/social factors — child care:					
Playgroup	6 (20)	27 (23)	1	1	1.24 (0.54)
Nursery	3 (10)	18 (15)	0.75 (0.17–3.39)	0.61 (0.13–2.89)	
School	21 (70)	73 (62)	1.29 (0.47–3.55)	1.25 (0.44–3.58)	

OR = odds ratio. LR = likelihood ratio. [a]Adjusted for significant predictors of outcome. Other variable assessed in models and shown not to predict outcome: asthma, eczema, exposure to smoke in the home, educational status of parents, history of breast feeding, past and current use of dummy, sibling having had otitis media.

be treated with caution (due to weaker evidence) — suggests that they may possibly benefit from immediate antibiotics in the medium term, but not in the longer term.

Strengths and limitations of this study
The main strengths of this study are the adequate long-term follow-up, the size of the study, the generalisable sample, and the pragmatic interventions and outcomes. Before discussing the detailed results, the potential limitations of this study will be outlined.

Selection and non-response bias. We have shown that low-recruiting doctors were apparently a little more unsure about recruiting younger children,[12] and the cohort contained few very young children. Thus, although there was no evidence that age predicted outcome in this cohort, it is more difficult to extrapolate the results to very young children. There was no evidence of significant differences in the characteristics of those who responded to follow-up questionnaires and those who did not.

Placebo effect. An open trial design and minimally intrusive outcomes (for example, no intrusive measures of compliance, or investigation) was chosen to assess realistic outcomes in everyday practice, but has the important disadvantage of a potential placebo effect. Although we minimised this using a structured advice sheet approach — which has been shown to abolish the antibiotic placebo effect in a previous trial[5] — a component of the placebo effect is possible. However, the effect if any is probably small: previous estimates from this study (for example, night disturbance and paracetamol consumption)[12] were very similar to the largest blinded trial performed in a similar study population,[13] and the estimates in this study demonstrate little or no placebo effect.

Outcomes. We wanted to measure outcomes reflecting parents' concerns — both of discomfort for their child and their child's functioning. Thus the study can be criticised for potential recall bias of episodes of earache, and by not including 'hard' outcomes such as tympanometry or audiometry — but the relationship of such outcomes to child discomfort, functioning and development is not clear-cut.[20] We have shown that the outcomes chosen are likely to be reliable, they are important to parents, and they reflect likely impact on health service utilisation by parents.[18]

Subsequent antibiotic use. Subsequent antibiotic use after the randomised episode could potentially

have altered the longer-term outcomes of the two prescribing strategies. In fact, controlling for subsequent antibiotic use did not alter the estimates.

Subgroup analysis. This study reports estimates of both the predictors of poor outcome, and also the effect of antibiotics in a clinical subgroup of a randomised trial (that is, a danger of type I error). These findings therefore require confirmation in further prospective studies.

Comparison with existing literature
Who is at risk of poor outcome? The most consistent predictor of poor outcome was the number of prior episodes of otitis media documented in the doctor's notes, which predicted episodes of earache reported since study entry after 1 year, and parental rating of function at both 3 months and 1 year. This is consistent with previous evidence,[21] which suggests that those with post-otitis media or secretory otitis media, past acute otitis media (AOM), and who were boys were less likely to have good outcome at 2 months.[21] We were unable to confirm other risk factors previously identified for adverse outcome such as sibling ear infection, use of a dummy, and age.[3]

Can poorer medium- and long-term outcomes be modified? For most children using a delayed prescribing strategy is not likely to have adverse longer-term consequences. The current study suggests that medium-term outcome may possibly be modified in children with recurrent ear infections — but with the important caveat about type I error above for secondary subgroup analysis. Furthermore, when longer-term outcomes are included (that is, from randomisation to 1 year), there is no longer an effect. A systematic review suggests prophylaxis has minimal effects,[22,23] but there is mixed evidence as to whether treating upper respiratory tract infections in otitis-prone children reduces subsequent otitis media in children with recurrent otitis media.[24,25] The difficulty of modifying longer-term outcomes is supported by previous research: when compared to children with no AOM, children with recurrent AOM had worse thresholds only at high frequencies when followed up to age 7 years.[26] The long-term outlook for most children with ear infections is good: adults who remember ear infections in childhood, are no more likely to suffer hearing impairment when compared to who do not remember ear infections.[27]

Implications for future research
Secondary analysis from this trial cohort highlights

the importance of performing a larger randomised controlled trial to assess the benefit of antibiotics and alternatives to antibiotics in the medium to longer term for children with recurrent otitis media.

Funding body
Paul Little is supported by the Medical Research Council (G108/322). The current study was supported by a grant from regional NHS responsive mode funding in the South West region

Ethics committee
Isle of White and Portsmouth (LReC number 12/96/484) also North and Mid Hampshire, Salisbury, Southampton and South West Hampshire

Competing interests
The authors have stated that there are none

Acknowledgements
We are grateful to the following doctors for their enthusiasm and help in recruitment: Doctors Newman, Taylor, Traynor, Tippett, Warner, Peace, Stephens, Glasspool, Stone, Webb, Snell, Devereux, Hoghton, Terry, Dickson, Nightingale, Richenbach, Bacon, Lupton, Padday, Cookson, Stanger, Glaysher, Bond, Baker, Barnsley, Jeffries, Willard, Carlisle, Hill, Collier, Cubitt, De Quincey, Over, White, Billington, Percival, Hollands, Glaysher, Stranger.

REFERENCES

1. Bain J. Controversies in therapeutics. Childhood otalgia. Justification for antibiotic use in general practice. *BMJ* 1990; **300:** 1006–1007.

2. Browning G. Controversies in therapeutics. Childhood otalgia: acute otitis media. Antibiotics not necessary in most cases. *BMJ* 1990; **300:** 1005–1006.

3. Froom J, Culpepper L, Jacobs M, *et al.* Antimicrobials for acute otitis media? A review from the international primary care network. *BMJ* 1997; **315:** 98–102.

4. Del Mar C, Glasziou P, Hayem M. Are antibiotics indicated as initial treatment for children with acute otitis media? A meta-analysis. *BMJ* 1997; **314:** 1526–1529.

5. Little PS, Williamson I, Warner G, *et al.* An open randomised trial of prescribing strategies for sore throat. *BMJ* 1997; **314:** 722–727.

6. Little PS, Gould C, Williamson I, *et al.* Reattendance and complications in a randomised trial of prescribing strategies for sore throat: the medicalising effect of prescribing antibiotics. *BMJ* 1997; **315:** 350–352.

7. Britten N, Ukoumunne O. The influence of patients' hopes of receiving a prescription on doctors' perceptions and the decision to prescribe: a questionnaire survey. *BMJ* 1997; **315:** 1506–1510.

8. MacFarlane J, Holmes W, MacFarlane R, Britten N. Influence of patients' expectations on antibiotics management of acute lower respiratory illness in general practice: questionnaire study. *BMJ* 1997; **315:** 1211–1214.

9. Arason V, Kristinsson K, Sigurdsson J, *et al.* Do antimicrobials increase the rate of penicillin resistant pneumococci in children? Cross sectional prevalence study. *BMJ* 1996; **313:** 387–391.

10. Van Buchem FL, Peeters MF, van't Hof MA. Acute otitis media a new treatment strategy. *BMJ* 1985; **290:** 1033–1037.

11. Pitts J. Shared decision making in the informed treatment of acute otitis media. *Practitioner* 1987; **231:** 1232–1233.

12. Little P, Gould C, Williamson I, *et al.* A pragmatic randomised controlled trial of two prescribing strategies for acute otitis media. *BMJ* 2001; **322:** 336–342.

13. Burke P, Bain J, Robinson D, Dunleavey J. Acute red ear in children: controlled trial of non-antibiotic treatment in general practice. *BMJ* 1991; **303:** 558–562.

14. Gates G, Northern J, Ferrer P, *et al.* Diagnosis and screening. *Ann Otol Rhinol Laryngol* 1989; **98(suppl 139):** 39–41.

15. Schwartz R, Rodriguez W, Brook I, Grundfast K. The febrile response in otitis media. *JAMA* 1981; **245:** 2057–2058.

16. Preston K. Pneumatic otoscopy: a review of the literature. *Issues In Compr Pediatr Nurs* 1998; **21(2):** 117–128.

17. Ruuskanen O, Heikkinen T. Otitis media: etiology and diagnosis. *Ped Inf Dis J* 1994; **13:** s23–s26.

18. Maw A, Tiwari R. Children with glue ear: how do they present? *Clin Otolaryngol Rhinol* 1988; **13:** 171–177.

19. Streiner DL, Norman GR. *Health measurement scales: a practical guide to their development and use.* Oxford: Oxford Medical Publications, 1995.

20. Williamson I, Sheridan C, Galker E, Lous J. A video-based performance in noise test for measuring audio-visual disability in young school children: test development, with validation by trained teachers, parents and audiometry as relative standards for disability. *Int J Pediatr Otorhinolaryngol* 1999; **49:** 127–133.

21. Froom J, Culpepper L, Bridges-Webb C, *et al.* Effect of patient characteristics and disease manifestations on the outcome of acute otitis media at 2 months. *Arch Fam Med* 1993; **2:** 841–846.

22. O'Neill P. Otitis media: a clinical review. *BMJ* 1999; **319:** 833–835.

23. Cantekin E. Where is the evidence? [rapid response] *BMJ* 1999; **319:** 833–835.

24. Prellner K, Fogle-Hansson M, Jorgensen F, *et al.* Prevention of recurrent acute otitis media in otitis-prone children by intermittent prophylaxis with penicillin. *Acta Otorhinolaryng* 1994; **114:** 182–187.

25. Autret-Leca E, Giraudeau B, Ployet M, Jonville-Bras A. Amoxicillin/clavulanic acid is ineffective at preventing otitis media in children with presumed viral upper respiratory infection: A randomised, double-blind equivalence, placebo-controlled trial. *Br J Clin Pharmacol* 2002; **54:** 652–656.

26. Sorri M, Maki-Torkko E, Alho O. Otitis media and long term follow-up of hearing. *Acta Otorhinolaryng* 1995; **115:** 193–195.

27. Stephenson H, Higson J, Haggard M. Binaural hearing in adults with histories of otitis media in childhood. *Audiology* 1995; **34:** 113–123.

CHAPTER 20

Family medicine development in Brazil

Gustavo Gusso

NOMINATED CLASSIC PAPER

James Macinko, Frederico C. Guanais, Maria de Fátima Marinho de Souza. Evaluation of the impact of the Family Health Program on infant mortality in Brazil, 1990–2002. *Journal of Epidemiology and Community Health*, 2006; 60(1): 13–19.

This article represented a milestone in the history of primary care in Brazil. Following the end of the dictatorship, a new national Constitution was inaugurated in 1988, and the Brazilian Unified Health System was implemented. In 1991 the Brazilian Community Health Worker Program started, and in 1994 the Family Health Program was launched.

The Brazilian Family Health Program involved doctors and represented a change in healthcare culture that was questioned by many important players. It challenged the common model of community-based polyclinics that used gynaecologists, paediatricians, and generalist physicians as the basis of the health team. Others questioned whether the role of community health workers was relevant. This article by James Macinko and colleagues represented a watershed.

Many commentators challenged this article when it was published. The most common criticism was that the infant mortality rate in Brazil had been decreasing since before the introduction of Family Health Teams. The authors had been very careful with this bias and had controlled for as many of the health determinants as possible. The authors discussed this possible limitation and clarified that they were not reviewing the role of individual health teams, but rather reviewing the Family Health Team strategy as a national policy for primary care. It was the population-level intervention of the Family Health Team strategy, rather than the interventions of individual teams, that was being assessed.

Although the paper does not discuss the importance of the contribution of one medical specialty over another, the Family Health Teams included doctors, nurses and community health workers. The model created the demand for family medicine in Brazil. The specialty of family medicine had been recognised in Brazil since 1981 but it was only after the launch of the Family Health Program that we saw an organised demand for family doctors in Brazil.

The conclusion from this research is that a commitment to teamwork and a strong national policy for Primary Health Care is probably more important than the specialty at the beginning. The Brazilian Family Health Team Strategy has been rolled out across the country and makes a major contribution to the delivery of universal health coverage to the 200 million people of Brazil. This globally recognised successful strategy is alive thanks to publications like this.

ABOUT THE LEAD AUTHOR OF THIS PAPER

James Macinko is Professor of Health Policy and Management and Community Health Sciences at the Jonathan and Karin Fielding School of Public Health. Prior to joining the faculty at UCLA in 2015, he was Associate Professor of Public Health and Health Policy at New York University and former director of the Master of Public Health programme. He is renowned for his research in Global Health with an emphasis on the impact of health reform and policy change, especially with a focus on the importance of primary care or family medicine. He was a Robert Wood Johnson Foundation Health and Society Scholar at the University of Pennsylvania from 2006 to 2008 and a Fulbright Scholar in Brazil in 2002. He speaks Portuguese, having spent some years working in Brazil, and many of his publications are about healthcare reforms in Brazil.

James' scientific career started with his PhD studies in Health and Social Policy at Johns Hopkins University where he worked with the late Professor Barbara Starfield, who became his mentor. He now leads a group of Brazilian researchers that focuses on the impact of the country's Family Health Team Strategy. He is one of the world's most qualified and fruitful researchers publishing about health reforms in Brazil.

ABOUT THE NOMINATOR OF THIS PAPER

Gustavo Gusso is a family doctor and part-time professor at the University of São Paulo in Brazil, where he coordinates the Family and Community Medicine residency programme. He graduated from the same university and carried out his residency at the Grupo Hospitalar Conceição where he studied with Carlos Grossman and Carmen Fernandes, among other family medicine leaders in Brazil.

> 'It is frustrating when we work hard just to prove the importance of family medicine. I now believe this is not the right approach. We must concentrate primarily on our patients, although sometimes we have to struggle for better recognition. I was lucky that at the end of my residency when I complained to Carlos Grossman, our "guru", he said, "You are too smug! Don't try to prove the importance of family medicine. If the world couldn't prove it, do you think you will?"'

Professor Gustavo Gusso, Brazil

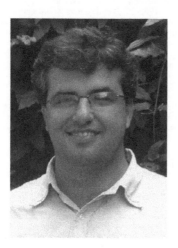

Attribution:

We attribute the original publication of *Evaluation of the impact of the Family Health Program on infant mortality in Brazil, 1990–2002* to *Journal of Epidemiology and Community Health*. With thanks to Laura Lacey and BMJ Journals.

EVIDENCE BASED PUBLIC HEALTH POLICY AND PRACTICE

Evaluation of the impact of the Family Health Program on infant mortality in Brazil, 1990–2002

James Macinko, Frederico C Guanais, Maria de Fátima Marinho de Souza

J Epidemiol Community Health 2006;**60**:13–19. doi: 10.1136/jech.2005.038323

Objective: To use publicly available secondary data to assess the impact of Brazil's Family Health Program on state level infant mortality rates (IMR) during the 1990s.
Design: Longitudinal ecological analysis using panel data from secondary sources. Analyses controlled for state level measures of access to clean water and sanitation, average income, women's literacy and fertility, physicians and nurses per 10 000 population, and hospital beds per 1000 population. Additional analyses controlled for immunisation coverage and tested interactions between Family Health Program and proportionate mortality from diarrhoea and acute respiratory infections.
Setting: 13 years (1990–2002) of data from 27 Brazilian states.
Main results: From 1990 to 2002 IMR declined from 49.7 to 28.9 per 1000 live births. During the same period average Family Health Program coverage increased from 0% to 36%. A 10% increase in Family Health Program coverage was associated with a 4.5% decrease in IMR, controlling for all other health determinants (p<0.01). Access to clean water and hospital beds per 1000 were negatively associated with IMR, while female illiteracy, fertility rates, and mean income were positively associated with IMR. Examination of interactions between Family Health Program coverage and diarrhoea deaths suggests the programme may reduce IMR at least partly through reductions in diarrhoea deaths. Interactions with deaths from acute respiratory infections were ambiguous.
Conclusions: The Family Health Program is associated with reduced IMR, suggesting it is an important, although not unique, contributor to declining infant mortality in Brazil. Existing secondary datasets provide an important tool for evaluation of the effectiveness of health services in Brazil.

See end of article for authors' affiliations

Correspondence to:
Professor J Macinko,
Department of Nutrition,
Food Studies, and Public
Health, New York
University, 35 West 4th
Street, 12th Floor, New
York, NY 10012-1172
USA; james.macinko@
nyu.edu

Accepted for publication
7 June 2005

The Brazilian unified health system (Sistema Único de Saúde or SUS in Portuguese) was created and structured on the principles of universal coverage and health as a right of all citizens, with an emphasis on decentralisation, equity, community participation, integration, shared financing among the different levels of government, and complementary participation by the private sector.[1][2] It was loosely patterned after the National Health Services of European countries like the United Kingdom.[3] Since 1990, Brazil has undergone considerable health reforms to implement this ambitious vision. The process of decentralisation, in particular, has advanced rapidly within the realm of primary health care.

The Family Health Program (Programa Saúde da Família or PSF in Portuguese) can be considered the main government effort to improve primary health care in Brazil. The PSF provides a broad range of primary health care services delivered by a team composed of one physician, one nurse, a nurse assistant, and (usually) four or more community health workers. In some places, the team also includes dental and social work professionals.[4][5] Each team is assigned to a geographical area and is then responsible for enrolling and monitoring the health status of the population living in this area, providing primary care services, and making referrals to other levels of care as required. Each team is responsible for an average of 3450 and a maximum of 4500 people. Physicians and nurses typically deliver services at health facilities placed within the community, while community agents provide health promotion and education services during household visits. As of 2004, the programme covered about 66 million people—nearly 40% of the entire population.[6]

Despite the considerable investments in the PSF programme to date, there has been little research into the extent to which these innovative features are associated with changes in health status at the national level while adequately controlling for other factors known to affect health.[7–11]

The objective of this study is to use publicly available datasets to evaluate the impact of the PSF on infant mortality over time, while controlling for other health determinants. We examine the period 1990–2002 because it includes three distinct periods: pre-PSF implementation (1990–1994), early PSF development (1995–1998), and late PSF expansion (1999–2002).

METHODS

The unit of analysis is the state. The state was used because reliable ecological data were available for the time period examined, there is a lower likelihood of random fluctuations in mortality and population size than there would be at a smaller level of analysis, and using state level aggregate data can attenuate possible "crossover" effects encountered when smaller units of analysis are used for measuring availability of medical care and mortality.[12] Including individual level data on PSF and non-PSF users would be desirable, but there is no existing dataset containing all the necessary variables for each state and year.

Data on infant mortality and other outcomes, PSF coverage (the proportion of the state population served by the PSF programme), and health resources are from the Brazilian Ministry of Health's web site.[13] Data on other health determinants are based on yearly population surveys conducted by the Brazilian Institute of Geography and Statistics

Abbreviations: IMR, infant mortality rate; PSF, Programa Saúde da Família; ARI, acute respiratory infections; VIF, variance inflation factor

Table 1 Mean values for Brazilian States 1990–2002 (n = 27)

Variable	Statistic	Year 1990	1996	2002	Change 1990–2002
Infant mortality rate (per 1000 live births)	mean	49.71	36.22*	28.91†	−20.79‡
	(SD)	(20.32)	(14.90)	(11.36)	
Coverage of Family Health Program (%)	mean	0.00	1.82*	36.06†	36.06‡
	(SD)	–	(3.08)	(17.90)	
Households with access to clean water supply (%)	mean	62.47	75.41*	82.13†	19.66‡
	(SD)	(21.82)	(17.59)	(15.07)	
Households with access to sewerage (%)	mean	39.73	47.57	54.05†	14.32‡
	(SD)	(23.26)	(23.73)	(21.44)	
Income per capita (in constant 2001 R$)	mean	284.26	307.58	323.72	39.46
	(SD)	(134.86)	(114.01)	(124.5)	
Female illiteracy rate (%)	mean	22.11	16.94*	13.60†	−8.51‡
	(SD)	(10.71)	(8.52)	(6.84)	
Fertility (average number children per woman)	mean	3.35	2.75*	2.40†	−0.95‡
	(SD)	(0.84)	(0.54)	(0.49)	
Physicians per 10000 population	mean	0.82	0.97*	1.07†	0.25‡
	(SD)	(0.55)	(0.62)	(0.66)	
Hospital beds per 1000 population	mean	3.06	3.01	2.40†	−0.65‡
	(SD)	(1.00)	(0.81)	(0.55)	
Nurses per 10000 population	mean	2.31	3.01*	4.74†	2.42‡
	(SD)	(2.55)	(2.51)	(2.21)	
Proportionate mortality from diarrhoea (% of all deaths of children under 5 years)	mean	12.27	7.32*	4.83†	−7.44‡
	(SD)	(4.20)	(2.98)	(2.47)	
Proportionate mortality from ARI (% of all deaths of children under 5 years)	mean	9.48	7.44*	5.32†	−3.49‡
	(SD)	(2.50)	(2.13)	(1.57)	
Immunisation coverage (TB)¶ (% of children under 5)	mean	NA	104.68	113.01†	13.27†
	(SD)	–	(14.68)	(8.48)	
Immunisation coverage (measles)¶ (% of children under 5)	mean	NA	76.10	96.59†	20.49†
	(SD)	–	(14.09)	(12.14)	

*Significant difference 1996 compared with 1990 (p<0.05). †Significant difference 2002 compared with 1996 (p<0.05). ‡Significant difference 2002 compared with 1990 (p<0.05). ¶Immunisation coverage may exceed 100%. NA, data not available; ARI, acute respiratory infections.

(IGBE) and developed for state level representativity by the Institute of Applied Economic Research (IPEA).[14 15]

The infant mortality rate (IMR) (expressed as the number of deaths of children under 1 year of age per 1000 live births in the same year) is used as the dependent variable. We use IMR in this study because the improvement of child health is a PSF programme priority. We use estimates of IMR that are adjusted for underreporting of child deaths in some areas of the country.[16 17]

Independent variables known to influence infant mortality include socioeconomic conditions (proportion of the population with access to adequate water supply and adequate sanitation installations, and income per capita in 2001 inflation adjusted Brazilian reais) women's development indicators (proportion of women over 15 who are illiterate, and the average number of children per woman), and health services indicators (physicians and nurses per 10 000 population, and hospital beds per 1000).[18 19]

About 10% of independent variable data were missing for one or two years for some states. Missing data were imputed using linear interpolation from within state time series.[20] Sensitivity tests using dummy variables to represent the pattern of missing values suggested that the they could be treated as missing at random.[21]

Statistical analyses

This study is a longitudinal analysis that uses panel data from all 27 Brazilian federative units (composed of the 26 states and the federal district, Brasília) for every year between 1990 and 2002. The study uses a fixed effects specification to correct for serial correlation of repeated measures and to control for time invariant unobserved or unobservable state characteristics.[22] An alternative approach, the random effects model, was rejected because of results of the Hausman test (p<0.001) that tested correlation between the regressors and error terms.[22]

One advantage of the fixed effects model over cross sectional analyses is that it is able to control for unmeasured time invariant characteristics of the state (such as geography, historical disadvantages, or local cultural practices) that might influence health outcomes.[23] We also include a year specific effect to control for unmeasured time variant characteristics such as new developments in technology or changes in national health policies that would affect all states during the period of the study. The disadvantage of the fixed effects approach is that the results obtained are conditional on the data used to estimate them; that is, results cannot be generalised to other years or states not included in the study.[23]

We performed a number of sensitivity tests including using robust (Huber/White/sandwich) standard errors, using Prais-Winsten regression to control for potential heteroskedasticity and AR-1 autocorrelation, and transforming the dependent variable to a logarithmic scale.[24] To control for potential multicollinearity, we transformed explanatory variables with high (over 10) variance inflation factors (VIFs) into dummy variables representing high (over 75th centile) values. The models with transformed models reduced average VIFs to less than six. We also tested models that weighted states by the number of live births. None of these alternative specifications significantly affected the sign, significance, or main conclusions reached with the fixed effects models, suggesting that the results presented here are robust.

To compare how variables changed over time, we calculate the mean values and standard deviations for 1990, 1996, and 2002 as well as the total change for each variable from 1990 to 2002. Differences in mean values between time periods were assessed using t tests. Results of regression models are presented as a series of nested models. The F test is used to assess whether the inclusion of an additional set of independent variables improved regression models. To compare the magnitude of the effects of the main explanatory variables on IMR, we present their marginal effects. This

Evaluation of the impact of the Family Health Program 15

Table 2 Results of fixed effects regression models of infant mortality rates for the 27 states of Brazil, 1990–2002

Variable	Model 1	Model 2	Model 3	Model 4
Family Health Program	−0.219**	−0.184**	−0.152**	−0.171**
(% of population)	(0.023)	(0.022)	(0.021)	(0.021)
Water access	−	−0.218**	−0.107**	−0.109**
(% population)		(0.039)	(0.04)	(0.040)
Sewerage access	−	0.037	0.038	0.051
(% population)		(0.028)	(0.026)	(0.026)
Mean income	−	0.011*	0.018**	0.015**
(in constant R$)		(0.005)	(0.005)	(0.005)
Female illiteracy	−	−	0.662**	0.630**
(% women >15 years)			(0.105)	(0.104)
Fertility	−	−	2.439**	2.378**
(mean number children/woman)			(0.866)	(0.881)
Physicians	−	−	−	−1.735
(per 10000 population)				(0.527)
Nurses	−	−	−	−0.423
(per 10000 population)				(0.239)
Hospital beds	−	−	−	−1.735**
(per 1000 population)				(0.527)
Constant	49.706**	58.697**	27.037**	35.465**
	(0.531)	(2.633)	(4.788)	(5.306)
Observations	351	351	351	351
Number of states	27	27	27	27
R^2 (within)	0.868	0.882	0.901	0.905
F test (model 2 v model 1)	−	12.07**	−	−
F test (model 3 v model 2)	−	−	29.46**	−
F test (model 4 v model 3)	−	−	−	4.53**

Standard errors in parentheses. Year and state fixed effects not shown. *Significant ($p<0.05$); **significant ($p<0.01$).

Table 3 Sensitivity tests for fixed effects regression models of infant mortality rates for the 27 states of Brazil, 1990–2002

Variable	Interaction effects Model 5	Immunisation coverage† Model 6	Lagged PSF (−1 year) Model 7	Stratified by region (N, NE ; S, SE, CW) Model 8‡	Model 9§
Family Health Program	−0.143**	−0.087**	−	−0.142**	−0.047**
(% of population)	(0.021)	(0.014)		(0.025)	(0.015)
Family Health Program	−	−	−0.194**	−	−
(1 year lag)			(0.023)		
Access to clean water	−0.103**	−0.114**	−0.116**	−0.097*	0.007
(% population)	(0.039)	(0.040)	(0.040)	(0.042)	(0.034)
Sewerage access	0.038	0.061**	0.059*	0.052	−0.002
(% population)	(0.026)	(0.019)	(0.025)	(0.028)	(0.021)
Mean income	0.012*	0.017**	0.017**	0.003	0.002
(in constant R$)	(0.005)	(0.005)	(0.005)	(0.006)	(0.003)
Female illiteracy	0.545**	0.509**	0.505**	0.385**	0.139
(% women >15 years)	(0.102)	(0.092)	(0.099)	(0.112)	(0.095)
Fertility	1.877*	0.625	2.785**	4.635**	3.718**
(mean number children/woman)	(0.859)	(0.898)	(0.913)	(1.147)	(1.132)
Physicians	−1.886	−0.719	−0.272	−5.966**	1.117
(per 10000 population)	(1.427)	(1.001)	(1.337)	(2.067)	(0.693)
Nurses	−0.422	0.133	−0.327	−0.434	0.523**
(per 10000 population)	(0.232)	(0.207)	(0.229)	(0.307)	(0.119)
Hospital beds	−1.416**	−1.634**	−2.017**	0.006	−0.790*
(per 1000 population)	(0.531)	(0.482)	(0.521)	(0.614)	(0.342)
High diarrhoea mortality	0.993*	−	−	−	−
(≥10% of child deaths)	(0.471)				
PSF×diarrhoea interaction	−0.136**	−	−	−	−
	(0.036)				
High ARI mortality	−1.659**	−	−	−	−
(≥9% of child deaths)	(0.465)				
PSF×ARI interaction	0.265	−	−	−	−
	(0.195)				
Tuberculosis immunisation	−	−0.001	−	−	−
(% of children covered)		(0.010)			
Measles immunisation	−	−0.008	−	−	−
(% of children covered)		(0.010)			
Constant	39.859**	35.846**	35.645**	76.133**	38.206**
	(5.201)	(5.531)	(5.316)	(6.583)	(5.297)
Observations	351	225	324	208	143
Number of states	27	27	27	16	11
R^2 (within)	0.913	0.899	0.902	0.944	0.979

Standard errors in parentheses; year and state fixed effects not shown. *Significant ($p<0.05$); **significant ($p<0.01$). †Covers the period 1994–2002 only (because of missing immunisation data). ‡Results for the 16 states in the north and north east regions only. §Results for the 11 states in the south, south east, and central west regions only.

Table 4 Marginal effects of main explanatory variables†

Independent variable	Marginal effects: percentage change in infant mortality associated with a 10% increase in the independent variable‡
Family Health Program (% of population covered)	−4.56** (−5.68 to −3.44)
Water access (% population covered)	−2.92** (−5.01 to −0.84)
Hospital beds (per 1000 population)	−1.35** (−2.16 to −0.55)
Female illiteracy (% women >15 years who are illiterate)	16.82** (11.38 to 22.26)
Fertility (mean number children/woman)	1.78** (0.49 to 3.08)
Mean income (in constant R$)	1.11** (0.37 to 1.85)

95% Confidence intervals errors in parentheses. **Significant (p<0.01). †Based on final model (model 4 from table 2); non-significant variables and fixed effects not shown. ‡Marginal effects evaluated at the mean of all other independent variables (predicted IMR = 37.441).

statistic represents the percentage change in IMR given a 1% change in the independent variable when all other values set at their mean.[25]

We also assessed several potential pathways by which the PSF might influence IMR. Each of these pathways has a particular limitation so they are presented separately from the main analyses. Firstly, it is possible that reduction in IMR could be attributable to improvements in immunisations independent of the PSF programme, so we test a model that includes childhood immunisation (measles and tuberculosis vaccinations). However, immunisation data are only available after 1995.

Secondly, deaths from diarrhoea and from acute respiratory infections (ARI) are important determinants of IMR in developing countries.[26] To test the impact of PSF expansion on these pathways we created dummy variables representing states in the highest 75th centile of under 5 year old deaths from both of these conditions (called "high diarrhoea deaths" and "high ARI deaths", respectively). We then created interaction terms between these binary variables and PSF coverage to test if PSF expansion was associated with changes in mortality from these conditions.

To assess temporality, we test the PSF variable with a one year lag—that is, we estimate the effect of a previous year's PSF coverage on this year's IMR.

Finally, because there are great differences in economic development, education, and infrastructure between the poorer north and north eastern regions of Brazil, as compared with the south, south east, and central west regions, we present analyses stratified by region (the poorer northern regions compared with the richer southern ones) to test whether the PSF effect might differ between them.

RESULTS

Table 1 presents descriptive statistics. By 2002, the IMR had declined to nearly half its 1990 rate and immunisation coverage reached over 95%. The PSF began expansion in the mid-1990s and covered more than a third of the Brazilian population by 2002. Child deaths from diarrhoea in 2002 were only a third of the 1990 rate, and deaths from acute respiratory infections were halved during the same period. Overall socioeconomic conditions also improved, although by 2002 barely 50% of the population had access to modern sewerage systems. Average income fluctuated each year and there was no significant increase over time. There was considerable progress in women's development: female illiteracy declined by a third, as did the average number of children per woman. Absolute rates of illiteracy are still high at 13%. In terms of health inputs, physicians and nurses

increased significantly, while the average number of hospital beds declined slightly.

Table 2 presents the results of the fixed effects analyses. Model 1 shows the bivariate relation between PSF and IMR: the larger the proportion of the state's population served by the PSF, the lower the expected IMR. Model 2 adds socioeconomic covariates to model 1. PSF coverage remains significant and negatively associated with IMR. In terms of covariates, access to water is negatively associated with IMR, while income is positively associated with it. Sewerage is not significant. The F test is statistically significant suggesting that addition of these covariates improves the explanatory power of model 2 over model 1.

Model 3 adds a set of variables related to women's health. Both female illiteracy and fertility rates are positively associated with infant mortality. The PSF coefficient remains significant and negative, and socioeconomic variables remain stable. Based on the results of the F test, model 3 is considered superior to the previous models.

Model 4 includes health system covariates. Physician and nurse supply are not significantly associated with IMR, but hospital beds per 1000 is associated. There is no change in any other covariate and PSF remains similar in magnitude, direction, and statistical significance. Results of the F test show that model 4 is superior to any previous models. The R^2 is 0.90 suggesting that the model explains up to 90% of the within state variation in IMR.

Table 3 presents sensitivity tests that further explore the relation between PSF and IMR at the state level. Model 5 tests the interaction terms between PSF coverage and states with high proportionate mortality from diarrhoea and ARI. The coefficient for high diarrhoea mortality is positive and significant, suggesting that states with higher proportionate mortality from diarrhoea also have higher IMR. The interaction variable for PSF×diarrhoea is significant and negative suggesting that as PSF coverage increases, the contribution of diarrhoea to infant mortality decreases. The results for ARI present a different pattern: states with a higher proportion of deaths from ARI also have lower IMR and the interaction between PSF coverage and ARI was not significant.

What is already known about the topic

There is evidence that comprehensive primary health care services can have a significant impact on improving child health, but most of this evidence does not assess longitudinal trends at the national level.

Model 6 tests the extent to which immunisation coverage contributes to lower IMR. The results show that increased vaccination coverage for BCG and for measles is not associated with IMR at the state level. The inclusion of immunisation rates into the model did not change the direction or significance of the PSF variable.

Model 7 tests a one year lagged PSF variable to assess whether a prior year's expansion in PSF coverage affects IMR in the following year. The lagged PSF variable is negative and significant and of a slightly higher magnitude than the contemporaneous PSF variable, suggesting a temporal relation between PSF coverage and reductions in IMR.

Models 8 and 9 present analyses stratified by geographical region. In model 9 (north), PSF coverage, access to clean water, and physicians per capita were associated with lower IMR, whereas female literacy and fertility has a positive association. In model 10 (south), PSF coverage and hospital beds were associated with lower IMR, while nurses per capita were associated with higher IMR.

Table 4 presents the marginal effects of the main explanatory variables included in the final model (model 4 in table 2). Marginal effects have been multiplied by 10 to give a measure of the percentage change in infant mortality associated with a 10% increase in the independent variable. Controlling for all other covariates, a 10% increase in PSF coverage was associated, on average, with a 4.6% decrease in IMR. Improving water access by 10% was associated with a 3% reduction, and increasing hospital beds only a 1.35% reduction. Female illiteracy was the most important determinant of infant mortality: decreasing female illiteracy by 10% could reduce IMR by a greater amount than all other variables combined. Higher fertility and income per capita had a modest, positive association with IMR.

DISCUSSION

The analyses presented here suggest that PSF coverage is independently associated with reductions in IMR: an increase in PSF coverage by 10% was associated with an average 4.6% decrease in IMR, controlling for other health determinants. Previous studies have emphasised the role of water supply, living conditions, and women's education on improving child health outcomes in Brazil.[27][28] Our results confirm these findings, but suggest that expansion of the PSF programme adds an important complementary explanation for the decrease in infant mortality in Brazil seen since the programme began in the mid-1990s.

Previous studies found no significant association between availability of physicians and reductions in child mortality, a result confirmed by our analyses. This finding could be in part because the number of physicians per capita is not necessarily associated with increased provision of primary health care. Most physicians in Brazil are specialty trained and thus provide services to a more limited population than would a primary care provider.[29] The finding of no relation between nurses and IMR reductions was not expected given

What this study adds

- This is the first study to assess the impact of Brazil's Family Health Program on infant mortality at the national level.
- The main determinants of infant mortality in Brazil include: primary care and hospital bed availability, clean water, income, women's literacy, and fertility.
- Family Health Program coverage was a significant contributor to improvements in infant mortality rates.

Policy implications

- A broad based approach to improving child health, with primary health care at its core, can make considerable improvements in health outcomes.
- Publicly available secondary datasets could be used more fully in Brazil to assess the effectiveness of public policies at the national and state levels.

that nurses are increasingly being deployed in primary care settings, and are the clinical backbone of the PSF.[9] One explanation is that the PSF effect could be related more to how health workers are deployed (that is, as a community based, integrated, multifunctional team) rather than the total number of health workers providing care.

The result that availability of hospital beds was associated with lower IMR is consistent with the fact that an important component of IMR is neonatal mortality (mortality within the first month of life); an outcome strongly influenced by the availability and quality of care during and after delivery, special care for low birthweight babies, and some aspects of prenatal care.[30] The other component of IMR, post-neonatal mortality, is more strongly associated with preventive and primary care such as breast feeding, oral rehydration therapy, immunisations, and treatment of respiratory and other infections.[31] Neonatal mortality has been linked to increased pre-term and low birthweight births and has become a more significant contributor to IMR in Brazil as post-neonatal mortality declined.[32][33] The PSF would be expected to have a direct influence on post-neonatal mortality, as well as indirect effect on neonatal mortality through promotion of maternal health and nutrition, initiation of prenatal care, and identification and referral of potentially high risk births to specialists.[34]

The finding of a positive association between income and IMR is surprising given the importance of socioeconomic development to improvements in IMR. In the case of Brazil, the observed relation probably reflects an increase in income inequalities, which are associated with higher child mortality.[35][36]

In the region stratified analyses, the effect of the PSF is reduced for the more developed south, south east and central west regions where IMR has been lower relative to the north and north east. The PSF variable is nevertheless negative and significant for both regions. Interestingly, physician supply became a significant predictor of lower IMR in the north and north east, probably reflecting the shortage of physicians in this area: physicians per 10 000 averaged 2.6 in the north region compared with 10.6 in the south east.[9]

This study explored several pathways through which the PSF might influence child health. The first of these is through reduction of deaths attributable to diarrhoea. The results of the interaction terms suggest that as PSF coverage increases, the contribution of diarrhoea deaths to IMR tends to decrease, suggesting one potential mechanism of PSF action.

The results from the ARI variables are more complex. The interaction term is not significant, but the dummy variable for "high ARI mortality" was significant and negative, suggesting that higher ARI mortality was associated with lower IMR. It may be that ARI deaths happen more frequently in children older than 1 year; we might have found a positive relation with the PSF if our outcome variable had been under 5 mortality rather than IMR. Regional differences may also help to explain this finding. An examination of the data by state shows that diarrhoea was persistently a larger problem in the north and north eastern parts of the country, while ARI seems to have been a larger problem in south, south east and central western regions in early and mid-late 1990s (where IMR was lower overall). But then in the late 1990s the proportion of ARI deaths declined rapidly in the south and overall rates became similar for both regions. This heterogeneous trend may not have been accurately captured in the regression analyses.

The fact that immunisation rates were not significant predictors of IMR was expected given the already high levels of coverage (over 90%) in most states.

Limitations

Because this study was carried out using ecological measures, we could not directly test whether the reductions in IMR occurred within families that visited the Family Health Program; to make that claim would be to commit an ecological fallacy. We believe there is a plausible causal chain linking PSF participation with better child health. There is evidence that Family Health Program clients regularly receive health education about breast feeding, use of oral rehydration therapy, immunisation, and infant growth monitoring.[7] There is also evidence that the PSF can provide quality primary care that is comprehensive, family oriented, longitudinal, and community oriented.[37] In a study of the PSF in eight large urban centres, more than three quarters of clients interviewed believed that child health services were of good quality and that the PSF was responsible for improvements in the health of the neighbourhood and their family.[7] Participation in the PSF programme within these large municipalities was associated with improved immunisation rates, breast feeding rates, and maternal management of diarrhoea and respiratory infections.[38] Preliminary evidence suggests that the PSF programme decreases financial barriers to access.[39] Finally, several studies have shown that in areas where the PSF or similar programmes have been implemented, infant mortality has actually declined.[11 40]

Although the results presented here seem to be robust to a number of different specifications, several limitations merit discussion.

Firstly, ecological analyses are prone to omitted variable problems. That is, there could be some latent, unmeasured variable (such as malnutrition) that is confounding the apparent relation between PSF and IMR. In this case, the existence of such a variable is unlikely given that we used a full model of health determinants, included state fixed effects to control for time invariant unobserved characteristics of states, included year fixed effects to control for unobserved factors that affect all states in each given year, and tested several pathways and alternative explanations. The high R^2 values of the regression models suggest that they do a good job explaining the variation in IMR.

Secondly, the implementation of the PSF can differ greatly from municipality to municipality and the programme itself has evolved over time. PSF expansion has not necessarily occurred in the most deprived municipalities and the distribution of PSF coverage is not uniform within states.[43] External factors, such as the availability of pharmaceuticals or access to needed specialty or hospital care can also undermine potential health gains derived from this model of primary care delivery.[41 42] Our study could not control for these limitations.

Conclusions

This study has shown the use of ecological analyses using publicly available secondary data for the evaluation of public health programmes. Despite the limitations presented by these analyses, they have the benefit of providing timely, policy relevant information on the performance of the Family

Health Program at the national level. The results showed that PSF expansion, along with other socioeconomic developments, were consistently associated with reductions in infant mortality. The policy implication is that a broad based approach to improving child health, with primary health care at its core, can make considerable improvements in outcomes. To more fully inform policy, future studies should assess the cost effectiveness of PSF expansion, its impact on adult health and equity, and estimate impacts at other levels of analysis (for example, municipal and individual levels).

. . . .
Authors' affiliations
J Macinko, Department of Nutrition, Food Studies, and Public Health, New York University, USA
F C Guanais, Robert F Wagner Graduate School of Public Service, New York University
M Marinho de Souza, Faculty of Medicine, University of São Paulo and University of Cuiabá; Secretariat of Health Surveillance, Ministry of Health of Brazil

Funding: this study was partially supported by the New York University Steinhardt School of Education and the Brazilian Ministry of Health. Frederico Guanais is supported by the National Council for Research and Development (CNPq). The conclusions presented in this paper represent the opinion of the authors alone.

Competing interests: none declared.

REFERENCES
1 **Brazil**. *Constitution of the Federative Republic of Brazil.* (In Portuguese). Brasília, Brazil, 1988.
2 **de Andrade LOM**, Pontes RJS, Martins Junior T. A descentralização no marco da Reforma Sanitária no Brasil. *Rev Panam Salud Publica* 2000;**8**:85–91.
3 **Abrantes Pego R**, Almeida C. [Theory and practice of the health systems reforms: the cases of Brazil and Mexico] (In Spanish). *Cad Saude Publica* 2002;**18**:971–89.
4 **Ministério da Saúde**. *Programa Saúde da Família.* Brasília, DF: Ministério da Saúde, 2001.
5 **Ministério da Saúde**. *Programa Agentes Comunitários de Saúde.* Brasília, DF: Ministério da Saúde, 2001.
6 **Sistema de Informação de Atenção Básica (SIAB)**. http://www.datasus.gov.br/siab/siab.htm, (accessed 23 May 23 2005).
7 **Escorel S**, Giovanella L, Mendonça MH, *et al. Avaliação da Implementação do Programa Saúde da Família em Dez Grande Centros Urbanos. Síntese dos Principais Resultados.* Brasília: Ministério da Saúde, Secretaria de Políticas de Saúde, 2002.
8 **Viana AL**, Pierantoni CR. *Indicadores de Monitoramento da Implementação do PSF em Grandes Centros Urbanos.* Brasília: Brazilian Ministry of Health, Department of Primary Care, 2002.
9 **Ministério da Saúde**. *Avaliação normativa do Programa Saúde da Família no Brasil.* Brasília: Sectária de Assistência à Saúde, Departamento de Atenção Básica, 2004.
10 **Conill EM**. [Primary care policies and health reforms: an evaluative approach based on an analysis of the Family Health Program in Florianopolis, Santa Catarina, Brazil, 1994–2000]. *Cad Saude Publica* 2002;**18**(suppl):191–202.
11 **Serra R**. *Uma avaliação empírica do impacto saúde da família sobre a saúde infantil no estado de São Paulo. Trabalho submetido ao Prêmio Economia da Saúde, IPEA.* Brasília: DF, 2005.
12 **Klein RJ**, Hawk SA. Health status indicators: definitions and national data. *Healthy People 2000 Stat Notes* 1992;**1**:1–7.
13 **Ministry of Health of Brazil**. Informações de Saúde. http://tabnet.datasus.gov.br/tabnet/tabnet.htm.
14 **Instituto de Pesquisa Econômica Aplicada (IPEA)**. Dados macroeconômicos e regionais. http://www.ipeadata.gov.br (accessed May 2005).
15 **Brazilian Institute of Geography and Statistics**. Banco multidimensional de estatísticas 2005. http://www.ibge.gov.br/.
16 **Szwarcwald CL**, Leal Medo C, de Andrade CL, *et al.* [Infant mortality estimation in Brazil: what do Ministry of Health data on deaths and live births say?]. *Cad Saude Publica* 2002;**18**:1725–36.
17 **Rede Interagencial de informações para a saúde (RIPSA)**. *Indicadores básicos para a saúde no Brasil.* Brasília, Brasil: Organização Panamericana da Saúde/OMS, 2002.
18 **Wang L**. Determinants of child mortality in LDCs. Empirical findings from demographic and health surveys. *Health Policy* 2003;**65**:277–99.
19 **Moore D**, Castillo E, Richardson C, *et al.* Determinants of health status and the influence of primary health care services in Latin America, 1990–98. *Int J Health Plann Manage* 2003;**18**:279–92.
20 **Allison P.** *Missing data.* Thousand Oaks, CA: Sage, 2002.
21 **Little RJ**, Rubin DB. *Statistical analysis with missing data.* New York: Wiley, 1987.
22 **Wooldridge J.** *Econometric analysis of cross section and panel data.* Cambridge, MA: The MIT Press, 2002.

23 **Hsiao C**. *Analysis of panel data*. 2nd ed. Cambridge: Cambridge University Press, 2003.

24 **Greene WH**. *Econometric analysis*. 5th ed. Upper Saddle River, NJ: Prentice Hall, 2003.

25 **Statacorp**. *Stata Statistical Software: release 8.0*. College Station, TX: Stata Corporation, 2003.

26 **Unicef**. *Facts for life*. 3rd ed. New York: United Nations Children's Fund, 2002.

27 **Sastry N**. Trends in socioeconomic inequalities in mortality in developing countries: the case of child survival in Sao Paulo, Brazil. *Demography* 2004;**41**:443–64.

28 **De Souza AC**, Petersont KE, Cufino E, *et al*. Underlying and proximate determinants of diarrhoea-specific infant mortality rates among municipalities in the state of Ceara, north-east Brazil: an ecological study. *J Biosoc Sci* 2001;**33**:227–44.

29 **Stein A**, Costa M, Busnello E, *et al*. Who in Brazil has a personal doctor? *Fam Pract* 1999;**16**:596–9.

30 **Martines J**, Paul VK, Bhutta ZA, *et al*. Neonatal survival: a call for action. *Lancet* 2005;**365**:1189–97.

31 **Starfield B**. Postneonatal mortality. *Annu Rev Public Health* 1985;**6**:21–40.

32 **Caldeira AP**, Franca E, Goulart EM. [Postneonatal infant mortality and quality of medical care: a case-control study]. *J Pediatr (Rio J)* 2001;**77**:461–8.

33 **Barros FC**, Victora CG, Barros AJ, *et al*. The challenge of reducing neonatal mortality in middle-income countries: findings from three Brazilian birth cohorts in 1982, 1993, and 2004. *Lancet* 2005;**365**:847–54.

34 **Shi L**, Macinko J, Starfield B, *et al*. Primary care, infant mortality, and low birth weight in the states of the USA. *J Epidemiol Community Health* 2004;**58**:374–80.

35 **Messias E**. Income inequality, illiteracy rate, and life expectancy in Brazil. *Am J Public Health* 2003;**93**:1294–6.

36 **Szwarcwald CL**, Andrade CL, Bastos FI. Income inequality, residential poverty clustering and infant mortality: a study in Rio de Janeiro, Brazil. *Soc Sci Med* 2002;**55**:2083–92.

37 **Macinko J**, Almeida C, dos SE, *et al*. Organization and delivery of primary health care services in Petropolis, Brazil. *Int J Health Plann Manage* 2004;**19**:303–17.

38 **Emond A**, Pollock J, Da Costa N, *et al*. The effectiveness of community-based interventions to improve maternal and infant health in the Northeast of Brazil. *Rev Panam Salud Publica* 2002;**12**:101–10.

39 **Goldbaum M**, Gianini RJ, Novaes HM, *et al*. [Health services utilization in areas covered by the family health program (Qualis) in Sao Paulo City, Brazil.]. *Rev Saúde Pública* 2005;**39**:90–9.

40 **Cufino Svitone E**, Garfield R, Vasconcelos MI, *et al*. Primary health care lessons from the northeast of Brazil: the Agentes de Saude Program. *Rev Panam Salud Publica* 2000;**7**:293–302.

41 **Chiesa AM**, Batista KBC. Desafios da implantação do Programa Saúde da Família em uma grande cidade: reflexões acerca da experiência de São Paulo/Challenges on the implementation of the Family Health Program in a great city: reflections on the experience São Paulo city. *Mundo Saúde (1995)* 2004;**28**:42–8.

42 **Franco AL**, Bastos AC, Alves VS. A relação médico-paciente no Programa Saúde da Família: um estudo em três municípios do Estado da Bahia, Brasil [The physician-patient relationship under the Family Health Program in three municipalities in Bahia State, Brazil]. *Cad Saúde Pública* 2005;**21**:246–55.

43 **Morsch E**, Chavannes N, van den Akker M, *et al*. The effects of the family health program in Ceará state, northeastern Brazil. *Arch Public Health* 2001;**59**:151–65.

CHAPTER 21

Global health, equity and primary care

Katherine Rouleau

NOMINATED CLASSIC PAPER

Barbara Starfield. Global health, equity, and primary care. *Journal of the American Board of Family Medicine*, 2007; 20(6): 511–13.

The paper is one of the first, and one of a notable few, to link family medicine directly to global health and equity. In contrast to the global health contributions of specialty disciplines, such as infectious diseases and paediatrics, it proposes a unique role for family medicine in strengthening health systems based on the demonstrated link between family medicine-centred health systems and greater equity, better outcomes and improved cost-efficiency. This is particularly relevant today as the global health community acknowledges the need to balance disease-focused and subpopulation-focused approaches with efforts to create health systems that are more accessible, more responsive, more resilient and ultimately more equitable for all. In this paper, Barbara Starfield calls for greater advocacy by 'world organisations of primary care physicians' in defining effective health systems globally.

The paper also highlights the inherent challenge facing family medicine of having diverse scopes of practice in different countries, mirroring the diverse health needs of populations. This diversity in scope is compounded by variations in the role of family medicine in relation to other health providers across settings. The paradox of a discipline united by common principles but articulated through varying scopes of activities remains a challenge today. As an increasing number of countries establish family medicine, the call to 'come to grips with defining an appropriate scope' has grown more urgent and deserves prompt collective attention.

In considering this paper's bold call for world organisations to 'become stronger advocates for primary care' we should acknowledge the steady voice provided by the World Organization of Family Doctors (WONCA) and the progress made. We further might consider adding to this the voices of global primary care research networks, family medicine teachers and experts from the global south, bringing together the global family medicine community to learn from each other and ensure that our discipline fulfils its potential.

ABOUT THE LEAD AUTHOR OF THIS PAPER

Barbara Starfield was a physician, a scholar and an advocate. She was trained as a paediatrician and a health services researcher at Johns Hopkins University in the United States of America. She led the Department of Health Policy and Management at that university from 1975 to 1994, and went on to produce foundational primary care research that still defines the field today. She demonstrated the relationship between primary care, including family medicine, and better outcomes, improved cost-efficiency and enhanced equity. In developing the Primary Care Assessment Tool (PCAT), she provided a much-needed framework to measure primary care across various settings. Through international consultations and collaboration, the impact of her work has extended well beyond the United States and North America.

In addition to being a consummate researcher, a brilliant academic and a gifted teacher, Professor Starfield was also a remarkable advocate. She co-founded the International Society of Inequity in Health, a scientific organisation focused on the identification and resolution of determinants that adversely and inequitably affect health. Through her extensive work, she consistently positioned individuals and populations at the centre of the healthcare equation. While the richness of her research outputs and impact are unequalled in the area of primary care and family medicine, the way in which she married stellar research, intelligent communication across boundaries, dedicated mentoring and bold advocacy sets her apart as a global family medicine icon.

ABOUT THE NOMINATOR OF THIS PAPER

Dr Katherine Rouleau is a Canadian family physician working in Toronto's inner city at St Michael's Hospital. She heads the Global Health programme of the Department of Family and Community Medicine at the University of Toronto and is the inaugural director of the Besrour Centre at the College of Family Physicians of Canada, a hub of a collaboration to advance family medicine globally.

'I invite new family physicians to consider, beyond our impact on individual health, our key role as a pathway to health equity. I see our community as

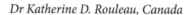

extending beyond our borders and urge us to find ways to come together across borders and culture to share, learn and contribute as a global family medicine community together to the health of all.'

Dr Katherine D. Rouleau, Canada

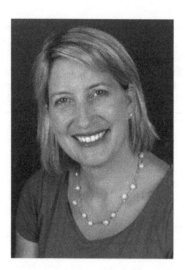

Attribution:

We attribute the original publication of *Global health, equity, and primary care* to the *Journal of the American Board of Family Medicine*. With thanks to Dr James C. Puffer, President and Chief Executive Officer of the American Board of Family Medicine and Phillip Lupo from the *Journal of the American Board of Family Medicine*.

COMMENTARY

Global Health, Equity, and Primary Care

Barbara Starfield, MD, MPH

Global health provides a special challenge for primary care and general practice, which will become increasingly important in the future as the prevalence of multimorbidity increases with increasing like-lihood of survival from acute manifestations of illness, as populations age, and as costs of care increase with increasing availability of technologic interventions. World organizations of primary care physicians need to take up the challenge before it becomes a crisis. (J Am Board Fam Med 2007;20:511–513.)

Interest in the health of other countries is not a new phenomenon. Late in the 19th century, Lord Chamberlain[1] made clear his view that global health meant "making the tropics safe for white men." In the 21st century, globalization is providing new imperatives largely because its effects on health are so pronounced,[2] occurring directly by means of increasing exposures to harmful social and environmental influences and indirectly through influences on health, economic, social, and health services.[3] Although definitions may vary depending on the particular interests of "global health practitioners," the definition provided by the US Institute of Medicine[4] provides a useful departure: "global health comprises health problems, issues, and concerns that transcend national boundaries, may be influenced by encounters or experiences in other countries, and are best addressed by cooperative efforts and solutions."

Despite common wisdom about the importance of commonly identified national characteristics, variability in health at any given level of country wealth or health professional supply is enormous,[5–7] providing evidence that differences in health cannot be a direct influence of these characteristics. Might there be a more consistent correlate?

The common focus of 20th century health systems on early identification and management of specific diseases was a by-product of the quest for single etiologies for clinical manifestations, fostered by epidemiologic evidence of environmental clusters of illnesses and the identification of disease-producing "germs." The 21st century era promises to be the era of pervasive effects of globalization, with interacting influences on health, increasing threats to equity in health, multiple co-occurring illnesses ("multimorbidity"), and increasing potential for adverse effects resulting from drug interactions, unnecessary interventions, and errors in providing services.

All these new challenges demand new approaches to organizing services: the disease-by-disease orientation is becoming increasingly dysfunctional. It must be replaced by a focus on people and populations with their unique combinations of illnesses and types of illnesses rather than specific diseases. Clustering of vulnerability, especially in deprived population groups, is associated with non-disease-specific symptoms and syndromes resulting from adverse social biological and environmental impacts. Multimorbidity is demanding not "chronic disease" management but, rather, a chronic care model in which person-focused primary care is the key element. The environment's impact on health and the effects of medical care itself are making it imperative to design services around the principle of rapid access to person-focused, comprehensive, and coordinated services provided over time to achieve early recognition and management for the multiplicity of conditions likely to be long-standing and eventually life-threatening. Known as "primary health care," such services are increasingly essential in meeting the health needs of all populations.[8,9]

This article was externally peer reviewed.
Submitted 25 July 2007; revised 6 August 2007; accepted 7 August 2007.
From Johns Hopkins University and Medical Institutions, Baltimore, MD.
Funding: none.
Conflict of interest: none declared.
Corresponding author: Barbara Starfield, Johns Hopkins University and Medical Institutions, 624 North Broadway, Room 452, Baltimore, MD 21205 (E-mail: bstarfie@jhsph.edu).

doi: 10.3122/jabfm.2007.06.070176

Barriers to the achievement of these goals may be thwarted by several characteristics of current health systems, particularly in some advanced industrialized nations with powerful hospital and specialist influences, the disease-oriented focus of major donors, and the lack of appreciation of the potential of primary care to foster effective and equitable health services at relatively low costs.[10] The imperative to maximize corporate market share and profit prevents societal action directed at equity goals ("reductions in disparities").[11]

Family medicine, acting on a global level, could play a major role in preparing for the new demands on health systems and services. A critical role is to develop a strong evidence base concerning the distribution of health problems, the way in which they present in community practice, and how they are modified by various types of interventions. Disease-oriented specialists cannot be the experts in how health problems are manifested in the community; the patients they see are not representative of the universe of patients with similar manifestations of problems.[12] Because of their training and experiences, they overestimate the likelihood of serious illness and therefore intervene excessively and unnecessarily in people who do not need their services. In their quest to find a specific disease and course of management, they are unable to deal with multimorbidity and the dangers of drug interactions for various syndromes and diseases.[13]

World family medicine must assume responsibility for changing outmoded hospital-based training.[14] The new imperative is to keep people away from hospitals by early, ongoing problem recognition and management in the community. Most diagnostic challenges, except for rare manifestations, are in the community, which is the most appropriate site for the training of health practitioners to provide ongoing care over time.

Another imperative for world family medicine is to come to grips with defining an appropriate scope for primary care practice. Countries, and areas within countries, vary widely in what problems are considered primary care problems.[15,16] Countries with a broader range of services within primary care achieve it by training family physicians with a broader range of skills. In countries such as the United States (where primary care general internist and general pediatrician primary care physicians are trained relatively narrowly in a disease-focused model), achieving greater comprehensiveness will require either an expansion of training experiences or the incorporation of other types of professionals into primary care teams. The new focus on "general practitioners with specialty interests" further threatens to reduce the breadth of primary care practice through its focus on specific types of problems with a loss of competence in dealing with the challenges of primary care problems.[17] Greater comprehensiveness (ie, breadth) of primary care practice, including services such as minor surgery, is associated with higher quality of primary care in general and better outcomes of care with lower costs.[10] It also reduces the likelihood of excessively costly, unnecessary, and potentially dangerous specialist referrals.[10,13] A wider range of focus allows health practitioners to better integrate all aspects of patient care rather than concentrating primarily on specific diagnoses and types of diagnoses. Although the range of services that are appropriately provided will depend on the needs of the population served, the frequency of particular types of diagnoses should determine which problems are in the province of primary care and which need referral to specialists for advice, guidance, and limited long-term management. Even though the range of services to be covered in primary care varies from area to area (as does the availability of primary care practitioners), principles for making decisions about the appropriate range of services in primary care need development by family physicians throughout the world.

Global health provides a special challenge for primary care and general practice, which will become increasingly important in the future as the prevalence of multimorbidity increases with increasing likelihood of survival from acute manifestations of illness, as populations age, and as costs of care increase with increasing availability of technologic interventions. World organizations need to become stronger advocates for primary care if the crisis in health system capacity is to be avoided.

References

1. Ming HT. Doctors in the east: when west meets east. Malaysia: Pelanduk Publications; 2001.
2. Gostin LO. Why rich countries should care about the world's least healthy people. JAMA 2007;298(1): 89–92.
3. Woodward D, Drager N, Beaglehole R, Lipson D. Globalization and health: a framework for analysis and action. Bull World Health Organ 2001;79(9): 875–81.

4. Institute of Medicine Board on International Health. America's vital interest in global health: protecting our people, enhancing our economy, and advancing our international interests. Washington, DC: National Academy Press; 1997.

5. Chen L, Evans T, Anand S, et al. Human resources for health: overcoming the crisis. Lancet 2004;364(9449):1984–90.

6. Karolinska Institute. Global health chart, 2004 [cited 2007 July 9]. Available from: www.whc.ki.se/index.php.

7. Economist Intelligence Unit. Healthcare international. 4th quarter 1999. London (UK): Economist Intelligence Unit; 1999.

8. Samarasekera U. Margaret Chan's vision for WHO. Lancet 2007;369(9577):1915–6.

9. American Academy of Family Physicians. Joint principles of the patient-centered medical home, March 2007 [cited 2 Aug 2007]. Available from: http:www.medicalhomeinfo.org/Joint%20Statement.pdf.

10. Starfield B, Shi L, Macinko J. Contribution of primary care to health systems and health. Milbank Q 2005;83(3):457–502.

11. Gilson L, Doherty J, Loewenson R, Francis V. Challenging inequity through health systems. Final report, Knowledge Network on Health Systems, June 2007. WHO Commission on the Social Determi-nants of Health. Johanesburg, South Africa: Centre for Health Policy, University of Witwatersrand; 2007.

12. Sox HC. Decision-making: a comparison of referral practice and primary care. J Fam Pract 1996;42(2):155–60.

13. Starfield B, Shi L, Grover A, Macinko J. The effects of specialist supply on populations' health: assessing the evidence. Health Aff 2005; W5:97–107. Available from: http://content.healthaffairs.org/cgi/reprint/hlthaff.w5.97v1.

14. Gibbon W. Medical schools for the health-care needs of the 21st century. Lancet 2007;369(9580):2211–3.

15. Bindman AB, Forrest CB, Britt H, Crampton P, Majeed A. Diagnostic scope of and exposure to primary care physicians in Australia, New Zealand, and the United States: cross sectional analysis of results from three national surveys. BMJ 2007;334(7606):1261–6.

16. Starfield B, Shi L. Policy relevant determinants of health: an international perspective. Health Policy 2002;60(3):201–18.

17. Starfield B, Gervas J. Comprehensiveness v special interests: Family medicine should encourage its clinicians to subspecialize: Negative. In: Kennealy T, Buetow S, editors. Ideological debates in family medicine. New York (NY): Nova Publishing; 2007.

CHAPTER 22

Dignity and the essence of medicine

Garth Manning

NOMINATED CLASSIC PAPER

Harvey Chochinov. Dignity and the essence of medicine: the A, B, C and D of dignity conserving care. *British Medical Journal*, 2007; 335(7612): 184–87.

In this paper, author Harvey Chochinov expressed concern that kindness, humanity and respect, what he called the core values of medical professionalism, were too often being overlooked in the time-pressured culture of modern healthcare. This article is more relevant than ever, prompting us to pause and reflect on how we manage our patients to preserve their dignity and to treat them as whole persons, rather than just disease entities.

Although written from a palliative care perspective, this philosophy has huge resonance within family medicine, where much of end-of-life care is managed. It emphasises the importance of putting ourselves in each patient's position. How would we be feeling in this patient's situation? How would we want to treated? How is our attitude towards our patient affecting him or her?

The *A, B, C and D of dignity conserving care* can make a huge difference to the patient and their experience. A is for Attitude, B for Behaviour, C for Compassion, and D for Dialogue. These provide a framework for clinicians to better incorporate humanity and kindness in the culture of patient care.

This paper had a huge effect on me, as it encapsulated so much of what I felt and believed in terms of whole-person, holistic care, which I regard as the essentials of family medicine. Like Atul Gawande in more recent times, Harvey Chochinov concisely but effectively made a compelling argument in favour of person-centred and integrated care, before those terms became current. This makes fascinating reading for any medical student or young doctor at the start of their career. I certainly regret not receiving such profound advice at the start of my own career.

ABOUT THE AUTHOR OF THIS PAPER

Harvey Chochinov is a Distinguished Professor of Psychiatry at the University of Manitoba in Canada, and Director of the Manitoba Palliative Care Research Unit. His seminal publications addressing psychosocial dimensions of palliation have helped define core competencies and standards of end-of-life care. He holds the only Canada Research Chair in Palliative Care, and is a member of the Governing Council of the Canadian Institutes of Health Research where he also chairs the Standing Committee on Ethics.

Harvey's work has explored various psychiatric dimensions of palliative medicine, such as depression, desire for death, will to live, and dignity at the end of life. He is the recipient of many prestigious awards and has presented at numerous international gatherings and is an active author and journal editor.

ABOUT THE NOMINATOR OF THIS PAPER

Dr Garth Manning qualified from Queens University Belfast in Northern Ireland in 1979 and undertook vocational training to become a specialist in general practice/family medicine. He has been working as an international consultant in primary health care development since 1994, working for several global organisations in many countries. In 1998 he was appointed as the first medical director of the International Development Programmes of the Royal College of General Practitioners in the United Kingdom. He has been chief executive officer of the World Organization of Family Doctors (WONCA) since 2012, based in Bangkok in Thailand.

> 'Look beyond the disease. Picture who the patient is, or has been, and consider how their disease process affects them, their families and the image of themselves. We can't prevent death, but we can make it as dignified as possible.'

> *Dr Garth Manning, Thailand*

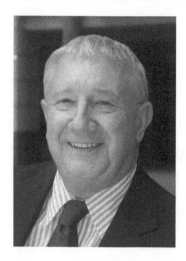

Attribution:

We attribute the original publication of *Dignity and the essence of medicine: the A, B, C and D of dignity conserving care* to *British Medical Journal*. With thanks to Editor in Chief, Fiona Godlee, and Laura Lacey.

Dignity and the essence of medicine: the A, B, C, and D of dignity conserving care

Kindness, humanity, and respect—the core values of medical professionalism—are too often being overlooked in the time pressured culture of modern health care, says **Harvey Chochinov**, and the A, B, C, and D of dignity conserving care can reinstate them

The late Anatole Broyard, essayist and former editor of the *New York Times Book Review*, wrote eloquently about the psychological and spiritual challenges of facing metastatic prostate cancer. "To the typical physician," he wrote, "my illness is a routine incident in his rounds while for me it's the crisis of my life. I would feel better if I had a doctor who at least perceived this incongruity… I just wish he would… give me his whole mind just once, be bonded with me for a brief space, survey my soul as well as my flesh, to get at my illness, for each man is ill in his own way."[1]

Broyard's words underscore the costs and hazards of becoming a patient. The word "patient" comes from the Latin *patiens*, meaning to endure, bear, or suffer, and refers to an acquired vulnerability and dependency imposed by changing health circumstances. Relinquishing autonomy is no small matter and can exact considerable costs.[2] These costs are sometimes relatively minor—for example, accepting clinic schedules or hospital routines. At other times, the costs seem incompatible with life itself. When patients experience a radical unsettling of their conventional sense of self[3] and a disintegration of personhood,[4] suffering knows few bounds. To feel sick is one thing, but to feel that who we are is being threatened or undermined—that we are no longer the person we once were—can cause despair affecting body, mind, and soul. How do healthcare providers influence the experience of patienthood, and what happens when this frame of reference dominates how they view people seeking their care?

Dignity and patienthood

Answering these questions begins with an examination of the relationship between patienthood and notions of dignity. Although the literature on dignity is sparse, it shows that "how patients perceive themselves to be seen" is a powerful mediator of their dignity.[5][6] In a study of patients with end stage cancer, perceptions of dignity were most strongly associated with "feeling a burden to others" and "sense of being treated with respect."[7] As such, the more that healthcare providers are able to affirm the patient's value—that is, seeing the person they are or were, rather than just the illness they have—the more likely that the patient's sense of dignity will be upheld. This finding, and the intimate connection between care provider's affirmation and

EDITORIAL, p 167

Harvey Max Chochinov
professor, department of
psychiatry, University of Manitoba,
CancerCare Manitoba, Winnipeg,
MB, Canada R3E 0V9
harvey.chochinov@cancercare.
mb.ca

Accepted: 15 May 2007

patient's self perception, underscores the basis of dignity conserving care.[8]

Yet, many healthcare providers are reticent to claim this particular aspect of care, which is variously referred to as spiritual care, whole person care, psychosocial care, or dignity conserving care.[9-12] This reluctance is often framed in terms of lack of expertise or concern about how much time this might consume. Yet, when personhood is not affirmed, patients are more likely to feel they are not being treated with dignity and respect.[13] Not being treated with dignity and respect can undermine a sense of value or worth.[5] Patients who feel that life no longer has worth, meaning, or purpose are more likely to feel they have become a burden to others, and patients

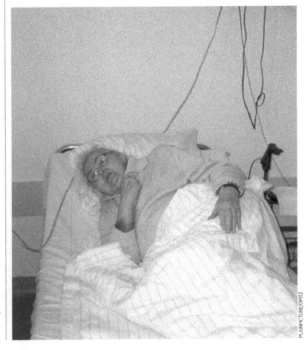

Box 1 | Attitudes

Questions to be asked

- How would I be feeling in this patient's situation?
- What is leading me to draw those conclusions?
- Have I checked whether my assumptions are accurate?
- Am I aware how my attitude towards the patient may be affecting him or her?
- Could my attitude towards the patient be based on something to do with my own experiences, anxieties, or fears?
- Does my attitude towards being a healthcare provider enable or disenable me to establish open and empathic professional relationships with my patients?

Actions to be taken

- Make a conscious effort to make these questions a part of your reflection on the care of each and every patient
- Discuss the issue of healthcare providers' attitudes and assumptions, and how they influence caring for patients, as a regular part of case reviews and clinical teaching
- Include ongoing professional development activities that have you challenge and question your attitudes and assumptions as they might affect patient care
- Create a culture among your colleagues and within your healthcare setting in which acknowledgement and discussion of these issues becomes a standard part of providing care

who feel they are little more than a burden may start to question the point of their continued existence.[14-16] Redressing the "incongruity" that Broyard raises—that is, the separation of humanity and compassion from healthcare delivery—requires that "treatment of disease takes its proper place in the larger problem of the care of the patient."[16]

The A, B, C, and D of dignity conserving care

The notion of dignity conserving care, while emerging primarily from palliative care, applies across the broad spectrum of medicine. Whether patients are young or old, and whatever their health problems, the core values of kindness, respect, and dignity are indispensable. Just as the simple "A, B, C" mnemonic (airway, breathing, and circulation) effectively summarises the fundamentals of critical care, an easily remembered core framework of dignity conserving care—the A, B, C, and D of dignity conserving care—may remind practitioners about the importance of caring for, as well as caring about, their patients.[16]

Attitude

"A"—attitude—underscores the need for healthcare providers first and foremost to examine their attitudes and assumptions towards patients. Attitude can be defined as an enduring, learnt predisposition to behave in a consistent way towards a given class of objects (or people), or a persistent mental or neural state of readiness to react to a certain class of objects (or people), not as they are but as they are conceived to be. The perceptions on which attitudes are based may or may not reflect the patient's reality. For instance, might an assumption of poor quality of life in a patient with longstanding disabilities lead to the withholding of life sustaining choices?[17] Might ageist assumptions mean that conversations about intimacy are rarely initiated?[18] Is a health worker more likely to assume intoxication in a confused, homeless patient, before considering whether they

have a metabolic disorder? Do people with chronic mental illness provoke assumptions about malingering or somatoform disorders, even before an appropriate medical examination has been done?

Examining attitudes and assumptions is a deeply personal task, requiring approaches suited to the individual (box 1). At a minimum, healthcare providers must ask some basic questions, meant to help them understand how attitudes and assumptions can influence the way they deal with patients. They are reminded that "what they believe about patients and their potential may affect them profoundly. The attitude of an expert is contagious and can become limiting."[19] As a case in point, inordinately high suicide rates were reported among Scandinavian patients with advanced cancer, who were offered no further treatment or contact with the healthcare system.[20] While the rationale for this may have been based on considerations of resource allocation or medical futility, the psychological and spiritual fallout is clear: people who are treated like they no longer matter will act and feel like they no longer matter. In other words, patients look at healthcare providers as they would a mirror, seeking a positive image of themselves and their continued sense of worth. In turn, healthcare providers need to be aware that their attitudes and assumptions will shape those all-important reflections.

Box 2 | Behaviours

Disposition

- Treat contact with patients as you would any potent and important clinical intervention
- Professional behaviours towards patients must always include respect and kindness
- Lack of curative options should never rationalise or justify a lack of ongoing patient contact

Clinical examination

- Always ask the patient's permission to perform a physical examination
- Always ask the patient's permission to include students or trainees in the clinical examination
- Although an examination may be part of routine care, it is rarely routine for the patient, so always, as far as possible, take time to set the patient at ease and show that you have some appreciation for what they are about to go through (for example, "I know this might feel a bit uncomfortable"; "I'm sorry that we have to do this to you"; "I know this is an inconvenience"; "This should only hurt for a moment"; "Let me know if you feel we need to stop for any reason"; "This part of the examination is necessary because . . .")
- Limit conversations with patients during an examination (aside from providing them with instruction or encouragement) until they have dressed or been covered appropriately

Facilitating communication

- Act in a manner that shows the patient that he or she has your full and complete attention
- Always invite the patient to have someone from his or her support network present, particularly when you plan to discuss or disclose complex or "difficult" information
- Personal issues should be raised in a setting that attempts to respect the patient's need for privacy
- When speaking with the patient, try to be seated at a comfortable distance for conversation, at the patient's eye level when possible
- Given that illness and changing health status can be overwhelming, offer patients and families repeated explanations as requested
- Present information to the patient using language that he or she will understand; never speak about the patient's condition within their hearing distance in terms that they will not be able to understand
- Always ask if the patient has any further questions and assure them that there will be other opportunities to pose questions as they arise

ANALYSIS

Box 3 | Compassion

Getting in touch with one's own feelings requires the consideration of human life and experience
- Reading stories and novels and observing films, theatre, art that portray the pathos of the human condition
- Discussions of narratives, paintings, and influential, effective role models
- Considering the personal stories that accompany illness
- Experiencing some degree of identification with those who are ill or suffering

Ways to show compassion
- An understanding look
- A gentle touch on the shoulder, arm, or hand
- Some form of communication, spoken or unspoken, that acknowledges the person beyond their illness.

Behaviour

A change, or at the very least an awareness, of one's attitudes can set the stage for modified behaviour—the "B" of dignity conserving care. Once healthcare providers are aware that they play an important role in mediating patients' dignity, several behaviours should logically follow (box 2). Healthcare providers' behaviour towards patients must always be predicated on kindness and respect. Small acts of kindness can personalise care and often take little time to perform.[21] Getting the patient a glass of water, helping them with their slippers, getting them their glasses or hearing aid, adjusting a pillow or their bed sheets, acknowledging a photograph, greetings card, or flowers—these behaviours convey a powerful message, indicating that the person is worthy of such attention. Such behaviour is particularly important when caring for patients with advanced disease "both because of the physical threats of dying and because of the challenge to our sense of self worth and self coherence."[22]

Box 4 | Dialogue

Acknowledging personhood
- "This must be frightening for you."
- "I can only imagine what you must be going through."
- "It's natural to feel pretty overwhelmed at times like these."

Knowing the patient
- "What should I know about you as a person to help me take the best care of you that I can?"
- "What are the things at this time in your life that are most important to you or that concern you most?"
- "Who else (or what else) will be affected by what's happening with your health?"
- "Who should be here to help support you?" (friends, family, spiritual or religious support network, etc)
- "Who else should we get involved at this point, to help support you through this difficult time?" (psychosocial services; group support; chaplaincy; complementary care specialists, etc)

Psychotherapeutic approaches
- Dignity therapy
- Meaning centred therapy
- Life review/reminiscence

One of the essential qualities of the clinician is interest in humanity, for the secret of the care of the patient is in caring for the patient

Certain communication behaviours, as outlined in box 2, enhance the trust and connection between patients and their healthcare providers. Certain intimacies of care require special mention—taking the time to ask patients their permission to perform an examination will make them feel less like a specimen to be poked and prodded and more like a person whose privacy is theirs to relinquish under mutually agreed conditions. This quality of professionalism and connectedness also increases the likelihood that patients will be forthright in disclosing personal information, which so often has a bearing on their ongoing care.

Compassion

Attitude and behaviour can be examined within the realm of the intellectual, but compassion, the "C" of dignity conserving care, requires a discourse about the healthcare provider's feelings. Compassion refers to a deep awareness of the suffering of another coupled with the wish to relieve it. Compassion speaks to feelings that are evoked by contact with the patient and how those feelings shape our approach to care. Like empathy (identification with and understanding of another's situation, feelings, and motives),[23] compassion is something that is felt, beyond simply intellectual appreciation. Healthcare providers arrive at compassion through various channels (see box 3). For some, compassion may be part of a natural disposition that intuitively informs patient care. For others, compassion slowly emerges with life experience, clinical practice, and the realisation that, like patients, each of us is vulnerable in the face of ageing and life's many uncertainties. Compassion may develop over time, and it may also be cultivated by exposure to the medical humanities (http://medhum.med.nyu.edu/), including the interdisciplinary field of humanities (literature, philosophy, ethics, history, and religion), social sciences (anthropology, cultural studies, psychology, sociology), and the arts (literature, theatre, film, and visual arts). Each of these will not speak to every healthcare provider, but they can offer insight into the human condition and the pathos and ambiguity that accompany illness.

Although the process of arriving at compassion can be difficult or complex, showing compassion often flows naturally and can be as quick and as easy as a gentle look or a reassuring touch. In fact, compassion can be conveyed by any form of communication—spoken or unspoken—that shows some recognition of the human stories that accompany illness. As Broyard stated in his wonderful way, "I'd like my doctor to scan me, to grope for my spirit as well as my prostate. Without some such recognition, I am nothing but my illness."[1]

Dialogue

Dialogue, the "D" of dignity conserving care, may be the most—and the least—important component of this framework. Through a genuine examination of attitudes that shape patient care, a change in behaviour that draws from these insights, and the awakening of compassion, many fundamental aims of dignity conserving care will already have been achieved. The practice of medicine requires the exchange of extensive information, within a partnership whose tempo is set by gathering, interpreting, and planning according to new and emerging details. As such, dialogue is a critical element of dignity conserving care. At its most basic, such dialogue must acknowledge personhood beyond the illness itself and recognise the emotional impact that accompanies illness (box 4).

Several psychotherapeutic approaches (dignity therapy,[24] meaning centred therapy,[25] life review or reminiscence[26]) engage patients in more extensive, formatted dialogue, with the intent of bolstering their sense of meaning, purpose, and dignity (see further reading in box).[27] Dialogue should routinely be used to acquaint the healthcare provider with aspects of the patient's life that must be known to provide the best care possible. Treating a patient's severe arthritis and not knowing their core identity as a musician; providing care to a woman with metastatic breast cancer and not knowing she is the sole carer for two young children; attempting to support a dying patient and not knowing he or she is devoutly religious—each of these scenarios is equivalent to attempting to operate in the dark. Obtaining this essential context should be a standard and indispensable element of dignity conserving care. It will also foster a sense of trust, honesty, and openness, wherein personal information and medical facts are woven into a continuous and rich dialogue informing care.

Conclusions

In his 1927 landmark paper "The care of the patient" Francis Peabody wrote: "One of the essential qualities of the clinician is interest in humanity, for the secret of the care of the patient is in caring for the patient."[16] The A, B, C, and D of dignity conserving care may provide clinicians with a framework to operationalise Peabody's sage insight and relocate humanity and kindness to their proper place in the culture of patient care. Easy to remember and empirically based, this framework may be readily applied to teaching, clinical practice, and standards at undergraduate and postgraduate levels and across all medical subspecialties, multidisciplinary teams, and allied health professions. For anyone privileged to look after patients, at whatever stage of the human life cycle, the duty to uphold, protect, and restore the dignity of those who seek our care embraces the very essence of medicine.

Funding: HMC is supported by funding from the Canadian Institutes of Health Research and the Canada Research Chairs programme; his work is also supported by CancerCare Manitoba Foundation.

Competing interests: None declared.

1 Broyard A. *Intoxicated by my illness: and other writings on life and death.* New York: Ballantine, 1992.
2 Murata H. Spiritual pain and its care in patients with terminal cancer: construction of a conceptual framework by philosophical approach. *Palliat Support Care* 2003;1:15-21.
3 Burt R. *Death is that man taking names: intersections of American

---

SUMMARY POINTS

Healthcare providers have a profound influence on how patients experience illness and on their sense of dignity

Dignity conserving care has an important effect on the experience of patienthood

The A, B, C, and D of dignity conserving care—attitude, behaviour, compassion, and dialogue—provide a framework to guide healthcare practitioners towards maintaining patients' dignity

This framework can be applied to teaching, clinical practice, and standards at undergraduate and postgraduate levels and across all medical subspecialties, multidisciplinary teams, and allied health professions

---

medicine, law, and culture. Berkeley: University of California Press, 2002.
4   Cassel EJ. The nature of suffering and the goals of medicine. *N Engl J Med* 1982;306:639-45.
5   Chochinov HM, Hack T, Hassard T, Kristjanson LJ, McClement S, Harlos M. Dignity in the terminally ill: a cross-sectional, cohort study. *Lancet* 2002;360:2026-30.
6   Chochinov HM. Dignity and the eye of the beholder. *J Clin Oncol* 2004;22:1336-40.
7   Chochinov HM, Krisjanson LJ, Hack TF, Hassard T, McClement S, Harlos M. Dignity in the terminally ill: revisited. *J Palliat Med* 2006;9:666-72.
8   Chochinov HM. Dignity-conserving care—a new model for palliative care: helping the patient feel valued. *JAMA* 2002;287:2253-60.
9   Mount B. Whole person care: beyond psychosocial and physical needs. *Am J Hosp Palliat Care* 1993;10:28-37.
10 Safran DJ. Defining the future of primary care: what can we learn from patients? *Ann Intern Med* 2003;138:248-55.
11 Murillo M, Holland JC. Clinical practice guidelines for the management of psychosocial distress at the end of life. *Palliat Support Care* 2004;2:65-77.
12 Chochinov HM, Hack T, Hassard T, Kristjanson LJ, McClement S, Harlos M. Dignity therapy: a novel psychotherapeutic intervention for patients near the end of life. *J Clin Oncol* 2005;23:5520-5.
13 Wilson KG, Curran D, McPherson CJ. A burden to others: a common source of distress for the terminally ill. *Cogn Behav Ther* 2005;34:115-23.
14 Chochinov HM. Burden to others in the terminally ill. *J Pain Symptom Manage* (in press).
15 McPherson CJ, Wilson KG, Murray MA. Feeling like a burden: exploring the perspectives of patients at the end of life. *Soc Sci Med* 2007;64:417-27.
16 Peabody FW. The care of the patient. *JAMA* 1927;88:876-82.
17 Stienstra D, Chochinov HM. Vulnerability, disability, and palliative end-of-life care. *J Palliat Care* 2006;22:166-74.
18 Lovell M. Caring for the elderly: changing perceptions and attitudes. *J Vasc Nurs* 2006;24:22-6.
19 Remen RN. The power of words: how the labels we give patients can limit their lives. *West J Med* 2001;175:353-4.
20 Louhivuori KA, Hakama J. Risk of suicide among cancer patients. *Am J Epidemiol* 1982;109:59-65.
21 Bollinger JL. Five dynamics in patienthood. *Bull Am Protestant Hosp Assoc* 1978;42:90-4.
22 Callahan D. Pursuing a peaceful death. *Hastings Center Report* 1993;23:33-8.
23 Spiro H. What is empathy and can it be taught? *Ann Int Med* 1992;116:843-6.
24 Chochinov HM, Hack T, Hassard T, Kristjanson LJ, McClement S, Harlos M. Dignity therapy: a novel psychotherapeutic intervention for patients near the end of life. *J Clin Oncol* 2005;23(24):5520-5.
25 Breitbart W. Spirituality and meaning in supportive care: spirituality-and meaning-centered group psychotherapy interventions in advanced cancer. *Support Care Cancer* 2002;10:272-80.
26 Bulter RN. The life review: an interpretation of reminiscence in the aged. *Psychiatry* 1963;26:65-76.
27 Chochinov HM, Cann B. Interventions to enhance the spiritual aspects of dying. *J Palliat Med* 2005;8:S103-15.

FURTHER READING

Block SD. Perspectives on care at the close of life. Psychological considerations, growth, and transcendence at the end of life: the art of the possible. *JAMA* 2001;285:2898-905.

Breitbart W, Gibson C, Poppito SR, Berg A. Psychotherapeutic interventions at the end of life: a focus on meaning and spirituality. *Can J Psychiatry* 2004;49:366-72.

Bauby J. *The diving bell and the butterfly: a memoir of life in death.* New York: Knopf, 1997.

Charon R. Narrative medicine: a model for empathy, reflection, profession, and trust. *JAMA* 2007;286:1897-1902.

Chochinov HM. Dying, dignity, and new horizons in palliative end-of-life care. *CA Cancer J Clin* 2006;56:84-103.

Lo B, Ruston D, Kates LW, Arnold RM, Cohen CB, Faber-Langendoen K, et al. Discussing religious and spiritual issues at the end of life: a practical guide for physicians. *JAMA* 2002;287:749-54.

Maguire P, Pitceathly C. Key communication skills and how to acquire them. *BMJ* 2002;325:697-700.

Sulmasy D. Spiritual issues in the care of dying patients: ". . . it's okay between me and God". *JAMA* 2006;296:1385-92.

Tulsky JA. Interventions to enhance communication among patients, providers, and families. *J Palliat Med* 2005;8(suppl 1):S95-102.

CHAPTER 23

Primary care: putting people first

Antoinette Perera

NOMINATED CLASSIC PAPER

Primary care: putting people first. *The World Health Report 2008. Primary Health Care – Now More Than Ever.* World Health Organization, 2008; chapter 3: 41–60.

This paper describes the many faces of family medicine, and how it works best when introduced at the interface between the population and a health system. The features described are the core principles of family medicine, viz. person-centredness, comprehensiveness and integration, and continuity of care, with a regular point of entry into the health system, and emphasises the need for building an enduring doctor–patient relationship. While the document references many papers from around the world describing research based in family medicine and general practice, the World Health Organization (WHO) chose to use the term 'generalist ambulatory care' rather than 'family medicine' or 'general practice'. Language is important and it is notable that the WHO has since started to use the term 'family medicine' to describe our medical discipline.

In the South Asia Region, where often only the 'specialist' doctors need mandatory training to deliver patient care, people often have no regular health provider or access to a referral system. This paper outlines the necessity for reorganisation of healthcare delivery: the necessary switch from specialised to generalist ambulatory care, with a doctor properly trained in family medicine and accountable for the health of a defined population.

The paper also emphasises the importance of a holistic approach and what represents 'good care', looking at each patient as a person. An apt quote is provided from Sir William Osler, 'It is much more important to know what sort of patient has a disease than what sort of disease a patient has'. I often use this same point when teaching my own medical students. It highlights the insufficient recognition of the human dimension in healthcare and a key aspect of what people value about healthcare: the satisfaction of an ill person being listened to and respected irrespective of his or her status.

This paper also provides examples of how a little reorganisation at a cost of few dollars can bring about far-reaching results. In fact I think that this paper is important not only now, but always.

ABOUT THE LEAD AUTHOR OF THIS PAPER

The World Health Organization (WHO) produces regular World Health Reports. This landmark report, published in 2008, was developed under the leadership of WHO Director-General, Dr Margaret Chan Fung Fu-chun OBE.

Born in Hong Kong in 1947, Dr Margaret Chan studied home economics and then medicine at the then University of Western Ontario in Canada, public health at the National University of Singapore, and management development at Harvard Business School. She was Director-General of Health Services in Hong Kong before being appointed as WHO Director-General in 2003. She was awarded Fellowship of the Faculty of Public Health Medicine of the Royal College of Physicians of the United Kingdom, and was honoured by Queen Elizabeth II by being appointed an Officer of the Order of the British Empire. Dr Chan has risen to great heights during her career and was nominated by *Forbes* as the 30th most powerful woman in the world in 2014.

Dr Chan has said she considers 'improvements in the health of the people of Africa and the health of women' to be key performance indicators of the WHO, and that she wants to focus the WHO's attention on 'the people in greatest need'. Dr Chan holds the view that universal health coverage, access to healthcare by everybody, is a 'powerful equaliser' and the most powerful concept of public health.

ABOUT THE NOMINATOR OF THIS PAPER

Antoinette Perera is Emeritus Professor and consultant to the Department of Family Medicine in the Faculty of Medical Sciences at University of Sri Jayewardenepura in Sri Lanka, and the current President of the College of General Practitioners of Sri Lanka. Antoinette says, 'Born in 1947, I am as old as Dr Chan. I loved family medicine from the time I started training and have taught many undergraduate and postgraduate students. I love teaching and research and my family practice. I am happily married, blessed with two sons and four granddaughters.'

'I have found that the family practice has given me the greatest contentment and satisfaction in life. It takes you into the hearts of people whose love cannot ever be bought. To all young doctors, I would like you to see beyond material gains, to the contentment in life which comes from commitment to your patients.'

Professor Antoinette Perera, Sri Lanka

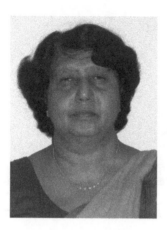

Attribution:

This paper is reprinted from *The World Health Report 2008. Primary Health Care – Now More Than Ever*, Chapter 3 (Primary care: putting people first): pages 41–60, copyright 2008. With thanks to the World Health Organization and Mrs Tatiana Titova of the WHO Press (Permissions) Office.

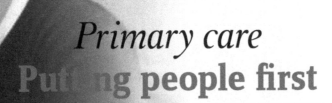

Primary care
Put ng **people first**

◆◆ *This chapter describes how primary care brings promotion and prevention, cure and care together in a safe, effective and socially productive way at the interface between the population and the health system. In short, what needs to be done to achieve this is "to put people first": to give balanced consideration to health and well-being as well as to the values and capacities of the population and the health workers[1]. The chapter starts by describing features of health care that, along with effectiveness and safety, are essential in ensuring improved health and social outcomes.*

Chapter 3

Good care is about people 42

The distinctive features of primary care 43

Organizing primary-care networks 52

Monitoring progress 56

41

The World Health Report **2008**   *Primary Health Care – Now More Than Ever*

These features are person-centredness, comprehensiveness and integration, and continuity of care, with a regular point of entry into the health system, so that it becomes possible to build an enduring relationship of trust between people and their health-care providers. The chapter then defines what this implies for the organization of health-care delivery: the necessary switch from specialized to generalist ambulatory care, with responsibility for a defined population and the ability to coordinate support from hospitals, specialized services and civil society organizations.

Good care is about people

Biomedical science is, and should be, at the heart of modern medicine. Yet, as William Osler, one of its founders, pointed out, "it is much more important to know what sort of patient has a disease than what sort of disease a patient has"[2]. Insufficient recognition of the human dimension in health and of the need to tailor the health service's response to the specificity of each community and individual situation represent major shortcomings in contemporary health care, resulting not only in inequity and poor social outcomes, but also diminishing the health outcome returns on the investment in health services.

Putting people first, the focus of service delivery reforms is not a trivial principle. It can require significant – even if often simple – departures from business as usual. The reorganization of a medical centre in Alaska in the United States, accommodating 45 000 patient contacts per year, illustrates how far-reaching the effects can be. The centre functioned to no great satisfaction of either staff or clients until it decided to establish a direct relationship between each individual and family in the community and a specific staff member[3]. The staff were then in a position to know "their" patients' medical history and understand their personal and family situation. People were in a position to get to know and trust their health-care provider: they no longer had to deal with an institution but with their personal caregiver. Complaints about compartmentalized and fragmented services abated[4]. Emergency room visits were reduced by approximately 50% and referrals to specialty care by 30%; waiting times

shortened significantly. With fewer "rebound" visits for unresolved health problems, the workload actually decreased and staff job satisfaction improved. Most importantly, people felt that they were being listened to and respected – a key aspect of what people value about health care[5,6]. A slow bureaucratic system was thus transformed into one that is customer-responsive, customer-owned and customer-driven[4].

In a very different setting, the health centres of Ouallam, a rural district in Niger, implemented an equally straightforward reorganization of their way of working in order to put people first. Rather than the traditional morning curative care consultation and specialized afternoon clinics (growth monitoring, family planning, etc.), the full range of services was offered at all times, while the nurses were instructed to engage in an active dialogue with their patients. For example, they no longer waited for women to ask for contraceptives, but informed them, at every contact, about the range of services available. Within a few months, the very low uptake of family planning, previously attributed to cultural constraints, was a thing of the past (Figure 3.1)[7].

People's experiences of care provided by the health system are determined first and foremost by the way they are treated when they experience a problem and look for help: by the responsiveness of the health-worker interface between population

Figure 3.1 The effect on uptake of contraception of the reorganization of work schedules of rural health centres in Niger

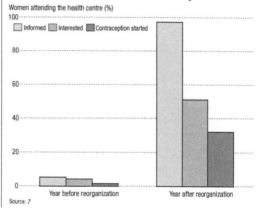

Source: 7

and health services. People value some freedom in choosing a health provider because they want one they can trust and who will attend to them promptly and in an adequate environment, with respect and confidentiality[8].

Health-care delivery can be made more effective by making it more considerate and convenient, as in Ouallam district. However, primary care is about more than shortening waiting times, adapting opening hours or getting staff to be more polite. Health workers have to care for people throughout the course of their lives, as individuals and as members of a family and a community whose health must be protected and enhanced[9], and not merely as body parts with symptoms or disorders that require treating[10].

The service delivery reforms advocated by the PHC movement aim to put people at the centre of health care, so as to make services more effective, efficient and equitable. Health services that do this start from a close and direct relationship between individuals and communities and their caregivers. This, then, provides the basis for person-centredness, continuity, comprehensiveness and integration, which constitute the distinctive features of primary care. Table 3.1 summarizes the differences between primary care and care provided in conventional settings, such as in clinics or hospital outpatient departments, or through the disease control programmes that shape many health services in resource-limited settings. The section that follows reviews these defining features of primary care, and describes how they contribute to better health and social outcomes.

The distinctive features of primary care

Effectiveness and safety are not just technical matters

Health care should be effective and safe. Professionals as well as the general public often over-rate the performance of their health services. The emergence of evidence-based medicine in the 1980s has helped to bring the power and discipline of scientific evidence to health-care decision-making[11], while still taking into consideration patient values and preferences[12]. Over the last decade, several hundred reviews of

Table 3.1 Aspects of care that distinguish conventional health care from people-centred primary care

Conventional ambulatory medical care in clinics or outpatient departments	Disease control programmes	People-centred primary care
Focus on illness and cure	Focus on priority diseases	Focus on health needs
Relationship limited to the moment of consultation	Relationship limited to programme implementation	Enduring personal relationship
Episodic curative care	Programme-defined disease control interventions	Comprehensive, continuous and person-centred care
Responsibility limited to effective and safe advice to the patient at the moment of consultation	Responsibility for disease-control targets among the target population	Responsibility for the health of all in the community along the life cycle; responsibility for tackling determinants of ill-health
Users are consumers of the care they purchase	Population groups are targets of disease-control interventions	People are partners in managing their own health and that of their community

effectiveness have been conducted[13], which have led to better information on the choices available to health practitioners when caring for their patients.

Evidence-based medicine, however, cannot in itself ensure that health care is effective and safe. Growing awareness of the multiple ways in which care may be compromised is contributing to a gradual rise in standards of quality and safety (Box 3.1). Thus far, however, such efforts have concentrated disproportionately on hospital and specialist care, mainly in high- and middle-income countries. The effectiveness and safety of generalist ambulatory care, where most interactions between people and health services take place, has been given much less attention[14]. This is a particularly important issue in the unregulated commercial settings of many developing countries where people often get poor value for money (Box 3.2)[15].

Technical and safety parameters are not the only determinants of the outcomes of health care. The disappointingly low success rate in preventing mother-to-child transmission (MTCT) of HIV in a study in the Côte d'Ivoire (Figure 3.2) illustrates that other features of the organization of health care are equally critical – good drugs are

---

Box 3.1 Towards a science and culture of improvement: evidence to promote patient safety and better outcomes

The outcome of health care results from the balance between the added value of treatment or intervention, and the harm it causes to the patient[16]. Until recently, the extent of such harm has been underestimated. In industrialized countries, approximately 1 in 10 patients suffers harm caused by avoidable adverse events while receiving care[17]: up to 98 000 deaths per year are caused by such events in the United States alone[18]. Multiple factors contribute to this situation[19], ranging from systemic faults to problems of competence, social pressure on patients to undergo risky procedures, to incorrect technology usage[20]. For example, almost 40% of the 16 billion injections administered worldwide each year are given with syringes and needles that are reused without sterilization[14]. Each year, unsafe injections thus cause 1.3 million deaths and almost 26 million years of life lost, mainly because of transmission of hepatitis B and C, and HIV[21].

Especially disquieting is the paucity of information on the extent and determinants of unsafe care in low- and middle-income countries. With unregulated commercialization of care, weaker quality control and health resource limitations, health-care users in low-income countries may well be even more exposed to the risk of unintended patient harm than patients in high-income countries. The World Alliance for Patient Safety[22], among others, advocates making patients safer through systemic interventions and a change in organizational culture rather than through the denunciation of individual health-care practitioners or administrators[23].

Box 3.2 When supplier-induced and consumer-driven demand determine medical advice: ambulatory care in India

"Ms. S is a typical patient who lives in urban Delhi. There are over 70 private-sector medical care providers within a 15-minute walk from her house (and virtually any household in her city). She chooses the private clinic run by Dr. SM and his wife. Above the clinic a prominent sign says "Ms. MM, Gold Medalist, MBBS", suggesting that the clinic is staffed by a highly proficient doctor (an MBBS is the basic degree for a medical doctor as in the British 2 system). As it turns out, Ms. MM is rarely at the clinic. We were told that she sometimes comes at 4 a.m. to avoid the long lines that form if people know she is there. We later discover that she has "franchised" her name to a number of different clinics. Therefore, Ms. S sees Dr. SM and his wife, both of whom were trained in traditional Ayurvedic medicine through a six-month long-distance course. The doctor and his wife sit at a small table surrounded, on one side, by a large number of bottles full of pills, and on the other, a bench with patients on them, which extends into the street. Ms. S sits at the end of this bench. Dr. SM and his wife are the most popular medical care providers in the neighbourhood, with more than 200 patients every day. The doctor spends an average of 3.5 minutes with each patient, asks 3.2 questions, and performs an average of 2.5 examinations. Following the diagnosis, the doctor takes two or three different pills, crushes them using a mortar and pestle, and makes small paper packets from the resulting powder which he gives to Ms. S and asks her to take for two or three days. These medicines usually include one antibiotic and one analgesic and anti-inflammatory drug. Dr. SM tells us that he constantly faces unrealistic patient expectations, both because of the high volume of patients and their demands for treatments that even Dr. SM knows are inappropriate. Dr. SM and his wife seem highly motivated to provide care to their patients and even with a very crowded consultation room they spend more time with their patients than a public sector doctor would. However, they are not bound by their knowledge […] and instead deliver health care like the crushed pills in a paper packet, which will result in more patients willing to pay more for their services"[24].

not enough. How services deal with people is also vitally important. Surveys in Australia, Canada, Germany, New Zealand, the United Kingdom and the United States show that a high number of patients report safety risks, poor care coordination and deficiencies in care for chronic conditions[25]. Communication is often inadequate and lacking in information on treatment schedules. Nearly one in every two patients feels that doctors only rarely or never asked their opinion about treatment. Patients may consult different providers for related or even for the same conditions which, given the lack of coordination among these providers, results in duplication and contradictions[25]. This situation is similar to that reported in other countries, such as Ethiopia[26], Pakistan[27] and Zimbabwe[28].

There has, however, been progress in recent years. In high-income countries, confrontation with chronic disease, mental health problems, multi-morbidity and the social dimension of disease has focused attention on the need for more comprehensive and person-centred approaches and continuity of care. This resulted not only from client pressure, but also from professionals who realized the critical importance of such

Figure 3.2 Lost opportunities for prevention of mother-to-child transmission of HIV (MTCT) in Côte d'Ivoire[29]: only a tiny fraction of the expected transmissions are actually prevented

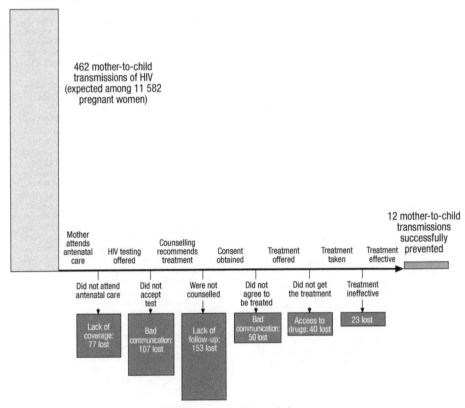

features of care in achieving better outcomes for their patients. Many health professionals have begun to appreciate the limitations of narrow clinical approaches, for example, to cardiovascular disease. As a result there has been a welcome blurring of the traditional boundaries between curative care, preventive medicine and health promotion.

In low-income countries, this evolution is also visible. In recent years, many of the programmes targeting infectious disease priorities have given careful consideration to comprehensiveness, continuity and patient-centredness. Maternal and child health services have often been at the forefront of these attempts, organizing a continuum of care and a comprehensive approach. This process has been consolidated through the joint UNICEF/WHO Integrated Management of Childhood Illness initiatives[30]. Their experience with programmes such as the WHO's Extended Programme for Immunization has put health professionals in many developing countries a step ahead compared to their high-income country colleagues, as they more readily see themselves responsible not just for patients, but also for population coverage. More recently, HIV/AIDS programmes have drawn the attention of providers and policy-makers to the importance of counselling, continuity of care, the complementarity of prevention, treatment and palliation and critically, to the value of empathy and listening to patients.

Understanding people: person-centred care

When people are sick they are a great deal less concerned about managerial considerations of productivity, health targets, cost-effectiveness and rational organization than about their own predicament. Each individual has his or her own way of experiencing and coping with health problems within their specific life circumstances[31]. Health workers have to be able to handle that diversity. For health workers at the interface between the population and the health services, the challenge is much more complicated than for a specialized referral service: managing a well-defined disease is a relatively straightforward technical challenge. Dealing with health problems, however, is complicated as people need to be understood holistically: their physical, emotional and social concerns, their past and their future, and the realities of the world in which they live. Failure to deal with the whole person in their specific familial and community contexts misses out on important aspects of health that do not immediately fit into disease categories. Partner violence against women (Box 3.3), for example, can be detected, prevented or mitigated by health services that are sufficiently close to the communities they serve and by health workers who know the people in their community.

People want to know that their health worker understands them, their suffering and the constraints they face. Unfortunately, many providers neglect this aspect of the therapeutic relation, particularly when they are dealing with disadvantaged groups. In many health services, responsiveness and person-centredness are treated as luxury goods to be handed out only to a selected few.

Over the last 30 years, a considerable body of research evidence has shown that person-centredness is not only important to relieve the patient's anxiety but also to improve the provider's job satisfaction[50]. The response to a health problem is more likely to be effective if the provider understands its various dimensions[51]. For a start, simply asking patients how they feel about their illness, how it affects their lives, rather than focusing only on the disease, results in measurably increased trust and compliance[52] that allows patient and provider to find a common ground on clinical management, and facilitates the integration of prevention and health promotion in the therapeutic response[50,51]. Thus, person-centredness becomes the "clinical method of participatory democracy"[53], measurably improving the quality of care, the success of treatment and the quality of life of those benefiting from such care (Table 3.2).

In practice, clinicians rarely address their patients' concerns, beliefs and understanding of illness, and seldom share problem management options with them[58]. They limit themselves to simple technical prescriptions, ignoring the complex human dimensions that are critical to the appropriateness and effectiveness of the care they provide[59].

Box 3.3 The health-care response to partner violence against women

Intimate partner violence has numerous well-documented consequences for women's health (and for the health of their children), including injuries, chronic pain syndromes, unintended and unwanted pregnancies, pregnancy complications, sexually transmitted infections and a wide range of mental health problems[32,33,34,35,36,37]. Women suffering from violence are frequent health-care users [38,39].

Health workers are, therefore, well placed to identify and provide care to the victims of violence, including referral for psychosocial, legal and other support. Their interventions can reduce the impact of violence on a woman's health and well-being, and that of her children, and can also help prevent further violence.

Research has shown that most women think health-care providers should ask about violence[40]. While they do not expect them to solve their problem, they would like to be listened to and treated in a non-judgemental way and get the support they need to take control over their decisions. Health-care providers often find it difficult to ask women about violence. They lack the time and the training and skills to do it properly, and are reluctant to be involved in judicial proceedings.

The most effective approach for health providers to use when responding to violence is still a matter of debate[41]. They are generally advised to ask all women about intimate partner abuse as a routine part of any health assessment, usually referred to as "screening" or routine enquiry[42]. Several reviews found that this technique increased the rate of identification of women experiencing violence in antenatal and primary-care clinics, but there was little evidence that this was sustained[40], or was effective in terms of health outcomes[43]. Among women who have stayed in shelters, there is evidence that those who received a specific counselling and advocacy service reported a lower rate of re-abuse and an improved quality of life[44]. Similarly, among women experiencing violence during pregnancy, those who received "empowerment counselling" reported improved functioning and less psychological and non-severe physical abuse, and had lower postnatal depression scores[45].

While there is still no consensus on the most effective strategy, there is growing agreement that health services should aim to identify and support women experiencing violence[46], and that health-care providers should be well educated about these issues, as they are essential in building capacity and skills. Health-care providers should, as a minimum, be informed about violence against women, its prevalence and impact on health, when to suspect it and how to best respond. Clearly, there are technical dimensions to this. For example, in the case of sexual assault, providers need to be able to provide the necessary treatment and care, including provision of emergency contraception and prophylaxis for sexually transmitted infections, including HIV where relevant, as well as psychosocial support. There are other dimensions too: health workers need to be able to document any injuries as completely and carefully as possible[47,48,49] and they need to know how to work with communities – in particular with men and boys – on changing attitudes and practices related to gender inequality and violence.

Table 3.2 Person-centredness: evidence of its contribution to quality of care and better outcomes

Improved treatment intensity and quality of life – Ferrer (2005)[54]
Better understanding of the psychological aspects of a patient's problems – Gulbrandsen (1997)[55]
Improved satisfaction with communication – Jaturapatporn (2007)[56]
Improved patient confidence regarding sensitive problems – Kovess-Masféty (2007)[57]
Increased trust and treatment compliance – Fiscella (2004)[52]
Better integration of preventive and promotive care – Mead (1982)[50]

Thus, technical advice on lifestyle, treatment schedule or referral all too often neglects not only the constraints of the environment in which people live, but also their potential for self-help in dealing with a host of health problems ranging from diarrhoeal disease[60] to diabetes management[61]. Yet, neither the nurse in Niger's rural health centre nor the general practitioner in Belgium can, for example, refer a patient to hospital without negotiating[62,63]: along with medical criteria, they have to take into account the patient's values, the family's values, and their lifestyle and life perspective[64].

Few health providers have been trained for person-centred care. Lack of proper preparation is compounded by cross-cultural conflicts, social stratification, discrimination and stigma[63]. As a consequence, the considerable potential of people to contribute to their own health through lifestyle, behaviour and self-care, and by adapting

---

Box 3.4 Empowering users to contribute to their own health

Families can be empowered to make choices that are relevant to their health. Birth and emergency plans[66], for example, are based on a joint examination between the expectant mother and health staff – well before the birth – of her expectations regarding childbirth. Issues discussed include where the birth will take place, and how support for care of the home and any other children will be organized while the woman is giving birth. The discussion can cover planning for expenses, arrangements for transport and medical supplies, as well as identification of a compatible blood donor in case of haemorrhage. Such birth plans are being implemented in countries as diverse as Egypt, Guatemala, Indonesia, the Netherlands and the United Republic of Tanzania. They constitute one example of how people can participate in decisions relating to their health in a way that empowers them[67]. Empowerment strategies can improve health and social outcomes through several pathways; the condition for success is that they are embedded in local contexts and based on a strong and direct relationship between people and their health workers[68]. The strategies can relate to a variety of areas, as shown below:

- developing household capacities to stay healthy, make healthy decisions and respond to emergencies – France's self-help organization of diabetics[69], South Africa's family empowerment and parent training programmes[70], the United Republic of Tanzania's negotiated treatment plans for safe motherhood[71], and Mexico's active ageing programme[72];
- increasing citizens' awareness of their rights, needs and potential problems – Chile's information on entitlements[73] and Thailand's Declaration of Patients' Rights[74];
- strengthening linkages for social support within communities and with the health system – support and advice to family caregivers dealing with dementia in developing country settings[75], Bangladesh's rural credit programmes and their impact on care-seeking behaviour[76], and Lebanon's neighbourhood environment initiatives[77].

---

professional advice optimally to their life circumstances is underutilized. There are numerous, albeit often missed, opportunities to empower people to participate in decisions that affect their own health and that of their families (Box 3.4). They require health-care providers who can relate to people and assist them in making informed choices. The current payment systems and incentives in community health-care delivery often work against establishing this type of dialogue[65]. Conflicts of interest between provider and patient, particularly in unregulated commercial settings, are a major disincentive to person-centred care. Commercial providers may be more courteous and client-friendly than in the average health centre, but this is no substitute for person-centredness.

Comprehensive and integrated responses
The diversity of health needs and challenges that people face does not fit neatly into the discrete diagnostic categories of textbook promotive, preventive, curative or rehabilitative care[78,79]. They call for the mobilization of a comprehensive range of resources that may include health promotion and prevention interventions as well as diagnosis and treatment or referral, chronic or long-term home care, and, in some models, social services[80]. It is at the entry point of the system, where people first present their problem, that the need for a comprehensive and integrated offer of care is most critical.

Comprehensiveness makes managerial and operational sense and adds value (Table 3.3). People take up services more readily if they know a comprehensive spectrum of care is on offer. Moreover, it maximizes opportunities for preventive care and health promotion while reducing unnecessary reliance on specialized or hospital care[81]. Specialization has its comforts, but the fragmentation it induces is often visibly counterproductive and inefficient: it makes no sense to monitor the growth of children and neglect the health of their mothers (and vice versa), or to treat someone's tuberculosis without considering their HIV status or whether they smoke.

Table 3.3 Comprehensiveness: evidence of its contribution to quality of care and better outcomes

Better health outcomes – Forrest (1996)[82], Chande (1996)[83], Starfield (1998)[84]
Increased uptake of disease-focused preventive care (e.g. blood pressure screen, mammograms, pap smears) – Bindman (1996)[85]
Fewer patients admitted for preventable complications of chronic conditions – Shea (1992)[86]

That does not mean that entry-point health workers should solve all the health problems that are presented there, nor that all health programmes always need to be delivered through a single integrated service-delivery point. Nevertheless, the primary-care team has to be able to respond to the bulk of health problems in the community. When it cannot do so, it has to be able to mobilize other resources, by referring or by calling for support from specialists, hospitals, specialized diagnostic and treatment centres, public-health programmes, long-term care services, home-care or social services, or self-help and other community organizations. This cannot mean giving up responsibility: the primary-care team remains responsible for helping people to navigate this complex environment.

Comprehensive and integrated care for the bulk of the assorted health problems in the community is more efficient than relying on separate services for selected problems, partly because it leads to a better knowledge of the population and builds greater trust. One activity reinforces the other. Health services that offer a comprehensive range of services increase the uptake and coverage of, for example, preventive programmes, such as cancer screening or vaccination (Figure 3.3). They prevent complications and improve health outcomes.

Comprehensive services also facilitate early detection and prevention of problems, even in the absence of explicit demand. There are individuals and groups who could benefit from care even if they express no explicit spontaneous demand, as in the case of women attending the health centres in Ouallam district, Niger, or people with undiagnosed high blood pressure or depression. Early detection of disease, preventive care to reduce the incidence of poor health, health promotion to reduce risky behaviour, and addressing social and other determinants of health all require the health service to take the initiative. For many problems, local health workers are the only ones who are in a position to effectively address problems in the community: they are the only ones, for example, in a position to assist parents with care in early childhood development, itself an important determinant of later health, well-being and productivity[87]. Such interventions require proactive health teams offering a comprehensive range of services. They depend on a close and trusting relationship between the health services and the communities they serve, and, thus, on health workers who know the people in their community[88].

Continuity of care

Understanding people and the context in which they live is not only important in order to provide a comprehensive, person-centred response, it also conditions continuity of care. Providers often behave as if their responsibility starts when a patient walks in and ends when they leave the premises. Care should not, however, be limited to the moment a patient consults nor be confined to the four walls of the consultation room. Concern for outcomes mandates a consistent and coherent approach to the management of the patient's problem, until the problem is resolved or the risk that justified follow-up has disappeared. Continuity of care is an important determinant of effectiveness, whether for chronic disease management, reproductive health, mental health or for making sure children grow up healthily (Table 3.4).

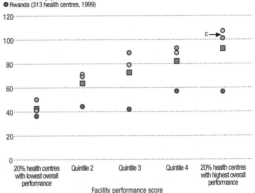

Figure 3.3 More comprehensive health centres have better vaccination coverage[a,b]

DPT3 vaccination coverage (%)
- Democratic Republic of the Congo (380 health centres, 2004)
- Madagascar (534 health centres, 2006)
- Weighted average of coverage in each country quintile
- Rwanda (313 health centres, 1999)

[a] Total 1227 health centres, covering a population of 16 million people.
[b] Vaccination coverage was not included in the assessment of overall health-centre performance across a range of services.
[c] Includes vaccination of children not belonging to target population.

Table 3.4 Continuity of care: evidence of its contribution to quality of care and better outcomes

Lower all-cause mortality – Shi (2003)[90], Franks (1998)[91], Villalbi (1999)[92], PAHO (2005)[93]
Better access to care – Weinick (2000)[94], Forrest (1998)[95]
Less re-hospitalization – Weinberger (1996)[96]
Fewer consultations with specialists – Woodward (2004)[97]
Less use of emergency services – Gill (2000)[98]
Better detection of adverse effects of medical interventions – Rothwell (2005)[99], Kravitz (2004)[100]

Continuity of care depends on ensuring continuity of information as people get older, when they move from one residence to another, or when different professionals interact with one particular individual or household. Access to medical records and discharge summaries, electronic, conventional or client-held, improves the choice of the course of treatment and of coordination of care. In Canada, for example, one in seven people attending an emergency department had medical information missing that was very likely to result in patient harm[101]. Missing information is a common cause of delayed care and uptake of unnecessary services[102]. In the United States, it is associated with 15.6% of all reported errors in ambulatory care[103]. Today's information and communication technologies, albeit underutilized, gives unprecedented possibilities to improve the circulation of medical information at an affordable cost[104], thus enhancing continuity, safety and learning (Box 3.5). Moreover, it is no longer the exclusive privilege of high-resource environments, as the Open Medical Record System demonstrates: electronic health records developed through communities of practice and open-source software are facilitating continuity and quality of care for patients with HIV/AIDS in many low-income countries[105].

Better patient records are necessary but not sufficient. Health services need to make active efforts to minimize the numerous obstacles to continuity of care. Compared to payment by capitation or by fee-for-episode, out-of-pocket fee-for-service payment is a common deterrent, not only to access, but also to continuity of care[107]. In Singapore, for example, patients were formerly not allowed to use their health savings account (Medisave) for outpatient treatment, resulting in patient delays and lack of treatment compliance for the chronically ill. This had become so problematic that regulations were changed. Hospitals are now encouraged to transfer patients with diabetes, high blood pressure, lipid disorder and stroke to registered general practitioners, with Medisave accounts covering ambulatory care[108].

Other barriers to continuity include treatment schedules requiring frequent clinic attendance that carry a heavy cost in time, travel expenses or lost wages. They may be ill-understood and patient motivation may be lacking. Patients may get lost in the complicated institutional environment of referral hospitals or social services. Such problems need to be anticipated and recognized at an early stage. The effort required from health workers is not negligible: negotiating the modalities of the treatment schedule with the patients so as to maximize the chances that it can be completed; keeping registries of clients with chronic conditions; and creating communication channels through home visits, liaison with community workers, telephonic reminders and text messages to re-establish interrupted continuity. These mundane tasks often make the difference between a successful outcome and a treatment failure, but are rarely rewarded. They are much easier to implement when patient and caregiver have clearly identified how and by whom follow-up will be organized.

A regular and trusted provider as entry point

Comprehensiveness, continuity and person-centredness are critical to better health outcomes. They all depend on a stable, long-term, personal relationship (a feature also called "longitudinality"[84]) between the population and the professionals who are their entry point to the health system.

Most ambulatory care in conventional settings is not organized to build such relationships. The busy, anonymous and technical environment of hospital outpatient departments, with their many specialists and sub-specialists, produce mechanical interactions between nameless individuals and an institution – not people-centred care. Smaller clinics are less anonymous, but the care they provide is often more akin to a commercial or administrative transaction that starts and ends with the consultation than to a responsive problem-solving exercise. In this regard, private clinics do not perform differently than public health centres[64]. In the rural areas of low-income countries, governmental health centres are usually designed to work in close relationship with the community they serve. The reality is often different. Earmarking of resources and staff for selected programmes is increasingly leading to fragmentation[109], while the lack of funds, the

pauperization of the health staff and rampant commercialization makes building such relationships difficult[110]. There are many examples to the contrary, but the relationship between providers and their clients, particularly the poorer ones, is often not conducive to building relationships of understanding, empathy and trust[62].

Building enduring relationships requires time. Studies indicate that it takes two to five years before its full potential is achieved[84] but, as the Alaska health centre mentioned at the beginning of this chapter shows, it drastically changes the way care is being provided. Access to the same team of health-care providers over time fosters the development of a relationship of trust between the individual and their health-care provider[97,111,112]. Health professionals are more likely to respect and understand patients they know

---

Box 3.5 Using information and communication technologies to improve access, quality and efficiency in primary care

Information and communication technologies enable people in remote and underserved areas to have access to services and expertise otherwise unavailable to them, especially in countries with uneven distribution or chronic shortages of physicians, nurses and health technicians or where access to facilities and expert advice requires travel over long distances. In such contexts, the goal of improved access to health care has stimulated the adoption of technology for remote diagnosis, monitoring and consultation. Experience in Chile of immediate transmission of electrocardiograms in cases of suspected myocardial infarction is a noteworthy example: examination is carried out in an ambulatory setting and the data are sent to a national centre where specialists confirm the diagnosis via fax or e-mail. This technology-facilitated consultation with experts allows rapid response and appropriate treatment where previously it was unavailable. The Internet is a key factor in its success, as is the telephone connectivity that has been made available to all health facilities in the country.

A further benefit of using information and communication technologies in primary-care services is the improved quality of care. Health-care providers are not only striving to deliver more effective care, they are also striving to deliver safer care. Tools, such as electronic health records, computerized prescribing systems and clinical decision aids, support practitioners in providing safer care in a range of settings. For example, in a village in western Kenya, electronic health records integrated with laboratory, drug procurement and reporting systems have drastically reduced clerical labour and errors, and have improved follow-up care.

As the costs of delivering health care continue to rise, information and communication technologies provide new avenues for personalized, citizen-centred and home-centred care. Towards this end, there has been significant investment in research and development of consumer-friendly applications. In Cape Town, South Africa, an "on cue compliance service" takes the names and mobile telephone numbers of patients with tuberculosis (supplied by a clinic) and enters them into a database. Every half an hour, the on cue server reads the database and sends personalized SMS messages to the patients, reminding them to take their medication. The technology is low-cost and robust. Cure and completion rates are similar to those of patients receiving clinic-based DOTS, but at lower cost to both clinic and patient, and in a way that interferes much less with everyday life than the visits to the clinic[106]. In the same concept of supporting lifestyles linked to primary care, network devices have become a key element of an innovative community programme in the Netherlands, where monitoring and communication devices are built into smart apartments for senior citizens. This system reduces clinic visits and facilitates living independently with chronic diseases that require frequent checks and adjustment of medications.

Many clinicians who want to promote health and prevent illness are placing high hopes on the Internet as the place to go for health advice to complement or replace the need to seek the advice of a health professional. New applications, services and access to information have permanently altered the relationships between consumers and health professionals, putting knowledge directly into people's own hands.

Table 3.5 Regular entry point: evidence of its contribution to quality of care and better outcomes

Increased satisfaction with services – Weiss (1996)[116], Rosenblatt (1998)[117], Freeman (1997)[124], Miller (2000)[125]
Better compliance and lower hospitalization rate – Weiss (1996)[116], Rosenblatt (1998)[117], Freeman (1997)[124], Mainous (1998)[126]
Less use of specialists and emergency services – Starfield (1998)[82], Parchman (1994)[127], Hurley (1989)[128], Martin (1989)[129], Gadomski (1998)[130]
Fewer consultations with specialists – Hurley (1989)[128], Martin (1989)[129]
More efficient use of resources – Forrest (1996)[82], Forrest (1998)[95], Hjortdahl (1991)[131], Roos (1998)[132]
Better understanding of the psychological aspects of a patient's problem – Gulbrandsen (1997)[55]
Better uptake of preventive care by adolescents – Ryan (2001)[133]
Protection against over-treatment – Schoen (2007)[134]

well, which creates more positive interaction and better communication[113]. They can more readily understand and anticipate obstacles to continuity of care, follow up on the progress and assess how the experience of illness or disability is affecting the individual's daily life. More mindful of the circumstances in which people live, they can tailor care to the specific needs of the person and recognize health problems at earlier stages.

This is not merely a question of building trust and patient satisfaction, however important these may be[114,115]. It is worthwhile because it leads to better quality and better outcomes (Table 3.5). People who use the same source of care for most of their health-care needs tend to comply better with advice given, rely less on emergency services, require less hospitalization and are more satisfied with care[98 116,117,118]. Providers save consultation time, reduce the use of laboratory tests and costs[95,119,120], and increase uptake of preventive care[121]. Motivation improves through the social recognition built up by such relationships. Still, even dedicated health professionals will not seize all these opportunities spontaneously[122,123].

The interface between the population and their health services needs to be designed in a way that not only makes this possible, but also the most likely course of action.

Organizing primary-care networks

A health service that provides entry point ambulatory care for health- and health-related problems should, thus, offer a comprehensive range of integrated diagnostic, curative, rehabilitative and palliative services. In contrast to most conventional health-care delivery models, the offer of services should include prevention and promotion as well as efforts to tackle determinants of ill-health locally. A direct and enduring relationship between the provider and the people in the community served is essential to be able to take into account the personal and social context of patients and their families, ensuring continuity of care over time as well as across services.

In order for conventional health services to be transformed into primary care, i.e. to ensure that these distinctive features get due prominence, they must reorganized. A precondition is to ensure that they become directly and permanently accessible, without undue reliance on out-of-pocket payments and with social protection offered by universal coverage schemes. But another set of arrangements is critical for the transformation of conventional care – ambulatory- and institution-based, generalist and specialist – into local networks of primary-care centres[135,136,137,138,139,140]:

■ bringing care closer to people, in settings in close proximity and direct relationship with the community, relocating the entry point to the health system from hospitals and specialists to close-to-client generalist primary-care centres;

■ giving primary-care providers the responsibility for the health of a defined population, in its entirety: the sick and the healthy, those who choose to consult the services and those who choose not to do so;

■ strengthening primary-care providers' role as coordinators of the inputs of other levels of care by giving them administrative authority and purchasing power.

Bringing care closer to the people

A first step is to relocate the entry point to the health system from specialized clinics, hospital outpatient departments and emergency services, to generalist ambulatory care in close-to-client settings. Evidence has been accumulating that this transfer carries measurable benefits in terms of relief from suffering, prevention of illness and death, and improved health equity. These findings hold true in both national and cross-national studies, even if all of the distinguishing features of primary care are not fully realized[31].

Generalist ambulatory care is more likely or as likely to identify common life-threatening conditions as specialist care[141,142]. Generalists adhere to clinical practice guidelines to the same extent as specialists[143], although they are slower to adopt them[144,145]. They prescribe fewer invasive interventions[146,147,148,149], fewer and shorter hospitalizations[127,133,149] and have a greater focus on preventive care[133,150]. This results in lower overall health-care costs[82] for similar health outcomes[146,151,152,153,154,155] and greater patient satisfaction[125,150,156]. Evidence from comparisons between high-income countries shows that higher proportions of generalist professionals working in ambulatory settings are associated with lower overall costs and higher quality rankings[157]. Conversely, countries that increase reliance on specialists have stagnating or declining health outcomes when measured at the population

level, while fragmentation of care exacerbates user dissatisfaction and contributes to a growing divide between health and social services[157,158,159]. Information on low- and middle-income countries is harder to obtain[160], but there are indications that patterns are similar. Some studies estimate that in Latin America and the Caribbean more reliance on generalist care could avoid one out of two hospital admissions[161]. In Thailand, generalist ambulatory care outside a hospital context has been shown to be more patient-centred and responsive as well as cheaper and less inclined to over-medicalization[162] (Figure 3.4).

The relocation of the entry point into the system from specialist hospital to generalist ambulatory care creates the conditions for more comprehensiveness, continuity and person-centredness. This amplifies the benefits of the relocation. It is particularly the case when services are organized as a dense network of small, close-to-client service delivery points. This makes it easier to have teams that are small enough to know their communities and be known by them, and stable enough to establish an enduring relationship. These teams require relational and organizational capacities as much as the technical competencies to solve the bulk of health problems locally.

Responsibility for a well-identified population

In conventional ambulatory care, the provider assumes responsibility for the person attending the consultation for the duration of the consultation and, in the best of circumstances, that responsibility extends to ensuring continuity of care. This passive, response-to-demand approach fails to help a considerable number of people who could benefit from care. There are people who, for various reasons, are, or feel, excluded from access to services and do not take up care even when they are in need. There are people who suffer illness but delay seeking care. Others present risk factors and could benefit from screening or prevention programmes (e.g. for cervical cancer or for childhood obesity), but are left out because they do not consult: preventive services that are limited to service users often leave out those most in need[163]. A passive, response-to-demand

Figure 3.4 Inappropriate investigations prescribed for simulated patients presenting with a minor stomach complaint, Thailand[a,b,162]

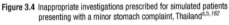

Patients for whom inappropriate investigations were prescribed (%)

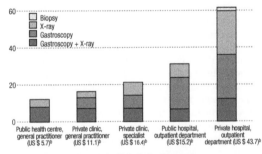

[a] Observation made in 2000, before introduction of Thailand's universal coverage scheme.
[b] Cost to the patient, including doctor's fees, drugs, laboratory and technical investigations.

approach has a second untoward consequence: it lacks the ambition to deal with local determinants of ill-health – whether social, environmental or work-related. All this represents lost opportunities for generating health: providers that only assume responsibility for their customers concentrate on repairing rather than on maintaining and promoting health.

The alternative is to entrust each primary-care team with the explicit responsibility for a well-defined community or population. They can then be held accountable, through administrative measures or contractual arrangements, for providing comprehensive, continuous and person-centred care to that population, and for mobilizing a comprehensive range of support services – from promotive through to palliative. The simplest way of assigning responsibility is to identify the community served on the basis of geographical criteria – the classic approach in rural areas. The simplicity of geographical assignment, however, is deceptive. It follows an administrative, public sector logic that often has problems adapting to the emergence of a multitude of other providers. Furthermore, administrative geography may not coincide with sociological reality, especially in urban areas. People move around and may work in a different area than where they live, making the health unit closest to home actually an inconvenient source of care. More importantly, people value choice and may resent an administrative assignment to a particular health unit. Some countries find geographical criteria of proximity the most appropriate to define who fits in the population of responsibility, others rely on active registration or patient lists. The important point is not how but whether the population is well identified and mechanisms exist to ensure that nobody is left out.

Once such explicit comprehensive responsibilities for the health of a well-identified and defined population are assigned, with the related financial and administrative accountability mechanisms, the rules change.

- The primary-care team has to broaden the portfolio of care it offers, developing activities and programmes that can improve outcomes, but which they might otherwise neglect[164]. This sets the stage for investment in prevention and promotion activities, and for venturing into areas that are often overlooked, such as health in schools and in the workplace. It forces the primary-care team to reach out to and work with organizations and individuals within the community: volunteers and community health workers who act as the liaison with patients or animate grassroots community groups, social workers, self-help groups, etc.

- It forces the team to move out of the four walls of their consultation room and reach out to the people in the community. This can bring significant health benefits. For example, large-scale programmes, based on home-visits and community animation, have been shown to be effective in reducing risk factors for neonatal mortality and actual mortality rates. In the United States, such programmes have reduced neonatal mortality by 60% in some settings[165]. Part of the benefit is due to better uptake of effective care by people who would otherwise remain deprived. In Nepal, for example, the community dynamics of women's groups led to the better uptake of care, with neonatal and maternal mortality lower than in control communities by 29% and 80%, respectively[166].

- It forces the team to take targeted initiatives, in collaboration with other sectors, to reach the excluded and the unreached and tackle broader determinants of ill-health. As Chapter 2 has shown, this is a necessary complement to establishing universal coverage and one where local health services play a vital role. The 2003 heatwave in western Europe, for example, highlighted the importance of reaching out to the isolated elderly and the dramatic consequences of failing to do so: an excess mortality of more than 50 000 people[167].

For people and communities, formal links with an identifiable source of care enhance the likelihood that long-term relationships will develop; that services are encouraged to pay more attention to the defining features of primary care; and that lines of communication are more intelligible. At the same time, coordination linkages can be formalized with other levels of care – specialists, hospitals or other technical services – and with social services.

The primary-care team as a hub of coordination

Primary-care teams cannot ensure comprehensive responsibility for their population without support from specialized services, organizations and institutions that are based outside the community served. In resource-constrained circumstances, these sources of support will typically be concentrated in a "first referral level district hospital". Indeed, the classic image of a health-care system based on PHC is that of a pyramid with the district hospital at the top and a set of (public) health centres that refer to the higher authority.

In conventional settings, ambulatory care professionals have little say in how hospitals and specialized services contribute – or fail to contribute – to the health of their patients, and feel little inclination to reach out to other institutions and stakeholders that are relevant to the health of the local community. This changes if they are entrusted with responsibility for a defined population and are recognized as the regular point of entry for that population. As health-care networks expand, the health-care landscape becomes far more crowded and pluralistic. More resources allow for diversification: the range of specialized services that comes within reach may include emergency services, specialists, diagnostic infrastructure, dialysis centres, cancer screening, environmental technicians, long-term care institutions, pharmacies, etc. This represents new opportunities, provided the primary-care teams can assist their community in making the best use of that potential, which is particularly critical to public health, mental health and long-term care[168].

The coordination (or gatekeeping) role this entails effectively transforms the primary-care pyramid into a network, where the relations between the primary-care team and the other institutions and services are no longer based only on top-down hierarchy and bottom-up referral, but on cooperation and coordination (Figure 3.5). The primary-care team then becomes the mediator between the community and the other levels

Figure 3.5 Primary care as a hub of coordination: networking within the community served and with outside partners[173,174]

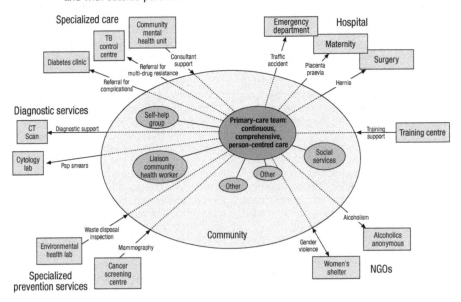

of the health system, helping people navigate the maze of health services and mobilizing the support of other facilities by referring patients or calling on the support of specialized services.

This coordination and mediation role also extends to collaboration with other types of organizations, often nongovernmental. These can provide significant support to local primary care. They can help ensure that people know what they are entitled to and have the information to avoid substandard providers[169,170]. Independent ombudsman structures or consumer organizations can help users handle complaints. Most importantly, there is a wealth of self-help and mutual support associations for diabetics, people living with handicaps and chronic diseases that can help people to help themselves[171]. In the United States alone, more than five million people belong to mutual help groups while, in recent years, civil society organizations dealing with health and health-related issues, from self-help to patient's rights, have been mushrooming in many low- and middle-income countries. These groups do much more than just inform patients. They help people take charge of their own situation, improve their health, cope better with ill-health, increase self-confidence and diminish over-medicalization[172]. Primary-care teams can only be strengthened by reinforcing their linkages with such groups.

Where primary-care teams are in a position to take on this coordinator role, their work becomes more rewarding and attractive, while the overall effects on health are positive. Reliance on specialists and hospitalization is reduced by filtering out unnecessary uptake, whereas patient delay is reduced for those who do need referral care, the duration of their hospitalization is shortened, and post-hospitalization follow-up is improved[83,128,129].

The coordination function provides the institutional framework for mobilizing across sectors to secure the health of local communities. It is not an optional extra but an essential part of the remit of primary-care teams. This has policy implications: coordination will remain wishful thinking unless the primary-care team has some form of either administrative or financial leverage. Coordination also depends on the different institutions'

recognition of the key role of the primary-care teams. Current professional education systems, career structure and remuneration mechanisms most often give signals to the contrary. Reversing these well-entrenched disincentives to primary care requires strong leadership.

Monitoring progress

The switch from conventional to primary care is a complex process that cannot be captured in a single, universal metric. Only in recent years has it been possible to start disentangling the effects of the various features that define primary care. In part, this is because the identification of the features that make the difference between primary care and conventional health-care delivery has taken years of trial and error, and the instruments to measure them have not been generalized. This is because these features are never all put into place as a single package of reforms, but are the result of a gradual shaping and transformation of the health system. Yet, for all this complexity, it is possible to measure progress, as a complement to the follow-up required for measuring progress towards universal coverage.

The first dimension to consider is the extent to which the organizational measures required to switch to primary care are being put into place.

- Is the predominant type of first-contact provider being shifted from specialists and hospitals to generalist primary-care teams in close proximity to where the people live?
- Are primary-care providers being made responsible for the health of all the members of a well-identified population: those who attend health services and those who do not?
- Are primary-care providers being empowered to coordinate the various inputs of specialized, hospital and social services, by strengthening their administrative authority and purchasing power?

The second dimension to consider is the extent to which the distinctive features of primary care are gaining prominence.

- Person-centredness: is there evidence of improvement, as shown by direct observation and user surveys?

- Comprehensiveness: is the portfolio of primary-care services expanding and becoming more comprehensive, reaching the full essential benefits package, from promotion through to palliation, for all age groups?
- Continuity: is information for individuals being recorded over the life-course, and transferred between levels of care in cases of referral and to a primary-care unit elsewhere when people relocate?
- Regular entry point: are measures taken to ensure that providers know their clients and vice versa?

This should provide the guidance to policy-makers as to the progress they are making with the transformation of health-care delivery. However, they do not immediately make it possible to attribute health and social outcomes to specific aspects of the reform efforts. In order to do so, the monitoring of the reform effort needs to be complemented with a much more vigorous research agenda. It is revealing that the Cochrane Review on strategies for integrating primary-health services in low- and middle-income countries could identify only one valid study that took the user's perspective into account[160]. There has been a welcome surge of research on primary care in high-income countries and, more recently, in the middle-income countries that have launched major PHC reforms. Nevertheless, it is remarkable that an industry that currently mobilizes 8.6% of the world's GDP invests so little in research on two of its most effective and cost-effective strategies: primary care and the public policies that underpin and complement it.

References

1. *People at the centre of health care: harmonizing mind and body, people and systems.* New Delhi, World Health Organization Regional Office for South-East Asia, Manila, World Health Organization Regional Office for the Western Pacific, 2007.
2. Osler W. *Aequanimitas.* Philadelphia PA, Blakiston, 1904.
3. Eby D. Primary care at the Alaska Native Medical Centre: a fully deployed "new model" of primary care. *International Journal of Circumpolar Health*, 2007, 66(Suppl. 1):4–13.
4. Eby D. Integrated primary care. *International Journal of Circumpolar Health*, 1998, 57(Suppl. 1):665–667.
5. Gottlieb K, Sylvester I, Eby D. Transforming your practice: what matters most. *Family Practice Management*, 2008, 15:32–38.
6. Kerssens JJ et al. Comparison of patient evaluations of health care quality in relation to WHO measures of achievement in 12 European countries. *Bulletin of the World Health Organization*, 2004 82:106–114.
7. Bossyns P, Miye M, Van Lerberghe W. Supply-level measures to increase uptake of family planning services in Niger: the effectiveness of improving responsiveness. *Tropical Medicine and International Health*, 2002, 7:383–390.
8. *The World Health Report 2000 – Health systems: improving performance.* Geneva, World Health Organization, 2000.
9. Mercer SW, Cawston PG, Bikker AP. Quality in general practice consultations: a qualitative study of the views of patients living in an area of high socio-economic deprivation in Scotland. *BMC Family Practice*, 2007, 8:22.
10. Scherger JE. What patients want. *Journal of Family Practice*, 2001, 50:137.
11. Sackett DL et al. Evidence based medicine: what it is and what it isn't. *British Medical Journal*, 1996, 312:71–72.
12. Guyatt G, Cook D, Haynes B. Evidence based medicine has come a long way: The second decade will be as exciting as the first. *BMJ*, 2004, 329:990–991.
13. Cochrane database of systematic reviews. The Cochrane Library, 2008 (http://www.cochrane.org, accessed 27 July 2008).
14. Iha A, ed. *Summary of the evidence on patient safety: implications for research.* Geneva, World Health Organization, The Research Priority Setting Working Group of the World Alliance for Patient Safety, 2008.
15. Smith GD, Mertens T. What's said and what's done: the reality of sexually transmitted disease consultations. *Public Health*, 2004, 118:96–103.
16. Berwick DM. The science of improvement. *JAMA*, 2008, 299:1182–1184.
17. Donaldson L, Philip P. Patient safety: a global priority. *Bulletin of the World Health Organization*, 2004, 82:892–893
18. Kohn LT, Corrigan JM, Donaldson MS, eds. *To err is human: building a safer health system.* Washington, DC, National Academy Press, Committee on Quality of Health Care in America, Institute of Medicine, 1999.
19. Reason J. Human error: models and management. *BMJ*, 2000, 320:768–770.
20. Kripalani S et al. Deficits in communication and information transfer between hospital-based and primary care physicians: implications for patient safety and continuity of care. *JAMA*, 2007, 297:831–841.
21. Miller MA, Pisani E. The cost of unsafe injections. *Bulletin of the World Health Organization*, 1999, 77:808–811.
22. *The purpose of a world alliance.* Geneva, World Health Organization, World Alliance for Patient Safety, 2008 (http://www.who.int/patientsafety/worldalliance/alliance/en/, accessed 28 July 2008).
23. Shortell SM, Singer SJ. Improving patient safety by taking systems seriously. *JAMA* 2008, 299:445–447.
24. Das J, Hammer JS, Kenneth LL. *The quality of medical advice in low-income countries.* Washington DC, The World Bank, 2008 (World Bank Policy Research Working Paper No. 4501; http://ssrn.com/abstract=1089272, accessed 28 Jul 2008).
25. Schoen C et al. Taking the pulse of health care systems: experiences of patients with health problems in six countries. *Health Affairs*, 2005 (web exclusive W 5-5 0 9 DOI 10.1377/hlthaff.W5.509).
26. Mekbib TA, Teferi B. Caesarean section and foetal outcome at Yekatit 12 hospital, Addis Abba, Ethiopia, 1987-1992. *Ethiopian Medical Journal*, 1994, 32:173–179.
27. Siddiqi S et al. The effectiveness of patient referral in Pakistan. *Health Policy and Planning*, 2001, 16:193–198.
28. Sanders D et al. Zimbabwe's hospital referral system: does it work? *Health Policy and Planning*, 1998, 13:359–370.
29. Data reported at World Aids Day Meeting, Antwerp, Belgium, 2000.
30. *The World Health Report 2005 – Make every mother and child count.* Geneva, World Health Organization, 2005.
31. Starfield B, Shi L, Macinko J. Contributions of primary care to health systems and health. *The Milbank Quarterly*, 2005, 83:457–502.
32. Heise L, Garcia-Moreno C. Intimate partner violence. In: Krug EG et al, eds. *World report on violence and health.* Geneva, World Health Organization, 2002.
33. Ellsberg M et al. Intimate partner violence and women's physical and mental health in the WHO multi-country study on women's health and domestic violence: an observational study. *Lancet*, 2008, 371:1165–1172.

34. Campbell JC. Health consequences of intimate partner violence. *Lancet*, 2002, 359:1331–1336.

35. Edleson JL. Children's witnessing of domestic violence. *Journal of Interpersonal Violence*, 1996, 14: 839–870.

36. Dube SR et al. Exposure to abuse, neglect, and household dysfunction among adults who witnessed intimate partner violence as children: implications for health and social services. *Violence and Victims*, 2002, 17: 3–17.

37. Åsling-Monemi K et al. Violence against women increases the risk of infant and child mortality: a case-referent study in Nicaragua. *Bulletin of the World Health Organization*, 2003, 81:10–18.

38. Bonomi A et al. Intimate partner violence and women's physical, mental and social functioning. *American Journal of Preventive Medicine*, 2006, 30:458-466.

39. National Centre for Injury Prevention and Control. *Costs of intimate partner violence against women in the United States*. Atlanta GA, Centres for Disease Control and Prevention, 2003.

40. Ramsay J et al. Should health professionals screen women for domestic violence? Systematic review. *BMJ*, 2002, 325:314–318.

41. Nelson HD et al. Screening women and elderly adults for family and intimate partner violence: a review of the evidence for the U.S. Preventive Services Task force. *Annals of Internal Medicine*, 2004, 140:387–403.

42. Garcia-Moreno C. Dilemmas and opportunities for an appropriate health-service response to violence against women. *Lancet*, 2002, 359:1509–1514.

43. Wathan NC, MacMillan HL. Interventions for violence against women. Scientific review. *JAMA*, 2003, 289:589–600.

44. Sullivan CM, Bybee DI. Reducing violence using community-based advocacy for women with abusive partners. *Journal of Consulting and Clinical Psychology*, 1999, 67:43–53.

45. Tiwari A et al. A randomized controlled trial of empowerment training for Chinese abused pregnant women in Hong Kong. *British Journal of Obstetrics and Gynaecology*, 2005, 112:1249–1256.

46. Taket A et al. Routinely asking women about domestic violence in health settings. *BMJ*, 2003, 327:673–676.

47. MacDonald R. Time to talk about rape. *BMJ*, 2000, 321:1034–1035.

48. Basile KC, Hertz FM, Back SE. *Intimate partner and sexual violence victimization instruments for use in healthcare settings*. 2008. Atlanta GA, Centers for Disease Control and Prevention, 2008.

49. *Guidelines for the medico-legal care of victims of sexual violence*. Geneva, World Health Organization, 2003.

50. Mead N, Bower P. Patient-centredness: a conceptual framework and review of the empirical literature. *Social Science and Medicine*, 51:1087–1110.

51. Stewart M. Towards a global definition of patient centred care. *BMJ*, 2001, 322:444–445.

52. Fiscella K et al. Patient trust: is it related to patient-centred behavior of primary care physicians? *Medical Care*, 2004, 42:1049–1055.

53. Marincowitz GJO, Fehrsen GS. *Caring, learning, improving quality and doing research: Different faces of the same process*. Paper presented at: 11th South African Family Practice Congress, Sun City, South Africa, August 1998.

54. Ferrer RL, Hambidge SJ, Maly RC. The essential role of generalists in health care systems. *Annals of Internal Medicine*, 2005, 142:691–699.

55. Gulbrandsen P, Hjortdahl P, Fugelli P. General practitioners' knowledge of their patients' psychosocial problems: multipractice questionnaire survey. *British Medical Journal*, 1997, 314:1014–1018.

56. Jaturapatporn D, Dellow A. Does family medicine training in Thailand affect patient satisfaction with primary care doctors? *BMC Family Practice*, 2007, 8:14.

57. Kovess-Masféty V et al. What makes people decide who to turn to when faced with a mental health problem? Results from a French survey. *BMC Public Health*, 2007, 7:188.

58. Bergeson D. A systems approach to patient-centred care. *JAMA*, 2006, 296:23.

59. Kravitz RL et al. Recall of recommendations and adherence to advice among patients with chronic medical conditions. *Archives of Internal Medicine*, 1993, 153:1869–1878.

60. Werner D et al. *Questioning the solution: the politics of primary health care and child survival, with an in-depth critique of oral rehydration therapy*. Palo Alto CA, Health Wrights, 1997.

61. Norris et al. Increasing diabetes self-management education in community settings. A systematic review. *American Journal of Preventive Medicine*, 2002, 22:39–66.

62. Bossyns P, Van Lerberghe W. The weakest link: competence and prestige as constraints to referral by isolated nurses in rural Niger. *Human Resources for Health*, 2004, 2:1.

63. Willems S et al. Socio-economic status of the patient and doctor-patient communication: does it make a difference. *Patient Eucation and Counseling*, 2005, 56:139–146.

64. Pongsupap Y. *Introducing a human dimension to Thai health care: the case for family practice*. Brussels, Vrije Universiteit Brussel Press. 2007.

65. *Renewing primary health care in the Americas. A Position paper of the Pan American Health Organization*. Washington DC, Pan American Health Organization, 2007.

66. Penny Simkin, PT. Birth plans: after 25 years, women still want to be heard. *Birth*, 34:49–51.

67. Portela A, Santarelli C. Empowerment of women, men, families and communities: true partners for improving maternal and newborn health. *British Medical Bulletin*, 2003, 67:59–72.

68. Wallerstein N. *What is the evidence on effectiveness of empowerment to improve health?* Copenhagen, World Health Organization Regional Office for Europe 2006 (Health Evidence Network report; (http://www.euro.who.int/Document/E88086.pdf, accessed 21-11-07).

69. Diabète-France.com – portail du diabète et des diabetiques en France, 2008 (http://www.diabete-france.com, accessed 30 July 2008).

70. Barlow J, Cohen E, Stewart-Brown SSB. Parent training for improving maternal psychosocial health. *Cochrane Database of Systematic Reviews*,2003, (4):CD002020.

71. Ahluwalia I. An evaluation of a community-based approach to safe motherhood in northwestern Tanzania. *International Journal of Gynecology and Obstetrics*, 2003, 82:231.

72. De la Luz Martínez-Maldonado M, Correa-Muñoz E, Mendoza-Núñez VM. Program of active aging in a rural Mexican community: a qualitative approach. *BMC Public Health*, 2007, 7:276 (DOI:10.1186/1471-2458-7-276).

73. Frenz P. *Innovative practices for intersectoral action on health: a case study of four programs for social equity*. Chilean case study prepared for the CSDH. Santiago, Ministry of Health, Division of Health Planning, Social Determinants of Health Initiative, 2007.

74. Paetthayasapaa. Kam Prakard Sitti Pu Paui, 2003? (http://www.tmc.or.th/, accessed 30 July 2008).

75. Prince M, Livingston G, Katona C. Mental health care for the elderly in low-income countries: a health systems approach. *World Psychiatry*, 2007, 6:5–13.

76. Nanda P. Women's participation in rural credit programmes in Bangladesh and their demand for formal health care: is there a positive impact? *Health Economics*, 1999, 8:415–428.

77. Nakkash R et al. The development of a feasible community-specific cardiovascular disease prevention program: triangulation of methods and sources. *Health Education and Behaviour*, 2003, 30:723–739.

78. Stange KC. The paradox of the parts and the whole in understanding and improving general practice. *International Journal for Quality in Health Care*, 2002, 14:267–268.

79. Gill JM. The structure of primary care: framing a big picture. *Family Medicine*, 2004, 36:65–68.

80. *Pan-Canadian Primary Health Care Indicator Development Project. Pan-Canadian primary health care indicators, Report 1, Volume 1*. Ottawa, Canadian Institute for Health Information 2008 (http:\www.cihi.ca).

81. Bindman AB et al. Primary care and receipt of preventive services. *Journal of General Internal Medicine*, 1996, 11:269–276.

82. Forrest CB, Starfield B. The effect of first-contact care with primary care clinicians on ambulatory health care expenditures. *Journal of Family Practice*, 1996, 43:40–48.

83. Chande VT, Kinane JM. Role of the primary care provider in expediting children with acute appendicitis. *Archives of Pediatrics and Adolescent Medicine*, 1996, 150:703–706.

84. Starfield B. *Primary care: balancing health needs, services, and technology*. New York, Oxford University Press 1998.

85. Bindman AB et al. Primary care and receipt of preventive services. *Journal of General Internal Medicine*, 1996, 11:269–276.

86. Shea S et al. Predisposing factors for severe, uncontrolled hypertension in an inner-city minority population. *New England Journal of Medicine*, 1992, 327:776–781.

87. Galobardes B, Lynch JW, Davey Smith G. Is the association between childhood socioeconomic circumstances and cause-specific mortality established? Update of a systematic review. *Journal of Epidemiology and Community Health*, 2008, 62:387–390.

88. *Guide to clinical preventive services, 2007*. Rockville MD, Agency for Healthcare Research and Quality, 2007 (AHRQ Publication No. 07-05100; http://www.ahrq.gov/clinic/pocketgd.htm).

89. Porignon D et al. *Comprehensive is effective: vaccination coverage and health system performance in Sub-Saharan Africa*, 2008 (forthcoming).

90. Shi L et al. The relationship between primary care, income inequality, and mortality in the United States, 1980–1995. *Journal of the American Board of Family Practice*, 2003, 16:412–422.

91. Franks P, Fiscella K. Primary care physicians and specialists as personal physicians. Health care expenditures and mortality experience. *Journal of Family Practice*, 1998, 47:105–109.

92. Villalbi JR et al. An evaluation of the impact of primary care reform on health. *Atenci'on Primaria*, 1999, 24:468–474.

93. *Regional core health data initiative.* Washington DC, Pan American Health Organization, 2005 (http://www.paho.org/English/SHA/coredata/tabulator/newTabulator.htm).

94. Weinick RM, Krauss NA. Racial/ethnic differences in children's access to care. *American Journal of Public Health,* 2000, 90:1771–1774.

95. Forrest CB, Starfield B. Entry into primary care and continuity: the effects of access. *American Journal of Public Health,* 1998, 88:1330–1336.

96. Weinberger M, Oddone EZ, Henderson WG. Does increased access to primary care reduce hospital readmissions? For The Veterans Affairs Cooperative Study Group on Primary Care and Hospital Readmission. *New England Journal of Medicine,* 1996, 334:1441–1447.

97. Woodward CA et al. What is important to continuity in home care? Perspectives of key stakeholders. *Social Science and Medicine,* 2004, 58:177–192.

98. Gill JM, Mainous AGI, Nsereko M. The effect of continuity of care on emergency department use. *Archives of Family Medicine,* 2000, 9:333–338.

99. Rothwell P. Subgroup analysis in randomised controlled trials: importance, indications, and interpretation, *Lancet,* 2005, 365:176–186.

100. Kravitz RL, Duan N, Braslow J. Evidence-based medicine, heterogeneity of treatment effects, and the trouble with averages. *The Milbank Quarterly,* 2004, 82:661–687.

101. Stiell A. et al. Prevalence of information gaps in the emergency department and the effect on patient outcomes. *Canadian Medical Association Journal,* 2003, 169:1023–1028.

102. Smith PC et al. Missing clinical information during primary care visits. *JAMA,* 2005, 293:565–571.

103. Elder NC, Vonder Meulen MB, Cassedy A. The identification of medical errors by family physicians during outpatient visits. *Annals of Family Medicine,* 2004, 2:125–129.

104. Elwyn G. Safety from numbers: identifying drug related morbidity using electronic records in primary care. *Quality and Safety in Health Care,* 2004, 13:170–171.

105. Open Medical Records System (OpenMRS) [online database]. Cape Town, South African Medical Research Council, 2008 (http://openmrs.org/wiki/OpenMRS, accessed 29 July 2008).

106. Hüsler J, Peters T. *Evaluation of the On Cue Compliance Service pilot: testing the use of SMS reminders in the treatment of tuberculosis in Cape Town, South Africa. Prepared for the City of Cape Town Health Directorate and the International Development Research Council (IDRC).* Cape Town, Bridges Organization, 2005.

107. Smith-Rohrberg Maru D et al. Poor follow-up rates at a self-pay northern Indian tertiary AIDS clinic. *International Journal for Equity in Health,* 2007, 6:14.

108. Busse R, Schlette S, eds. *Focus on prevention, health and aging, and health professions.* Gütersloh, Verlag Bertelsmann Stiftung, 2007 (Health policy developments 7/8).

109. James Pfeiffer International. NGOs and primary health care in Mozambique: the need for a new model of collaboration. *Social Science and Medicine,* 2003, 56:725–738.

110. Jaffré Y, Olivier de Sardan J-P. *Une médecine inhospitalière. Les difficiles relations entre soignants et soignés dans cinq capitales d'Afrique de l'Ouest.* Paris, Karthala, 2003.

111. Naithani S, Gulliford M, Morgan M. Patients' perceptions and experiences of "continuity of care" in diabetes. *Health Expectations,* 2006, 9:118–129.

112. Schoenbaum SC. The medical home: a practical way to improve care and cut costs. *Medscape Journal of Medicine ,* 2007, 9:28.

113. Beach MC. Are physicians' attitudes of respect accurately perceived by patients and associated with more positive communication behaviors? *Patient Education and Counselling,* 2006, 62:347–354 (Epub 2006 Jul 21).

114. Farmer JE et al. Comprehensive primary care for children with special health care needs in rural areas. *Pediatrics,* 2005, 116:649–656.

115. Pongsupap Y, Van Lerberghe W. Patient experience with self-styled family practices and conventional primary care in Thailand. *Asia Pacific Family Medicine Journal,* 2006, Vol 5.

116. Weiss LJ, Blustein J. Faithful patients: the effect of long term physician–patient relationships on the costs and use of health care by older Americans. *American Journal of Public Health,* 1996, 86:1742–1747.

117. Rosenblatt RL et al. The generalist role of specialty physicians: is there a hidden system of primary care? *JAMA,*1998, 279:1364–1370.

118. Kempe A et al. Quality of care and use of the medical home in a state-funded capitated primary care plan for low-income children. *Pediatrics,* 2000, 105:1020–1028.

119. Raddish MS et al. Continuity of care: is it cost effective? *American Journal of Managed Care,* 1999, 5:727–734.

120. De Maeseneer JM et al. Provider continuity in family medicine: does it make a difference for total health care costs? *Annals of Family Medicine,* 2003, 1:131–133.

121. Saver B. Financing and organization findings brief. *Academy for Research and Health Care Policy,* 2002, 5:1–2.

122. Tudiver F, Herbert C, Goel V. Why don't family physicians follow clinical practice guidelines for cancer screening? *Canadian Medical Association Journal,* 1998, 159:797–798.

123. Oxman AD et al. No magic bullets: a systematic review of 102 trials of interventions to improve professional practice. *Canadian Medical Association Journal,* 1995, 153:1423–1431.

124. Freeman G, Hjortdahl P. What future for continuity of care in general practice? *British Medical Journal,* 1997, 314: 1870–1873.

125. Miller MR et al. Parental preferences for primary and specialty care collaboration in the management of teenagers with congenital heart disease. *Pediatrics,* 2000, 106:264–269.

126. Mainous AG III, Gill JM. The importance of continuity of care in the likelihood of future hospitalization: is site of care equivalent to a primary clinician? *American Journal of Public Health,* 1998, 88:1539–1541.

127. Parchman ML, Culler SD. Primary care physicians and avoidable hospitalizations. *Journal of Family Practice,* 1994, 39:123–128.

128. Hurley RE, Freund DA, Taylor DE. Emergency room use and primary care case management: evidence from four medicaid demonstration programs. *American Journal of Public Health,* 1989, 79: 834–836.

129. Martin DP et al. Effect of a gatekeeper plan on health services use and charges: a randomized trial. *American Journal of Public Health,* 1989, 79:1628–1632.

130. Gadomski A, Jenkins P, Nichols M. Impact of a Medicaid Primary Care Provider and Preventive Care on pediatric hospitalization. *Pediatrics,* 1998, 101:E1 (http://pediatrics.aappublications.org/cgi/reprint/101/3/e1, accessed 29 July 2008).

131. Hjortdahl P, Borchgrevink CF. Continuity of care: influence of general practitioners' knowledge about their patients on use of resources in consultations. *British Medical Journal,* 1991, 303:1181–1184.

132. Roos NP, Carriere KC, Friesen D. Factors influencing the frequency of visits by hypertensive patients to primary care physicians in Winnipeg. *Canadian Medical Association Journal,* 1998, 159:777–783.

133. Ryan S et al. The effects of regular source of care and health need on medical care use among rural adolescents. *Archives of Pediatric and Adolescent Medicine,* 2001, 155:184–190.

134. Schoen C et al. Towards higher-performance health systems: adults' health care experiences in seven countries, 2007. *Health Affairs,* 2007, 26:w717–w734.

135. Saltman R, Rico A, Boerma W, eds. *Primary care in the driver's seat? Organizational reform in European primary care.* Maidenhead, England, Open University Press, 2006 (European Observatory on Health Systems and Policies Series).

136. Nutting PA. Population-based family practice: the next challenge of primary care. *Journal of Family Practice,* 1987, 24:83–88.

137. *Strategies for population health: investing in the health of Canadians.* Ottawa, Health Canada, Advisory Committee on Population Health, 1994.

138. Lasker R. *Medicine and public health: the power of collaboration.* New York, New York Academy of Medicine, 1997.

139. Longlett SK, Kruse JE, Wesley RM. Community-oriented primary care: historical perspective. *Journal of the American Board of Family Practice,* 2001,14:54–563.

140. *Improving health for New Zealanders by investing in primary health care.* Wellington, National Health Committee, 2000.

141. Provenzale D et al. Gastroenterologist specialist care and care provided by generalists – an evaluation of effectiveness and efficiency. *American Journal of Gastroenterology,* 2003, 98:21-8.

142. Smetana GW et al. A comparison of outcomes resulting from generalist vs specialist care for a single discrete medical condition: a systematic review and methodologic critique. *Archives of Internal Medicine,* 2007, 167:10–20.

143. Beck CA et al. Discharge prescriptions following admission for acute myocardial infarction at tertiary care and community hospitals in Quebec. *Canadian Journal of Cardiology,* 2001, 17:33–40.

144. Fendrick AM, Hirth RA, Chernew ME. Differences between generalist and specialist physicians regarding Helicobacter pylori and peptic ulcer disease. *American Journal of Gastroenterology,* 1996, 91:1544–1548.

145. Zoorob RJ et al. Practice patterns for peptic ulcer disease: are family physicians testing for H. pylori? *Helicobacter,* 1999, 4:243–248.

146. Rose JH et al. Generalists and oncologists show similar care practices and outcomes for hospitalized late-stage cancer patients. For SUPPORT Investigators (Study to Understand Prognoses and Preferences for Outcomes and Risks for Treatment). *Medical Care,* 2000, 38:1103–1118.

147. Krikke EH, Bell NR. Relation of family physician or specialist care to obstetric interventions and outcomes in patients at low risk: a western Canadian cohort study. *Canadian Medical Association Journal,* 1989, 140:637–643.

148. MacDonald SE, Voaklander K, Birtwhistle RV. A comparison of family physicians' and obstetricians' intrapartum management of low-risk pregnancies. *Journal of Family Practice,* 1993, 37:457–462.

149. Abyad A, Homsi R. A comparison of pregnancy care delivered by family physicians versus obstetricians in Lebanon. *Family Medicine,* 1993 25:465–470.

150. Grunfeld E et al. Comparison of breast cancer patient satisfaction with follow-up in primary care versus specialist care: results from a randomized controlled trial. *British Journal of General Practice*, 1999, 49:705–710.

151. Grunfeld E et al. Randomized trial of long-term follow-up for early-stage breast cancer: a comparison of family physician versus specialist care. *Journal of Clinical Oncology*, 2006, 24:848–855.

152. Scott IA et al. An Australian comparison of specialist care of acute myocardial infarction. *International Journal for Quality in Health Care*, 2003, 15:155–161..

153. Regueiro CR et al. A comparison of generalist and pulmonologist care for patients hospitalized with severe chronic obstructive pulmonary disease: resource intensity, hospital costs, and survival. For SUPPORT Investigators (Study to Understand Prognoses and Preferences for Outcomes and Risks of Treatment). *American Journal of Medicine*, 1998, 105:366–372.

154. McAlister FA et al. The effect of specialist care within the first year on subsequent outcomes in 24,232 adults with new-onset diabetes mellitus: population-based cohort study. *Quality and Safety in Health Care*, 2007, 16:6–11.

155. Greenfield S et al. Outcomes of patients with hypertension and non-insulin dependent diabetes mellitus treated by different systems and specialties. Results from the medical outcomes study. *Journal of the American Medical Association*, 1995, 274:1436–1444.

156. Pongsupap Y, Boonyapaisarnchoaroen T, Van Lerberghe W. The perception of patients using primary care units in comparison with conventional public hospital outpatient departments and "prime mover family practices": an exit survey. *Journal of Health Science*, 2005, 14:3.

157. Baicker K, Chandra A. Medicare spending, the physician workforce, and beneficiaries' quality of care. *Health Affairs*, 2004 (Suppl. web exclusive: W4-184–197).

158. Shi, L. Primary care, specialty care, and life chances. *International Journal of Health Services*, 1994, 24:431–458.

159. Baicker K et al. Who you are and where you live: how race and geography affect the treatment of Medicare beneficiaries. *Health Affairs*, 2004 (web exclusive: VAR33–V44).

160. Briggs CJ, Garner P. Strategies for integrating primary health services in middle and low-income countries at the point of delivery. *Cochrane Database of Systematic Reviews*, 2006, (3):CD003318.

161. *Estudo regional sobre assistencia hospitalar e ambulatorial especializada na America Latina e Caribe*. Washington DC, Pan American Health Organization, Unidad de Organización de Servicios de Salud, Area de Tecnología y Prestación de Servicios de Salud, 2004.

162. Pongsupap Y, Van Lerberghe W. Choosing between public and private or between hospital and primary care? Responsiveness, patient-centredness and prescribing patterns in outpatient consultations in Bangkok. *Tropical Medicine and International Health*, 2006, 11:81–89.

163. *Guide to clinical preventive services, 2007*. Rockville MD, Agency for Healthcare Research and Quality, 2007 (AHRQ Publication No. 07-05100; http://www.ahrq.gov/clinic/pocketgd.htm).

164. Margolis PA et al. From concept to application: the impact of a community-wide intervention to improve the delivery of preventive services to children. *Pediatrics*, 2001, 108:E42.

165. Donovan EF et al. Intensive home visiting is associated with decreased risk of infant death. *Pediatrics*, 2007, 119:1145–1151.

166. Manandhar D et al. Effect of a participatory intervention with women's groups on birth outcomes in Nepal: cluster-randomised controlled trial. *Lancet*, 364:970–979.

167. Rockenschaub G, Pukkila J, Profili MC, eds. *Towards health security. A discussion paper on recent health crises in the WHO European Region*. Copenhagen, World Health Organization Regional Office for Europe, 2007

168. *Primary care. America's health in a new era*. Washington DC, National Academy Press Institute of Medicine, 1996.

169. Tableau d'honneur des 50 meilleurs hôpitaux de France. Palmarès des Hôpitaux. *Le Point*, 2008 (http://hopitaux.lepoint.fr/tableau-honneur.php, accessed 29 July 2008).

170. Davidson BN, Sofaer S, Gertler P. Consumer information and biased selection in the demand for coverage supplementing Medicare. *Social Science and Medicine*, 1992, 34:1023–1034.

171. Davison KP, Pennebaker JW, Dickerson SS. Who talks? The social psychology of illness support groups. *American Psychology*, 2000, 55:205–217.

172. Segal SP, Redman D, Silverman C. Measuring clients' satisfaction with self-help agencies. *Psychiatric Services*, 51:1148–1152.

173. Adapted from Wollast E, Mercenier P. Pour une régionalisation des soins. In: Groupe d'Etude pour une Réforme de la Médecine. *Pour une politique de la santé*. Bruxelles, Editions Vie Ouvrière/La Revue Nouvelle, 1971.

174. Criel B, De Brouwere V, Dugas S. *Integration of vertical programmes in multi-function health services*. Antwerp, ITGPress, 1997 (Studies in Health Services Organization and Policy 3).

CHAPTER 24

The paradox of primary care

Andrew Bazemore

NOMINATED CLASSIC PAPER

Kurt C. Stange, Robert L. Ferrer. The paradox of primary care. *Annals of Family Medicine*, 2009; 7(4): 293–99.

This paper clearly and succinctly outlines the primary care paradox – that (1) when measured at the level of individual diseases, most studies suggest that primary care physicians provide poorer-quality care than do specialists, while (2) primary care is associated with greater value at the level of the whole person, and lower costs, better health and quality, and greater equity, at the level of populations.

This critical appraisal reminds us of the perils of measurement as healthcare systems shift to paying for value. When focused principally on measures at the disease level, as most health systems currently are, one risks continued undervaluing of the primary care function and overemphasis on specialty care.

In this paper the authors reveal how the interplay of reductionist and ecological fallacies affects current healthcare outcome evaluations. Disease-specific research is prone to the reductionist fallacy, whereby outcome measurements focus solely on the treatment of a specific disease. Primary care research, on the other hand, can fall prey to the ecological fallacy, whereby conclusions about individual diseases are drawn from population data. The value of primary care and specialty care is then obscured because each research enterprise gauges outcomes based on its own one-dimensional evaluation scheme.

The authors argue that it is crucial to understand that healthcare should integrate information from disease to whole person to population levels, thereby maximising the value of healthcare and necessitating integration of both specialty care and primary care. As they note, in order to achieve an ideal system, critical attention is required to the integration of primary and specialty care, and research is desperately needed to enable measurement of the real value of primary care, and its benefits to whole-person and population health.

ABOUT THE LEAD AUTHOR OF THIS PAPER

Kurt Stange is a family doctor and public health physician, practising at Neighborhood Family Practice, a federally qualified community health centre in Cleveland, Ohio, in the United States of America. He is also the Gertrude Donnelly Hess, MD Professor of Oncology Research, and Professor of Family Medicine, Epidemiology & Biostatistics, Oncology and Sociology at Case Western Reserve University. He is also an American Cancer Society Clinical Research Professor.

Kurt serves as editor for the peer-reviewed, indexed, primary care research journal, the *Annals of Family Medicine*, and directs the multi-site Center for Research in Family Practice and Primary Care, one of three research centres funded by the American Academy of Family Physicians. He is actively engaged in ongoing basic and applied research that aims to understand the core structures and processes of primary care practice and their effect on preventive service delivery and patient outcomes, and to discover new methods of enhancing the comprehensive, integrative and relationship-centred generalist approach to patient care. He is a Past-President of the North American Primary Care Research Group, and a member of the Institute of Medicine of the National Academy of Sciences.

ABOUT THE NOMINATOR OF THIS PAPER

Dr Andrew Bazemore, MD MPH, is a practising family physician, and Director of the Robert Graham Center for Policy Studies in Washington DC in the United States of America. He has published over 140 peer-reviewed publications, book chapters, and monographs, and serves on faculties of Georgetown University, George Washington University, University of Cincinnati, and the Virginia Commonwealth University.

'Embrace your generalist instincts and curiosity, look for patterns within and across your patients, panel and population, and commit yourself to scholarship and leadership on behalf of each. You are trained to operate and serve at the centre of "Communities of Solution" for health.'

Dr Andrew Bazemore, United States of America

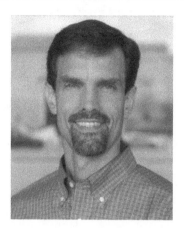

Attribution:

We attribute the original publication of *The paradox of primary care* to *Annals of Family Medicine*. With thanks to Joshua Freeman, Stephanie Hanaway, Mindy Cleary and Doug Henley at the American Academy of Family Physicians.

EDITORIAL

The Paradox of Primary Care

Kurt C. Stange, MD, PhD, Editor; Robert L. Ferrer, MD, MPH, Associate Editor

Ann Fam Med 2009;7:293-299. doi:10.1370/afm.1023.

THE PROBLEM

Despite rising costs, health care often is of poor quality.[1-4] Current solutions to improving quality may do more harm than good if they focus more on diseases than on people.[2,5-9] Efforts to improve the parts (evidence-based care of specific diseases)[10-13] may not necessarily improve the whole (the health of people and populations).[14-18]

Expanding access to specialty care has been proposed as both a source[19-21] of and a solution[22,23] for deficiencies in quality of care. Primary care is touted as an essential building block of a high-value health care system[24-28] even as it is undermined by systems attempting to improve the quality, effectiveness, and value of their health care.[4,29-32] These contradictions plague improvement efforts in health care systems around the world, particularly the United States. This article, the third in a series to understand and improve health care, attempts to define and unravel the paradox of primary care. To make sense of this and other paradoxes affecting health care and health, it is useful to begin by considering different levels of analysis and thinking inclusively about seemingly contradictory evidence.

DIFFERENT LEVELS OF ANALYSIS YIELD DIFFERENT VIEWS

Quality of health care most commonly is measured by the application of disease-specific, evidence-based process-of-care guidelines.[33-36] This evidence fairly consistently shows that primary care clinicians deliver poorer quality care than specialists.[37-67]

Evidence from the Medical Outcomes Study assesses care of patients with several chronic diseases. The study finds that patients' functional health status outcomes are similar for care rendered by specialists and generalists but that generalists use fewer resources.[68,69] Similar outcome at lower cost represents higher value.[70]

A growing number of studies show that for patients with chronic somatic and/or mental illness, shared care between specialists and generalists is optimal.[23,71-83]

In further contrast, ecological studies comparing states in the United States find that a greater supply of generalists and a lower supply of specialists is associated with greater quality of care on multiple disease-specific quality measures.[21,84] Ecological studies comparing westernized countries show that more primary care (and perhaps its associated societal values and public health systems) is associated with better population health with lower cost and greater equity.[85-92]

NAMING THE PARADOX

Thus, the paradox is that compared with specialty care or with systems dominated by specialty care, primary care is associated with the following: (1) apparently poorer quality care for individual diseases, yet (2) similar functional health status at lower cost for people with chronic disease, and (3) better quality, better health, greater equity, and lower cost for whole people and populations.

INTERPRETATION

Two possible explanations might explain this paradox.

Studies Are Flawed; There Is No Paradox

First, is it possible that one or all groups of these studies are fatally flawed, and there is no paradox.

Each of the bodies of work cited has inherent limitations. Studies of disease-specific quality of care typically use as outcomes evidence-based guidelines based on clinical trials that largely exclude patients with comorbid conditions.[93,94] Thus, measures of quality may inadequately reflect population morbidity and may not be applicable to most people.[94] Unmeasured confounding and selection biases appear to explain part, but not all, of the observed differences between specialty and primary care.[42,95] Nonetheless, the face validity of disease-specific studies is high, as it is implausible that, compared with generalists, specialists would know less about their disease of interest or would be less likely to follow guidelines based on evidence derived from the types of patients they typically see.[37]

The selection factors involved in the Medical Outcomes Study have been well-articulated, as has the judgment that "no one is likely to ever do a better job."[70] This study is unique in comparing care at the level of functional health status of the whole person.

Studies of shared care are limited by focusing on care of patients with chronic and recurrent illness, where conjoint generalist-specialist care is most likely to be helpful. Although largely internally valid, their generalizability to other populations is not known.

Just as the studies of care of individual diseases may be prone to the reductionist fallacy, population-level studies are prone to the ecological fallacy. In health care the reductionist fallacy is making attributions about whole people, systems, and populations from studies of individual diseases. The ecological fallacy is making attributions about individual diseases or people based on whole-person or group data.[96-99] As discussed below, it is likely that reductionist and ecological analyses represent separate but interacting truths.

Different Levels of Analysis May Reveal a Complex and Interrelated Whole

A second possible explanation is that the paradox of primary care is a function of different levels of observation, with different levels revealing varied aspects of complex and interrelated factors.

A key barrier to understanding has been the failure to recognize that the driving forces for health outcomes differ by level of analysis. At the level of specific diseases, technical quality of care may be a major determinant of narrowly focused disease markers of clinical success or failure.

At the population level, however, access to care and appropriateness of care (including avoiding overtreatment),[100] two functions to which a strong primary care function contributes, may be major outcome drivers. For example, improved access to primary care for veterans led to significant improvements in health outcomes.[101] Appropriateness of care can suffer in areas with a high concentration of specialists,[21,102] as clinicians working at the level of specific diseases do what they were trained to do without the benefits of the generalist approach described in the prior article in this series.[103]

At the person level, primary care may be particularly important for those with multimorbidity, social deprivation, poorly defined or as-yet undiagnosed illness, or situations in which personal context is important.[104-110] Specialty care is especially important for those needing particular medical knowledge or procedural expertise for which higher volume sometimes is associated with better outcomes.[111] Specialty care may be most important for individuals whose needs are dominated by a particular disease, especially if that disease is uncommon. For most people, and probably for almost everyone over time, a combination of continuing primary care and selective specialty care is needed.[72-74,112,113] Provision of the majority of care through ongoing person-focused, contextualized primary care relationships can allow care to be integrated and prioritized across acute and chronic illness, preventive, psychosocial, and family care.[103,114] That health care is not organized this way in the United States[115,116] may be an important factor in the high cost and low performance of the US health care system compared with other systems based on primary care.[19,24,30]

Not only the forces driving the outcomes, but also the important outcomes themselves may differ by level of analysis. People generally are more interested in how health care helps them accomplish what is important in their lives than they are in how it affects their disease numbers.[117-119] In addition, important outcomes for systems and populations, such as optimizing specialists' case mix or improving equity,[120] are measurable only at the system or population level. Thus, the value of primary care accrues not only from the services provided to individual patients but also from the improved functioning of health care systems,[121] and possibly from freeing resources to be spent on public health and the social determinants of health.[122] Unfortunately, this value is not captured in current performance measures,[119] and efforts to improve quality often place the resource burden on the primary care front line, whereas the benefits accrue to the individual patient, the health care system, and society.

IMPLICATIONS

The implications of the primary care paradox are multiple:

- It is important to simultaneously understand and value quality of care at the level of specific illnesses, whole people, communities, and populations. These different levels may have different drivers of process and outcome. Currently, whole-person and community foci are undervalued, resulting in adverse consequences for the cost, effectiveness, and equity of health care.
- Systems of care are needed that value *both* generalist *and* specialist care and that foster their integration.
- Systems that integrate care both horizontally for individuals, communities, and populations and vertically for specific diseases are most likely to provide the greatest value.[18,123,124] Currently, vertical integration of care for disease is rewarded and supported to a greater degree than horizontal integration of

care for people and populations. This imbalance is a source of the dysfunction of the health care system.

Some of these implications may seem obvious; however, we often do not act as though they are obvious or even apparent. The natural human tendency to simplify problems, focusing on easily conceptualized and measured components,[125] can lead us to act in unintentionally damaging[126] ways that overlook what is clear when a broader perspective is taken.

Thus, it is possible that pay-for performance schemes may not improve the health of the population if they lead to a narrow focus on improving process measures for specific diseases without also creating incentives for the much more difficult-to-measure integration of care of the whole person and the development of systems that foster relationships which integrate narrow and broad knowledge to personalize care.[5,8,13,103,127,128]

Evidence-based assessments of quality tend to be based on measures of central tendency from clinical trials that systematically exclude the majority of people with comorbid conditions.[94] The resulting reductionistically biased interventions may achieve their goal. achieve their goal of improving the narrow quality measure but fail in the larger goals of improving the functional health of the individual and providing health care value to the population.

It is easier to conceptualize and measure the value of specialism[22,129] than of generalism.[103] Specialism fits with the reductionistic understanding of disease and medical care that is dominant in Western countries.[17,130] Generalism is better understood with broader conceptualizations of health based on systems and complexity theories.[131-137] The added value of a generalist approach most likely involves integrative functions based on an inclusive focus and an ability to prioritize care within a relationship-centered, whole-person, community-based context, fostering connections to more narrowly focused care when it is needed.[103,114] These properties affect the performance of other health system components, including efficiency and equity.[19,92]

An important insight from the paradox of primary care is to distinguish among complex diseases, complex patients, and complex populations. People with a single complex disease, for which successful management requires narrowly focused expertise with uncommon presentations or complicated treatment regimens, are the domain of the specialist. Complex patients, characterized by multiple chronic illnesses and competing priorities, often derive the greatest value from shared care, with selective specialist care integrated by primary care. Complex populations, such as those with large variations in wealth, education, culture, access to health care, or remoteness from health services, will rely heavily on a robust system of primary health

care and public health to achieve equity in health outcomes.[138] Care at all levels (diseases, patients, and populations) is best integrated by a generalist approach that prioritizes and personalizes care.[103] Personalization means actually knowing the person over time in their family and community contexts.[24] This contrasts with the current corruption and debasement of the term *personalized* to mean knowing the person's genome sufficiently to tailor pharmacotherapy.[139-141]

One task of health systems is to learn how to support the most effective and efficient care, and where possible, to measure outcomes for complex diseases, patients, and populations. Narrowly defined performance measures are likely to miss performance gaps for complex populations when poor access is the culprit rather than poor technical quality. Conversely, detecting overservice will be important for groups with high access and resources, as overservice is a substantial contributor to poor outcomes.[100,142-144] For complex patients, in whom the treatment burden for multiple illnesses may create a new set of functional limitations, more global outcomes measures may be necessary. Creating the lenses to rectify current distortions in health services' evaluative vision is an urgent priority.[119]

Understanding the paradox of primary care and acting on that wisdom can help us to develop systems that maximize the value of health care for individuals and for the population. The next article in this series will address how the components of health care fit together to create value.[145]

CONCLUSION

The primary care paradox is the observation that primary care physicians provide poorer quality care of specific diseases than do specialists; yet primary care is associated with higher value health care at the level of the whole person, and better health, greater equity, lower costs, and better quality of care at the level of populations.

This paradox shows that current disease-specific scientific evidence is inadequate for conceptualizing, measuring, and paying for health care performance. Unraveling the paradox of primary care depends on understanding the added value of integrating, prioritizing, contextualizing, and personalizing health care across acute and chronic illness, psychosocial issues and mental health, disease prevention, and optimization of health and meaning. This added value is hard to see in assessments at the level of diseases. The added value is readily apparent, however, at the level of whole people and populations.

Systems development is needed to integrate the complementary strengths of primary and specialty care to avoid unintended negative health and societal consequences from fragmenting efforts to improve the quality of health care. Research is needed to understand and support the complex and high-value but poorly comprehended generalist function.

To read or post commentaries in response to this article, see it online at http://www.annfamed.org/cgi/content/full/7/4/293.

Key words: Primary health care; quality of care; cost of care; health; health care, value

Funding support: Dr Stange is supported in part by a Clinical Research Professorship from the American Cancer Society. Dr Ferrer is supported during the writing of this article by a Robert Wood Johnson Foundation Generalist Physician Faculty Scholar award.

Acknowledgments: The authors are grateful to David Aron, Larry Green, Chris van Weel, Paul Thomas, the UCLA/Rand Robert Wood Johnson Foundation Clinical Scholars, Robert Brook, and Fiona Walter, who contributed helpful comments on earlier versions of this work.

References

1. McGlynn EA, Asch SM, Adams J, et al. The quality of health care delivered to adults in the United States. *N Engl J Med.* 2003; 348(26):2635-2645.

2. Marshall MN, Romano PS, Davies HT. How do we maximize the impact of the public reporting of quality of care? *Int J Qual Health Care.* 2004;16(Suppl 1):i57-i63.

3. Institute of Medicine. Committee on Quality of Helath Care in America. *Crossing the Quality Chasm: A New Health System for the 21st Century.* Washington, DC: National Academy Press; 2001.

4. Geyman JP. *Health Care in America : Can Our Ailing System be Healed?* Boston, MA: Butterworth-Heinemann; 2002.

5. Casalino LP. The unintended consequences of measuring quality on the quality of medical care. *N Engl J Med.* 1999;341(15):1147-1150.

6. McGlynn EA. Intended and unintended consequences: what should we really worry about? *Med Care.* 2007;45(1):3-5.

7. Ash JS, Sittig DF, Poon EG, Guappone K, Campbell E, Dykstra RH. The extent and importance of unintended consequences related to computerized provider order entry. *J Am Med Inform Assoc.* 2007;14(4):415-423.

8. Roland M. Pay-for-performance: too much of a good thing? A conversation with Martin Roland. Interview by Robert Galvin. *Health Aff (Millwood).* 2006;25(5):w412-w419.

9. Watts IT, Wenck B. Financing and the quality framework. *Aust Fam Physician.* 2007;36(1-2):32-34.

10. Downing A, Rudge G, Cheng Y, Tu YK, Keen J, Gilthorpe MS. Do the UK government's new Quality and Outcomes Framework (QOF) scores adequately measure primary care performance? A cross-sectional survey of routine healthcare data. *BMC Health Serv Res.* 2007;7:166.

11. Doran T, Fullwood C, Gravelle H, et al. Pay-for-performance programs in family practices in the United Kingdom. *N Engl J Med.* 2006;355(4):375-384.

12. Wald DS. Problems with performance related pay in primary care. *BMJ.* 2007;335(7619):523.

13. McDonald R, Harrison S, Checkland K, Campbell SM, Roland M. Impact of financial incentives on clinical autonomy and internal motivation in primary care: ethnographic study. *BMJ.* 2007;334 (7608):1357.

14. Ham C. Integrating Care: Lessons from the front line. The Nuffield Trust. 2008. http://nuffieldtrust.nvisage.uk.com/publications/ detail.asp?id=0&PRid=383. Accessed May 19, 2009.

15. Stange KC. The paradox of the parts and the whole in understanding and improving general practice. *Int J Qual Health Care.* 2002;14(4):267-268.

16. De Maeseneer J, van Weel C, Egilman D, Mfenyana K, Kaufman A, Sewankambo N. Strengthening primary care: addressing the disparity between vertical and horizontal investment. *Br J Gen Pract.* 2008;58(546):3-4.

17. Stange KC. The problem of fragmentation and the need for integrative solutions. *Ann Fam Med.* 2009;7(2):100-103.

18. Thomas P, Meads G, Moustafa A, Nazareth I, Stange KC., Donnelly Hess G. Combined vertical and horizontal integration of health care-a goal of practice based commissioning. *Qual. Primary Care.* 2008;16(6):425-432.

19. Starfield B, Shi LY, Macinko J. Contribution of primary care to health systems and health. *Milbank Q.* 2005;83(3):457-502.

20. Starfield B, Shi L, Grover A, Macinko J. The effects of specialist supply on populations' health: assessing the evidence. *Health Aff (Millwood).* 2005;(Suppl Web Exclusives):W5-97-W95-107.

21. Baicker K, Chandra A. Medicare spending, the physician workforce, and beneficiaries' quality of care. *Health Aff (Millwood).* 2004;(Suppl Web Exclusives):W184-197.

22. Goldman L. The value of cardiology. *N Engl J Med.* 1996;335(25): 1918-1919.

23. Surís X, Cerdà D, Ortiz-Santamaría V, et al. A rheumatology consultancy program with general practitioners in Catalonia, Spain. *J Rheumatol.* 2007;34(6):1328-1331.

24. Donaldson MS, Yordy KD, Lohr KN, Vanselow NA, eds. *Primary Care America's Health in a New Era.* Washington DC: National Academy Press; 1996.

25. Chan M. Return to Alma-Ata. *Lancet.* 2008;372(9642):865-866.

26. Lawn JE, Rohde J, Rifkin S, Were M, Paul VK, Chopra M. Alma-Ata 30 years on: revolutionary, relevant, and time to revitalise. *Lancet.* 2008;372(9642):917-927.

27. Gunn JM, Palmer VJ, Naccarella L, et al. The promise and pitfalls of generalism in achieving the Alma-Ata vision of health for all. *Med J Aust.* 2008;189(2):110-112.

28. Gunn J, Naccarella L, Palmer V, Kokanovic R, Pope C, Lathlean J. What is the place of generalism in the 2020 primary health care team? Australian Primary Health Care Research Institute. 2008. http://www.anu.edu.au/aphcri/Domain/Workforce/Perkins_25_ final.pdf. Accessed May 12, 2009.

29. Bodenheimer T. Primary care—will it survive? *N Engl J Med.* 2006; 355(9):861-864.

30. Starfield B. Is US health really the best in the world? *JAMA.* 2000; 284(4):483-485.

31. Lewin S, Lavis JN, Oxman AD, et al. Supporting the delivery of cost-effective interventions in primary health-care systems in low-income and middle-income countries: an overview of systematic reviews. *Lancet.* 2008;372(9642):928-939.

32. Rohde J, Cousens S, Chopra M, et al. 30 years after Alma-Ata: has primary health care worked in countries? *Lancet.* 2008;372(9642): 950-961.

33. Marshall M, Campbell S, Hacker J, Roland M, eds. *Quality Indicators For General Practice: A Practical Guide to Clinical Quality Indicators For Primary Care Health Professional and Managers.* Lake Forest, IL: Royal Society of Medicine Press, Ltd; 2002.

34. Marshall MN, Shekelle PG, McGlynn EA, Campbell S, Brook RH, Roland MO. Can health care quality indicators be transferred between countries? *Qual Saf Health Care.* 2003;12(1):8-12.

35. McGlynn EA. Selecting common measures of quality and system performance. *Med Care.* 2003;41(1)(Suppl):I39-I47.

36. McGlynn EA. An evidence-based national quality measurement and reporting system. *Med Care.* 2003;41(1)(Suppl):I8-I15.

37. Harrold LR, Field TS, Gurwitz JH. Knowledge, patterns of care, and outcomes of care for generalists and specialists. *J Gen Intern Med.* 1999;14(8):499-511.

38. Vollmer WM, O'Hollaren M, Ettinger KM, et al. Specialty differences in the management of asthma. A cross-sectional assessment of allergists' patients and generalists' patients in a large HMO. *Arch Intern Med.* 1997;157(11):1201-1208.

39. Tseng FY, Lai MS. Effects of physician specialty on use of antidiabetes drugs, process and outcomes of diabetes care in a medical center. *J Formos Med Assoc.* 2006;105(10):821-831.

40. Stone VE, Mansourati FF, Poses RM, Mayer KH. Relation of physician specialty and HIV/AIDS experience to choice of guideline-recommended antiretroviral therapy. *J Gen Intern Med.* 2001;16(6):360-368.

41. Solomon DH, Bates DW, Panush RS, Katz JN. Costs, outcomes, and patient satisfaction by provider type for patients with rheumatic and musculoskeletal conditions: a critical review of the literature and proposed methodologic standards. *Ann Intern Med.* 1997;127(1):52-60.

42. Smetana GW, Landon BE, Bindman AB, et al. A comparison of outcomes resulting from generalist vs specialist care for a single discrete medical condition: a systematic review and methodologic critique. *Arch Intern Med.* 2007;167(1):10-20.

43. Simon GE, Von Korff M, Rutter CM, Peterson DA. Treatment process and outcomes for managed care patients receiving new antidepressant prescriptions from psychiatrists and primary care physicians. *Arch Gen Psychiatry.* 2001;58(4):395-401.

44. Shah BR, Hux JE, Laupacis A, Zinman B, Zwarenstein M. Deficiencies in the quality of diabetes care: comparing specialist with generalist care misses the point. *J Gen Intern Med.* 2007;22(2):275-279.

45. Shah BR, Hux JE, Laupacis A, Zinman B, Booth GL. Use of vascular risk-modifying medications for diabetic patients differs between physician specialties. *Diabet Med.* 2006;23(10):1117-1123.

46. Shackelford DP, Griffin D, Hoffman MK, Jones DED. Influence of specialty on pathology resource use in evaluation of cervical dysplasia. *Obstet Gynecol.* 1999;94(5 Pt 1):709-712.

47. Schreiber TL, Elkhatib A, Grines CL, O'Neill WW. Cardiologist versus internist management of patients with unstable angina: treatment patterns and outcomes. *J Am Coll Cardiol.* 1995;26(3):577-582.

48. Pugh MJ, Anderson J, Pogach LM, Berlowitz DR. Differential adoption of pharmacotherapy recommendations for type 2 diabetes by generalists and specialists. *Med Care Res Rev.* 2003;60(2):178-200.

49. Provenzale D, Ofman J, Gralnek I, Rabeneck L, Koff R, McCrory D. Gastroenterologist specialist care and care provided by generalists—an evaluation of effectiveness and efficiency. *Am J Gastroenterol.* 2003;98(1):21-28.

50. Nash IS, Corrato RR, Dlutowski MJ, O'Connor JP, Nash DB. Generalist versus specialist care for acute myocardial infarction. *Am J Cardiol.* 1999;83(5):650-654.

51. Melniker LA, Leo PJ. Comparative knowledge and practice of emergency physicians, cardiologists, and primary care practitioners regarding drug therapy for acute myocardial infarction. *Chest.* 1998;113(2):297-305.

52. McAlister FA, Majumdar SR, Eurich DT, Johnson JA. The effect of specialist care within the first year on subsequent outcomes in 24,232 adults with new-onset diabetes mellitus: population-based cohort study. *Qual Saf Health Care.* 2007;16(1):6-11.

53. Levetan CS, Passaro MD, Jablonski KA, Ratner RE. Effect of physician specialty on outcomes in diabetic ketoacidosis. *Diabetes Care.* 1999;22(11):1790-1795.

54. Ko CW, Kelley K, Meyer KE. Physician specialty and the outcomes and cost of admissions for end-stage liver disease. *Am J Gastroenterol.* 2001;96(12):3411-3418.

55. Janson S, Weiss K. A national survey of asthma knowledge and practices among specialists and primary care physicians. *J Asthma.* 2004;41(3):343-348.

56. Indridason OS, Coffman CJ, Oddone EZ. Is specialty care associated with improved survival of patients with congestive heart failure? *Am Heart J.* 2003;145(2):300-309.

57. Go AS, Rao RK, Dauterman KW, Massie BM. A systematic review of the effects of physician specialty on the treatment of coronary disease and heart failure in the United States. *Am J Med.* 2000;108(3):216-226.

58. Gabriel SE, Wagner JL, Zinsmeister AR, Scott CG, Luthra HS. Is rheumatoid arthritis care more costly when provided by rheumatologists compared with generalists? *Arthritis Rheum.* 2001;44(7):1504-1514.

59. Foody JM, Rathore SS, Wang YF, et al. Physician specialty and mortality among elderly patients hospitalized with heart failure. *Am J Med.* 2005;118(10):1120-1125.

60. Federman DG, Concato J, Kirsner RS. Comparison of dermatologic diagnoses by primary care practitioners and dermatologists. A review of the literature. *Arch Fam Med.* 1999;8(2):170-172.

61. Dohmen K, Shirahama M, Shigematsu H, Irie K, Ishibashi H. Impact of hepatologists to extend survival of hepatocellular carcinoma patients with cirrhosis: a comparison with non-hepatologists. *Hepatogastroenterology.* 2004;51(56):564-569.

62. Diette GB, Skinner EA, Nguyen TT, Markson L, Clark BD, Wu AW. Comparison of quality of care by specialist and generalist physicians as usual source of asthma care for children. *Pediatrics.* 2001;108(2):432-437.

63. Chin MH, Zhang JX, Merrell K. Specialty differences in the care of older patients with diabetes. *Med Care.* 2000;38(2):131-140.

64. Casale PN, Jones JL, Wolf FE, Pei Y, Eby LM. Patients treated by cardiologists have a lower in-hospital mortality for acute myocardial infarction. *J Am Coll Cardiol.* 1998;32(4):885-889.

65. Backer V, Nepper-Christensen S, Nolte H. Quality of care in patients with asthma and rhinitis treated by respiratory specialists and primary care physicians: a 3-year randomized and prospective follow-up study. *Ann Allergy Asthma Immunol.* 2006;97(4):490-496.

66. Anderson JJ, Ruwe M, Miller DR, Kazis L, Felson DT, Prashker M. Relative costs and effectiveness of specialist and general internist ambulatory care for patients with 2 chronic musculoskeletal conditions. *J Rheumatol.* 2002;29(7):1488-1495.

67. Wierzchowiecki M, Poprawski K, Nowicka A, Kandziora M, Piatkowska A. [Knowledge of primary care physicians, cardiologists from cardiology clinics, internal and cardiology department physicians about chronic heart failure diagnosis and treatment] [In Polish]. *Pol Merkur Lekarski.* 2005;18(104):210-215.

68. Greenfield S, Rogers W, Mangotich M, Carney MF, Tarlov AR. Outcomes of patients with hypertension and non-insulin dependent diabetes mellitus treated by different systems and specialties. Results from the medical outcomes study. *JAMA.* 1995;274(18):1436-1444.

69. Greenfield S, Nelson EC, Zubkoff M, et al. Variations in resource utilization among medical specialties and systems of care. Results from the medical outcomes study. *JAMA.* 1992;267(12):1624-1630.

70. Rosenblatt RA. Specialists or generalists. On whom should we base the American health care system? *JAMA.* 1992;267(12):1665-1666.

71. Ahmed A, Allman RM, Kiefe CI, et al. Association of consultation between generalists and cardiologists with quality and outcomes of heart failure care. *Am Heart J.* 2003;145(6):1086-1093.

72. Katon W, Von Korff M, Lin E, et al. Collaborative management to achieve treatment guidelines. Impact on depression in primary care. *JAMA.* 1995;273(13):1026-1031.

73. Katon WJ, Von Korff M, Lin EH, et al. The Pathways Study: a randomized trial of collaborative care in patients with diabetes and depression. *Arch Gen Psychiatry.* 2004;61(10):1042-1049.

74. Lafata JE, Martin S, Morlock R, Divine G, Xi H. Provider type and the receipt of general and diabetes-related preventive health services among patients with diabetes. *Med Care.* 2001;39(5):491-499.

75. Willison DJ, Soumerai SB, McLaughlin TJ, et al. Consultation between cardiologists and generalists in the management of acute myocardial infarction: implications for quality of care. *Arch Intern Med.* 1998;158(16):1778-1783.

76. Ouwens M, Wollersheim H, Hermens R, Hulscher M, Grol R. Integrated care programmes for chronically ill patients: a review of systematic reviews. *Int J Qual Health Care.* 2005;17(2):141-146.

77. Kodner DL. Whole-system approaches to health and social care partnerships for the frail elderly: an exploration of North American models and lessons. *Health Soc Care Community.* 2006;14(5):384-390.

78. Graber AL, Elasy TA, Quinn D, Wolff K, Brown A. Improving glycemic control in adults with diabetes mellitus: shared responsibility in primary care practices. *South Med J.* 2002;95(7):684-690.

79. Callahan CM, Boustani MA, Unverzagt FW, et al. Effectiveness of collaborative care for older adults with Alzheimer disease in primary care: a randomized controlled trial. *JAMA.* 2006;295(18):2148-2157.

80. Kaasa S, Jordhøy MS, Haugen DF. Palliative care in Norway: a national public health model. *J Pain Symptom Manage.* 2007;33(5):599-604.

81. Conceição C, Van Lerberghe W, Ramos V, Hipólito F, Ferrinho P. A case study of team work and performance-linked payment of family physicians in Portugal. *Cah Sociol Demogr Med.* 2007;47(3):293-313.

82. Meulepas MA, Jacobs JE, Smeenk FW, et al. Effect of an integrated primary care model on the management of middle-aged and old patients with obstructive lung diseases. *Scand J Prim Health Care.* 2007;25(3):186-192.

83. Blaauwbroek R, Tuinier W, Meyboom-de Jong B, Kamps WA, Postma A. Shared care by paediatric oncologists and family doctors for long-term follow-up of adult childhood cancer survivors: a pilot study. *Lancet Oncol.* 2008;9(3):232-238.

84. Roetzheim RG, Gonzalez EC, Ramirez A, Campbell R, van Durme DJ. Primary care physician supply and colorectal cancer. *J Fam Pract.* 2001;50(12):1027-1031.

85. Starfield B. *Primary Care: Balancing Health Needs, Services, and Technology.* Rev ed. New York, NY: Oxford University Press; 1998.

86. Starfield B, Shi LY, Macinko J. Contribution of primary care to health systems and health. *Milbank Q.* 2005;83(3):457-502.

87. Shi L, Macinko J, Starfield B, Politzer R, Wulu J, Xu J. Primary care, social inequalities, and all-cause, heart disease, and cancer mortality in US counties, 1990. *Am J Public Health.* 2005;95(4):674-680.

88. Shi L, Macinko J, Starfield B, Wulu J, Regan J, Politzer R. The relationship between primary care, income inequality, and mortality in US States, 1980-1995. *J Am Board Fam Pract.* 2003;16(5):412-422.

89. Shi L, Macinko J, Starfield B, et al. Primary care, infant mortality, and low birth weight in the states of the USA. *J Epidemiol Community Health.* 2004;58(5):374-380.

90. Shi L, Starfield B. The effect of primary care physician supply and income inequality on mortality among blacks and whites in US metropolitan areas. *Am J Public Health.* 2001;91(8):1246-1250.

91. Starfield B. New paradigms for quality in primary care. *Br J Gen Pract.* 2001;51(465):303-309.

92. Starfield B. Primary care and equity in health: The importantce to effectiveness and equity of responsiveness to people's needs. *Humanity Soc.* In press.

93. Fortin M, Soubhi H, Hudon C, Bayliss EA, van den Akker M. Multimorbidity's many challenges. *BMJ.* 2007;334(7602):1016-1017.

94. Fortin M, Dionne J, Pinho G, Gignac J, Almirall J, Lapointe L. Randomized controlled trials: do they have external validity for patients with multiple comorbidities? *Ann Fam Med.* 2006;4(2):104-108.

95. Hartz A, James PA. A systematic review of studies comparing myocardial infarction mortality for generalists and specialists: lessons for research and health policy. *J Am Board Fam Med.* 2006;19(3):291-302.

96. Susser M. The logic in ecological: II. The logic of design. *Am J Public Health.* 1994;84(5):830-835.

97. Susser M. The logic in ecological: I. The logic of analysis. *Am J Public Health.* 1994;84(5):825-829.

98. Koopman JS, Longini IM Jr. The ecological effects of individual exposures and nonlinear disease dynamics in populations. *Am J Public Health.* 1994;84(5):836-842.

99. Schwartz S. The fallacy of the ecological fallacy: the potential misuse of a concept and the consequences. *Am J Public Health.* 1994;84(5):819-824.

100. Franks P, Clancy CM, Nutting PA. Gatekeeping revisited—protecting patients from overtreatment. *N Engl J Med.* 1992;327(6):424-429.

101. Rubenstein LV, Yano EM, Fink A, et al. Evaluation of the VA's Pilot Program in Institutional Reorganization toward Primary and Ambulatory Care: Part I, Changes in process and outcomes of care. *Acad Med.* 1996;71(7):772-783.

102. Tu JV, Naylor CD, Kumar D, DeBuono BA, McNeil BJ, Hannan EL. Coronary artery bypass graft surgery in Ontario and New York State: which rate is right? Steering Committee of the Cardiac Care Network of Ontario. *Ann Intern Med.* 1997;126(1):13-19.

103. Stange KC. The generalist approach. *Ann Fam Med.* 2009;7(3):198-203.

104. McWhinney IR, Freeman T. *Textbook of Family Medicine.* 3rd ed. New York, NY: Oxford University Press; 2009.

105. McWhinney IR. 'An acquaintance with particulars...'. *Fam Med.* 1989;21(4):296-298.

106. Flocke SA, Stange KC, Zyzanski SJ. The impact of insurance type and forced discontinuity on the delivery of primary care. *J Fam Pract.* 1997;45(2):129-135.

107. Kahana E, Stange KC, Meehan R, Raff L. Forced disruption in continuity of primary care: the patients' perspective. *Sociol Focus.* 1997;30:172-181.

108. Nutting PA, Goodwin MA, Flocke SA, Zyzanski SJ, Stange KC. Continuity of primary care: to whom does it matter and when? *Ann Fam Med.* 2003;1(3):149-155.

109. Thomas P. *Integrating Primary Health Care: Leading, Managing, Facilitating.* Oxford, UK: Radcliffe Publishing; 2006.

110. Mainous AG III, Goodwin MA, Stange KC. Patient-physician shared experiences and value patients place on continuity of care. *Ann Fam Med.* 2004;2(5):452-454.

111. Halm EA. C. L, Chassin MR. *How is Volume Related to Quality in Health Care? A Systematic Review of the Medical Literature. Interpreting the Volume-Outcome Relationship in the Context of Health Care Quality.* Washington, DC: National Academy of Science; 2000:27-62.

112. Ahmed A, Allman RM, Kiefe CI, et al. Association of consultation between generalists and cardiologists with quality and outcomes of heart failure care. *Am Heart J.* 2003;145(6):1086-1093.

113. Katon W, Russo J, Von Korff M, et al. Long-term effects of a collaborative care intervention in persistently depressed primary care patients. *J Gen Intern Med.* 2002;17(10):741-748.

114. Stange KC, Jaén CR, Flocke SA, Miller WL, Crabtree BF, Zyzanski SJ. The value of a family physician. *J Fam Pract.* 1998;46(5):363-368.

115. Starfield B, Lemke KW, Herbert R, Pavlovich WD, Anderson G. Comorbidity and the use of primary care and specialist care in the elderly. *Ann Fam Med.* 2005;3(3):215-222.

116. Valderas JM, Starfield B, Forrest CB, Sibbald B, Roland M. Ambulatory care provided by office-based specialists in the United States. *Ann Fam Med.* 2009;7(2):104-111.

117. Howie JG, Heaney DJ, Maxwell M. Measuring quality in general practice. Pilot study of a needs, process and outcome measure. *Occas Pap R Coll Gen Pract.* 1997;Feb(75)i-xii[1-32].

118. Howie JG, Heaney D, Maxwell M. Quality, core values and the general practice consultation: issues of definition, measurement and delivery. *Fam Pract.* 2004;21(4):458-468.

119. Heath I, Rubinstein A, Stange KC, van Driel ML. Quality in primary health care: a multidimensional approach to complexity. *BMJ.* 2009;338:b1242.

120. Ferrer RL. Pursuing equity: contact with primary care and specialist clinicians by demographics, insurance, and health status. *Ann Fam Med.* 2007;5(6):492-502.

121. Ferrer RL, Hambidge SJ, Maly RC. The essential role of generalists in health care systems. *Ann Intern Med.* 2005;142(8):691-699.

122. World Health Organization. Commission on Social Determinants of Health—Final Report. 2008. http://www.who.int/social_determinants/final_report/en/index.html. Accessed Jan 30, 2009.

123. De Maeseneer J, van Weel C, Egilman D, Mfenyana K, Kaufman A, Sewankambo N. Strengthening primary care: addressing the disparity between vertical and horizontal investment. *Br J Gen Pract.* 2008;58(546):3-4.

124. Stange KC. Polyclinics must integrate health care vertically AND horizontally [Editorial]. *Lond J Prim Care* 2008;1:42-44.

125. Miles RW. Fallacious reasoning and complexity as root causes of clinical inertia. *J Am Med Dir Assoc.* 2007;8(6):349-354.

126. May R. Forecast. *New Sci.* 2006;192(2578):49.

127. McDonald R, Harrison S, Checkland K. Incentives and control in primary health care: findings from English pay-for-performance case studies. *J Health Organ Manag.* 2008;22(1):48-62.

128. Campbell SM, McDonald R, Lester H. The experience of pay for performance in English family practice: a qualitative study. *Ann Fam Med.* 2008;6(3):228-234.

129. Committee of the American College of Rheumatology Council on Health Care Research. Role of specialty care for chronic diseases: a report from an ad hoc committee of the American College of Rheumatology. *Mayo Clin Proc.* 1996;71(12):1179-1181.

130. Koestler A, Smythies JR, eds. *Beyond Reductionism: New Perspectives on the Life Sciences.* Boston, MA: Houghton Mifflin Co; 1971.

131. Stange KC, Miller WL, McWhinney I. Developing the knowledge base of family practice. *Fam Med.* 2001;33(4):286-297.

132. Sturmberg JP. Systems and complexity thinking in general practice. Part 2: application in primary care research. *Aust Fam Physician.* 2007;36(4):273-275.

133. Sturmberg JP. Systems and complexity thinking in general practice: part 1 - clinical application. *Aust Fam Physician.* 2007;36(3):170-173.

134. McDaniel R, Driebe DJ. Complexity science and health care management. In: Blair JD, Myron DG, Savage GT, eds. *Advances in Health Care Management.* Vol 2. Stamford, CT: JAI Press; 2000:11-36.

135. Stacey RD. *Complexity and Creativity in Organizations.* 1st ed. San Francisco, CA: Berrett-Koehler Publishers; 1996.

136. Plsek PE, Greenhalgh T. Complexity science: The challenge of complexity in health care. *BMJ.* 2001;323(7313):625-628.

137. Plsek PE, Wilson T. Complexity, leadership, and management in healthcare organisations. *BMJ.* 2001;323(7315):746-749.

138. Meads G. *Primary Care in the Twenty-First Century.* Seattle, WA: Radcliffe; 2006.

139. Ferrara J. Personalized medicine: challenges in assessing and capturing value in the commercial environment. *Expert Rev Mol Diagn.* 2006;6(2):129-131.

140. Langreth R, Waldholz M. New era of personalized medicine: targeting drugs for each unique genetic profile. *Oncologist.* 1999; 4(5):426-427.

141. Kalow W. Pharmacogenetics and pharmacogenomics: origin, status, and the hope for personalized medicine. *Pharmacogenomics J.* 2006;6(3):162-165.

142. Brook RH, Kamberg CJ, Mayer-Oakes A, Beers MH, Raube K, Steiner A. Appropriateness of acute medical care for the elderly: an analysis of the literature. *Health Policy.* 1990;14(3):225-242.

143. Wennberg JE, Fisher ES, Goodman DC, Skinner JB. Tracking the care of patients with severe chronic illness: the Dartmouth Atlas of Health Care 2008. The Dartmouth Institute of Health Policy and Clinical Practic Center for Health Policy Research. 2008. http://www.dartmouthatlas.org/atlases/2008_Chronic_Care_Atlas.pdf. Accessed May 23, 2009.

144. Kohn LT, Corrigan JM, Donaldson MS, eds. *To Err is Human. Building a Safer Health System.* Washington, DC: National Academy Press; 2000.

145. Stange KC. A science of connectedness. *Ann Fam Med.* (forthcoming).

CHAPTER 25

Social accountability and medical education

Allyn Walsh

NOMINATED CLASSIC PAPER

Charles Boelen and Bob Woollard. Social accountability and accreditation: a new frontier for educational institutions. *Medical Education*, 2009: 43: 887–94.

This paper raised important issues around the accountability of medical education institutions and medical educators. In strongly worded language, the authors describe the failure of educational programmes to affect what is described as a global crisis in human resource development in the healthcare sector. These issues include: a lack of healthcare staff; inadequate proportions of specialties with respect to priority healthcare needs; a chronic dearth of primary healthcare staff; the migration of health professionals to more socially and financially attractive working environments; the underserving of rural areas; a general deficit of effective action towards disease prevention and health promotion; and little mobilisation of citizens to assume responsibility for protecting their own health.

What does this mean in practice? The authors point out that excellent medical institutions and medical schools must show how their activities and graduates are making a difference to people's well-being. This means not just passing academic exams but showing how they pay attention to workforce needs and career choices. They argue that by adapting norms and accreditation standards that reflect social accountability, educational institutions can be measured and rewarded for their capacity to meet the healthcare needs of society. The authors went on to lead the development of a global consensus document on Social Accountability of Medical Schools.

Since this paper was published in 2009, it has greatly influenced accreditation standards in Canada, where the Association of Faculties of Medicine of Canada has described a social accountability mandate, and has also developed the Charles Boelen International Social Accountability Award. The Global Standards for Postgraduate Family Medicine Education of the World Organization of Family Doctors (WONCA) were heavily influenced by the paper, and incorporate themes of social accountability. The paper has been cited by landmark documents such as the 2010 Lancet Commission on *Health professionals for a new century: transforming education to strengthen health systems in an interdependent world*, and has had global influence on the goals of many medical institutions and the selection of medical students.

ABOUT THE AUTHORS OF THIS PAPER

Charles Boelen is a medical doctor from Belgium who specialised in public health, epidemiology, health system management and education of health professionals. He is considered a world expert in the social accountability of academic institutions, primary healthcare professionals, and healthcare reform. During a career of 30 years with the World Health Organization, Charles developed worldwide human resources development projects in coordination with Ministries of Health and Higher Education, professional associations and academic institutions. He co-chairs the Global Consensus for Social Accountability of Medical Schools with Bob Woollard.

Bob Woollard is a family doctor who was Head of the Department of Family Practice at the University of British Columbia in Canada. He works extensively on the issue of the social accountability of medical schools and is currently involved in the development of a new medical school founded on these principles in Nepal. He is also working in East Africa on social accountability, primary care and accreditation systems, and has recently completed a five-year, five-university project on localised poverty reduction in rural Vietnam.

ABOUT THE NOMINATOR OF THIS PAPER

Dr Allyn Walsh is a Canadian family physician and Professor in the Department of Family Medicine at McMaster University in Canada. She has been chair of the World Organization of Family Doctors (WONCA) Working Party on Education, and in 2016 became president of the Canadian Association for Medical Education. She has led the development of many national and international activities aimed at enhancing family medicine education.

> 'We are so honoured and privileged to be family doctors. Savour each moment when you realise that simply by being present and listening, you are helping

someone heal. Enjoy the ambiguity and uncertainty of the clinical problems, for they keep us engaged, interested, and learning. Our work has such meaning!'

Dr Allyn Walsh, Canada

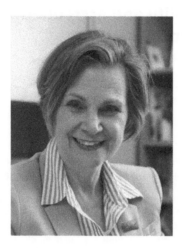

Attribution:

We attribute the original publication of *Social accountability and accreditation: a new frontier for educational institutions* to *Medical Education*, published by Wiley. Original copyright Blackwell Publishing Ltd 2009. With thanks to Paulette Goldweber at Wiley, and Karen Eccles at Medical Education.

social accountability

Social accountability and accreditation: a new frontier for educational institutions

Charles Boelen[1] & Bob Woollard[2]

CONTEXT An association with *excellence* should be reserved for educational institutions which verify that their actions make a difference to people's well-being. The graduates they produce should not only *possess* all of the competencies desirable to improve the health of citizens and society, but should also *use* them in their professional practice. Four principles enunciated by the World Health Organization refer to the type of health care to which people have a right, from both an individual and a collective standpoint: *quality, equity, relevance* and *effectiveness*. Therefore, social, economic, cultural and environmental determinants of health must guide the strategic development of an educational institution.

DISCUSSION Social responsibility implies accountability to society for actions intended to serve it. In the health field, social accountability involves a commitment to respond as best as possible to the priority health needs of citizens and society. An educational institution should verify its impact on society by following basic principles of quality, equity, relevance and effectiveness, and by active participation in health system development. Its social accountability should be measured in three interdependent domains concerning health personnel: conceptualisation, production and utilisability. An educational institution that fully assumes the position of a responsible partner in the health care system and is dedicated to the public interest deserves a label of excellence.

CONCLUSIONS As globalisation is reassessed for its social impact, societies will seek to justify their investments with more solid evidence of their impact on the public good. Medical schools should be prepared to be judged accordingly. There is an urgent need to foster the adaptation of accreditation standards and norms that reflect social accountability. Only then can educational institutions be measured and rewarded for their real capacity to meet the pressing health care needs of society.

Medical Education 2009: 43: 887–894
doi:10.1111/j.1365-2923.2009.03413.x

[1]International Consultant in health systems and personnel, Sciez-sur-Léman, France
[2]Department of Family Practice, University of British Columbia, Vancouver, British Columbia, Canada

Correspondence: Bob Woollard, Department of Family Practice, Suite 320, 5950 University Boulevard, Vancouver, British Columbia V6T 1Z3, Canada. Tel: 00 1 604 731 4688; Fax: 00 1 604 827 4184; E-mail: Woollard@familypractice.ubc.ca

C Boelen & B Woollard

INTRODUCTION

An educational institution that aspires to *excellence* in the production of health care professionals should be granted that status not only when its graduates possess all of the competencies desirable to improve the health of citizens and society, but when they are able to use them in their professional practice. Although medical schools are not presently held to account for the ways in which their graduates are used, and serve, their societies, such an accounting may be required in the future. Educational institutions are increasingly requested to be more explicit about their outputs of professional practitioners and the impact of their presence on social well-being. We may expect policies in higher education and health care to foster such an approach, providing there is political will to improve coordination between the identification of people's health needs, health care system management and educational strategies. In return, educational institutions must use their autonomy and resources to make the best use of their innovative potential to meet these challenges.

Over the last half-century, the quality of education of health care professionals has progressively improved through a series of educational advances.[1] These have included among other things: planning of educational programmes by objectives; problem-based learning; training in multi-professional teams; early immersion in the community and first-line health care services; the adoption of a 'learner-centred' approach; faculty development; educational research; and, more recently, extensive use of informatics and the Internet. Moreover, in many instances norms used for the evaluation and accreditation of educational institutions take these developments into account.

Although these are all very useful, these innovations have not materially contributed to correcting the global crisis affecting human resources development in the health care sector.[2] This crisis is exemplified by an appalling inventory of contributory factors, which include: a quantitative lack of health care staff; inadequate proportions of specialties with respect to priority health care needs; a chronic dearth of primary health care staff; the migration of health professionals to more socially and financially attractive working environments; the underserving of rural areas; a general deficit of effective action towards disease prevention and health promotion; little mobilisation of citizens to assume responsibility for protecting their own health; poor incentives to work in partnership with the social sector for a more effective impact on the social determinants of health; a drifting towards the merchandising of services at the expense of professional ideals; lessening trust in health professionals by administration and the public, and the de-motivation of health care professionals. If we add the professional migration patterns aggravating the already inequitable distribution of health care human resources, we present a context of severe global challenge for medical schools.

How can they cope with such a crisis? To what extent can an educational institution help mitigate the crisis through its education, research and service missions? It is imperative that the design, implementation and follow-up of educational programmes be established in a manner that ensures they are relevant to the needs of citizens and society as a whole and are closely related to the process of national health development. Because health policy has an influence on the spectrum of competencies that health care professionals need to possess, the institution must have an interest in such policy. This proactive posture of the institution should be clearly enunciated in its mission statement and institutional objectives. Moreover, its strategic development plan should be formulated with due regard to evolutionary trends in the health care system and the projected needs of health care personnel, in both qualitative and quantitative terms. Educational programmes should be adjusted accordingly.

There is an expectation that the other partners in social accountability (policy makers, health service managers, health professionals and the public) are equally committed to anticipation, adaptation and quality assurance.

WHAT SOCIAL ACCOUNTABILITY IMPLIES

The World Health Organization (WHO) defines the social accountability of medical schools as representing: 'the obligation to direct their education, research and service activities towards addressing the priority health concerns of the community, region, or nation they have a mandate to serve. The priority health concerns are to be identified jointly by governments, health care organisations, health professionals and the public.'[3] From this, two features of social accountability emerge: altruism and integration. Altruism focuses primarily on society's well-being and integration is an integral part of the social canvas.

© Blackwell Publishing Ltd 2009. MEDICAL EDUCATION 2009; **43**: 887–894

Two groups of principles may serve as frames of reference: humanistic principles, which are relative to people's protection, and systemic principles, which are relative to the relationship of the institution with the health care system.

Humanistic principles

Four principles, enunciated by WHO, refer to the type of health care to which people have a right, from both an individual and a collective standpoint: *quality*, *equity*, *relevance* and *effectiveness*. The principle of quality seeks to provide the citizen with the best possible measures to protect, restore and promote a state of physical, mental and social well-being. The principle of equity tries to ensure that every citizen has full access to health care services and does not face any form of discrimination. The principle of relevance seeks a response to priority health care needs and the provision of special attention to the most vulnerable individuals or groups in society. The principle of effectiveness refers to the utilisation of health care resources, both human and material, in a manner that serves the public interest in the most effective and efficient way.

Systemic principles

These principles relate to the understanding of the complexity of a health care system and to the capacity to find a most useful place in it. The institution is likely to improve its effectiveness if it works in partnership with other stakeholders in the system, namely, policy makers, health system managers, health care professionals and civil society. In order to implement the humanistic principles outlined above, each of these stakeholders has a coordinated role to play. For instance, the policy maker should frame a long-term vision of a health care system which is coherent and integrated; the health system manager should ensure an allocation of resources that is consistent with this vision; the health care professional should acquire competences to deliver the appropriate range of services, and the citizen should assume greater responsibility in protecting his or her own health and that of the community. All partners should adapt their roles and act in synergy to strengthen the system and its human resources for health.[4]

To be fully socially accountable, an institution needs to claim the right to question whether its 'products' (graduates, service models or research findings) are being used in the best interest of the public. Social accountability entails a duty to venture into a field

over which the institution has no formal authority, namely, the functioning of the health care system. We suggest that, taking humanistic and systemic principles as references, a label of excellence should be reserved exclusively for institutions which are designed to make an impact on society.

EXCELLENCE IN IMPACT

By questioning its raison d'être and the final impact of its work, such an institution undertakes a higher order of social accountability. Achieving such an undertaking requires the institution to address a number of interconnected issues: the prioritisation of needs; the system characteristics necessary to facilitate the greatest impact of its graduates; health promotion; required competences; career supports, and impact analysis, etc. These issues need to be addressed by the institution in order to establish and orient its mission. The institution in isolation cannot find all the answers. As a 'producer' of professionals, it must enter into a series of relationships with the social institutions that will utilise its output. At the same time, it must realise that needs are in constant evolution and thus its curriculum and goals must be in a state of constant adjustment. The series of relationships, information gathering, feedback loops and effectors of change needed for this require that the institution recognise principles of complexity in its plans and actions.[5–7] Thus linear relationships of cause and effect need to be replaced by the creation of explicit, adaptable processes that define desired outputs and measure actual outputs while adjusting to the needs of the system their graduates are entering. This is no small task.

Achieving the desired impact requires an initial definition of the type of graduates desired. Desirable profiles, with their spectra of competencies, have been described in models suggested by the WHO (i.e. the 'Five-Star Doctor'), the UK General Medical Council (i.e. 'Tomorrow's Doctor'), the Royal College of Physicians and Surgeons of Canada (i.e. in CanMEDS), and by promoters of the concept of 'professionalism'.[8–11] However, even if such graduates are achieved, if their competencies are not formally recognised and fairly rewarded by the health care system, their desired impact will not be achieved. The graduates will either be underemployed or will revert to the kinds of practices that *are* incentivised. The educational institution must therefore initiate a frank conversation between those who design health policies, those who organise health care services and

C Boelen & B Woollard

those who create job opportunities and support services requiring the acquired competencies.

Partnership is productive within an institution if common interest prevails over private interests. The threat is real if the members of one partner focus on their own interests and ignore the wider social perspective. Within medical education the focus on acquiring biomedical information and technology skills often directs students away from developing the skills and attitudes required to understand and address the true determinants of health in their patients. It should not come as a surprise that most of the creativeness in medical education concentrates on curriculum content and learning methods rather than on the social purpose and moral obligations of the curriculum. In brief, a lot of emphasis is placed on processes and not enough on impact.

This disappointment is not new! At the beginning of last century, Abraham Flexner was mandated by the Carnegie Foundation to undertake a review of the quality of North American medical schools. Aware of lack of equity in the US health care system, he recommended that Afro-American students should benefit from excellent medical education in order to contribute to raising the health status of their communities. Flexner dared to make a correlation between good medical education and population health. Achieving a positive impact on the health of citizens through improved medical education was indeed the prime motive for the exercise. Unfortunately this expectation fell short as the reform of medical schools conducted by his successors consisted of strengthening the scientific nature of the curriculum but little else.[12] History has demonstrated the result: blocks of education in the basic sciences became a compulsory passage before students were allowed any contact with patients and the social environment; the introduction of the social sciences and humanities is limited and late; disciplines and departments guard their autonomy jealously; vertical teaching is enhanced at the expense of the integrated teaching best suited to address complex health issues, and the public health sciences have been marginalised. These were unintended consequences of good intentions. The lack of assessment of the impact of graduates and the evolving needs of society have tended to isolate the institution from the living environment. This model has remained distressingly~prevalent worldwide for over a century and continues to inspire parameters for the accreditation of medical schools. This represents an historical missed opportunity for the academe to set as its raison d'être its impact on social well-being.[13]

EXPRESSIONS OF SOCIAL ACCOUNTABILITY

Social accountability requires that the actions of a medical school begin and be grounded in the identification of societal needs. The meeting of those needs is the desired end. We suggest that the beginning and end of this complex process are connected through a cascade of three specific, although interdependent, domains concerning the health professionals they produce: conceptualisation, production and usability (Fig. 1).

The domain of *conceptualisation* involves the collaborative design of the kind of professional needed and the system that will utilise his or her skills. The domain of *production* involves the main components of training and learning. The domain of *usability* involves initiatives taken by the institution to ensure that its trained professionals are put to their highest and best use.

The term 'usability' is preferred to the terms 'utilisation' or 'usefulness'. Graduates may indeed be utilised and useful as soon as they are employed in any health care structure, even if they only partially apply the spectrum of competencies in which they have been trained. By contrast, the notion of usability refers to the degree of concordance between their acquired competencies and their opportunities to practise them. Therefore, the domain of usability should reflect processes initiated by the institution to ensure that the profile of a health professional on which the training was based is properly valued in the future working environment.

There may be a mismatch between an institution applying this conceptualisation–production–usability (CPU) model and the health system if there are not enough job opportunities for health professionals educated to respond to the public interest. A sustainable series of partnerships is necessary if feedback loops of CPU activities are to be built. Social accountability cannot be entirely fulfilled if all of the

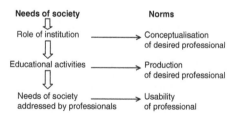

Figure 1 Needs of society and norms

© Blackwell Publishing Ltd 2009. MEDICAL EDUCATION 2009; **43**: 887–894

main actors do not share a common set of values and an effective, although complex, system through which to express those common values.

Table 1 presents a general framework from which specific norms, indicators and criteria can be drawn to orient an educational institution towards greater social relevance. It covers three domains and 11 sections for a total of 31 items. A certain degree of redundancy among items is unavoidable because of the inherent structure of the model.

One of the major concerns in the design of the CPU model is to ensure consistency among the three domains of conceptualisation, production and usability. Here are some illustrations:

- the value of equity mentioned at item 1.1, which the institution declares is one of the founding principles, is referred to in items of section 5 (Educational programme) and in items 10.1 and 10.2 of section 10 (Employment);
- there is a link between item 1.3 (Health system), advocating that an educational institution should be an integral part of a health system (provided it is oriented to meet the needs of citizens and society), and an engagement with health management in a given geographical area in partnership with other actors (items 2.2 and 2.3), and between the utilisation of this area for field operations in education, research and service delivery (section 4), and, finally, the verification of effects (items 11.1 and 11.2), and
- the same concern for consistency is demonstrated when the institution undertakes to train a certain type of health professional (items 1.4 and 2.4), designs an educational programme (item 5.1), evaluates the acquisition of competencies (item 6.3) and verifies the effects on practice (item 10.3).

An illustration of how the CPU model could be used concretely, with examples relative to the different items, will be addressed in another paper.

RELATING TO CURRENT EVALUATION AND ACCREDITATION SYSTEMS

Since the introduction of norms for evaluating and accrediting medical schools in North America by the Liaison Committee on Medical Education (LCME), through the different national initiatives inspired by these and until the more recent publication of international standards by the World Federation of

Medical Education (WFME), the main emphasis has been put on the domain of production, and only minor interest shown in the domains of conceptualisation and usability[14–16] (Table 2).

In 1995, the WHO, in its advocacy role for socially responsive health policies, recommended that principles of social accountability be taken into account in the quality assurance of medical education. The WHO did not make concrete proposals regarding norms and nor did it explicitly encourage countries to avail themselves of revised accreditation systems.[17,18]

Recently, international groups such as the Network towards Unity for Health, via a task force on 'social accountability and accreditation',[19] the Conférence Internationale des Doyens des Facultés de Médecine d'Expression Française (International Organisation of Deans of Francophone Medical Schools, CIDMEF), via its council for evaluation,[20] and the Société Internationale Francophone d'Education Médicale (International Francophone Society of Medical Education, SIFEM), through its working group for 'society and health',[21] have began to support this direction for action. Similarly, the Foundation for the Advancement of International Medical Education and Research (FAIMER), the mandate of which is to develop medical education expertise worldwide, stresses the need for medical education to demonstrate tangible effects for the improvement of the health of populations.[22] Moreover, national health policy analysts, specialised groups in the development of human resources for health, and the United Nations, through Millennium Development Goals, add their support for such a reorientation.[23,24]

Many national and regional efforts are underway to establish accreditation systems. There is a pressing need to launch an initiative that embraces standards based on social accountability before institutions and countries become too firmly engaged in adopting accreditation approaches that do not optimally reflect obligations to society.

TRENDS AND OPPORTUNITIES

As globalisation is reassessed for its social impact, societies will seek to justify their investments with more solid evidence of the impact of these investments on the public good. Medical schools should be prepared to be judged accordingly. Arguments in favour of the CPU model based on ethical, democratic, economic and political issues are presented below.

C Boelen & B Woollard

Table 1 The conceptualisation–production–usability model

Conceptualisation

1 References

    1.1 Values: explicit reference to values (i.e. quality, equity, relevance, effectiveness)

    1.2 Population: reference to population features and priority health needs

    1.3 Health system: reference to health system development for greater coherence and integration

    1.4 Health personnel: reference to qualitative and quantitative needs (see 1.1, 1.2, 1.3)

2 Engagements

    2.1 Mandate: mission and institutional objectives consistent with References

    2.2 Field: involvement in health management of a territory and given population

    2.3 Partnership: institutionalised partnership with key stakeholders, locally and nationally

    2.4 Expected outcome: definition/justification of profile (list of competencies) (see References above)

3 Governance

    3.1 Strategic planning: engagements incorporated in a widely accepted development plan

    3.2 Management: validation, co-ordination and evaluation of implementation of plan

    3.3 Resources: mobilisation of internal and external resources consistent with Engagements (see 2)

Production

4 Field operations: education, research and services activities consistent with Engagements (see 2)

5 Educational programme

    5.1 Objectives and content: consistent with profile of health professional (see 2.4)

    5.2 Curriculum structure: early and longitudinal exposure to priority health issues in the community

    5.3 Learning process: solving complex health problems, both for individuals and communities

    5.4 Practicals: sites prioritising primary health care and linkage with other levels of health service

6 Students

    6.1 Recruitment: equal opportunity and priority to students from underserved communities

    6.2 Career: orientation and assistance to access jobs related to priority health issues

    6.3 Evaluation: reference to the entire spectrum of competencies (see 2.4)

7 Teachers

    7.1 Source: involvement of a variety of teachers from the health and social sectors

    7.2 Abilities: teachers serving as role models, in reference to the profile (see 2.4)

    7.3 Support: training and incentives to improve abilities in public health and medical education

8 Research: related to health system management (see References, section 1, and Usability, sections 10, 11)

9 Service: excellence in primary health care services (see Usability, sections 10, 11)

Usability

10 Employment

    10.1 Job opportunities: advocacy and partnership for emergence of priority health professions

    10.2 Settlement: retention and distribution of graduates according to needs (see 1.1, 1.2)

    10.3 Quality of services: maintenance of competences of graduates (see 2.4)

    10.4 Practice: improving working conditions at primary health care level (see sections 4, 9, 10)

11 Impact

    11.1 Partnership: relationship with stakeholders for improved management of health system

    11.2 Effects on health: risk reduction and health promotion in the field (see 2.2, 2.3, 4)

    11.3 Promotion: dispatching results on usability to decision-making bodies, both local and national

© Blackwell Publishing Ltd 2009. MEDICAL EDUCATION 2009; **43**: 887–894

Table 2 Societal needs and medical education norms

	Conceptualisation	Production	Usability
Current norms	+	+++	+
Desired norms	+++	+++	+++

Ethical issues: causes and consequences

The aim to minimise risks (first, do not harm) in human endeavours that affect people's health is older than the legacy of Hippocrates. Society demands this cautionary principle of its practitioners and, increasingly, of the institutions that produce them. Further, society demands that a relationship be established between decisions for actions and the long-term effects of those actions. Although a direct correlation between educational strategies and population health is not easily demonstrable, proxies exist. We can differentiate a socially accountable institution from one that is not.[1,3] We should also provide evidence that the educational programmes of socially accountable institutions result in the education of health professionals who are responsive to society's priority health care needs.

Democratic issues: openness and transparency

Areas that used to be reserved for experts are increasingly accessible to the public. Wide access to information and the more critical attention of citizens lead to questioning of the management of any institution. The explicit recognition of a socially accountable institution will reassure both its students and the wider public.

Economic issues: results and support

Greater transparency will induce comparisons among institutions. Accreditation norms based on principles of social accountability will enable public authorities, funding agencies and civil society to more knowledgably support those institutions with the capacity for a higher social impact.

Political issues: system approach and enhanced synergies

Good governance of institutions will be defined increasingly by these institutions' capacity to take into account the complexity of the socio-political environment and to take advantage of opportunities to build sustainable partnerships with other institutions with similar or complementary missions. We may anticipate that political authorities will attribute excellence and provide resources preferentially to institutions that show an aptitude to create synergies that induce greater coherence and performance of the health care system.

CONCLUSIONS

Accreditation systems, properly designed and mandated, can be powerful forces for quality and change in any complex system. This is particularly true of the institutions of medical education. Accreditation can support countries in their regulatory obligation to institutionalise quality assurance approaches and guide individual institutions in their development. Therefore, it is very important to pay close attention to developments in this area. There is an urgent need to foster the adaptation of accreditation standards and norms that reflect social accountability. Only then can educational institutions be measured and rewarded for their real capacity to meet the pressing health care needs of society.

Contributors: the authors worked together in an iterative process to conceptualise, execute and revise this paper.
Acknowledgements: none.
Funding: none.
Conflicts of interest: none.
Ethical approval: not applicable.

REFERENCES

1 Woollard R. Caring for a common future: medical schools' social accountability. *Med Educ* 2006;**40**:301–11.
2 Joint Learning Initiative. *Human Resources for Health: Overcoming the Crisis.* Cambridge, MA: President and Fellows of Harvard College 2004.
3 Boelen C, Heck J. *Defining and measuring the social accountability of medical schools.* Geneva: World Health Organization 1995. http://whqlibdoc.who.int/hq/1995/WHO_HRH_95.7_fre.pdf. [Accessed 15 November 2008.]
4 Boelen C. *Towards unity for health: challenges and opportunities for partnership in health development.* Geneva: World Health Organization 2000. http://whqlibdoc.who.int/hq/2000/WHO_EIP_OSD_2000.9.pdf. [Accessed 15 November 2008.]
5 Waldrop M. *Complexity: the Emerging Science at the Edge of Order and Chaos.* New York, NY: Simon & Schuster 1992.

6 Mennin S. Small-group problem-based learning as a complex adaptive system. *Teach Teacher Educ* 2007;**23**:303–13.

7 Glouberman S, Zimmerman B. Complicated and complex systems: what would successful reform of Medicare look like? *Commission on the Future of Health Care in Canada* Discussion Paper No. 8, Government of Canada, July 2002.

8 World Health Organization. *Doctors for Health. Doctors for Health. A WHO global strategy for reorienting medical education and medical practice for Health for All.* Geneva: WHO 1996 (WHO/HRH/96.1).

9 General Medical Council. *Tomorrow's Doctors: Recommendations on Undergraduate Medical Education.* London: GMC 2003. http://www.gmc-uk.org/education/undergraduate/tomdoc.pdf. [Accessed 15 November 2008.]

10 Frank JR, ed. *The CanMEDS 2005 Physician Competency Framework. Better Physicians. Better Care.* Ottawa, ON: Royal College of Physicians and Surgeons of Canada 2005. http://crmcc.medical.org/canmeds/canMEDS2005/index.php. [Accessed 15 November 2008.]

11 American Board of Internal Medicine Foundation, American College of Physicians Foundation, European Federation of Internal Medicine. Medical Professionalism in the New Millennium. A Physician Charter. *Ann Intern Med* 2002;**163**:243–6.

12 Flexner A. *Medical education in the United States and Canada. A report to the Carnegie Foundation for the Advancement of Teaching.* New York, NY: Carnegie Foundation (Bulletin No. 4) 1910.

13 Boelen C. A new paradigm for medical schools a century after Flexner's report. *Bull World Health Organ* 2002;**80**:592–3.

14 Liaison Committee on Medical Education. *Functions and structure of a medical school. Standards for accreditation of medical education programmes leading to the MD degree.* 2008. http://www.lcme.org/functions2008jun.pdf. [Accessed 15 November 2008.]

15 World Federation for Medical Education. *Basic Medical Education Standards. WFME global standards for quality improvement.* Copenhagen: WFME 2003. http://www.wfme.com. [Accessed 15 November 2008.]

16 Karle H. International recognition of basic medical education programmes. *Med Educ* 2008;**42**:12–7.

17 Boelen C, Bandanarayake R, Bouhuijs PAJ, Page GG, Rothman AI. *Towards the assessment of quality in medical education.* Geneva: World Health Organization 1992 (WHO/HRH/92.7).

18 Gastel B, Wilson MP, Boelen C, eds. Toward a global consensus on the quality of medical education: serving the needs of populations and individuals. Proceedings of the 1994 WHO/Educational Commission for Foreign Medical Graduates Invitational Conference, Geneva, 3–4 October 1994. *Acad Med* 1995;**70** (Suppl 7):1–90.

19 World Health Organization Network towards Unity for Health. The Network towards Unity for Health. http://www.the-networktufh.org. [Accessed 15 November 2008.]

20 Conférence Internationale des Doyens de Facultés de Médecine d'Expression Française. *Politique et méthodologie d'évaluation des facultés de médecine et des programmes d'études médicales.* Bordeaux: CIDMEF 2006. http://www.cidmef.u-bordeaux2.fr. [Accessed 15 November 2008.]

21 Société Internationale Francophone d'Education Médicale. *Facultés de médecine et besoins de santé. Vers de nouvelles normes d'évaluation/accréditation.* Grenoble, France: SIFEM 2007. http://www.sifem.net/SanteSociete.php. [Accessed 15 November 2008.]

22 Foundation for the Advancement of International Medical Education and Research. *Improving world health through education.* Philadelphia, USA: FAIMER. http://www.faimer.org. [Accessed 15 November 2008.]

23 World Health Organization. *Global Health Workforce Alliance. Strategic Plan.* Geneva: WHO 2006. http://www.who.int/workforcealliance. [Accessed 15 November 2008.]

24 United Nations. *Millennium Development Goals.* http://www.un.org/milleniumgoals/index.shtml. [Accessed 15 November 2008.]

Received 1 January 2009; accepted for publication 16 April 2009

© Blackwell Publishing Ltd 2009. MEDICAL EDUCATION 2009; **43**: 887–894

CHAPTER 26

Family medicine in Africa

Shabir Moosa

NOMINATED CLASSIC PAPER

Bob Mash, Steve Reid. Statement of consensus on family medicine in Africa. *African Journal of Primary Health Care & Family Medicine*, 2010; 2(1).

This article is important firstly because it is a consensus statement that came from a three-day long participatory process with group discussions involving almost 300 participants, mostly family physicians and mostly from across Africa.

There was an attempt to bring the group discussions together into a coherent whole document, in a very democratic manner, but there is considerable repetition. This serves to underline this participatory process as well as highlight important ideas shared by family physicians from across Africa. These ideas resonate throughout sections of the consensus statement and are important for the rest of the world.

The statement highlights the context of family physicians working in areas with limited resources, and the need to find a balance between equity and quality in healthcare. It also highlights the plight of women affected by global inequity. The response of family physicians should be to stress universal access, not just as an ideal, but also as an ethos of both practice and training. There is considerable emphasis on family physicians playing an advocacy role and leading social accountability, especially in training. African family physicians also see themselves as integral to rational primary healthcare systems that address the needs of the entire population.

Very importantly, the role of the family physicians, in the light of resource constraint, is to locate themselves between district hospitals and small clinics, and within a very strong team-based approach with appropriate task shifting. This shapes their role to be more than just providing clinical services, and includes strong clinical leadership to ensure overall service quality. Family doctors need to look at how they might reconfigure team-based practice for defined communities to ensure the best outcomes including the quality and cost-effectiveness of care.

Lastly, the document emphasises that patient-centred services are not sufficient for health but need the family physician to address the needs of defined communities in an empowering approach.

While Africa will long suffer this yoke of limited resources, the rest of the world is also fast approaching a dire situation with spiralling healthcare expenditures and growing marginalisation of the poor. The document not only presents a strongly contextualised response to the crisis in national health systems in Africa, but also opens up many questions worthy of further exploration globally.

ABOUT THE LEAD AUTHORS OF THIS PAPER

Bob Mash is committed to the development and contribution of primary care doctors and family physicians to health systems in an African context. In the early 1990s, before the fall of Apartheid, he worked with community health workers to offer primary care in townships on the edge of Cape Town in South Africa. Subsequently he worked in the public sector as a family physician in Khayelitsha, a large Xhosa community in Cape Town. In 1997 Bob joined Stellenbosch University where he introduced their first clinical rotation in family medicine and primary care for final year medical students. Subsequently he developed a Masters of Medicine in Family Medicine degree by web-based distance education, which has enabled many African doctors to become family physicians. He obtained his PhD on mental disorders in primary care. He is the editor of the *Handbook of Family Medicine* and the *South African Family Practice Manual*, which have become essential textbooks for training in sub-Saharan Africa. He is now Professor and Head of Family Medicine and Primary Care at Stellenbosch University. Recently he became Editor-in-Chief of the *African Journal of Primary Health Care & Family Medicine* and has been actively supporting the growth of PRIMAFAMED, an educational and research network of Departments of Family Medicine in nations across sub-Saharan Africa.

Steve Reid is a family physician with extensive experience in clinical practice, education and research in the field of rural health in South Africa. He established the Vocational Training Programme for rural doctors at McCord Hospital in Durban and was then appointed director of a research unit called the Centre for Health and Social Studies (CHESS) at the University of Natal, and with his team pursued a number of training and operational research projects in rural districts around KwaZulu-Natal, focused on the strengthening of the district health system. In 2001 the Centre was renamed the Centre for Rural Health, and Steve was appointed Associate Professor in the University of KwaZulu-Natal, with responsibility for community-based education and rural health. He teaches undergraduate and postgraduate students in public health, family medicine and health promotion, around the theme of Community-Oriented Primary Care.

ABOUT THE NOMINATOR OF THIS PAPER

Shabir Moosa is a family physician in the Department of Family Medicine at the University of Witwatersrand in Johannesburg, South Africa. He has a PhD on the emergence of family medicine in Africa. He has a background in rural private practice. He is currently Secretary of the WONCA Africa Executive and involved in developing community practice models for national health insurance.

> 'An expanded family physician role, with clinical teamwork, can address the spiral in healthcare expenditure and the growing marginalisation of millions of people across the world. Every young family doctor needs to understand the sociopolitical world better and explore the strong social activist within to make the world a better place for all.'

Dr Shabir Moosa, South Africa

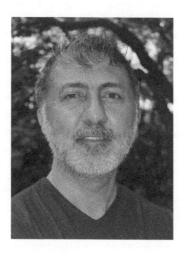

Attribution:

We attribute the original publication of *Statement of consensus on family medicine in Africa* to *African Journal of Primary Health Care & Family Medicine* and the World Organization of Family Doctors (WONCA). With thanks to Bob Mash and Steve Reid.

Conference Report

STATEMENT OF CONSENSUS ON FAMILY MEDICINE IN AFRICA

Authors:
Robert (Bob) Mash[1]
Steve Reid[2]

Affiliations:
[1]Division of Family
Medicine and Primary
Care, Stellenbosch
University, Tygerberg
campus, South Africa

[2]Faculty of Health Sciences,
University of Cape Town,
South Africa

Correspondence to:
Robert (Bob) Mash

email:
rm@sun.ac.za

Postal address:
Division of Family
Medicine and Primary
Care, Stellenbosch
University, PO Box 19063,
Tygerberg 7505,
South Africa

Keywords:
Family Medicine; regional
definition; statement of
consensus; sub-Saharan
Africa; WONCA

Dates:
Received: 10 Dec. 2009
Accepted: 26 Jan. 2010
Published: 12 Mar. 2010

How to cite this article:
Mash R, Reid S. Statement
of consensus on Family
Medicine in Africa. Afr
J Prm Health Care Fam
Med. 2010;2(1), Art. #151,
4 pages. DOI: 10.4102/
phcfm.v2i1.151

**This article is available
at:**
http://www.phcfm.org

© 2010. The Authors.
Licensee: OpenJournals
Publishing. This work
is licensed under the
Creative Commons
Attribution License.

ABSTRACT

Family Medicine is an emerging speciality in sub-Saharan Africa and yet potential interest in the contribution of Family Medicine to health, primary care and district health services is limited by the lack of a regional definition. Governments, health departments and academic institutions would benefit from a clearer understanding of Family Medicine in an African context.

The 2nd African Regional WONCA (World Organisation of Family Doctors) Conference, held in Rustenberg, South Africa in October 2009, engaged participants from sub-Saharan Africa in the development of a consensus statement on Family Medicine. The consensus statement agreed to by the conference defined the contribution of Family Medicine to equity, quality and primary health care within an African context, as well as the role and training requirements of the family physician. Particular attention was given to the contribution of women in Family Medicine.

INTRODUCTION

Points of recognition

The participants at the 2nd African Regional WONCA (World Organisation of Family Doctors) Conference that was held in Rustenburg, South Africa from 25 to 28 October 2009 noted the following:

- the universal and recognised human right to health
- the gross inequalities and disparities in health status and health care within Africa, as well as between Africa and the rest of the world
- the limitation of resources for health care in Africa
- the strength of extended family values, interdependence and community accountability and the continuity between individual, family and community systems in Africa
- the variety of perceptions and beliefs with regard to health care that stem from Africa's cultural, religious and ethnic diversity
- gender inequality and the status of girls' and women's health directly influence the health of families and communities; gender is an important social determinant of health
- the Millennium Development Goal targets to be achieved by 2015
- the significant value of Family Medicine to the quality and equity of health services in many countries around the world
- the support of WONCA, governments, academic institutions, non-governmental organisations, donors and other stakeholders in Family Medicine.

The recognition of these points led to the development of an eight-tiered statement of consensus on the role of Family Medicine in Africa.

STATEMENT OF CONSENSUS

1. The contribution of Family Medicine to equity in health care

1.1. Family Medicine, a core contributor to primary health care, is critical to the achievement of equitable health outcomes for all.
1.2. All people should have equal access to health care. In particular, access should not be limited by the inability to pay, or the lack of health care providers or facilities. Care should be focused on people and not specific diseases, as is the situation with regard to the funding of vertical health programmes. Access should not be limited by geography, culture, gender, religion, administration, policy or disability.
1.3. In order to deliver better health outcomes for all, the principles of Family Medicine should be shared by the whole primary health care team. They include the family physician, the general practitioner, the clinical nurse practitioner, the midwife, mid-level workers (including clinical/medical officers and assistants) and community-based health workers.
1.4. Training institutions should be socially accountable in adequately preparing health workers with the correct knowledge, attitudes and competencies, so that they are able to play their part in the primary care team.
1.5. Family Medicine should advocate for social and health policies that promote equitable health care. For example, health funding should be allocated according to the health needs of the population and incentives should be provided to attract health workers to underserved communities in order to improve the quality of care.
1.6. Family Medicine should advocate for the resolution of conflicts and promote peace as a fundamental prerequisite for the provision of equitable health care.
1.7. Family Medicine should practice cost-effective care in order to attain maximum value from limited resources.
1.8. Family Medicine should contribute to quality care that is not threatened by commercialisation, or by weak services in the public sector.
1.9. Family Medicine should empower people in communities to tackle the social determinants of ill-health.

2. Family Medicine and primary health care

2.1 The concept of comprehensive primary health care and the principles of Family Medicine overlap considerably and should be considered together.

African Journal of Primary Health Care & Family Medicine

Article #151

2.2. The World Health Organization resolutions on strong decentralised district health systems need to be implemented in Africa.

2.3. The clinical practice of Family Medicine is integral to the district health system and includes care at community, clinic, health centre and hospital levels.

2.4. Family Medicine should strive to create an integrated system of health care that includes private, faith-based and traditional health care providers and supports inter-sectoral collaboration and active community participation.

2.5. Family Medicine should be delivered by a team with the appropriate skills mix and strong teamwork.

2.6. Family Medicine plays a clear gate-keeping role in referring patients to the rest of the health care system.

2.7. Public–private partnerships that are socially accountable (e.g. not for profit) have the potential to improve health care outcomes in terms of service delivery, teaching and research.

2.8. All governments in Africa should create viable frameworks to support health for all through the inclusion of family physicians in primary health care teams.

3. The role of the family physician in Africa

3.1. In an African context, the family physician is a clinical leader and consultant in the primary health care team, ensuring primary, continuing, comprehensive, holistic and personalised care of high quality to individuals, families and communities.

3.2. The family physician in Africa operates according to the principles of comprehensive person-centred care, with a family and community orientation, responding to undifferentiated illness and acting as a consultant to the primary health care team.

3.3. The role of the family physician in Africa involves a comprehensive set of skills adapted to the circumstances, local needs, available resources, facilities and the competency and limitations of the practitioner.

3.4. The family physician has a commitment and responsibility to a defined population to whom they are accountable through its representative structure.

3.5. The family physician's role requires close collaboration and teamwork with other members of the primary health care team, especially in the light of specific challenges, such as the insufficient numbers of health care workers.

3.6. The limited human, financial and material resources which exist necessitate skills appropriate to the situation. The family physician's responsibility as consultant and gate-keeper encompasses the economic, effective and efficient use of available resources (human, financial and informational), as well as the ability to prioritise.

3.7. The family physician is also a life-long scholar, which includes a commitment to life-long learning, research and audit, and a responsibility for the continuing education of the primary health care team and community.

3.8. The family physician is an interdisciplinary player, with a pivotal role in the coordination of the primary health care team, including leadership in clinical governance and patient referrals.

3.9. Cultural competency – in relation to language, gender, traditions and religious beliefs – is an essential attribute.

3.10. The family physician must play an advocacy role, both through daily example and through their institutions, by actively identifying with, and advocating for, the poor and marginalised.

3.11. The family physician should generate social and managerial accountability and transparency in terms of effective and efficient health care delivery.

3.12. Family physicians have a responsibility for health resource and service management based on their clinical understanding and should have direct access to District Health Management Teams.

3.13. The family physician may focus on various areas of special interest at different times in their career. At the same time, they must remain competent across a broad scope of practice as a generalist.

4. The African context and community

4.1. Family Medicine is community-based and must be embedded in all settings within the District Health System.

4.2. Family Medicine practice should always be community-oriented and context-specific. The starting point is a defined community. Family physicians' care for individuals is informed by their community orientation, with their community role arising out of their clinical role. Community-oriented primary care is one tool that family physicians can use to make the link between individual and community care.

4.3. Family physicians must consistently be aware of, and continue to address, the priority health needs of the community.

4.4. Family physicians are committed to improving the health of all the people in the communities they serve, not just those who are able to access care. They must be recognised and rewarded for the quality of care and the improved health of all members of the community.

4.5. Context is critical for training and should, to a large extent, determine the curriculum. Family physicians must be provided with the appropriate contextual training that will enable them to identify and address community needs.

4.6. Family physicians must understand, be sensitive to, and work within, the culture of the community, as well as the ongoing changes to this culture. Family physicians must respect the family and community values of the people they serve, encouraging those that support positive health outcomes.

4.7. Family physicians must work with, and in, teams that are defined by the context, as team members and not only as leaders. They play a supportive and consultative role in the primary health care team.

4.8. Appropriate resources must be allocated for community-based training, research and practice.

5. Quality of Family Medicine practice in Africa

5.1. Family Medicine regards good clinical governance and quality of primary health care as fundamental to the profession. This will be achieved through sound training and maintained by continuous, peer-reviewed, medical education that is formally accredited.

5.2. Family physicians should perform regular reviews and audits to enable reflection on their work and service, building on strengths and correcting weaknesses in the primary health care system on a regular basis.

5.3. Appropriate tools and systems for the evaluation of Family Medicine practice need to be developed, and indicators defined to benchmark practice in Africa. This should be based on key domains of quality, which include cost effectiveness, safety, equity, continuity of care and patient satisfaction.

5.4. It is recognised that maintaining the quality of services requires well-motivated family physicians working within an environment that provides adequate human and physical resources.

5.5. Quality service must be rewarded.

5.6. The practice of Family Medicine should, as far as possible, be evidence-based.

6. Family physician training in sub-Saharan Africa

6.1. Training should take place in all the District Health Services where teachers of Family Medicine function, with in-patient, out-patient, and outreach programmes.

Article #151   African Journal of Primary Health Care & Family Medicine

6.2. Both full-time residential and part-time training programmes may be necessary to maximise training opportunities.

6.3. Teaching sites must be of sufficient size, with a 'critical mass' of trainers to create teaching and practice centres of excellence.

6.4. Experience in the management of chronic disease and undifferentiated illness should be part of the training throughout the programme.

6.5. Research must be included in all graduate programmes.

6.6. Training should include cross-cutting themes of specific relevance to Family Medicine, such as communication and consultation skills, reflective practice, holistic care, health systems management, and how to teach.

6.7. Training should be outcome- and competency-based.

6.8. Training should have a strong academic (university-based) foundation.

6.9. The principles of Family Medicine should be introduced early in undergraduate medical training and continue throughout the training.

6.10. Internship programmes should include rotations with exposure to family physicians and Family Medicine registrars.

6.11. Length of postgraduate Family Medicine training should be sufficient to teach core competencies and prepare for life-long learning. The length of the program must take into account the local postgraduate university requirements.

6.12. All relevant stakeholders (e.g. Ministries of Health and Education, Medical Councils, and professional organisations) should ideally be involved from the start of Family Medicine training programmes.

6.13. Trained and qualified family physicians should have consultant status and be remunerated at the same level as other specialists.

6.14. Family physicians should be locally produced and of international standard.

6.15. The family physician should be involved in the training of medical personnel in the public and the private sectors. Private-sector facilities may form part of the training sites for undergraduate students.

6.16. The family physician should collaborate with general practitioners in the development of clinical guidelines.

6.17. Training of family physicians should include an understanding of traditional health practices and integrative medicine.

6.18. Training should have equivalent length to other specialities, especially with the need for procedural skills in an African context.

6.19. Training should allow registrarship in Family Medicine during community service.

6.20. Training should be outcome-based and the location of training will depend on the learning opportunities offered.

6.21. The rotation of a specific registrar must depend on their prior skills and competency.

7. Women in Family Medicine in Africa

7.1. WONCA Africa Region commits to uphold: the Hamilton Equity regulations, the Ten Steps to Gender Equity, and the by-law changes pertaining to equity within the governance and activities of the organisation, as proposed by the WONCA Working Party on Women and Family Medicine – recommended by the WONCA Executive, and due to be approved by WONCA World Council.

7.2. All family physicians need to be advocates for gender equality; female practitioners should act as role models for girls in general, as well as for female patients and colleagues.

7.3. The Life Care Model adopted by WONCA internationally should be promoted in Africa (see Table 1).

7.4. Leadership amongst female family physicians should be promoted and supported at all levels, leading to proportional representation in leadership positions within the next 5 years.

7.5. A network of female family physicians should be developed.

7.6. Gender-based research and empowerment of female researchers should be promoted.

8. Nomenclature

8.1. The term 'family doctor' should be understood as referring to the following: family physician, general practitioner, or medical officer.

8.2. A family physician has postgraduate training in Family Medicine. The term 'family physician' should be the nomenclature in Africa.

8.3. A medical officer is a generalist in the public sector, without postgraduate training.

DEVELOPMENT PROCESS

The consensus statement was the result of a participatory process which culminated in an African Regional WONCA conference. In the year preceding the conference, a number of initiatives prepared the ground for the development of a consensus statement. These initiatives included:

- May 2008: Publication of a study, 'Exploring the key principles of Family Medicine in sub-Saharan Africa: International Delphi consensus process', that enabled an expert panel to reach consensus on the key principles of Family Medicine.[1]

- Primafamed Conference, Kampala, Uganda, 17–22 November 2008: 'Improving the quality of Family Medicine training in sub-Saharan Africa'. This conference enabled dialogue between family physicians in sub-Saharan Africa. The initial conference themes and plans for discussion papers emerged from the dialogue at this conference.

- Discussion papers on all the key themes (except Women in Family Medicine, which was a late submission) were written and published in the WONCA Regional Conference brochure, as well as on the WONCA website. These discussion papers were designed to stimulate initial thinking and debate at the conference.

- The WONCA Working Party on Women in Family Practice held a pre-conference workshop during which their recommendations were generated.

- The conference was attended by 294 participants from various African countries and elsewhere (see acknowledgements). The conference was designed around eight themes that had been previously identified at the regional Primafamed Conference and by the scientific committee.

TABLE 1
The Life Care Model

Motivate and empower every girl-child towards a professional career.

Address equity in university selection, enrolment and in terms of admission policies.

Be flexible, where appropriate, in extending the academic training period.

Create a grandmother clause for general practitioners who missed the new formal family medicine training due to family responsibilities.

Lobby for the removal of an age limit for postgraduate studies and scholarships.

'Stay-at-home' family physicians to be targeted for ongoing continuing professional development.

Revise public service standing orders to be gender sensitive, such as appropriate flexible working hours and placements near families.

In terms of promotion, defined family responsibility activities should be considered, possibly using a points system.

Sexual harassment policies be developed and implemented.

Security precautions for remote travel, night work and other vulnerable situations should be provided.

Gender-based violence against female family physicians must be acknowledged as a risk, recognised and managed.

After retirement, female family physicians to be employed as resource persons.

African Journal of Primary Health Care & Family Medicine

Article #151

These themes were:

1. African context and community
2. Primary health care and health systems
3. Training in Family Medicine
4. Ensuring quality of care
5. Role and scope of practice of the family practitioner
6. Equity and Family Medicine
7. Private practice, faith-based hospitals and private–public partnerships
8. African family values and women in Family Medicine.

Key note speakers, in addition to the discussion papers on each theme, were included in the conference programme to stimulate dialogue. The conference itself was designed as a participatory process, whereby all the participants signed up to a small group of their choice which focused on one of the conference theme areas. Each small group consisting of a maximum of 20 people, met twice over a total period of 4 hours and, after deliberation, created a 250 word statement on their theme, to be included as a paragraph in the final conference statement. Each group was led by a facilitator and utilised a modified nominal group technique to prioritise the group's recommendations. Facilitators who led groups on the same theme gave feedback to one another halfway through the small group process and, at the end, combined their recommendations into one joint paragraph.

The final paragraphs on each theme were presented to a plenary session and discussed by all the conference participants. Participants in the plenary session had the opportunity to suggest amendments and additions to the wording of the paragraphs. Following this, the revised paragraphs were voted on, point by point by a show of hands in the final plenary session. If the total number of those who abstained, or those who disagreed with a point in the statement was more than 25% of those present in the final plenary session, then the point was excluded from the final consensus statement (see Table 2). The reason for rejection was not clarified, but, in addition to disagreement with the concept, may also have been because of poor wording or duplication elsewhere.

ACKNOWLEDGEMENTS

The following people contributed to the development of the consensus statement at the WONCA conference:

- Editors and co-ordinators of the consensus process: Mash B (South Africa), Reid S (South Africa).
- Scientific committee: Reid S (Chairman), Chandia J, Mash B, Ndimande J, Ogunbanjo G, Steinberg J, van Deventer C.
- Facilitators of small groups: Bevins B (Kenya), Chege P (Kenya), Dahlman B (Kenya), Downing R (Kenya), Thigiti J (Kenya), Couper I (South Africa), Govender S (South Africa), Hugo J (South Africa), Mabuza H (South Africa), Moosa S (South Africa), Ndimande J (South Africa), Reid S (South Africa), Steinberg H (South Africa), van Deventer C (South Africa), Mugisha N (Uganda).

There were a total of 294 participants from the following countries: Belgium, Botswana, Democratic Republic of the Congo, Denmark, Finland, Ghana, India, Kenya, Lesotho, Mozambique, Namibia, Nigeria, South Africa, Rwanda, Sudan, Tanzania, Uganda, United Kingdom, USA, Zambia, and Zimbabwe.

REFERENCES

1. Mash R, Downing R, Moosa S, de Maeseneer J. Exploring the key principles of Family Medicine in sub-Saharan Africa: International Delphi consensus process SA Fam Pract. 2008:50(3);60–65.

Article #151

African Journal of Primary Health Care & Family Medicine

TABLE 2
Rejected statements

Family Medicine can and will improve equity and quality of service delivery with a comprehensive approach and the essential human element.

The family physician is complemented by and collaborates with other generalists and specialists.

The family physician in Africa has a leading role in surgical, procedural and emergency care, at the district hospital level.

Faith-based hospitals tend to survive difficult times (e.g. wars) and are therefore fairly stable education and training sites.

Traditional health practitioners, as defined by WHO, form an integral part of the primary health care team in Africa.

A general practitioner is a generalist in independent private practice, without postgraduate training.

A medical officer is a generalist, in private-sector or public-sector practice, without postgraduate training.

CHAPTER 27

Multimorbidity

Amanda Howe

NOMINATED CLASSIC PAPER

Karen Barnett, Stewart Mercer, Michael Norbury, Graham Watt, Sally Wyke, Bruce Guthrie. Epidemiology of multimorbidity and implications for health care, research, and medical education: a cross-sectional study. *The Lancet*, 2012: 380(9836): 37–43.

This paper won the 'Research Paper of the Year' award in 2013 from the Royal College of General Practitioners in the United Kingdom. It combines rigorous analysis and extensive data collection from 1.75 million patients, asking a really important research question: do people from lower socioeconomic backgrounds suffer more co-morbidity (multiple illnesses)? The short answer is yes – they get sicker younger, more frequently have several illnesses, lose more years of healthy life, and get mental illness earlier too. It also makes the important point that doctors and teams who work in poorer communities will have higher workloads, and will need better resourcing if they are to meet the demands of their sicker population.

The paper has a really strong 'family medicine' worldview – it looks at people rather than single diseases, and frames its intention to ensure these findings inform government and health services. It challenges us to change a demand-led service, where fitter richer adults take up the bulk of doctor and nurse time, to one that is needs-led, where efforts are made to target the most 'at risk' groups with preventive care at an early stage. The paper also demonstrates what amazing research can be done by large-scale data pooling across practices with almost a third of the Scottish population contributing to the study through data from their family practice records.

The funding came from the Scottish government, so this was a partnership model between academics and politicians aiming to answer important population health questions, and demonstrating the value of primary care research to policy-makers.

This paper matters because it tells us a huge amount about the consequences of socioeconomic inequality and the adverse effects of some social determinants of health. It is highly technical work, but clearly written, and with important messages for patients, clinicians and policy-makers. It also shows us that family practice is a crucial setting for research into population health.

ABOUT THE AUTHORS OF THIS PAPER

This paper was published as part of a programme of research on multimorbidity led by Professor Stewart Mercer from Glasgow University, and was funded by the Chief Scientist Office of the Scottish Government from 2009 to 2104. The team included Professor Bruce Guthrie from the University of Dundee, who led the epidemiology work, and Professors Graham Watt and Sally Wyke, also from Glasgow University. Stewart Mercer leads the Scottish School of Primary Care Multimorbidity Research theme, and is internationally recognised for his research on multimorbidity. Bruce Guthrie is an academic general practitioner (GP) who leads the Scottish Primary Care Research Network, and is internationally recognised for his work on primary care quality and safety. Graham Watt is an academic GP, who led the development of the 'GPs at the Deep End' group, and is internationally recognised for his work on deprivation and the 'inverse care law'. Sally Wyke is a primary care social scientist and Deputy Director of the Institute of Health and Wellbeing at Glasgow University, and is internationally recognised for her work on the application of social science to complex interventions. Dr Karen Barnett is a post-doctoral researcher who did much of the analysis and initial drafting, and Dr Mike Norbury was an 'early career' GP on an academic fellowship who assisted with the literature and writing up.

ABOUT THE NOMINATOR OF THIS PAPER

Professor Amanda Howe is President of WONCA (2016–2018), a family doctor, Professor of Primary Care and International Director at the Norwich Medical School at the University of East Anglia in the United Kingdom. She became involved in academic work while running a general practice in a very deprived community in the north of England, and values good research for its help with patients' needs.

> 'Family doctors need to support research done through their own communities, because it allows us to discover answers to real-world problems. By making the extra effort to collect data, collaborate with academics, and learn how to produce and evaluate new knowledge, we find the evidence we need to explain what is happening to our patients – and make the case for their needs.'

Professor Amanda Howe OBE, United Kingdom

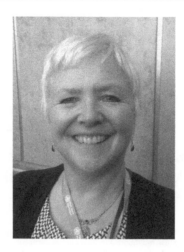

Attribution:

'Special Credit'. Reprinted with permission from Elsevier (*The Lancet*, 2012: 380 (9836): 37–43). With thanks to Lakshmi Priya and the publisher.

Articles

Epidemiology of multimorbidity and implications for health care, research, and medical education: a cross-sectional study

Karen Barnett, Stewart W Mercer, Michael Norbury, Graham Watt, Sally Wyke, Bruce Guthrie

Summary

Background Long-term disorders are the main challenge facing health-care systems worldwide, but health systems are largely configured for individual diseases rather than multimorbidity. We examined the distribution of multimorbidity, and of comorbidity of physical and mental health disorders, in relation to age and socioeconomic deprivation.

Methods In a cross-sectional study we extracted data on 40 morbidities from a database of 1 751 841 people registered with 314 medical practices in Scotland as of March, 2007. We analysed the data according to the number of morbidities, disorder type (physical or mental), sex, age, and socioeconomic status. We defined multimorbidity as the presence of two or more disorders.

Findings 42·2% (95% CI 42·1–42·3) of all patients had one or more morbidities, and 23·2% (23·08–23·21) were multimorbid. Although the prevalence of multimorbidity increased substantially with age and was present in most people aged 65 years and older, the absolute number of people with multimorbidity was higher in those younger than 65 years (210 500 vs 194 996). Onset of multimorbidity occurred 10–15 years earlier in people living in the most deprived areas compared with the most affluent, with socioeconomic deprivation particularly associated with multimorbidity that included mental health disorders (prevalence of both physical and mental health disorder 11·0%, 95% CI 10·9–11·2% in most deprived area vs 5·9%, 5·8%–6·0% in least deprived). The presence of a mental health disorder increased as the number of physical morbidities increased (adjusted odds ratio 6·74, 95% CI 6·59–6·90 for five or more disorders vs 1·95, 1·93–1·98 for one disorder), and was much greater in more deprived than in less deprived people (2·28, 2·21–2·32 vs 1·08, 1·05–1·11).

Interpretation Our findings challenge the single-disease framework by which most health care, medical research, and medical education is configured. A complementary strategy is needed, supporting generalist clinicians to provide personalised, comprehensive continuity of care, especially in socioeconomically deprived areas.

Funding Scottish Government Chief Scientist Office.

Lancet 2012; **380**: 37–43

Published Online
May 10, 2012

DOI:10.1016/S0140-6736(12)60240-2

See Comment page 7

Quality, Safety and Informatics Research Group, Population Health Sciences Division, University of Dundee, Dundee, UK (K Barnett PhD, M Norbury MBChB, Prof B Guthrie PhD); Institute of Health and Wellbeing, General Practice and Primary Care (Prof S W Mercer PhD, Prof G Watt MD), and Institute of Health and Wellbeing, College of Social Sciences (Prof S Wyke PhD), University of Glasgow, Glasgow, UK

Correspondence to:
Prof Bruce Guthrie, Quality, Safety and Informatics Research Group, Population Health Sciences Division, University of Dundee, Dundee DD2 4BF, UK
b.guthrie@dundee.ac.uk

Introduction

Management of the rising prevalence of long-term disorders is the main challenge facing governments and health-care systems worldwide.[1] Although individual diseases dominate health-care delivery, medical research, and medical education, people with multimorbidity—those with two or more chronic morbidities—need a broader approach. Use of many services to manage individual diseases can become duplicative and inefficient, and is burdensome and unsafe for patients because of poor coordination and integration.[2–4] Multimorbidity becomes progressively more common with age[5–7] and is associated with high mortality,[8] reduced functional status,[9,10] and increased use of both inpatient and ambulatory health care.[2,7] Estimates of the prevalence of multimorbidity vary widely; most studies have counted small numbers of morbidities, frequently based on self-reports, and focused on either older people or hospital populations.[11]

Although the association between socioeconomic status and prevalence of individual chronic diseases is well established,[12,13] few studies have examined the association between multimorbidity and socioeconomic status.[6,7,14] In the most deprived 10% of the Scottish population, men

have life expectancies 13 years shorter, and women 9 years shorter, than do those in the most affluent 10%. The most deprived people spend twice as many years in poor health before they die than do the most affluent (10·3 years vs 5·5 years for men; 14·4 years vs 6·0 years for women).[15]

Better understanding of the epidemiology of multimorbidity is necessary to develop interventions to prevent it, reduce its burden, and align health-care services more closely with patients' needs. We aimed to use a large, representative primary medical care electronic database to examine the distribution of multimorbidity in relation to age and socioeconomic deprivation, and the relation between comorbidity of physical and mental health disorders and deprivation.

Methods

Study design and participants

Our study is a cross-sectional analysis of a national dataset held by the Primary Care Clinical Informatics Unit at the University of Aberdeen, UK. The dataset consisted of complete copies of clinical data for all registered patients from 314 medical practices caring for about a third of the Scottish population. The UK National Health Service (NHS) requires registration with a medical practice to access health-care services for people living at home or in nursing care homes. The NHS National Research Ethics Service had previously approved the anonymous use of these data for research purposes, therefore this study did not need individual ethics approval.

Data collection

At the time of data extraction, participating practices systematically used electronic medical records for registration of patients, morbidity recording, and prescriptions. The data for this analysis are from all patients who were alive and permanently registered with a participating practice on March 31, 2007. The dataset included age, sex, and socioeconomic status, and is representative of all Scottish patients.[16] Deprivation of the area in which a

See Online for appendix

	n (%)	Mean number of morbidities (SD)*	Percentage (95% CI) with multimorbidity†	Percentage (95% CI) with physical-mental health comorbidity†
All patients	1751841 (100%)	0·96 (1·56)	23·2% (23·1–23·2)	8·34% (8·3–8·4)
Sex				
Female	884420 (50·5%)	1·09 (1·65)	26·2% (26·1–26·3)	10·2% (10·2–10·3)
Male	867421 (49·5%)	0·84 (1·46)	20·1% (20·0–20·1)	6·4% (6·4–6·5)
Age, years				
0–24	479156 (27·4%)	0·16 (0·44)	1·9% (1·9–2·0)	0·5% (0·5–0·6)
25–44	508389 (29·0%)	0·50 (0·92)	11·3% (11·2–11·4)	5·7% (5·6–5·7)
45–64	473127 (27·0%)	1·18 (1·50)	30·4% (30·2–30·5)	12·4% (12·3–12·5)
65–84	254600 (14·5%)	2·60 (2·09)	64·9% (64·7–65·1)	17·5% (17·4–17·7)
≥85	36569 (2·1%)	3·62 (2·30)	81·5% (81·1–81·9)	30·8% (30·3–31·3)
Deprivation decile				
1 (affluent)	163283 (9·3%)	0·82 (1·42)	19·5% (19·3–19·6)	5·9% (5·8–6·0)
2	171296 (9·8%)	0·83 (1·44)	19·9% (19·7–20·1)	6·2% (6·1–6·3)
3	165199 (9·4%)	0·92 (1·50)	22·2% (22·0–22·4)	7·0% (6·9–7·1)
4	207129 (11·8%)	0·95 (1·54)	23·0% (22·9–23·2)	7·5% (7·4–7·7)
5	198419 (11·3%)	1·02 (1·60)	24·5% (24·3–24·7)	8·6% (8·5–8·7)
6	198526 (11·3%)	0·97 (1·57)	23·4% (23·2–23·5)	8·4% (8·3–8·5)
7	186083 (10·6%)	1·00 (1·59)	24·4% (24·2–24·6)	9·1% (9·0–9·2)
8	147836 (8·4%)	1·00 (1·59)	24·2% (24·0–24·4)	9·3% (9·2–9·5)
9	164386 (9·4%)	1·09 (1·70)	26·3% (26·1–26·5)	10·7% (10·6–10·9)
10 (deprived)	149684 (8·5%)	1·01 (1·65)	24·1% (23·9–24·4)	11·0% (10·9–11·2)
Number of disorders				
0	1012980 (57·8%)	..	..	..
1	333365 (19·0%)	..	..	..
2	167518 (9·6%)	..	..	22·2% (22·0–22·4)
3	99487 (5·7%)	..	..	36·1% (35·8–36·4)
4	60417 (3·4%)	..	..	44·8% (44·4–45·2)
5	35641 (2·0%)	..	..	52·1% (51·6–52·6)
6	20507 (1·2%)	..	..	59·0% (58·3–59·7)
7	11080 (0·6%)	..	..	65·7% (64·8–66·6)
≥8	10846 (0·6%)	..	..	73·9% (73·1–74·7)

*Differences between means within each variable differed significantly p<0·0001 (t test for independent samples for sex; one-way ANOVA for age-group and deprivation) †Differences between categories within each variable differed significantly p<0·0001 (χ² test for 2×n tables).

Table 1: Demography, multimorbidity, and physical–mental health comorbidity

patient lived was used to define socioeconomic status, and was measured by Carstairs score (grouped into tenths of the distribution), which uses census and other routine data, and is widely used for research.[17]

No standard approach for the measurement of multimorbidity exists, and selection and definition of morbidities to include is inevitably partly subjective and dependent on the data available. We specifically sought to include morbidities recommended as core for any multimorbidity measure by a systematic review,[11] diseases in the quality and outcomes framework (QOF) of the UK general practice contract,[18] and long-term disorders identified as important by NHS Scotland.[19] We selected 40 such morbidities, which were defined by Read codes (the clinical coding system used in UK general practice to record patient findings and procedures in health-care IT systems) and prescription data. When possible, we based our morbidity definitions on QOF business rules[18] and Read code groups for long-term disorders (as defined by NHS Scotland).[19] When coding definitions were unavailable or did not apply to the available routine data, the clinicians in our team (BG, SM, MN, and GW) agreed new definitions by discussion. The appendix provides further detail of definitions and the 40 morbidities included. As in most other studies, we defined multimorbidity as the presence of two or more of these 40 morbidities in one patient.[11] To specifically examine comorbidity of physical and mental health disorders, we also defined each morbidity as either a physical or mental health disorder.

Statistical analyses

We used frequencies, percentages, cross tabulations, and graphical display for descriptive analysis. We did a *t* test to analyse differences in mean number of morbidities between men and women and one-way ANOVA for differences across age groups and deprivation deciles. We applied the χ^2 test to measure differences in prevalence of multimorbidity and physical–mental health comorbidity between variables. We used binary logistic regression to examine associations between physical and mental health comorbidities, restricting the analysis to those aged 16 years and older because mental health morbidities in children are rare. Since the association with age is roughly quadratic in adults, we also fitted a term for age-squared. We reported unadjusted and adjusted odds ratios (ORs) and 95% CIs. We did all analyses with PASW Statistics (version 18).

Role of the funding source

The sponsor of the study had no role in study design, data collection, data analysis, data interpretation, or writing of the report, or the decision to submit for publication. The corresponding author had full access to all the data in the study and had final responsibility for the decision to submit for publication.

Results

We analysed data from 1751841 patients (about a third of the Scottish population) from 314 Scottish medical practices. Table 1 shows the demographic characteristics of the study population, the proportion of those with multimorbidity, and the proportion with physical and mental health comorbidity. Men and women were equally represented, as were all deprivation deciles. 42·2% (95% CI 42·1–42·3) of the population had one or more chronic morbidities, 23·2% (23·1–23·2) had multimorbidity, and 8·3% (8·3–8·4) had physical and mental health comorbidity. Of people with at least one morbidity, 54·9% (54·8–55·0) had multimorbidity and 19·8% (19·8–19·9) had physical and mental health comorbidity. Most people with common chronic morbidities had at least two, and frequently more, other disorders (appendix).

The number of morbidities and the proportion of people with multimorbidity increased substantially with age (table 1). By age 50 years, half of the population had at least one morbidity, and by age 65 years most were multimorbid (figure 1). However, in absolute terms, more people with multimorbidity were younger than 65 years than 65 years and older (210500 vs 194966), although older people had more morbidities on average (table 1).

The crude prevalence of multimorbidity increased modestly with the deprivation of the area in which patients lived (19·5%, 95% CI 19·3–19·6, in the most affluent areas vs 24·1%, 23·9–24·4, in the most deprived; difference 4·6%, 95% CI 4·3–4·9; table 1). However, this finding should be interpreted with caution because the population in more deprived areas was, on average, younger (median age 37 years [IQR 21–53] in the most deprived areas vs 42 years [IQR 22–58] in the most affluent areas). People living in more deprived areas were more likely to be multimorbid than were those living in the most affluent areas at all ages, apart from those aged 85 years and older (figure 2). Young and middle-aged adults living in the most deprived areas had rates of multimorbidity equivalent to those aged 10–15 years older in the most affluent areas (figure 2 and appendix).

8·3% (95% CI 8·3–8·4) of all patients, and 36·0% (35·9–36·2) of people with multimorbidity, had both a physical and a mental health disorder. The prevalence of physical and mental health comorbidity was higher in women than in men, and was substantially higher in older people than in younger people (table 1). Although older people were much more likely to have physical–mental health comorbidity, the absolute numbers were greater in younger people (90139 people <65 years vs 55912 people ≥65 years). The crude socioeconomic gradient in physical–mental health comorbidity was greater than that for any multimorbidity, with a near doubling in prevalence in the most deprived versus the most affluent areas (table 1; difference 5·1%, 95% CI 4·9–5·3). In the logistic regression analysis with the presence of any mental health

disorder as the outcome (table 2), we noted a non-linear association with age, so we included an age-squared term in the model. The predicted probability of having a mental health disorder increased with age up until about age 60 years, and then decreased (data not shown). Men were less likely to have a mental health disorder than were women, and those in the most deprived decile were more than twice as likely to have a mental health disorder than were those in the most affluent decile (adjusted OR 2·28, 95% CI 2·21–2·32). The presence of a mental health disorder was strongly associated with the number of physical disorders that an individual had—eg, people with five or more disorders had an OR of 6·74 (95% CI

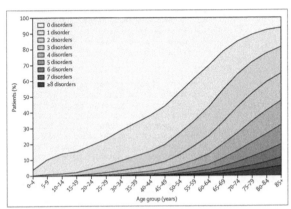

Figure 1: Number of chronic disorders by age-group

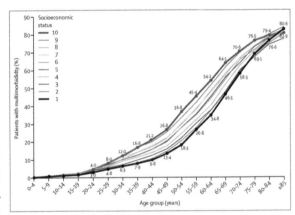

Figure 2: Prevalence of multimorbidity by age and socioeconomic status
On socioeconomic status scale, 1=most affluent and 10=most deprived.

Articles

6·59–6·90) compared with those with none (table 2). Figure 3 shows the consistent and large socioeconomic gradient in the presence of any mental health disorder by number of physical disorders.

Despite the most affluent people being on average 2–5 years older at onset of morbidity (dependent on the

	Any mental health disorder (unadjusted OR, 95% CI)	Any mental health disorder (adjusted OR, 95% CI)*
Male (vs female)	0·66 (0·66–0·67)	0·71 (0·70–0·71)
Age†	1·64 (1·62–1·66)	1·64 (1·62–1·66)
Age squared†	0·972 (0·971–0·974)	0·954 (0·953–0·955)
Deprivation decile		
1 (affluent)	1	1
2	1·07 (1·05–1·10)	1·08 (1·05–1·11)
3	1·21 (1·18–1·24)	1·17 (1·15–1·20)
4	1·32 (1·29–1·35)	1·26 (1·23–1·29)
5	1·52 (1·49–1·57)	1·44 (1·41–1·47)
6	1·53 (1·50–1·56)	1·48 (1·45–1·52)
7	1·66 (1·63–1·70)	1·60 (1·56–1·63)
8	1·78 (1·74–1·82)	1·75 (1·71–1·79)
9	2·00 (1·96–2·05)	1·91 (1·87–1·96)
10 (deprived)	2·19 (2·15–2·24)	2·28 (2·21–2·32)
Number of physical disorders		
0	1	1
1	2·09 (2·06–2·11)	1·95 (1·93–1·98)
2	3·16 (3·12–3·21)	2·95 (2·90–3·00)
3	4·07 (4·00–4·14)	3·91 (3·83–3·98)
4	4·88 (4·78–4·98)	4·85 (4·74–4·96)
≥5	6·43 (6·31–6·56)	6·74 (6·59–6·90)

*All adjusted for other listed variables in model. †ORs are per 10-year increase in age.

Table 2: **Odds ratios (OR) for any mental health disorder by age, sex, socioeconomic status, and number of physical disorders**

disorder), comorbidities of people diagnosed with coronary heart disease, diabetes, chronic obstructive pulmonary disease, or cancer were more common in people living in deprived areas, with the exception of dementia and atrial fibrillation, in which a small reverse gradient was seen (figure 4). People living in deprived areas were much more likely to have chronic obstructive pulmonary disease, depression, and painful disorders as comorbidities than other disorders (figure 4).

Discussion

By contrast with the assumptions implicit in health-care organisation, our analysis of a large, nationally representative primary care dataset shows that multimorbidity is common, and that most of those with a long-term disorder are multimorbid. The strong association of multimorbidity with age is well recognised, but three other aspects of our findings are new or less well described. First, although the prevalence of multimorbidity is much higher in older people than in young or middle-aged people, more than half of people with multimorbidity and nearly two-thirds with physical–mental health comorbidity were younger than 65 years.[20] Second, although age had the strongest association with multimorbidity, we noted a substantial excess of multimorbidity in young and middle-aged adults living in the most deprived areas who had the same prevalence of multimorbidity as people aged about 10–15 years older living in the most affluent areas.[14] Whether this excess of multimorbidity in socioeconomically deprived people is a result of a concentration of common causes such as smoking, which would be amenable to preventive interventions affecting several diseases, or an accumulation of disparate causes, which would be harder to prevent, is unclear. Third, our study agrees with previous work showing that mental health disorders, particularly depression, are more prevalent in people with increasing numbers of physical disorders,[21,22] but it also shows that this association has a consistent social gradient. This data strongly suggests that clinicians working in highly deprived areas treating patients with common physical disorders have a greater number of both physical and mental health disorders to manage simultaneously than do their colleagues working in the most affluent areas, with substantially more depression in particular. Additionally, women had higher rates of multimorbidity than did men, and consistently higher rates of mental health disorders. Detailed examination of this finding was beyond the scope of our broad descriptive analysis, but would be useful in future research.

The study used a large primary-care database that is representative of the wider population. Because we used routine data, our study shares the limitations of other multimorbidity studies, particularly reliance on the quality of data recording. Some morbidities are probably under-recorded, implying that the findings underestimate the true prevalence of multimorbidity. Furthermore, no standard method for measuring multimorbidity exists.

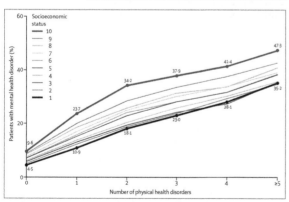

Figure 3: **Physical and mental health comorbidity and the association with socioeconomic status**
On socioeconomic status scale, 1=most affluent and 10=most deprived.

We used standardised definitions of individual morbidities when possible and, unlike most previous studies, we have explicitly reported the assumptions and limitations of our approach to make the design open to critique (appendix). We included 40 morbidities, which is substantially more than most similar studies, and incorporated those recommended as core disorders for any multimorbidity measure by the most recent systematic review at the time of our study.[11] We included morbidities that are not always thought of as clear-cut diseases because these morbidities play an important part in patients' ill health.

Our analysis weights all disorders equally, with a simple count to define multimorbidity, although the effect of multimorbidity on individuals will vary with the combination and severity of disorders. Older people typically have more morbidities and lower functional status, whereas multimorbidity in younger people is more often associated with combinations of physical and mental health disorders. Challenges presented by both age groups will probably call for different organisation of care to meet patients' needs.

People with multimorbidity have poorer functional status, quality of life, and health outcomes, and are higher users of ambulatory and inpatient care than are those without multimorbidity.[2,8–10] Although the quality of health care that they receive might be better than that for individuals with only one disorder, at least partly because of greater contact with health services,[23] people with multimorbidity have more difficulties with fragmentation of care and medical error because much specialist care is focused on treatment of one disease.[4] Improvement in the continuity and coordination of care for people with multimorbidity is a key challenge for health-care systems worldwide, and each patient needs a dedicated clinician to take responsibility for care coordination.[24]

The right clinician to take overall responsibility for people with multimorbidity will depend on individual circumstances.[24] For patients in whom one disease is dominant or comorbidities are closely related, a specialist will often be the best choice. For most multimorbid patients, however, a generalist service is needed. Geriatricians have a key role in provision of care for the frailest elderly patients with predominantly physical disorders, but in most countries most elderly people will be treated in primary care. Our data show that people younger than 65 years have as much multimorbidity as do older people, and that physical–mental health comorbidity is very common. For this younger age group, no equivalent to the geriatrician exists, and specialists are often reluctant to provide care or coordination outside their area of expertise. Person-centred approaches, together with longlasting doctor–patient relationships, should help clinicians and patients when making decisions that have to balance biotechnical rationales with patients' circumstances, priorities, and preferences.[25] A strong, generalist primary care system based around an

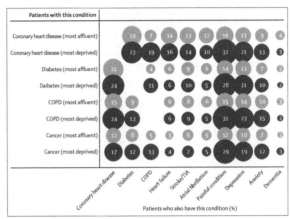

Figure 4: Selected comorbidities in people with four common, important disorders in the most affluent and most deprived deciles
COPD=chronic obstructive pulmonary disease. TIA=transient ischaemic attack.

appropriately skilled multiprofessional team is the most obvious way to deliver this holistic, longitudinal care for most people with multiple disorders, and should seek to maximise quality of life and minimise future disability and morbidity.[3,25]

Countries with strong primary health-care systems have better health outcomes and lower health-care costs than do those without,[3,25] but primary care is weak and underdeveloped worldwide, and even countries with strong primary care systems face substantial challenges from ageing populations and increasing multimorbidity. Training for primary medical care is typically shorter than that for specialists, and—if present at all—training in geriatrics is only one of several components, with little structured training for most clinical disciplines focused on the organisation and delivery of systematic chronic disease management and care coordination. Undergraduate and postgraduate training and continuous professional development need reshaping to develop knowledge and skills in the management and coordination of longitudinal care.[24,25]

Clinical evidence and guidelines are largely created for individual diseases, and most randomised trials exclude multimorbid and elderly people.[26] Therefore, more externally valid trials examining effectiveness in more representative populations are needed to complement existing efficacy trials in highly selected populations.[27] Additionally, clinical guidelines rarely account for multimorbidity or help clinicians to prioritise recommendations from several guidelines.[27,28] A result is that patients with multimorbidity might be prescribed several drugs, each of which is recommended by a disease-specific guideline, but the overall drug

Articles

Panel: Research in context

Systematic review

We assessed the 39 measures of multimorbidity identified in Diederichs and colleagues'[11] 2010 systematic review, and searched Medline for relevant reports published in English after August, 2009, with the keywords "multimorbidity" and "multi-morbidity", selecting reports that described the measurement or prevalence of multimorbidity. Diederichs and colleagues'[11] review reported major variation in how multimorbidity was defined (ie, the nature and number of morbidities included, and how they were weighted), the way in which data were collected (eg, by survey self-report, by research interview, or from clinical databases), and the populations studied (ranging from random community samples to specialist referral populations in hospitals). The estimated prevalence of multimorbidity in the studies reviewed varied substantially, and our study therefore sought to use a representative primary care population in a health system with universal registration with one primary care provider, include large numbers of morbidities in the count, and include all of the recommended core disorders for any multimorbidity measure. We specifically explored how multimorbidity varied with socioeconomic deprivation, which has previously been little studied, and examined physical–mental health comorbidity in particular, because this combination is the most discordant in terms of health-service organisation.

Interpretation

Multimorbidity is the norm for people with chronic disease, and although its prevalence increases with age, more than half of all people with multimorbidity are younger than 65 years. The most socioeconomically deprived young and middle-aged people have substantially more multimorbidity than do their most affluent peers. Prevalence of mental health disorders in an individual increases with the number of physical disorders that they have, and this association is stronger in younger people and has a consistent socioeconomic gradient. The appropriate management of long-term disorders is a key challenge for health systems internationally. Existing health systems are dominated by single-disease approaches that are increasingly inappropriate, and need to be complemented by strengthening generalism in both specialist and primary care. Physical and mental health care is particularly divided, despite the prevalence of physical–mental comorbidity. Research is needed into how multimorbidity develops (including the extent to which many disorders are driven by one cause, or whether they occur independently), its associations with a range of outcomes (including quality of life, functional status, health-service use, quality of care, and mortality), how preventable these outcomes are and how to intervene to minimise them, and how best to organise health care to address the needs of people with multimorbidity.

burden is difficult for patients to manage and potentially harmful.[28] Evidence of how best to deliver care to people with several disorders in middle age is scarce, although this drawback is beginning to be addressed, particularly for people with both depression and a physical disorder—one of the most common comorbidities—which is associated with poor physical and mental health outcomes.[21,29]

The representative nature of our data means that they are indicative of the higher rates of socioeconomic deprivation and lower life expectancy in Scotland than in most developed countries. However, our findings are consistent with multimorbidity studies from other countries that have used primary care or population data, included reasonable numbers of morbidities, and examined socioeconomic inequalities.[5-7] We believe that they will therefore broadly apply in other countries,

although the relations in our study might be weaker or stronger, and the age of onset of multimorbidity will probably vary with population life expectancy. In relation to the challenges to health-care delivery, this study shows the concentration of multimorbidity in deprived areas, but has not examined the concentration of multimorbidity and other issues within families, the concentration of such families within practices, or the concentration of practices within areas.[14,30] Strengthening of primary care in such deprived areas is a particular priority.

As health systems evolve to address the emerging challenges of long-term care, widening inequality, and financial constraints, multimorbidity is becoming the norm rather than the exception. Existing approaches focusing on patients with only one disease dominate most medical education, clinical research, and hospital care, but increasingly need to be complemented by support for the work of generalists, mainly but not exclusively in primary care, providing continuity, coordination, and above all a personal approach for people with multimorbidity. This approach is most needed in socioeconomically deprived areas, where multimorbidity happens earlier, is more common, and more frequently includes physical–mental health comorbidity.

Contributors

BG, SWM, SW, and GW conceived the study and obtained the funding. All authors contributed to the analysis, which was mainly done by KB and BG. KB and MN wrote the first draft, and all authors contributed to the writing of the final report.

Conflicts of interest

We declare that we have no conflicts of interest.

Acknowledgments

We thank the Chief Scientist Office of the Scottish Government Health Directorates (Applied Research Programme Grant ARPG/07/1), which funded the work; the Scottish School of Primary Care, which part supported SWM's post and the development of the Applied Research Programme; and the Primary Care Clinical Informatics Unit at the University of Aberdeen, which provided the data contained herein. The views in this publication are not necessarily the views of the University of Aberdeen, its agents, or employees. We thank Katie Wilde and Fiona Chaloner of the University of Aberdeen, who did the initial data extraction and management.

References

1 WHO. Global status report on noncommunicable diseases 2010: description of the global burden of NCDs, their risk factors and determinants. Geneva: World Health Organization, 2011. http://www.who.int/nmh/publications/ncd_report2010/en/ (accessed Dec 22, 2011).

2 Wolff J, Starfield B, Anderson G. Prevalence, expenditures, and complications of multiple chronic conditions in the elderly. *Arch Intern Med* 2002; **162:** 2269–76.

3 Starfield B, Shi L, Macinko J. Contribution of primary care to health systems and health. *Milbank Q* 2005; **83:** 457–502.

4 Schoen C, Osborn R. 2010 Commonwealth Fund international health policy survey. http://www.commonwealthfund.org/Surveys/2010/Nov/2010-International-Survey.aspx (accessed Dec 22, 2011).

5 van den Akker M, Buntinx F, Metsemakers JFM, Roos S, Knottnerus JA. Multimorbidity in general practice: prevalence, incidence, and determinants of co-occurring chronic and recurrent diseases. *J Clin Epidemiol* 1998; **51:** 367–75.

6 Walker A. Multiple chronic diseases and quality of life: patterns emerging from a large national sample, Australia. *Chronic Illn* 2007; **3:** 202–18.

Articles

7   Salisbury C, Johnson C, Purdy S, Valderas JM, Montgomery A. Epidemiology and impact of multimorbidity in primary care: a retrospective cohort study. *Br J Gen Pract* 2011; **582**: e12–21.

8   Gijsen R, Hoeymans N, Schellevis F, Ruwaard D, Satariano W, Bos G. Causes and consequences of comorbidity: a review. *J Clin Epidemiol* 2001; **54**: 661–74.

9   Kadam U, Croft P, for the North Staffordshire GP Consortium Group. Clinical multimorbidity and physical function in older adults: a record and health status linkage study in general practice. *Fam Pract* 2007; **24**: 412–19.

10   Fortin M, Lapointe L, Hudon C, Vanasse A, Ntetu A, Maltais D. Multimorbidity and quality of life in primary care: a systematic review. *Health Qual Life Outcomes* 2004; **2**: 51.

11   Diederichs C, Berger K, Bartels D. The measurement of multiple chronic diseases—a systematic review on existing multimorbidity indices. *J Gerontol A Biol Sci Med Sci* 2011; **66**: 301–11.

12   Eachus J, Williams M, Chan P, et al. Deprivation and cause specific morbidity: evidence from the Somerset and Avon survey of health. *BMJ* 1996; **312**: 287–92.

13   Marmot M. Social determinants of health inequalities. *Lancet* 2005; **365**: 1099–104.

14   Mercer SW, Watt GCM. The inverse care law: clinical primary care encounters in deprived and affluent areas of Scotland. *Ann Fam Med* 2007; **5**: 503–10.

15   The Scottish Government. Long-term monitoring of health inequalities. Edinburgh, Scotland: The Scottish Government, 2010.

16   Elder R, Kirkpatrick M, Ramsay W, et al. Measuring quality in primary medical services using data from SPICE. Edinburgh, Scotland: NHS National Services Scotland, 2007.

17   Carstairs V, Morris R. Deprivation and health in Scotland. Aberdeen: Aberdeen University Press, 1991.

18   NHS—Primary Care Commissioning. QOF implementation: business rules v 16.0, updated December 2009. http://www.pcc.nhs.uk/145/ (accessed Dec 22, 2011).

19   Information Services Division, NHS National Services Scotland. Measuring long-term conditions in Scotland, June 2008. http://www.isdscotland.org/isd/5658.html (accessed Dec 22, 2011).

20   Taylor A, Price K, Gill T, et al. Multimorbidity—not just an older person's issue: results from an Australian biomedical study. *BMC Public Health* 2010; **10**: 718.

21   Gunn J, Ayton D, Densley K, et al. The association between chronic illness, multimorbidity and depressive symptoms in an Australian primary care cohort. *Soc Psychiat Epidemiol* 2012; **47**: 175–84.

22   Moussavi S, Chatterji S, Verdes E, Tandon A, Patel V, Ustun B. Depression, chronic diseases, and decrements in health: results from the World Health Surveys. *Lancet* 2007; **370**: 851–58.

23   Higashi T, Wenger NS, Adams JL, et al. Relationship between number of medical conditions and quality of care. *N Engl J Med* 2007; **356**: 2496–504.

24   Guthrie B, Saultz JW, Freeman GK, Haggerty JL. Continuity of care matters. *BMJ* 2008; **337**: a867.

25   WHO. The World Health Report 2008: primary healthcare, now more than ever. Geneva, Switzerland: World Health Organization, 2008.

26   Van Spall HGC, Toren A, Kiss A, Fowler RA. Eligibility criteria of randomized controlled trials published in high-impact general medical journals: a systematic sampling review. *JAMA* 2007; **297**: 1233–40.

27   van Weel C, Schellevis FG. Comorbidity and guidelines: conflicting interests. *Lancet* 2006; **367**: 550–51.

28   Boyd CM, Darer J, Boult C, Fried LP, Boult L, Wu AW. Clinical practice guidelines and quality of care for older patients with multiple comorbid diseases. *JAMA* 2005; **294**: 716–24.

29   Katon WJ, Lin EHB, Von Korff M, et al. Collaborative care for patients with depression and chronic illnesses. *N Engl J Med* 2010; **363**: 2611–20.

30   Watt G. The inverse care law today. *Lancet* 2002; **360**: 252–54.

CHAPTER 28

The impact of primary care and the importance of indicators

Kate Anteyi

NOMINATED CLASSIC PAPER

Leiyu Shi. The impact of primary care: a focused review. *Scientifica*, 2012; Article ID 432892: 1–22.

This paper reviewed primary care definitions, primary care measurement, primary care practice, primary care and health, primary care and quality, primary care and cost, primary care and equity, primary care and health centres, and primary care and healthcare reform in both developed and developing countries.

The paper demonstrates that primary care is associated with enhanced access to healthcare services, better health outcomes, and a decrease in hospitalisation and use of emergency department visits. Primary care can also help counteract the negative impact of poor economic conditions on health.

The paper further demonstrated that primary care is imperative for building a strong healthcare system that ensures positive health outcomes, effectiveness and efficiency, and health equity.

The research included in this review paper showed that many countries in the world have embraced primary care, using a variety of structures and models. Lessons from these countries could serve as case studies, especially for healthcare systems in Africa, which currently face an imbalance between specialty and primary care as well as a significant shortage and inequitable distribution in the primary care workforce. It can also guide in structuring family medicine training in Africa, using models that meet local needs.

The reviewed research suggests the need to increase the supply of primary care physicians in both developing and developed countries. This is still important as the need for primary care physicians continues to increase, especially in Africa. There is also need to increase the critical mass of family medicine training institutions in Africa.

While different types of indicators and tools have been developed to measure the function of primary care, the performance of providers and facilities, and the quality of care delivered, the need for more indicators and more data continues. Patient-centred measurements are gradually replacing disease-specific measurements to yield more accurate assessments of primary care. Further research is needed to evaluate what models of primary care can produce the best health outcomes for individual countries.

ABOUT THE AUTHOR OF THIS PAPER

Leiyu Shi is Director of the Johns Hopkins Primary Care Policy Center and Professor of Health Policy & Health Services Research at Johns Hopkins Bloomberg School of Public Health. Professor Leiyu has a global reputation for his research into primary care, health disparities, and vulnerable populations. He has studied the association between primary care and health outcomes, particularly the role of primary care in mediating the adverse impact of income inequality on health outcomes. He has also researched community health centres that serve vulnerable populations, including their sustainability, provider recruitment and retention experiences, financial performance, experience under managed care, and quality of care.

ABOUT THE NOMINATOR OF THIS PAPER

Dr Kate Anteyi is a family physician and Chief Consultant at the Health and Human Services Secretariat of the Federal Capital Territory, in Abuja, Nigeria, where she is involved in family practice, administration, research and coordinating residency training in family medicine. She has a commitment to the role of women family doctors in leadership, equity and quality of care. She is a member of the working party for women and family medicine of the World Organization of Family Doctors (WONCA). Kate has also led research into the association between gender and health equity in primary care.

> 'My message to new physicians is to practise patient-centred care. To medical educators in Africa, structure family medicine training using models that meet local needs. And to primary care researchers, focus on patient-centred measurements that yield more accurate assessment of primary care, and

evaluate which models of primary care produce the best health outcomes for various countries.'

Dr Kate Anteyi, Nigeria

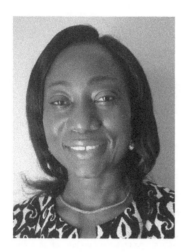

Attribution:

We attribute the original publication of *The impact of primary care: a focused review* to *Scientifica*, and thank Professor Leiyu Shi for permission to reproduce this paper.

Hindawi Publishing Corporation
Scientifica
Volume 2012, Article ID 432892, 22 pages
http://dx.doi.org/10.6064/2012/432892

Review Article
The Impact of Primary Care: A Focused Review

Leiyu Shi

Johns Hopkins Bloomberg School of Public Health, 624 North Broadway, Baltimore, MD 21205, USA

Correspondence should be addressed to Leiyu Shi, lshi@jhsph.edu

Received 27 September 2012; Accepted 8 November 2012

Academic Editors: K. Eriksson, A. P. Giardino, G. Mastrangelo, and P. J. Schluter

Copyright © 2012 Leiyu Shi. This is an open access article distributed under the Creative Commons Attribution License, which permits unrestricted use, distribution, and reproduction in any medium, provided the original work is properly cited.

Primary care serves as the cornerstone in a strong healthcare system. However, it has long been overlooked in the United States (USA), and an imbalance between specialty and primary care exists. The objective of this focused review paper is to identify research evidence on the value of primary care both in the USA and internationally, focusing on the importance of effective primary care services in delivering quality healthcare, improving health outcomes, and reducing disparities. Literature searches were performed in PubMed as well as "snowballing" based on the bibliographies of the retrieved articles. The areas reviewed included primary care definitions, primary care measurement, primary care practice, primary care and health, primary care and quality, primary care and cost, primary care and equity, primary care and health centers, and primary care and healthcare reform. In both developed and developing countries, primary care has been demonstrated to be associated with enhanced access to healthcare services, better health outcomes, and a decrease in hospitalization and use of emergency department visits. Primary care can also help counteract the negative impact of poor economic conditions on health.

1. Introduction

Primary care serves as the cornerstone for building a strong healthcare system that ensures positive health outcomes and health equity [1, 2]. In the past century, there has been a transition in healthcare from focusing on disease-oriented etiologies to examining the interacting influences of factors rooted in culture, race/ethnicity, policy, and environment. Such a transition called for person/family-focused and community-oriented primary care services to be provided in a continuous and coordinated manner in order to meet the health needs of the population. In 2001, the World Health Organization (WHO) proposed a global goal of achieving universal primary care in the six domains established by the 1978 Alma-Ata Declaration: first contact, longitudinality, comprehensiveness, coordination, person or family-centeredness, and community orientation. These six attributes, agreed upon internationally, have proved effective in identifying breadth of primary care services and monitoring primary care quality [3–6].

However, despite near consensus around the world that primary care is a critical component of any healthcare system, there is a considerable imbalance between primary and specialty care in the United States (USA) and many other parts of the world. For example, in the USA, in 2008, among 954,224 total doctors of medicine, 784,199 were actively practicing and 305,264 were practicing in primary care specialties (32% of the total and 39% of actively practicing physicians) [7]. The proportion of specialists was over 60% of all patient care physicians.

The major driving force behind the increasing number of medical specialists is the development of medical technology. The rapid advances in medical technology continuously expanded the diagnostic and therapeutic options at the disposal of physician specialists. The majority of patients, significantly freed from financial constraints thanks to third-party insurance payment, have turned to physicians who can provide them with the most up-to-date, sophisticated treatment. Hence, the rapid advance of medical technology contributes to the demand for specialty services and provides an impetus for further specialty development.

In addition, significantly higher insurance reimbursement for specialists relative to primary care physicians also contributes to the current imbalance. Under the resource-based relative value scale (RBRVS), implemented for US Medicare physician payment, primary care physicians continue to receive lower payments than specialists for comparable work because physician payments are based on historically determined, estimated practice costs as well as total work effort [8, 9]. Moreover, many insurance companies will pay for hospital-based complex diagnostic and invasive procedures using high technology, but not for routine preventive visits and consultations. Such practices not only encourage medical students' career choices in subspecialties and practicing physicians' provision of intensive specialty services, but also discourage the provision of important primary care services and deter patients from early care-seeking behavior.

Specialist physicians enjoy other benefits as well. Not only do specialists earn significantly higher incomes than primary care physicians, but also they are more likely to have predictable work hours and enjoy higher prestige both among their colleagues and from the public at large [10, 11]. Problems typically cited in recruiting primary care physicians include longer working hours during the day as well as on call, less financial reward for service, and less access to the highly technological approaches to diagnosis which is an important part of the medical center approach to patient care [12]. Among factors affecting medical students' career choice, society's perception of value, intellectual challenge, and lifestyle factors (e.g., hours worked) were ranked as very important along with financial reward [13–15]. The medical education environment, organized according to specialties and controlled largely by those who have achieved their leadership positions by demonstrating their ability in narrow scientific or clinical areas, emphasizes technology intensive procedures, and tertiary care settings also deter the choice by students of primary care specialties [16, 17].

Perhaps the most important reason for this imbalance is the lack of appreciation for the true value of primary care. Relative to disease-specific research, primary care-oriented studies have been relatively few. Their dissemination and recognition within the medical field are also problematic. Policymakers and the general public also have little knowledge of the efficacy of primary care, its impact on individual and population health, and its role in today's healthcare delivery. These realities have led to superfluous political commitments and the disengagement of related sectors [18, 19]. A WHO 2000 report announced that primary care has failed to serve as the foundation of care for all people [2].

The objective of this focused review paper is to present the research findings regarding the efficacy of primary care so that the value of primary care can be better appreciated. Specifically, it will demonstrate the importance of effective primary care services in delivering quality healthcare, improving health outcomes, and reducing disparities.

2. Methods

Literature searches were performed in PubMed using the following key search terms: primary care (also general practice, family medicine) and quality, performance, health outcome, and health equity. The search was limited to English language journals. The titles and abstracts of all papers identified by the electronic search were inspected. Papers that failed to

satisfy the inclusion criteria were discarded. The resulting references were required to be related to primary care quality and outcome studies. Articles focusing on clinical procedures were excluded since the focus of this paper was on the general characteristics of primary care. Additional important articles were subsequently located by examining the bibliographies of the retrieved articles. The content areas to be reviewed include the following: primary care definitions, primary care measurement, primary care practice, primary care and health, primary care and quality, primary care and cost, primary care and equity, primary care and health centers, and primary care and healthcare reform.

2.1. Primary Care Definitions. The terms "primary care" and "primary healthcare" describe two different concepts. The former, primary care, refers to family medicine services typically provided by physicians to individual patients and is person-oriented, longitudinal care [20]. Primary healthcare, in contrast, is a broader concept intended to describe both individual-level care and population-focused activities that incorporate public health elements. In addition, primary healthcare may include broader societal policies such as universal access to healthcare, an emphasis on health equity, and collaboration within and beyond the medical sector [20].

Primary care plays a central role in a healthcare delivery system. Other essential levels of care include secondary and tertiary care, which encompass different roles within the health spectrum. Compared to primary care, secondary and tertiary care services are more complex and specialized, and the types of care are further distinguished according to duration, frequency, and level of intensity. Secondary care is usually short-term, involving sporadic consultation from a specialist to provide expert opinion and/or surgical or other advanced interventions that primary care physicians (PCPs) are not equipped to perform. Secondary care thus includes hospitalization, routine surgery, specialty consultation, and rehabilitation. Tertiary care is the most complex level of care, needed for conditions that are relatively uncommon. Typically, tertiary care is institution-based, highly specialized, and technology-driven. Much of tertiary care is rendered in large teaching hospitals, especially university-affiliated teaching hospitals. Examples include trauma care, burn treatment, neonatal intensive care, tissue transplants, and open heart surgery. In some instances, tertiary treatment may be extended, and the tertiary care physician may assume long-term responsibility for the bulk of the patient's care. It has been estimated that 75% to 85% of people in a general population require only primary care services in a given year; 10% to 12% require referrals to short-term secondary care services; 5% to 10% use tertiary care specialists [21].

Since its introduction in 1961, the term primary care has been defined in various ways, often using one or more of the following categories of classification [4, 22–24]. These categories include the following.

(i) The care provided by certain clinicians, the Clinton administration's Health Security Act, for example, specified primary care as family medicine, general internal medicine, general pediatrics, and obstetrics and gynecology. Some experts and groups have also included nurse practitioners and physician assistants.

(ii) A set of activities whose functions act as the boundaries of primary care—such as curing or alleviating common illnesses and disabilities.

(iii) A level of care or setting—an entry point to a system that also includes secondary care (by community hospitals) and tertiary care (by medical centers and teaching hospitals).

(iv) A set of attributes, as in the 1978 IOM definition—care that is accessible, comprehensive, coordinated, continuous, and accountable—or as defined by Starfield [4]—care that is characterized by first contact, accessibility, longitudinality, and comprehensiveness.

(v) A strategy for organizing the healthcare system as a whole—such as community-oriented primary care, which gives priority and resources to community-based healthcare while placing less emphasis on hospital-based, technology-intensive, and acute-care medicine.

Definitions of primary care often focus on the type or level of services, such as prevention, diagnostic and therapeutic services, health education and counseling, and minor surgery. Although primary care specifically emphasizes these services, many specialists also provide the same spectrum of services. For example, the practice of most ophthalmologists has a large element of prevention, as well as diagnosis, treatment, followup, and minor surgery. Similarly, most cardiologists are engaged in health education and counseling. Hence, according to some experts, primary care should be more appropriately viewed as an approach to providing healthcare, rather than as a set of specific services [21].

The World Health Organization (WHO) describes primary care as essential healthcare based on practical, scientifically sound, and socially acceptable methods and technology made universally accessible to individuals and families in the community by means acceptable to them and at a cost that the community and the country can afford to maintain at every stage of their development in a spirit of self-reliance and self-determination. It forms an integral part of both the country's health system (of which it is the central function) and a main focus of the overall social and economic development of the community. It is the first level of contact for individuals, the family, and the community with the national health system, bringing healthcare as close as possible to where people live and work, and constitutes the first element of a continuing healthcare process [25].

Others define primary care as the health services rendered by providers acting as the principal point of consultation for patients within a healthcare system [26, 27]. This provider could be a primary care physician, such as a general practitioner or family physician, or (depending on the locality, health system organization, and the patient's discretion) a pharmacist, a physician assistant, a nurse practitioner, a nurse (as is common in the United Kingdom), a clinical officer (such as in parts of Africa), or an Ayurvedic or other

traditional medicine professionals (such as in parts of Asia). Depending on the nature of the health condition, patients may then be referred for secondary or tertiary care.

Perhaps the most comprehensive definition of primary care was given by Starfield in her landmark book *Primary care: balancing health needs, services and technology* [4]; Starfield defined primary care as the provision of integrated, accessible healthcare services by clinicians who are accountable for addressing a large majority of personal healthcare needs, developing a sustained partnership with patients, and practicing in the context of family and community. She summarized the following characteristics of primary care (pp. 19–34).

(i) Integrated care is intended to encompass the provision of comprehensive, coordinated, and continuous services that provide a seamless process of care. Integration combines information about events occurring in disparate settings and levels of care as well as over time, preferably throughout the life span.

(ii) Comprehensive care addresses any health problem at any given stage of a patient's life cycle.

(iii) Coordinated care ensures the provision of a combination of health services and information to meet a patient's needs. It also refers to the connection between, or the rational ordering of, those services, including the resources of the community.

(iv) Continuous care is a characteristic that refers to care over time by a single individual or team of healthcare professionals ("clinician continuity") as well as to effective and timely maintenance and communication of health information (events, risks, advice, and patient preferences) ("record continuity").

(v) Accessible care refers to the ease with which a patient can initiate an interaction for any health problem with a clinician (e.g., by phone or at a treatment location) and includes efforts to eliminate barriers such as those posed by geography, administrative hurdles, financing, culture, and language.

(vi) Healthcare services refer to an array of services that are performed by healthcare professionals or under their direction, for the purpose of promoting, maintaining, or restoring health. The term refers to all settings of care (such as hospitals, nursing homes, physicians' offices, intermediate care facilities, schools, and homes).

(vii) A clinician is an individual who uses a recognized scientific knowledge base and has the authority to direct the delivery of personal health services to patients.

(viii) Accountability is applied to primary care clinicians and the systems in which they operate. These clinicians and systems are responsible to their patients and communities for addressing a large majority of personal health needs through a sustained partnership with a patient in the context of a family and community and for (1) quality of care, (2) patient satisfaction, (3) efficient use of resources, and (4) ethical behavior.

(ix) A majority of personal healthcare needs refer to the essential characteristic of primary care clinicians: that they receive all problems that patients bring—unrestricted by problem or organ system—and have the appropriate training to manage a large majority of those problems, involving other practitioners for further evaluation or treatment when appropriate. Personal healthcare needs include physical, mental, emotional, and social concerns that involve the functioning of an individual.

(x) Sustained partnership refers to the relationship established between the patient and clinician with the mutual expectation of continuation over time. It is predicated on the development of mutual trust, respect, and responsibility.

(xi) A patient is an individual who interacts with a clinician either because of real or perceived illness or for health promotion and disease prevention.

(xii) Context of family and community refers to an understanding of the patient's living conditions, family dynamics, and cultural background. Community refers to the population served, whether they are patients or not. It can refer to a geopolitical boundary (a city, county, or state), members of a health plan, or neighbors who share values, experiences, language, religion, culture, or ethnic heritage.

2.2. Primary Care Measurement. Measurement enables assessment of the performance of a healthcare delivery system and individual providers. Additionally, measurement facilitates efforts to improve accountability, quality, appropriate use of resources, and patient outcomes and to lower the risk of adverse events [28]. Measurement is also increasingly tied to healthcare financing through pay-for-performance programs. As the USA attempts to emphasize primary care functions through aspects of the Patient Protection and Affordable Care Act [29], measurement of primary care will take on even greater importance. Shi notes that assessments of the quality of primary care patients receive should consider the four dimensions of primary care: the first contact experience, longitudinality, coordination, and comprehensiveness [30].

Researchers can use various types of indicators depending on the goal of measurement [28]. Indicators can provide some sense of the structure, process, or outcome of care, can be used to measure activity, performance, and quality, and can help determine whether the care is being provided according to guidelines specified by an expert body or consensus [28].

The Primary Care Assessment Tool (PCAT) is a collection of questionnaires, developed by Johns Hopkins Primary Care Policy Center under the leadership of the late Dr. Barbara Starfield, that assess whether a healthcare provider or system is achieving the four core functions of primary

care (first contact, longitudinality, comprehensiveness, and coordination) and three supplementary aspects of primary care (family centeredness, community orientation, and cultural competence). The first PCAT-adult questionnaire was developed and validated in the USA [31, 32] but its validity and reliability have been demonstrated in other countries, such as in Brazil [33] and Spain [34]. Several forms of the PCAT exist, varying in length and target population. For example, while the Primary Care Assessment Tool-Adult Edition's (PCAT-AE) original form includes 74 items assessing adult patient experiences with primary care [31, 32] a short 10-item version, the PCAT10-AE has also been used and integrated into a national population health survey [34]. A PCAT assessing the primary care experiences of children has been developed as well [33, 35]. In addition to these questionnaires targeting patients, versions of the PCAT have been developed that also survey providers and administrators of facilities, providing another perspective on the provision of primary care [36].

In addition to the PCAT collection of survey instruments, researchers have used other surveys to measure aspects of primary care provision from the patient and provider perspective in the USA and in international settings. These include the Health Tracking Physician Survey [37], the International Health Policy Survey [38], and the Ambulatory Care Experiences Survey [39]. Other studies have used claims data [40, 41] and medical record review [40, 42–44] to assess the quality, performance, and cost-effectiveness of primary care in various settings.

Medical experts have defined standards of practice for assessment of providers or facilities in terms of whether they are practicing according to recommended guidelines [38, 44]. For example, a survey fielded in five countries determined that the USA performed well in delivering preventive care according to clinical guidelines [38], hypothesizing that this result might be due to third party insurers' increasing emphasis on quality measurement using tools such as the National Committee for Quality Assurance's (NCQA) Healthcare Effectiveness Data and Information Set (HEDIS). In addition to HEDIS, other indicators, such as the Diabetes Quality Improvement Project [40], have been developed to support measurement of the quality of care provided in a primary care setting for a particular condition. Many measures of performance and quality in the healthcare setting are disease-specific. Given primary care's emphasis on patient-centered and comprehensive care, these disease-specific measures may not be most useful for the primary care context. Other measurement efforts attempt to move beyond condition-specific indicators. Hospitalization for ambulatory care sensitive conditions (ACSC), defined as "diagnoses for which timely and effective outpatient care can help to reduce the risk of hospitalization" [45], has been proposed as a way to assess access to care and as an outcome measure of the effectiveness of prior primary care intervention [41]. However, research has shown that ACSC-related hospitalizations may occur too infrequently and be too difficult to link with previous receipt of primary care to serve as a viable outcome measure [41]. On the other hand, increased access to healthcare services is accomplished through expanded insurance coverage, thus also enabling greater financial access to hospital resources. Therefore, studies using preventable hospitalizations as outcome measures to examine the impacts of primary care access should consider how that improved access is being facilitated [46]. Another survey attempting to identify good indicators asked physicians about the types of patient outcomes that they value as good indicators of primary care providers' performance; respondents identified nineteen indicators related to patients' physical functioning, physical pain, physical symptoms besides pain, clinical indicators, emotional distress, health behaviors, and general quality of life.

Other literature examines the measurement of primary care with respect to unique populations, particular models of care, or atypical settings [39, 47, 48]. One challenge is measuring care provided to complex patients (patients with multiple chronic conditions), given that disease-specific measures are ill-suited for this population [48]. Therefore, indicators of the continuity and coordination aspects of primary care provision are particularly important for assessing the quality of care this complex population experiences [48]. Given the increasing emphasis on patient-centered medical homes (PCMH), measuring the impact of multidisciplinary teams (in contrast to individual providers) may better elucidate the patient experience of care in PCMH settings [39]. However, NCQA standards to assess medical homes may not be appropriate for all practice settings; for example, the military health system confronts different challenges when establishing medical homes related to deployment and the frequent movement of patients and providers [47].

Finally, the facilitators and barriers to implementing quality measurement in primary care were systematically reviewed in a study on primary care in Canada [49]. Content analysis of the 57 English-language articles published between 1996 and 2005 identified seven common categories of facilitators and barriers for implementing innovations, guidelines, and quality indicators. The authors found that successful implementation of quality measures can occur but that success depends on the interaction of multiple factors, including measurement characteristics, promotional messages, implementation strategies, resources, the intended adopters, and the intraorganizational and interorganizational contexts. Research has also found that the nature of the relationship between the patient and PCP impacts patients' perception of the quality of care they are receiving [50] and correlates positively with measures of primary care provider performance [51]. However, while the quality of care patients receive may be heavily impacted by the strength of connection patients feel with their providers, research has found that patients generally do not feel well connected to their PCPs [51].

In summary, primary care measurement includes tools that assess many aspects of care: the extent to which a primary care setting fulfills the major components of primary care; the performance of the provider or facility; the quality of care patients receive; how facets of care delivery, such as various models of care, team approaches, and different settings, impact care. Tools to collect data include primary data collection from surveys and secondary analysis using claims data and medical chart abstraction. Given the nature of primary care practice, indicators that are patient-centered rather than disease-specific are likely going to be increasingly important in enabling a more accurate assessment of the care patients receive.

2.3. Primary Care Practice. Many countries place great emphasis on primary care and have developed strong primary care infrastructures [52–54]. Examples include Britain's National Health Service (NHS), which established Primary Care Trusts (PCT) that integrate primary and hospital-based care and comprise the bulk of the NHS budget [52, 55]. Canada has a more balanced primary care-specialist physician ratio than the USA with only 10% more specialists than primary care physicians, in contrast to over 50% more in the USA [56]. Developing countries, like Brazil and Thailand, have also implemented national-level strategies to increase access to primary care services [57, 58].

An increasingly popular model for orienting the healthcare system to primary care is the gatekeeper model, which requires patients to select a primary care physician (PCP) and then obtain referrals through that PCP to specialists [59]. However, gatekeeper models may meet resistance from medical professionals and consumers in some countries [60]. Therefore, efforts to promote gate keeping in a healthcare system should consider gradual, incentive-driven approaches [60].

In conjunction with acting, in some systems, as gatekeepers to more specialized services, PCPs also may serve as patients' point of first contact with the healthcare system. Many countries have expanded access to primary care by establishing call centers, flexible hours, and clinics. Spain, for example, has sought to make care accessible both in financial and geographic terms, by enacting universal insurance coverage and striving to make healthcare facilities available within fifteen minutes to every person in need [61].

Continuity of care is also promoted through structures such as medical homes or well-developed health information technology (health IT) systems [59]. In Spain, for example, nearly every resident has an identification card that enables providers to access their medical history and relevant information at an appointment or emergency [61]. These countries have also sought to raise the status of primary care by establishing the discipline as a specialty within medicine and instituting reforms to payment systems [59].

Team-based models of providing primary care and the connections of these models with quality are becoming increasingly important as insurers use pay-for-performance incentives in payment schemes [62]. In order to support high-functioning teams, the associations between team-level job satisfaction and performance should be explored, a relationship which may be affected by the status and support enjoyed by the PCPs in a setting [62]. Research also suggests that the functioning level of primary care teams may affect patient outcomes, with those patients cared for by high functioning primary care teams experiencing better health outcomes [63]. Team-based approaches to primary care may also facilitate integration of mental health and primary care. As an example, the USA-based Intermountain Healthcare's mental health integration system includes PCPs, psychiatrists, nurses, family members, and other parties to integrate mental health services into the usual practice of primary care [64].

Scope of practice, the extent of health insurance coverage in a region, ease of coordination with other sectors, and myriad other factors impact the way in which primary care is practiced in a country, region, or individual practice. Countries that have enacted reforms that build on their existing primary care infrastructures can serve as case studies for the USA, where the ongoing implementation of the Patient Protection and Affordable Care Act (ACA) seeks to enhance the role of primary care in the US healthcare system.

Currently, in contrast to some of its industrialized peers, the US healthcare system is much more heavily skewed toward specialty care [56, 58]. Although 51.3% of office visits were to primary care physicians in 2008, only about one-third of practicing physicians specialize in primary care [65]. A combination of primary care physicians, nurse practitioners (NPs), and physician assistants (PAs) comprise the estimated 400,000 primary care providers in the USA, with physicians contributing the largest portion (74%) [66]. Scopes of practice for NPs and PAs have broadened in many states in recent years, enabling these providers to take on more responsibilities in the provision of care. However, the distribution of primary care providers in the USA is uneven, with 5,902 communities designated as primary care health professional shortage areas [67].

Changes to the Medicare fee schedule (which had previously favored specialists in reimbursement rates) [68], support for Title VII health professions training programs [69, 70], and the recent ACA are some examples of policies that have attempted to strengthen the role of primary care within the US healthcare system. Some experts have suggested that the ACA and the aging population will place an increased burden on the primary care workforce in the USA, contributing to a severe workforce shortage in the future [71]. Although about one-third of practicing physicians work in primary care, less than a fourth of current medical school graduates are pursuing careers in primary care fields, and many primary care physicians are projected to retire in coming years, raising additional concerns that the future US primary care workforce will be unable to respond to the growing demand for primary care [72]. A factor contributing to the small percentage of graduating medical students that pursue residencies in primary care is the significantly lower salaries in these fields, a trend that has continued despite some efforts to reduce this disparity [71, 73].

Similarly, in order to incentivize providers to accept patients newly eligible for Medicaid under the reforms, the ACA temporarily raises reimbursement for PCPs serving Medicaid patients to the same level as Medicare reimbursements [74]. However, a study found that those states that have a low supply of PCPs serving Medicaid enrollees already have higher reimbursement levels [74]. Therefore, this increase may have little effect in increasing the supply of PCPs available to care for disadvantaged groups, such as the Medicaid population.

In order to address these fears, more research is needed on the capabilities and capacities of the current PCP workforce, as well as projections about how it will change over time. Indeed, a 2011 Robert Wood Johnson Foundation (RWJF) report observes that workforce projections are complicated [66]. The report cautions that although the workforce is likely to be strained by the country's changing demographics and increasing demand under the ACA, other clinicians, such as NPs and PAs, in addition to new team-based models of care, may change primary care workforce needs in unanticipated ways [66]. Nevertheless, the irregular distribution of providers in the USA remains a significant issue that is likely to continue inhibiting access to primary care services among particular segments of the population and in certain geographic regions [66].

Next steps and future directions have been identified to strengthen the primary care infrastructure abroad and in the USA. To start, there has been increasing interest in exploring how primary care and public health might better coordinate in order to support population health improvement efforts [75, 76]. A review of literature on the coordination of primary care with public health suggests that combinatory efforts can lead to improvements in the management of chronic diseases, control of communicable diseases, and in maternal and child health [76]. In addition, there is need for additional clarification on the unique roles of primary care and public health and the ways in which these sectors can work together [77].

In the USA in particular, new models of delivering care through patient-centered medical homes (PCMHs) and accountable care organizations (ACOs) require team-based approaches to care with a heavy emphasis on primary care. As previously discussed, some experts suggest that the shift to these models for delivering care will require an increased supply of primary care providers [58] whereas others note that little is definitively known about how these models of care will impact provider productivity [66]. This renewed interest in improving primary care capacity has led to some recommended initiatives for enhancing the stature of primary care in the USA, including increasing Title VII funding to better support the education of primary care providers that agree to practice in underserved communities [69, 70]; addressing salary disparities between PCPs and specialists by changing Medicare's resource-based relative value scale to give more equal reimbursement, which also influences private insurance reimbursement rates [78]; exploring the role that other primary care providers, such as NPs and PAs, can play in reducing burdens on primary care physicians [66]. Additional research is obviously needed; topics that should be examined include the methods and tools for conducting research on primary care, clinical issues of relevance to the practice of primary care, primary care service delivery, health systems (including the social and political factors affecting primary care provision), and how to improve the education and training of primary care providers [54].

2.4. Primary Care and Health. Logically, primary care is seen as an important medical specialty and healthcare necessity because it is assumed to have a positive impact on health outcomes; the USA and most other countries believe that increasing the quality and quantity of primary care services will lead to better population health. A number of ecological studies have examined the relationship between primary care infrastructure and health outcomes internationally [79-83] as well as in the USA at various levels of geographic units [84, 85]. Studies conducted in industrialized countries, such as member nations of the Organization for Economic Cooperation and Development (OECD), do indicate that stronger primary care systems are generally associated with better population health outcomes including lower mortality rates, rates of premature death and hospitalizations for ambulatory care sensitive conditions, and higher infant birth weight, life expectancy, and satisfaction with the healthcare system [79, 80, 82, 86]. Studies in the USA have also indicated that greater primary care availability in a community is correlated with both better health outcomes [87] and a decrease in utilization of more expensive types of health services, such as hospitalizations and emergency department (ED) visits [88].

Experiences in the international context suggest that primary care-oriented healthcare delivery systems can produce better health outcomes [52-55] in addition to counteracting, to some extent, the negative impact of poor economic conditions on health [57]. Reforms of healthcare systems to emphasize primary care generally are associated with improved health outcomes, including evidence from several countries in Latin America and Asia [83]. However, given that these reforms typically included multiple components, attributing change in population health to any one aspect of the reform is difficult [83]. Increasing primary care availability in low- and middle-income countries also correlates with improved health; however, many of these studies are limited to child and infant health outcomes [81]. Additionally, much of the research in this setting consists of observational studies rather than more rigorous research designs, and studies may also use different definitions of what constitutes a "primary care system" or "program" [81].

In a review of US primary care and its relationship with health outcomes, Starfield et al. [89] note that there may be several mechanisms of primary care that explain this positive association with population health: (1) better access to health services; (2) improved quality of care; (3) emphasis on prevention; (4) the identification and early management of conditions; (5) the combined impact of many characteristics of solid primary care systems; (6) reduction in unnecessary specialist care [89, 90].

Primary care and health service use were also studied in the USA using an interactional analysis instrument to characterize patient-centered care in the primary care setting and examine its relationship with healthcare utilization [91]. A total of 509 adult patients at a university medical center were randomized into groups receiving care by family physicians or general internists. An adaptation of the Davis Observation Code was used to measure patient-centered practices; the main outcome measures of the study were the patients' use of medical services and accrued charges over one year. The results indicated that higher amounts of patient-centered care were related to a significantly decreased annual number of visits to specialty providers, less frequent hospitalizations,

and fewer laboratory and diagnostic tests. Total medical charges for the year were also significantly reduced.

Another US study examined the relationship between physician-patient connectedness and measures of physician performance [51]. 155,590 patients who made one or more visits to a study practice from 2003 to 2005 in the Massachusetts General Hospital adult primary care network were identified, and a validated algorithm was used to connect patients to physicians or practices. Performance measures, including breast, cervical, and colorectal cancer screening in eligible patients, hemoglobin A1C measurement and control in patients with diabetes, and low-density lipoprotein cholesterol measurement and control in patients with diabetes and coronary artery disease, were used to examine clinical performance. The results indicated that physician-connected patients were significantly more likely than practice-connected patients to receive guideline-consistent care. Receipt of preventive care varied more by whether patients were more or less connected to a primary care physician than by race or ethnicity, which are often cited as major determinants of healthcare usage.

The role of primary care in referral was studied in a multicountry project in Europe and Australia [92]. The study compared weight loss achieved through standard treatment in primary care versus weight loss achieved after referral by the primary care team to a commercial provider in the community. In this parallel group, nonblinded, randomized controlled trial, 772 overweight, and obese adults were recruited by primary care practices in Australia, Germany, and the UK to receive either 12 months of standard care, as defined by national treatment guidelines or 12 months of free membership in a commercial program; analysis was by intention to treat amongst the population who completed the 12-month assessment. The results showed that the participants referred to community-based commercial providers lost more than twice as much weight over the year as compared to those who received standard care. These results indicate that referral to a commercial weight loss program that provides regular weighing, advice about diet and physical activity, motivation, and group support can offer a clinically useful early intervention for weight management in overweight and obese people and can be delivered on a large scale as well. However, it also demonstrates that primary care physicians and teams have limits in the scope and quality of interventions they can provide; in this case, the primary care team provided better care through the referral to an outside company than through the team-managed care seen as standard.

The impact of primary care outreach was tested in a Canadian study [93] using a randomized, controlled trial design to evaluate the impact of a provider-initiated primary care outreach intervention as compared with usual care among older adults at risk of functional decline. The sample was comprised of 719 patients enrolled with 35 family physicians in five primary care networks in Hamilton, Ontario, Canada. The 12-month intervention, provided by experienced home care nurses from 2004 to 2006, consisted of a comprehensive initial assessment using the Resident Assessment Instrument for home care, collaborative care planning with patients, their families, and family physicians, health promotion activities, and referral to community health and social support services. The primary outcome measures were quality adjusted life years (QALYs), use and costs of health and social services, functional status, self-rated health, and mortality. The results for the mean difference in QALYs, overall cost of prescription drugs and services, and changes over 12 months in functional status and self-rated health were not statistically significant. Therefore, the results of this study do not support adoption of this particular preventive primary care intervention for this target population of high-risk older adults.

Another study conducted in Pittsburgh, Pennsylvania, examined the role of nurses in primary care [94]. This study evaluated findings from a trial treatment for behavioral problems in 163 clinically referred children from six primary care offices in Pittsburgh. Participants were randomized to be treated in either the on-site, nurse-administered intervention (PONI) in primary care or enhanced usual care (EUC) characterized by on-site diagnostic assessment and facilitated referral to a local mental health provider. The main outcomes were measured by standardized rating scales. The results showed that children randomized to the PONI intervention were significantly more likely to access their assigned treatment, received more direct treatment, adjunctive services, and a longer duration of treatment, and had greater levels of sibling participation than children assigned to receive EUC. These findings indicate that a psychosocial intervention for behavioral problems delivered by nurses in a primary care setting is feasible, improves access to mental health services, and has some clinical efficacy. Options for enhancing clinical outcomes may include multifaceted collaborative care interventions in the pediatric practice.

The impact of primary care on chronic disease management is the subject of much research. For example, a USA-based study examined the impact of a multifaceted intervention on cholesterol management in primary care practices [95]. The study used a practice-based trial to test the hypothesis that a multifaceted intervention consisting of guideline dissemination enhanced by a computerized decision support system (CDSS) would improve primary care physician adherence to the Third Adult Treatment Panel (ATP III) guidelines and improve the management of cholesterol levels. A total of 61 primary care families and internal medicine practices in North Carolina enrolled in the trial; 29 received the Third Adult Treatment Panel (ATP III) intervention and 32 received an alternate intervention (JNC-7). The ATP III providers received a personal digital assistant providing the Framingham risk scores and ATP III-recommended treatment. They examined 5,057 baseline and 3,821 follow-up medical records. The study reports the positive effect on screening of lipid levels and appropriate management of lipid level test results and concludes that a multifactorial intervention, including personal digital assistant-based decision support, may improve primary care physician adherence to the ATP III guidelines.

In a US study that focused on diabetes disease management, researchers used a randomized, controlled trial to examine the relationships among patient characteristics, labor inputs, and improvement in glycosylated hemoglobin (A1C) level in a primary care-based diabetes disease management program (DDMP) [96]. A total of 217 patients with type 2 diabetes mellitus and poor glucose control were enrolled. The results showed that patients in the intervention group had significantly greater improvement in A1C level than the control group that received no additional disease management support. In multivariate analysis, no significant differences in A1C level improvement were observed when stratified by age, race/ethnicity, income, or insurance status, and no interaction effect was observed between any covariate and intervention status. Labor inputs were similar regardless of age, race/ethnicity, sex, or education and may reflect the nondiscriminatory nature of providing algorithm-based disease management care.

The role of primary care in preventive care has also been studied. In a study conducted in Spain on physical activity promotion by general practitioners, researchers sought to assess the effectiveness of a physical activity promotion program at 11 Spanish public primary care centers using 6-, 12-, and 24-month follow-up measurements [97]. They recruited 4,317 individuals (2,248 intervention and 2,069 control), and fifty-six general practitioners (GPs) were randomly assigned to intervention or standard care (control) groups. The primary outcome measure was the change in self-reported physical activity from baseline. The results indicated that general practitioners were effective at increasing the level of physical activity among their inactive patients during the initial six months of an intervention but the effect leveled off at 12 and 24 months. Only the subgroup of patients receiving repeat prescriptions of physical activity maintained gains over the long term.

Many people suffering from mental health issues also receive health services in a primary care setting [98]. In the USA, an evaluation of a Department of Veterans Affairs (VA) program establishing primary care clinics in underserved communities found that while these clinics did improve access to more general health services, without a specialty mental healthcare component, they did not effectively expand access to mental health services [99]. Research is mixed on whether psychotherapy and counseling in the primary care setting is cost-effective but it does suggest that patients may be more open to these strategies than to antidepressant prescriptions, and psychotherapy may be more effective in treating depression than counseling [98]. Research has found that while counseling in primary care is associated with short-term improvement and patient satisfaction, there is little evidence of its effectiveness, in comparison to usual care, in treating depression in the long run [100].

An overview of low- and middle-income countries found that 14 countries, including China, with comprehensive primary care (defined as >80% skilled birth attendance rates) experienced health gains compared with countries with more selective primary care approaches. These health improvements seemed to "depend on progression to comprehensive primary care with a reliable referral system linking to functioning facilities" [101, p. 958]. However, the study looked at countries as a whole and so could not account for within-country variation, and additionally, the study defined countries as having comprehensive primary care based only upon their skilled birth attendance rates, and other primary care attributes were not considered.

In the USA, a growing body of research has focused on the impact of primary care supply, infrastructure, and models of care on health outcomes. A review of studies assessing the relationship between supply of PCPs and various outcomes, such as all-cause and disease-specific mortality, life expectancy, low birth weight, and self-rated health, found correlations at the state, county, and MSA levels [84]. Research also indicates that local supply of PCPs per capita, using radii around zip codes to define service areas, is associated positively with patient receipt of preventive health services and that this local primary care availability mediates, to some extent, the impact of socioeconomic factors on the receipt of preventive care [102]. In addition, according to one study, Medicaid-enrolled children who have access to high quality, family-centered primary care have both lower nonurgent and urgent hospitalization rates [103].

However, methodological challenges exist in conducting research linking PCP supply to population health. When doing these analyses, the ratio of primary care to specialist physicians may be a more appropriate measure than just physician supply [85]. For example, while a correlation exists between the PCP supply and health outcomes, there is no association between specialist supply and health outcomes [89, 90]. Therefore, using a measure of physician supply per capita, without consideration of the balance of primary care and specialist physicians, may skew findings.

In response to this policy-relevant research, next steps have included proposals to increase the supply of primary care physicians in the USA. Findings suggest that increasing the supply of PCPs by just one unit per 10,000 physicians might improve health outcomes by 0.66% to as much as 10.8%, depending on the outcome considered [84].

Further research is needed on which models of care produce the best health outcomes. While past research has indicated team-based care produces better outcomes in some settings, few studies have examined the use of teams in primary care practice [104].

Other issues will also continue to affect the relationship between primary care and health. Many experts believe that primary care will have to change practice models to improve patient outcomes and physician job satisfaction, as demonstrated in many of the previously mentioned researches. However, others have also argued that in order to revitalize primary care in the USA, major system-level change is needed, especially in the way that primary care physicians are compensated relative to specialists [105].

2.5. Primary Care and Quality. Ease of access, the clinical quality of the care, interpersonal aspects of care, continuity, and coordination all are important elements to consider when assessing primary care quality [106].

Research exploring access has found that factors can impede or facilitate access, such as the availability of after-hours care, the length of office wait time, travel time to an appointment, lack of a specific PCP at the site of primary care,

and lower perceived flexibility in selecting a PCP [5, 107]. Level of access to primary care impacts other facets of quality as well. For example, improved access to primary care may also improve the continuity of care for patients with depression [108]. An evaluation of a PCP access program found that better access led to reduced emergency department use in the long term [109]. Family-centered primary care may also lower rates of nonurgent emergency department visits and hospitalizations for certain populations [110]. However, a relationship between other measures of quality of primary care and urgent hospitalizations has not been established [110, 111].

The structure of the primary care delivery system may also affect levels of access and quality. For example, one New Zealand study comparing nonprofit and for-profit primary care practices found that the nonprofit practices in the study offered increased access at a lower cost in addition to offering a more expansive array of services and instituting written policies related to quality management [112]. In the USA, patients may experience differing levels of quality of primary care depending on insurance type. In an analysis comparing quality of primary care across various managed care models (i.e., managed indemnity, point of service, staff-model HMO, etc.), managed indemnity models performed best on quality of primary care measures, followed by point of service and network-model HMO structures [113]. The motivations within the delivery system can affect patient care as well; in a study of the impact of pay-for-performance initiatives on the quality of primary care received by patients with chronic conditions, researchers found a positive quality association for patients with two of the three conditions studied [114].

US Medicare recipients have a choice between private managed care plans (through the Medicare Advantage program) and the traditional government-managed fee for service (FFS) plan. Research indicates that while most quality performance measures are superior in the traditional FFS program, enrollees in some private plans may have better financial access to care [115]. Research has also sought to identify the most appropriate site for delivering primary care to low-income populations in the USA; these studies have mixed findings, with vaccination rates higher in hospital outpatient settings but fewer delays in receiving care in physicians' offices [116]. Structural features of primary care practices, such as having an electronic health record (EHR) and holding regular meetings devoted to discussing quality issues, can also be associated with higher performance on Healthcare Effectiveness Data and Information Set (HEDIS) measures [117]. Much research has examined EHRs and other health IT systems in hospitals or acute care settings, but these tools can facilitate quality improvement efforts in primary care settings as well [118]. Researchers have also found that health IT infrastructure facilitates provision of care for chronic conditions in line with the Chronic Care Model [119]. However, there remain significant challenges in the implementation of IT due to lack of reimbursement by insurance plans and the learning curve experienced by practitioners with the new technology [120].

Another component of primary care quality is continuity, defined as person-focused care over time. The following factors may affect the extent to which continuity can be achieved: appointment wait time length, the insurance status of patient, and after-hours care availability [5]. A review of studies conducted in 6 countries regarding primary care quality suggests that better continuity may decrease hospitalizations and ED visits, lowering healthcare costs [121].

In order to facilitate quality improvement in the primary care context, information is needed on appropriate benchmarks that can be used to evaluate performance in primary care-specific settings. Wessell et al. [122] identify Achievable Benchmarks of Care (ABCs) for 54 quality indicators based on data collected through the Practice Partner Research Network (PPRNet) demonstration. Twenty-five to 99% of the PCPs participating in the PPRNet demonstration met the ABCs [122]. A New Zealand effort identified 28 evidence-based, population-focused indicators that may be used to assess quality of primary care in five categories: smoking cessation, prescribing practices, chronic disease management, preventive health, and quality of data [123]. Furthermore, many of these indicators are already available from the data routinely collected in health IT systems [123].

Patient evaluations of the quality of care they receive in primary care settings can be appropriate complements to other measures of quality [106]. Patient assessments may be particularly useful for evaluating the quality of access, the practitioner-patient relationship, continuity, and coordination [106]. While findings from patient assessments, commonly conducted through questionnaires, may inform quality improvement efforts, it is not clear that the information gleaned from patients assessments can be successfully translated into actual improvements in the quality of care [106]. One study found that patient-reported satisfaction with quality of care among the elderly was not a good predictor of the effectiveness of the care these patients received [124]. However, ratings of coordination of care did have a relationship with survival time among the higher utilizers [124].

Studies conducted in the international setting have assessed how emphasis on primary care quality may impact health outcomes, and whether specialists or PCPs provide better quality of care for chronic conditions. The results were mixed. Improvements in health outcomes for diabetes type 2 patients in Norway may reflect special emphasis on improving diabetes care in primary care practices [125]. Research in Taiwan has found that patients with a PCP or a usual source of care (USC) experience superior primary care quality, including better access, coordination, family centeredness, continuity, and cultural competence [126, 127]. In Britain, an evaluation comparing the quality of diabetes care provided in specialist diabetes clinics to that provided by primary care clinics found no long-term difference in the rates of improvement in HbA1c, cholesterol, and blood pressure over time [128]. In contrast, a Danish study found that patients suffering from asthma or rhinitis experience superior care quality from respiratory specialists as opposed to PCPs [129]. In a study in Canada looking at asthmatic patients participating in an intervention designed to improve access to primary care, intervention patients did initially have better access in comparison to those patients without the

primary care intervention [130]. However, after 12 months, there was no difference between the two groups [130]. In Canada, a small-scale preventive primary care outreach program targeting the elderly included home care, collaborative planning between patients, families and physicians, and referral to appropriate social support and community resources; the program, however, had no significant positive findings and no relationship with the functional status and self-rated health of participants [93].

Medical, contextual (specific to the medical encounter), and policy evidence is needed to further research on quality in primary care [131]. Cross-country comparisons may elucidate how broader systems-level factors impact primary care quality. Future studies should be undertaken to examine primary care reforms; how financing mechanisms impact PCP cooperation and workforce issues; the relationship between balance of primary and specialty care; the patient's role; community-oriented care; equity in access and outcomes [132].

In the USA specifically, Friedberg et al. [133] categorize the focus of proposed policy interventions intended to strengthen primary care and improve healthcare quality into three categories: (1) supply of PCPs; (2) the set of functions and services provided by a usual source of care; (3) the orientation of the health system. Based on a review of the evidence, these authors suggest that policy prescriptions should focus on reorienting the health system in the USA to emphasize and reward primary care provision and support providers' capacity for practicing primary care through such interventions as health IT, the Chronic Care Model, and team-based approaches to delivering care [133]. Although experts disagree over whether the current supply of PCPs impacts the overall quality of healthcare, some policy prescriptions for emphasizing primary care in the USA focus on increasing PCP supply by making the career more attractive through better wages [134] and through funding of Title VII Section 747, which supports workforce development [69, 70]. Grumbach and Mold also propose circulating a primary care version of an agricultural extension agent to disseminate the latest knowledge and clinical guidelines, improve the quality of care provided by PCPs, and strengthen the country's primary care infrastructure [135]. In addition, increased collaboration between primary care and public health may improve quality and health outcomes by refocusing family medicine on population or community health rather than just individuals [136]. In addition to these proposals, some point out that more policy actions should be devoted to distributing primary care resources more fairly and evenly [137]. Low-income, deprived communities are burdened by higher morbidity and mortality rates and, therefore, should receive more health services [137].

2.6. Primary Care and Cost. One consequence of having many specialists is the possibility that specialist care has contributed to increasing the volume of intensive, expensive, and invasive medical services and therefore the costs of healthcare [138–144]. Higher surgeon supply has been found to increase the demand for initial contacts with surgeons

[145]. Many now frequently performed operations, such as coronary artery bypass, hip replacement, carotid endarterectomy, arthroscopy, laparoscopy, and heart and liver transplantation, were little known and hardly ever performed 50 years ago. Today, they are both fairly common and expensive.

Technological developments also drive up healthcare costs [146]. Systematic comparison across industrialized countries shows that the USA has higher rates of coronary surgery, diagnostic imaging, neurosurgery, treatment for end-stage renal disease, and cancer chemotherapy than any other country [147, 148]. As the disease prevalence for these conditions is still relatively low, an excess of specialists in these areas may lead to the performance of unnecessary procedures. The Congressional Subcommittee on Oversight and Investigations estimated that nationwide there were 2.4 million unnecessary operations performed annually, resulting in a cost of $3.9 billion and 11,900 deaths [149, 150]. Overall, primary care services are less costly than specialty services because they are less technology-intensive.

An economic analysis was conducted in the UK to assess the cost-effectiveness of Quality and Outcomes Framework (QOF) payments, which is an attempt to improve the quality of primary care in the UK through the use of financial rewards [151]. The study used 2004/2005 data on the QOF performance of all English primary care practices. Cost-effectiveness evidence was collected for a subset of nine QOF indicators with direct therapeutic impact. The authors found that the proportional changes required to make QOF payments cost-effective varied widely between the indicators. It showed that QOF incentive payments are likely to be a cost-effective use of resources for a high proportion of primary care practices, and incentive payments are likely to be a good value for the NHS.

Health policy experts suggest that systems, models, and providers oriented toward primary care may achieve lower healthcare costs, a top priority in the USA [52, 133]. The bulk of the evidence suggests that PCPs order fewer diagnostic tests and procedures than specialists, leading to lower costs [133]. In addition, having a usual source of care (defined as a primary care function, not explicitly as a PCP) is correlated with lower use of healthcare resources and lower rates of nonurgent emergency department visits, thus also decreasing costs [152]. On a systems level, regions of the USA with a higher PCP to specialist ratio experience not only better health outcomes but also lower costs [152]. Comparative analyses have found that other countries with health systems oriented toward primary care, on average, also have lower costs and better population health outcomes [152].

In addition to these more macro-level demonstrations of relationships between the primary care system and healthcare spending, cost-effectiveness studies and other forms of cost analyses can inform efforts to strengthen and improve primary care delivery [153]. One area of research explores what settings produce the best value or the highest quality care for the lowest costs. The community health center (CHC) program delivers primary care for vulnerable populations in areas identified by the Department of Health and Human Services' Health Resource and Services Administration as medically underserved [67]. A review of the literature on CHCs indicates that these centers provide quality primary care at low cost to especially disadvantaged populations [154]. However, the authors note that few studies have used formal cost-effectiveness methods to compare the value of CHCs to the value achieved in other primary care settings [154]. One recent study using Medicaid claims data to compare CHCs to other primary care settings found that while hospital outpatient departments and CHCs have similar costs, private physician practices actually have somewhat lower costs [155].

Some suggest that certain models of care may also lower costs. Staub, for instance, has argued that larger primary care group practices can apply management and technology innovations more fluidly than smaller practices, lowering the costs associated with these kinds of changes [156]. Others have looked to the patient-centered medical home (PCMH) as one model that shows promise in reducing healthcare spending. While the literature to date generally supports an association between the improved access and coordination of the PCMH model and reduced hospitalizations and ED visits, other predicted effects, such as decreased use of unnecessary tests, procedures, and referrals, have not yet been demonstrated [157]. One example of an integrated program, the Geisinger Health System's Proven Health Navigator (PHN), has led to cost savings of 4.3% to 7.1% [158]. The program's success in reducing costs may be an inspiration to other integrated delivery systems or primary care practices seeking to adopt the PCMH model [158]. Friedman et al. [152] also observe that health professionals who are not PCPs can perform primary care functions, an important consideration for the team-oriented PCMH model. Research suggests that care by nonphysicians, like physician assistants (PAs), for example, may be less costly than care by physicians [159].

Access to care may also impact costs. One study assessed a low-cost primary care physician access program's impact on ED use, noting that while the increased access may have prompted patients to change where they sought care for nonurgent purposes, the study could not demonstrate statistically significant cost savings [109]. This study and the evaluation of the Geisinger PCMH suggest that primary care interventions may require long periods of time to demonstrate financial savings [109, 158]. An eight-year study assessing the impact of a primary care case management (PCCM) program in Iowa's Medicaid program did demonstrate reductions in costs due to shifting expenses from the hospital to outpatient setting [160]. These savings increased over time, reinforcing what other studies suggest: these desired significant cost savings may take time to achieve [160]. Chernew et al. [161] explored how PCP/specialist supply influences cost, and the findings indicated that increasing the PCP supply may accrue a short-term advantage but does not address long-term problems. Although the proportion of the workforce comprised of PCPs in contrast to specialists likely affects healthcare expenditures, balancing the workforce in favor of PCPs may do little to curb the rate of growth in healthcare spending and thus will not reduce overall costs [161].

PCCM programs, like the one implemented for the Iowa Medicaid program, use the gatekeeper approach, in which patients select a PCP and are then required to obtain referrals through this PCP to see specialists, reducing unnecessary specialist appointments and procedures and therefore reducing healthcare costs. The PCP also may coordinate care for a panel of patients in a cost-effective manner [160].

Another intervention that has been touted as a potential way to reduce the costs of medical care in the USA is health IT. Research indicates that health IT systems may yield financial gains for PCPs by reducing drug expenditures, reducing utilization of expensive tests in favor of other equally useful diagnostic methods, and decreasing billing mistakes [162]. One study of the implementation of an electronic medical record (EMR) system in primary care clinics found cost savings that increased over time [162].

Other lines of research explore the cost-effectiveness of particular interventions conducted in the primary care setting [42, 98, 100, 163, 164]. For example, studies have explored the cost-effectiveness of different techniques designed to increase cancer screenings [42, 163], diabetes self-management programs [164], mental health interventions [98, 100], smoking cessation treatment [165], and lifestyle counseling and interventions [166], all within the primary care setting. This type of research seeks to inform quality improvement efforts in primary care with cost-effectiveness information. Ideally, PCPs could use this information to provide both higher quality and more efficient care.

2.7. Primary Care and Equity. Better primary care is also associated with more equitable distribution of health within a population [89, 90, 167, 168]. The annual National Healthcare Disparities Report in the USA [169] stated that equitable primary care eliminates disparities "related to preventive services and management of common chronic diseases typically delivered in primary care settings" [170]. Primary care providers deliver a disproportionate share of ambulatory care to disadvantaged populations. Improved access to primary care was associated with reduced mortality rates, better health outcomes, and lower costs [6, 171–175]. A higher proportion of PCPs in a given area has also been shown to lead to lower spending on healthcare [161]. Additionally, an increase of one primary care physician per a population of 10,000 is associated with a reduction of 1.44 deaths, a 2.5% reduction in infant mortality, and a 3.2% reduction of low birthweight on average in the population [167, 168, 176–179]. Such associations hold even in the presence of income inequality and other health determinants [172–175]. Adults who have PCPs as their regular source of care experience lower mortality and incur reduced healthcare costs [6].

Research has also shown that primary care may play an important role in mitigating the adverse health effects of income inequality [180–183]. Specifically, research has demonstrated associations between income inequality and self-rated health and primary care and self-rated health [181]. Therefore, the pathway through which income inequality impacts health may be partly attenuated by primary care [182]. Access to quality primary care may have the largest impact on health in areas with the highest levels of income inequality [182]. However, socioeconomic status may also reduce to some extent the impact of primary care on health

[182]. The relationship between race, income inequality, primary care availability, and health is complicated; in stratified analyses of the impacts of primary care and income inequality on mortality, Shi and Starfield [183] found while independent associations between primary care and mortality and income inequality and mortality persisted after controlling for other socioeconomic variables among white Americans, the relationship between primary care physician supply and mortality lost its statistical significance with the inclusion of other socioeconomic factors in the model.

Primary care availability may also be more strongly correlated with health outcomes in areas with greater levels of income inequality, suggesting that expanding primary care availability in these areas may have a substantial impact on population health [180]. However, only certain specialties under the umbrella of primary care may have this impact. For example, family medicine has been found to have the strongest inverse relationship with mortality [172–175]. These findings have been consistent in examinations of mortality at the state level [172–175], at the county level [167, 168], in comparisons of urban and nonurban areas [167, 168], and in stratifications by race [167, 168].

In the USA, racial and ethnic minorities face greater difficulty accessing regular primary care than white Americans and use hospitals more often than private clinics as usual sources of care [184]. Challenges included long wait times and difficulty obtaining timely appointments [184]. Addressing these barriers and ensuring more equitable access to high quality primary care may translate into reduced disparities in self-rated health status [176–178].

Access to primary care may have the greatest impact on health status for racial and ethnic minorities living in poverty [176–178]. However, research exploring why racial and ethnic minorities in the USA receive fewer preventive services determined that while frequency of visits to primary care physicians likely explains a small portion of the disparity, factors related to poverty are significantly more important [185]. While some research has suggested that physician-patient racial concordance may positively affect the quality of care racial/ethnic minority patients receive, other research has not borne out these conclusions [186].

A US study looking at the Latino population aimed to identify subgroup variations in having a patient-centered medical home, the PCMH's impact on disparities, and factors associated with Latinos having a PCMH in the USA [187]. The 2005 Medical Expenditure Panel Survey (MEPS) Household Component that sampled 24,000 adults, including 6,200 Latinos, was used in this analysis. Self-reports of preventive care and patient experiences were also examined. The results showed that white (57.1%) and Puerto Rican (59.3%) adults were most likely to have a PCMH, while Mexican/Mexican Americans (35.4%) and Central and South Americans (34.2%) were least likely. Much of this disparity was caused by lack of access to a regular provider. Respondents with a PCMH had higher rates of preventive care and positive patient experiences. Disparities in care were eliminated or reduced for Latinos with PCMHs. The regression models showed that private insurance, which is less common among Latinos than whites, was an important predictor of having a PCMH. These findings indicate that eliminating healthcare disparities will require assuring access to a PCMH and that addressing differences in healthcare coverage that contribute to lower rates of Latino access to the PCMH will also reduce disparities.

As seen in the previous study, insurance status is associated with access to primary care and the quality of that care [30]. The uninsured have greater difficulty accessing good primary care than the insured; among the insured, those with private insurance have better access to quality primary care than the publicly insured [30]. Those with health maintenance organization (HMO) plans have more comprehensive care but poorer measures of longitudinal and coordinated care than those in fee for service (FFS) plans [30].

Children also experience racial and ethnic disparities in access to and quality of primary care [188]. Stevens and Shi propose the following research agenda to explore health disparities in children further: (1) conduct research using more racial and ethnic granularity rather than categorizing groups superficially; (2) explore the role of language in contributing to health disparities; (3) consider cultural influences; (4) examine how health systems-level policies and factors contribute to disparities [188]. Recent attention has focused on how models, such as the patient-centered medical home, may improve quality of care for children. Yet research on the association between race and ethnicity and having a medical home has determined that minority children have lower odds of having healthcare experiences that contain features of the medical home, such as having a usual provider, a provider who spends sufficient time with him or her, and a provider who communicates well [189].

One unique population on which there is little literature is the migrant worker population. Part of the reason for this gap in research is the difficulty in determining how many migrant workers are living currently in the USA [190]. Although the federally qualified health center (FQHC) program currently provides primary care to an estimated 20% of agricultural workers, most migrant workers face significant structural barriers to accessing adequate primary healthcare [190].

The Patient Protection and Affordable Care Act may impact disparities in access to and quality of primary care by expanding insurance coverage and funding for FQHCs and the National Health Service Corps, which repays loans to physicians and health professionals practicing in shortage areas [191]. In addition, it includes innovations like the community-based collaborative care networks, which support low-income populations in accessing medical homes [191].

2.8. Primary Care and Health Centers. Creation of community health centers (CHCs)—formerly called neighborhood health centers—was authorized during the 1960s under the Johnson administration's War on Poverty program, seeking to address healthcare needs in medically underserved regions of the USA. The federal government determines the medically underserved designation to indicate a shortage of primary care providers and delivery settings, as well as poor health

indicators for the population. Such areas are often characterized by economic, geographic, or cultural barriers that limit access to primary care for a large segment of the population. CHCs are required by law to locate in medically underserved areas and provide services to anyone seeking care, regardless of insurance status or ability to pay. Hence, CHCs are a primary care safety net for the nation's poor and uninsured in both inner city and rural areas.

CHCs operate under the Bureau of Primary Health Care (BPHC), Health Resources and Services Administration (HRSA), US Department of Health and Human Services (DHHS). Under Section 330 of the Public Health Service Act, CHCs receive some federal funds to provide primary care and services that improve access for disadvantaged populations, such as low-income groups, racial and ethnic minorities, public housing residents, the homeless [192], and migrant workers [190]. CHCs are private, nonprofit organizations that nonetheless depend heavily on funding through the Medicaid program and federal grants. Private-pay patients are charged on sliding-fee scales, determined by the patients' income.

CHCs tailor their services to family-oriented primary and preventive healthcare and dental services [193]. These centers have developed considerable expertise managing the healthcare needs of underserved populations. Many have developed systems of care that include outreach programs, case management, transportation, translation services, alcohol and drug abuse screening and treatment, mental health services, health education, and social services.

CHCs are governed by an executive director or administrator, have a medical director, and are staffed by multidisciplinary teams of clinicians. The typical CHC employs 6 PCPs, 8 nurses, and 3 NPPs. Some clinics also have dentists, mental health practitioners, and pharmacists on site. Other members of these teams may include case managers and education specialists [193].

In 2009, CHCs served 18.8 million individual patients in 74 million patient visits. The majority of groups that utilize CHCs are vulnerable populations—92% of patients were below the 200% federal poverty level and 38% were uninsured. Among special populations, more than 1 million homeless individuals, 865,000 migrant/seasonal farmworkers, and 165,000 residents from public housing were seen through the program [194].

Expanding the services of CHCs was a central element of President Bush's plan for expanding healthcare access to the uninsured and underserved. In 2002, the Bush Administration proposed a $1.5 billion budget to continue a long-term strategy that would fund 1,200 new and expanded CHC sites over 5 years and serve an additional 6.1 million patients [193]. The Obama Administration continued this growth through the American Recovery and Reinvestment Act of 2009, which allocated $2 billion to CHCs to expand their patient populations, create new jobs, and meet the increasing demand for primary care services [7].

Components of the Patient Protection and Affordable Care Act of 2010 that affect CHCs involve payment protections and initiatives to develop teaching health centers. The law ensures that CHCs are not underpaid for the services they provide and adds preventive services to the Medicare

14

payment system, while eliminating Medicare payment caps. Additionally, the law allows for a Title VII grant program to develop residency programs in CHCs to teach the next generation of primary care providers [195]. This may be especially important because, although the ACA has increased CHC funding, health centers still face challenges in recruiting employees and maintaining financial viability. Rural centers, in particular, face personnel recruitment barriers [196, 197]. Research suggests that physicians who have exposure to medically underserved communities such as inner cities or rural areas of the country may be more inclined to practice in health centers located in these environments, making ACA efforts to offer residency training in these environments particularly prudent [198]. In addition to difficulties recruiting medical staff, CHCs have also faced fiscal challenges through the years. In the last several decades, as state Medicaid programs have increasingly relied upon managed care organizations to reduce costs, CHCs have engaged with managed care in order to maintain the important revenue obtained through Medicaid reimbursement [199]. However, research has found that CHC involvement with managed care also is associated with financial instability and serving fewer homeless and uninsured patients [199]. Therefore, federal funding of these centers remains imperative.

Because the majority of the population served by CHCs belongs to vulnerable groups (i.e., low income, minorities, homeless), studies show potential for CHCs to help bridge the disparities faced by these populations [200–203]. A large body of research suggests that CHCs increase access to primary care for these populations [192, 193, 204, 205], reduce hospitalizations [192], and provide high quality care for these particularly challenging populations when compared to other providers and settings [172–175, 196, 197, 206]. In addition, CHCs may reduce disparities by race/ethnicity, income, or insurance status [31, 32, 176–178, 205, 207, 208]. Studies also suggest that the quality of care these populations receive at CHCs is the same as the quality provided by other primary care providers and that health center patients may incur lower inpatient costs [155, 209].

However, some disparities persist among health center patients. For example, the uninsured report poorer primary care experiences than Medicaid enrollees utilizing CHCs [205]. Generally, however, CHCs are an important avenue for accessing primary care for Medicaid and uninsured patients [193].

2.9. Primary Care and Healthcare Reform. A number of industrialized countries have embarked on healthcare reforms aimed, at least in part, at strengthening their primary care delivery systems. For example, a primary care reform in Quebec, Canada, was studied to see if/how patients' perceptions of the quality of care changed [210]. The study used a before-and-after comparison of the perceptions of patients to evaluate how primary care reform affected patients' experiences in primary care. A random sample of 1,046 participants from five family medicine groups (FMGs) in two regions of Quebec completed both the baseline and follow-up

questionnaires. The authors found that perceptions of relational and informational continuity increased significantly, whereas organizational and first-contact accessibility and service responsiveness did not change significantly. Perception of physician-nurse coordination remained unchanged, but perception of primary care physician-specialist coordination decreased significantly. The proportion of participants reporting visits with nurses and reporting use of FMGs' emergency services increased significantly from baseline to followup. The findings showed that the reorganization of primary care services resulted in considerable changes in care practices, leading to improvements in patients' continuity of care but not to improvements in accessibility of care.

Another recent study assessed changes in patient experiences of primary care during health service reforms in England between 2003 and 2007 [211]. The researchers conducted a cross-sectional study of family practices in which questionnaires were sent to serial samples of patients in 42 representative general practices in England. Up to 12 patients with a confirmed diagnosis of each chronic illness (coronary heart disease, diabetes, or asthma) were randomly sampled in each practice. In addition, a random sample of 200 adult patients (excluding patients who reported any long-term condition) in each practice were also mailed a questionnaire. The results show that were no significant changes in quality of care reported by either group of patients between 2003 and 2007 regarding communication, nursing care, coordination, and overall satisfaction. Some aspects of access improved significantly for patients with chronic disease, but not for the patients without a long-term condition. The findings indicate that there were modest improvements in access to care for patients with chronic illness, but overall, patients now find it somewhat harder to obtain care, affecting care continuity. This outcome may be related to incorrect incentives to provide rapid appointments or to the increased number of specialized clinics in primary care. This research indicates that the possibility of unintended effects needs to be considered when introducing pay for performance schemes.

The impact of China's New Rural Cooperative Medical Scheme (NCMS) and its implications for rural primary healthcare were evaluated in a study that performed a difference-in-difference analysis to determine whether China's NCMS has corrected distortions in rural primary care and whether the policy has affected the operation and use of village health clinics [212]. A total of 160 village primary care clinics and 8,339 individuals within 25 rural counties across five Chinese provinces were involved in this study. The study sought to evaluate the effect of NCMS by using individual level and village clinic level data collected in 2004 (shortly after the introduction of the scheme in selected regions) and in 2007 (after the dramatic expansion of the scheme across most rural areas). For individuals, NCMS is not clearly related to the use of medical care, but it may have redirected patients away from specialized facilities to village clinics. On the clinic level, NCMS has increased clinics' weekly patient flow and gross income, but not annual net revenue. Increases in patient flow and gross, but not net, clinic income may reflect desirable reductions in the provision of specialized, high profit services and rates of drug sales.

3. Conclusion

Primary care is imperative for building a strong healthcare system that ensures positive health outcomes, effectiveness and efficiency, and health equity. It is the first contact in a healthcare system for individuals and is characterized by longitudinality, comprehensiveness, and coordination. It provides individual and family-focused and community-oriented care for preventing, curing or alleviating common illnesses and disabilities, and promoting health.

Many countries in the world have embraced primary care, using a variety of structures and models. Lessons from these countries could serve as case studies for the US healthcare system, which currently faces an imbalance between specialty and primary care as well as a significant shortage and inequitable distribution in the primary care workforce. Different types of indicators and tools have been developed to measure the function of primary care, the performance of providers and facilities, quality of care, and so forth, but the need for more indicators and more data continues. Patient-centered measurements are gradually replacing disease specific measurements to yield more accurate assessment of primary care.

In both developed and developing countries, primary care has been demonstrated to be associated with enhanced access to healthcare services, better health outcomes, and a decrease in hospitalization and use of emergency department visits. Primary care can also help counteract the negative impact of poor economic conditions on health. Therefore, research suggests the need to increase the supply of primary care physicians in the USA. Further research is also needed to evaluate what models of primary care can produce the best health outcomes.

There are many factors determining quality of care, such as ease of access (including availability of after-hours care, length of office wait time, travel time to an appointment, and flexibility in selecting a PCP), clinical quality, interpersonal aspects, continuity, structure through which primary care is delivered, and insurance coverage. Although studies in international settings have compared quality of care in primary care and specialty care settings, the results were mixed, and further research is needed to elucidate how system-level factors, and certain policies may influence quality in the USA.

In addition, research has indicated that countries and regions more oriented to primary care have lower healthcare costs but better health outcomes, although further studies using formal cost-effectiveness methods need to be conducted. Cost-effectiveness of primary care has been tentatively established through a few interventions conducted in primary care settings, and adoption of health information systems in primary care settings may further yield financial gains.

Furthermore, better primary care is correlated with more equitable distribution of health within a population and can mitigate the adverse effects of income inequality, which is especially important in the USA where racial and ethnic minorities face greater difficulties accessing regular primary care. This in turn emphasizes the significant role of CHCs in the USA in providing primary care services

to vulnerable groups and reducing disparities. CHCs in the USA are primary care facilities that provide family-oriented services to meet the healthcare needs of medically underserved populations. However, difficulties in recruiting primary care providers and maintaining financial viability are major challenges to the sustainability of CHCs, which subsequently influences primary care services available to and health outcomes for these underserved populations. Additionally, research on health disparities in children and migrant workers is still lacking and needs further attention.

Lastly, healthcare reforms aimed at strengthening the primary care system have been implemented in a number of countries, both developed and developing, and have generally proven to improve the healthcare system as a whole. The Patient Protection and Affordable Care Act (ACA) also emphasizes primary care in the USA. Future assessments focusing on the impact of the ACA on primary care, health outcomes, healthcare costs, and health disparities should be conducted to serve as an empirical basis for policy making in the future.

Acknowledgment

The author would like to acknowledge the research assistantship provided by Alene Kennedy, Hannah Sintek, and Xiaoyu Nie.

References

[1] J. E. Lawn, J. Rohde, S. Rifkin, M. Were, V. K. Paul, and M. Chopra, "Alma-Ata 30 years on: revolutionary, relevant, and time to revitalise," *The Lancet*, vol. 372, no. 9642, pp. 917–927, 2008.

[2] J. J. Hall and R. Taylor, "Health for all beyond 2000: the demise of the Alma-Ata Declaration and primary health care in developing countries," *Medical Journal of Australia*, vol. 178, no. 1, pp. 17–20, 2003.

[3] World Health Organisation, "The World Health Report 2008: Primary Health Care, Now more than ever," 2008, http://www.who.int/whr/2008/whr08_en.pdf.

[4] B. Starfield, *Primary Care: Balancing Health Needs, Services and Technology*, Oxford University Press, New York, NY, USA, 1998.

[5] C. B. Forrest and B. Starfield, "Entry into primary care and continuity: the effects of access," *American Journal of Public Health*, vol. 88, no. 9, pp. 1330–1336, 1998.

[6] P. Franks and K. Fiscella, "Primary care physicians and specialists as personal physicians: health care expenditures and mortality experience," *Journal of Family Practice*, vol. 47, no. 2, pp. 105–109, 1998.

[7] U. S. Department of Health and Human Services, "Health Resources and Services Administration (HRSA)," 2011, About Health Centers: Program Requirements, http://bphc.hrsa.gov/about/requirements/index.html.

[8] Physician Payment Review Commission, *Annual Report To Congress*, Physician Payment Review Commission, Washington, DC, USA, 1993.

[9] W. C. Hsiao, D. L. Dunn, and D. K. Verrilli, "Assessing the implementation of physician-payment reform," *New England Journal of Medicine*, vol. 328, no. 13, pp. 928–933, 1993.

[10] M. E. Samuels and L. Shi, *Physician Recruitment and Retention: A Guide For Rural Medical Group Practice*, Medical Group Management Association Press, Englewood, Colo, USA, 1993.

[11] R. A. Rosenblatt and D. M. Lishner, "Surplus or shortage? Unraveling the physician supply conundrum," *Western Journal of Medicine*, vol. 154, no. 1, pp. 43–50, 1991.

[12] P. O. Kohler, "Specialists/primary care professionals: striking a balance," *Inquiry*, vol. 31, no. 3, pp. 289–295, 1994.

[13] D. G. Kassebaum and P. L. Szenas, "Factors influencing the specialty choices of 1993 medical school graduates," *Academic Medicine*, vol. 69, no. 2, pp. 163–170, 1994.

[14] M. P. Rosenthal, J. J. Diamond, H. K. Rabinowitz et al., "Influence of income, hours worked, and loan repayment on medical students' decision to pursue a primary care career," *Journal of the American Medical Association*, vol. 271, no. 12, pp. 914–917, 1994.

[15] R. Steinbrook, "Money and career choice," *New England Journal of Medicine*, vol. 330, no. 18, pp. 1311–1312, 1994.

[16] AAMC, "Medical education may deter grads from choosing primary care careers," AAMC Weekly Report 1, 1990.

[17] J. E. Verby, J. P. Newell, S. A. Andresen, and W. M. Swentko, "Changing the medical school curriculum to improve patient access to primary care," *Journal of the American Medical Association*, vol. 266, no. 1, pp. 110–113, 1991.

[18] M. I. Roemer, "Priority for primary health care: its development and problems," *Health Policy and Planning*, vol. 1, no. 1, pp. 58–66, 1986.

[19] G. Walt and P. Vaughan, "Primary health care approach: how did it evolve?" *Tropical Doctor*, vol. 12, no. 4, part 1, pp. 145–147, 1982.

[20] L. K. Muldoon, W. E. Hogg, and M. Levitt, "Primary care (PC) and primary health care (PHC): what is the difference?" *Canadian Journal of Public Health*, vol. 97, no. 5, pp. 409–411, 2006.

[21] B. Starfield, "Is primary care essential?" *The Lancet*, vol. 344, no. 8930, pp. 1129–1133, 1994.

[22] J. J. Alpert and E. Charney, "The education of physicians for primary care," Publ. No. (HRA) 74-3113, DHEW, Washington, DC, USA, 1973.

[23] J. Fry, Ed., *Primary Care*, Heineman, London, UK, 1980.

[24] J. H. Abramson and S. L. Kark, "Community-oriented primary care: meaning and scope," in *Community Oriented Primary Care—New Directions For Health Services*, pp. 21–59, National Academy Press, Washington, DC, USA, 1983.

[25] World Health Organization (WHO), *Primary Health Care*, WHO, Geneva, Switzerland, 1978.

[26] R. Thomas-MacLean, D. Tarlier, M. Ackroyd-Stolarz, and M. Steward, "No cookie-cutter response: conceptualizing primary health care," http://www.uwo.ca/fammed/csfm/tutor-phc/documentation / trainingpapers / TUTOR_Definitio_%20of_primar_%20health_care.pdf.

[27] World Health Organization, *Definition of Terms*, 2011.

[28] S. M. Campbell, J. Braspenning, A. Hutchinson, and M. Marshall, "Research methods used in developing and applying quality indicators in primary care," *Quality and Safety in Health Care*, vol. 11, no. 4, pp. 358–364, 2002.

[29] L. Tobler, "A primary problem: more patients under federal health reform with fewer primary care doctors spell trouble," *State Legislatures*, vol. 36, no. 10, pp. 20–24, 2010.

[30] L. Shi, "Type of health insurance and the quality of primary care experience," *American Journal of Public Health*, vol. 90, no. 12, pp. 1848–1855, 2000.

[31] L. Shi, J. Regan, R. M. Politzer, and J. Luo, "Community health centers and racial/ethnic disparities in healthy life," *International Journal of Health Services*, vol. 31, no. 3, pp. 567–582, 2001.

[32] L. Shi, B. Starfield, and J. Xu, "Validating the adult primary care assessment tool," *Canadian Family Physician*, vol. 50, pp. 161W–175W, 2001.

[33] E. Harzheim, B. Starfield, L. Rajmil, C. Álvarez-Dardet, and A. T. Stein, "Internal consistency and reliability of Primary Care Assessment Tool (PCATool-Brasil) for child health services," *Cadernos de Saude Publica*, vol. 22, no. 8, pp. 1649–1659, 2006.

[34] K. B. Rocha, M. Rodríguez-Sanz, M. I. Pasarín, S. Berra, M. Gotsens, and C. Borrell, "Assessment of primary care in health surveys: a population perspective," *European Journal of Public Health*, vol. 22, no. 1, pp. 14–19, 2012.

[35] S. Berra, K. B. Rocha, M. Rodríguez-Sanz et al., "Properties of a short questionnaire for assessing Primary Care experiences for children in a population survey," *BMC Public Health*, vol. 11, article no. 285, 2011.

[36] J. L. Haggerty, R. Pineault, M. D. Beaulieu et al., "Practice features associated with patient-reported accessibility, continuity, and coordination of primary health care," *Annals of Family Medicine*, vol. 6, no. 2, pp. 116–123, 2008.

[37] S. P. Deshpande and J. Demello, "A comparative analysis of factors that hinder primary care physicians' and specialist physicians' ability to provide high-quality care," *Health Care Manager*, vol. 30, no. 2, pp. 172–178, 2011.

[38] C. Schoen, R. Osborn, P. T. Huynh et al., "Primary care and health system performance: adults' experiences in five countries," *Health Affairs*, pp. W4-487–W4-503, 2004.

[39] H. P. Rodriguez, W. H. Rogers, R. E. Marshall, and D. G. Safran, "Multidisciplinary primary care teams: effects on the quality of clinician-patient interactions and organizational features of care," *Medical Care*, vol. 45, no. 1, pp. 19–27, 2007.

[40] P. Hollander, D. Nicewander, C. Couch et al., "Quality of care of medicare patients with diabetes in a metropolitan fee-for-service primary care integrated delivery system," *American Journal of Medical Quality*, vol. 20, no. 6, pp. 344–352, 2005.

[41] J. F. Steiner, P. A. Braun, P. Melinkovich et al., "Primary-care visits and hospitalizations for ambulatory-care-sensitive conditions in an inner-city health care system," *Ambulatory Pediatrics*, vol. 3, no. 6, pp. 324–328, 2003.

[42] T. N. Chirikos, L. K. Christman, S. Hunter, and R. G. Roetzheim, "Cost-effectiveness of an intervention to increase cancer screening in primary care settings," *Preventive Medicine*, vol. 39, no. 2, pp. 230–238, 2004.

[43] A. Kempe, B. Beaty, B. P. Englund, R. J. Roark, N. Hester, and J. F. Steiner, "Quality of care and use of the medical home in a state-funded capitated primary care plan for low-income children," *Pediatrics*, vol. 105, no. 5, pp. 1020–1028, 2000.

[44] C. Ulmer, D. Lewis-Idema, A. von Worley et al., "Assessing primary care content: four conditions common in community health center practice," *Journal of Ambulatory Care Management*, vol. 23, no. 1, pp. 23–38, 2000.

[45] J. Billings, L. Zeitel, J. Lukomnik, T. S. Carey, A. E. Blank, and L. Newman, "Impact of socioeconomic status on hospital use in New York City," *Health Affairs*, vol. 12, no. 1, pp. 162–173, 1993.

Scientifica 17

[46] S. Saha, R. Solotaroff, A. Oster, and A. B. Bindman, "Are preventable hospitalizations sensitive to changes in access to primary care? The case of the Oregon health plan," *Medical Care*, vol. 45, no. 8, pp. 712–719, 2007.

[47] R. C. Marshall, M. Doperak, M. M. Milner et al., "Patient-Centered medical home: an emerging primary care model and the military health system," *Military Medicine*, vol. 176, no. 11, pp. 1253–1259, 2011.

[48] A. Y. Chen, S. M. Schrager, and R. Mangione-Smith, "Quality measures for primary care of complex pediatric patients," *Pediatrics*, vol. 129, no. 3, pp. 433–445, 2012.

[49] D. Addington, T. Kyle, S. Desai, and J. Wang, "Facilitators and barriers to implementing quality measurement in primary mental health care: systematic review," *Canadian Family Physician*, vol. 56, no. 12, pp. 1322–1331, 2010.

[50] R. Saitz, N. J. Horton, D. M. Cheng, and J. H. Samet, "Alcohol counseling reflects higher quality of primary care," *Journal of General Internal Medicine*, vol. 23, no. 9, pp. 1482–1486, 2008.

[51] S. J. Atlas, R. W. Grant, T. G. Ferris, Y. Chang, and M. J. Barry, "Patient-physician connectedness and quality of primary care," *Annals of Internal Medicine*, vol. 150, no. 5, pp. 325–335, 2009.

[52] T. Rice, "Lessons from across the pond. U.K.'s NHS gets better outcomes at less cost by emphasizing primary-care docs," *Modern Healthcare*, vol. 40, no. 37, p. 17, 2010.

[53] B. Starfield, "Primary care in Canada: coming or going?" *HealthcarePapers*, vol. 8, no. 2, pp. 58–67, 2008.

[54] J. W. Beasley, B. Starfield, C. van Weel, W. W. Rosser, and C. L. Haq, "Global health and primary care research," *Journal of the American Board of Family Medicine*, vol. 20, no. 6, pp. 518–526, 2007.

[55] J. de Maeseneer, P. Hjortdahl, and B. Starfield, "Fix what's wrong, not what's right, with general practice in Britain," *British Medical Journal*, vol. 320, no. 7250, pp. 1616–1617, 2000.

[56] B. Starfield, "Reinventing primary care: lessons from Canada for the United States," *Health Affairs*, vol. 29, no. 5, pp. 1030–1036, 2010.

[57] C. S. Mendonça, E. Harzheim, B. B. Duncan, L. N. Nunes, and W. Leyh, "Trends in hospitalizations for primary care sensitive conditions following the implementation of Family Health Teams in Belo Horizonte, Brazil," *Health Policy and Planning*, vol. 27, no. 4, pp. 348–355, 2012.

[58] R. L. Phillips Jr. and A. W. Bazemore, "Primary care and why it matters for U.S. health system reform," *Health Affairs*, vol. 29, no. 5, pp. 806–810, 2010.

[59] S. Willcox, G. Lewis, and J. Burgers, "Strengthening primary care: recent reforms and achievements in Australia, England, and the Netherlands," Issue Brief. Commonwealth Fund, pp. 1–19, 2011.

[60] H. Tabenkin and R. Gross, "The role of the primary care physician in the Israeli health care system as a "gatekeeper"—the viewpoint of health care policy makers," *Health Policy*, vol. 52, no. 2, pp. 73–85, 2000.

[61] J. Borkan, C. B. Eaton, D. Novillo-Ortiz, P. R. Corte, and A. R. Jadad, "Renewing primary care: lessons learned from the Spanish health care system," *Health Affairs*, vol. 29, no. 8, pp. 1432–1441, 2010.

[62] J. R. Kimberly, "The relationship between job satisfaction of primary care team members and quality of care: a comment on Mohr et al," *American Journal of Medical Quality*, vol. 26, no. 1, pp. 8–9, 2011.

[63] D. W. Roblin, D. H. Howard, J. Ren, and E. R. Becker, "An evaluation of the influence of primary care team functioning on the health of Medicare beneficiaries," *Medical Care Research and Review*, vol. 68, no. 2, pp. 177–201, 2011.

[64] B. Reiss-Brennan, "Can mental health integration in a primary care setting improve quality and lower costs? A case study," *Journal of Managed Care Pharmacy*, vol. 12, supplement 1, no. 2, pp. S14–S20, 2006.

[65] Agency for Healthcare Research and Quality, *Primary Care Workforce Facts and Stats No. 1: The Number of Practicing Primary Care Physicians in the United States*, Agency for Healthcare Research and Policy, Rockville, Md, USA, 2011, http://www.ahrq.gov/research/pcwork1.htm.

[66] E. O'Neil and C. Dower, "Primary care health workforce in the United States," *The Synthesis Project Research Synthesis Report*, no. 22, article 72579, 2011.

[67] Health Resources and Services Administration, "Shortage designation: Health Professional Shortage Areas and Medically Underserved Areas/Populations," http://bhpr.hrsa.gov/shortage/.

[68] B. Starfield and T. Oliver, "Primary care in the United States and its precarious future," *Health and Social Care in the Community*, vol. 7, no. 5, pp. 315–323, 1999.

[69] P. P. Reynolds, "A legislative history of federal assistance for health professions training in primary care medicine and dentistry in the United States, 1963–2008," *Academic Medicine*, vol. 83, no. 11, pp. 1004–1014, 2008.

[70] P. P. Reynolds, "Why we need to restore primary care generalist training as the centerpiece of federal policy," *Academic Medicine*, vol. 83, no. 11, pp. 993–995, 2008.

[71] R. Cardarelli, "The primary care workforce: a critical element in mending the fractured US health care system," *Osteopathic Medicine and Primary Care*, vol. 3, article 11, 2009.

[72] Agency for Healthcare Research and Quality, *Primary Care Workforce Facts and Stats: Overview*, Agency for Healthcare Research and Policy, Rockville, Md, USA, 2012, http://www.ahrq.gov/research/pcworkforce.htm.

[73] M. H. Ebell, "Future salary and US residency fill rate revisited," *Journal of the American Medical Association*, vol. 300, no. 10, pp. 1131–1132, 2008.

[74] P. J. Cunningham, "State variation in primary care physician supply: implications for health reform Medicaid expansions," *Research Briefs*, no. 19, pp. 1–11, 2011.

[75] S. Powell, A. Towers, and P. Milne, "The public health view on closing the gap between public health and primary care," *Family Practice*, vol. 25, supplement 1, pp. i17–i19, 2009.

[76] R. Martin-Misener, R. Valaitis et al., "A scoping literature review of collaboration between primary care and public health," *Primary Health Care Research & Development*, vol. 13, no. 4, pp. 327–346.

[77] M. Stevenson Rowan, W. Hogg, and P. Huston, "Integrating public health and primary care," *Healthc Policy*, vol. 3, no. 1, pp. e160–e181, 2007.

[78] M. D. Schwartz, "Health care reform and the primary care workforce bottleneck," *Journal of General Internal Medicine*, vol. 27, no. 4, pp. 469–472, 2012.

[79] B. Starfield and L. Shi, "Policy relevant determinants of health: an international perspective," *Health Policy*, vol. 60, no. 3, pp. 201–218, 2002.

[80] J. Macinko, B. Starfield, and L. Shi, "The contribution of primary care systems to health outcomes within Organization

for Economic Cooperation and Development (OECD) countries, 1970–1998," *Health Services Research*, vol. 38, no. 3, pp. 831–865, 2003.

[81] J. Macinko, B. Starfield, and T. Erinosho, "The impact of primary healthcare on population health in low- and middle-income countries," *Journal of Ambulatory Care Management*, vol. 32, no. 2, pp. 150–171, 2009.

[82] M. Niti and T. P. Ng, "Avoidable hospitalisation rates in Singapore, 1991–1998: assessing trends and inequities of quality in primary care," *Journal of Epidemiology and Community Health*, vol. 57, no. 1, pp. 17–22, 2003.

[83] M. E. Kruk, D. Porignon, P. C. Rockers, and W. van Lerberghe, "The contribution of primary care to health and health systems in low- and middle-income countries: a critical review of major primary care initiatives," *Social Science and Medicine*, vol. 70, no. 6, pp. 904–911, 2010.

[84] J. Macinko, B. Starfield, and L. Shi, "Quantifying the health benefits of primary care physician supply in the United States," *International Journal of Health Services*, vol. 37, no. 1, pp. 111–126, 2007.

[85] B. Starfield and L. Shi, "Commentary: primary care and health outcomes: a health services research challenge," *Health Services Research*, vol. 42, no. 6, pp. 2252–2256, 2007.

[86] B. . Starfield, "Primary care and health: a cross-national comparison," in *Generalist Medicine and the U.S. Health System*, S. L. Isaacs and J. R. Knickman, Eds., chapter 11, pp. 187–196, Robert Wood Johnson, Princeton, NJ, USA, 2004.

[87] C. H. Chang, T. A. Stukel, A. B. Flood, and D. C. Goodman, "Primary care physician workforce and medicare beneficiaries' health outcomes," *Journal of the American Medical Association*, vol. 305, no. 20, pp. 2096–2105, 2011.

[88] S. J. Kravet, A. D. Shore, R. Miller, G. B. Green, K. Kolodner, and S. M. Wright, "Health care utilization and the proportion of primary care physicians," *American Journal of Medicine*, vol. 121, no. 2, pp. 142–148, 2008.

[89] B. Starfield, L. Shi, and J. Macinko, "Contribution of primary care to health systems and health," *Milbank Quarterly*, vol. 83, no. 3, pp. 457–502, 2005.

[90] B. Starfield, L. Shi, A. Grover, and J. Macinko, "The effects of specialist supply on populations' health: assessing the evidence," *Health Affairs*, pp. W5-97–W5-107, 2005.

[91] K. D. Bertakis and R. Azari, "Patient-centered care is associated with decreased health care utilization," *Journal of the American Board of Family Medicine*, vol. 24, no. 3, pp. 229–239, 2011.

[92] S. A. Jebb, A. L. Ahern, A. D. Olson et al., "Primary care referral to a commercial provider for weight loss treatment versus standard care: a randomised controlled trial," *The Lancet*, vol. 378, no. 9801, pp. 1485–1492, 2011.

[93] J. Ploeg, K. Brazil, B. Hutchison et al., "Effect of preventive primary care outreach on health related quality of life among older adults at risk of functional decline: randomised controlled trial," *British Medical Journal*, vol. 340, p. c1480, 2010.

[94] D. J. Kolko, J. V. Campo, K. Kelleher, and Y. Cheng, "Improving access to care and clinical outcome for pediatric behavioral problems: a randomised trial of a nurse-administered intervention in primary care," *Journal of Developmental and Behavioral Pediatrics*, vol. 31, no. 5, pp. 393–404, 2010.

[95] A. G. Bertoni, D. E. Bonds, H. Chen et al., "Impact of a multifaceted intervention on cholesterol management in primary care practices guideline adherence for heart health randomized trial," *Archives of Internal Medicine*, vol. 169, no. 7, pp. 678–686, 2009.

[96] R. O. White, D. A. DeWalt, R. M. Malone, C. Y. Osborn, M. P. Pignone, and R. L. Rothman, "Leveling the field: addressing health disparities through diabetes disease management," *American Journal of Managed Care*, vol. 16, no. 1, pp. 42–48, 2010.

[97] G. Grandes, A. Sanchez, I. Montoya, R. Sanchez-Pinilla, and J. Torcal, "Two-year longitudinal analysis of a cluster randomized trial of physical activity promotion by general practitioners," *PLoS One*, vol. 6, no. 3, Article ID e18363, 2011.

[98] J. E. Bosmans, D. J. F. van Schaik, M. C. de Bruijne et al., "Are psychological treatments for depression in primary care cost-effective?" *Journal of Mental Health Policy and Economics*, vol. 11, no. 1, pp. 3–15, 2008.

[99] R. Rosenheck, "Primary care satellite clinics and improved access to general and mental health services," *Health Services Research*, vol. 35, no. 4, pp. 777–790, 2000.

[100] N. Rowland, P. Bower, C. Mellor, P. Heywood, and C. Godfrey, "Effectiveness and cost effectiveness of counselling in primary care," *Cochrane Database of Systematic Reviews*, no. 3, p. CD001025, 2001.

[101] J. Rohde, S. Cousens, M. Chopra et al., "30 years after Alma-Ata: has primary health care worked in countries?" *The Lancet*, vol. 372, no. 9642, pp. 950–961, 2008.

[102] T. Continelli, S. McGinnis, and T. Holmes, "The effect of local primary care physician supply on the utilization of preventive health services in the United States," *Health and Place*, vol. 16, no. 5, pp. 942–951, 2010.

[103] D. C. Brousseau, M. H. Gorelick, R. G. Hoffmann, G. Flores, and A. B. Nattinger, "Primary care quality and subsequent emergency department utilization for children in wisconsin medicaid," *Academic Pediatrics*, vol. 9, no. 1, pp. 33–39, 2009.

[104] K. Grumbach and T. Bodenheimer, "Can health care teams improve primary care practice?" *Journal of the American Medical Association*, vol. 291, no. 10, pp. 1246–1251, 2004.

[105] D. W. Bates, "Primary care and the US health care system: what needs to change?" *Journal of General Internal Medicine*, vol. 25, no. 10, pp. 998–999, 2010.

[106] P. Bower, "Measuring patients' assessments of primary care quality: the use of self-report questionnaires," *Expert Review of Pharmacoeconomics and Outcomes Research*, vol. 3, no. 5, pp. 551–560, 2003.

[107] C. B. Forrest, L. Shi, S. von Schrader, and J. Ng, "Managed care, primary care, and the patient-practitioner relationship," *Journal of General Internal Medicine*, vol. 17, no. 4, pp. 270–277, 2002.

[108] L. I. Solberg, A. L. Crain, J. M. Sperl-Hillen, M. C. Hroscikoski, K. I. Engebretson, and P. J. O'Connor, "Effect of improved primary care access on quality of depression care," *Annals of Family Medicine*, vol. 4, no. 1, pp. 69–74, 2006.

[109] A. G. Zahradnik, "Does providing uninsured adults with free or low-cost primary care influence their use of hospital emergency departments?" *Journal of Health and Human Services Administration*, vol. 31, no. 2, pp. 240–258, 2008.

[110] J. L. Raphael, M. Mei, D. C. Brousseau, and T. P. Giordano, "Associations between quality of primary care and health care use among children with special health care needs," *Archives of Pediatrics and Adolescent Medicine*, vol. 165, no. 5, pp. 399–404, 2011.

[111] D. C. Brousseau, R. G. Hoffmann, A. B. Nattinger, G. Flores, Y. Zhang, and M. Gorelick, "Quality of primary care and subsequent pediatric emergency department utilization," *Pediatrics*, vol. 119, no. 6, pp. 1131–1138, 2007.

Scientifica

19

[112] P. Crampton, P. Davis, R. Lay-Yee, A. Raymont, C. B. Forrest, and B. Starfield, "Does community-governed nonprofit primary care improve access to services? Cross-sectional survey of practice characteristics," *International Journal of Health Services*, vol. 35, no. 3, pp. 465–478, 2005.

[113] D. G. Safran, W. H. Rogers, A. R. Tarlov et al., "Organizational and financial characteristics of health plans: are they related to primary care performance?" *Archives of Internal Medicine*, vol. 160, no. 1, pp. 69–76, 2000.

[114] S. Campbell, D. Reeves, E. Kontopantelis, E. Middleton, B. Sibbald, and M. Roland, "Quality of primary care in England with the introduction of pay for performance," *New England Journal of Medicine*, vol. 357, no. 2, pp. 181–190, 2007.

[115] D. G. Safran, I. B. Wilson, W. H. Rogers, J. E. Montgomery, and H. Chang, "Primary care quality in the Medicare program: comparing the performance of medicare health maintenance organizations and traditional fee-for-service Medicare," *Archives of Internal Medicine*, vol. 162, no. 7, pp. 757–765, 2002.

[116] E. Grossman, A. T. R. Legedza, and C. C. Wee, "Primary care for low-income populations: comparing health care delivery systems," *Journal of Health Care for the Poor and Underserved*, vol. 19, no. 3, pp. 743–757, 2008.

[117] M. W. Friedberg, K. L. Coltin, D. G. Safran, M. Dresser, A. M. Zaslavsky, and E. C. Schneider, "Associations between structural capabilities of primary care practices and performance on selected quality measures," *Annals of Internal Medicine*, vol. 151, no. 7, pp. 456–463, 2009.

[118] K. B. Baldwin, "Evaluating quality of primary care using the electronic medical record," *Journal for Healthcare Quality*, vol. 28, no. 6, pp. 40–47, 2006.

[119] J. van Lieshout, M. Goldfracht, S. Campbell, S. Ludt, and M. Wensing, "Primary care characteristics and population-orientated health care across Europe: an observational study," *British Journal of General Practice*, vol. 61, no. 582, pp. e22–e30, 2011.

[120] D. A. Ludwick and J. Doucette, "Adopting electronic medical records in primary care: lessons learned from health information systems implementation experience in seven countries," *International Journal of Medical Informatics*, vol. 78, no. 1, pp. 22–31, 2009.

[121] C. J. Hsiao and C. Boult, "Effects of quality on outcomes in primary care: a review of the literature," *American Journal of Medical Quality*, vol. 23, no. 4, pp. 302–310, 2008.

[122] A. M. Wessell, H. A. Liszka, P. J. Nietert, R. G. Jenkins, L. S. Nemeth, and S. Ornstein, "Achievable benchmarks of care for primary care quality indicators in a practice-based research network," *American Journal of Medical Quality*, vol. 23, no. 1, pp. 39–46, 2008.

[123] B. Gribben, G. Coster, M. Pringle, and J. Simon, "Quality of care indicators for population-based primary care in New Zealand," *New Zealand Medical Journal*, vol. 115, no. 1151, pp. 163–166, 2002.

[124] J. W. Mold, F. Lawler, K. J. Schauf, and C. B. Aspy, "Does patient assessment of the quality of the primary care they receive predict subsequent outcomes? An Oklahoma physicians resource/research network (OKPRN) study," *Journal of the American Board of Family Medicine*, vol. 24, no. 5, pp. 511–523, 2011.

[125] J. G. Cooper, T. Claudi, A. K. Jenum et al., "Quality of care for patients with type 2 diabetes in primary care in Norway is improving," *Diabetes Care*, vol. 32, no. 1, pp. 81–83, 2009.

[126] J. Tsai, L. Shi, W. L. Yu, L. M. Hung, and L. A. Lebrun, "Physician specialty and the quality of medical care experiences in the context of the Taiwan National Health Insurance System," *Journal of the American Board of Family Medicine*, vol. 23, no. 3, pp. 402–412, 2010.

[127] J. Tsai, L. Shi, W. L. Yu, and L. A. Lebrun, "Usual source of care and the quality of medical care experiences: a cross-sectional survey of patients from a taiwanese community," *Medical Care*, vol. 48, no. 7, pp. 628–634, 2010.

[128] H. Ismail, J. Wright, P. Rhodes, and A. Scally, "Quality of care in diabetic patients attending routine primary care clinics compared with those attending GP specialist clinics," *Diabetic Medicine*, vol. 23, no. 8, pp. 851–856, 2006.

[129] V. Backer, S. Nepper-Christensen, and H. Nolte, "Quality of care in patients with asthma and rhinitis treated by respiratory specialists and primary care physicians: a 3-year randomized and prospective follow-up study," *Annals of Allergy, Asthma and Immunology*, vol. 97, no. 4, pp. 490–496, 2006.

[130] D. D. Sin, N. R. Bell, and S. F. Man, "Effects of increased primary care access on process of care and health outcomes among patients with asthma who frequent emergency departments," *American Journal of Medicine*, vol. 117, no. 7, pp. 479–483, 2004.

[131] M. L. van Driel, A. I. de Sutter, T. C. M. Christiaens, and J. M. de Maeseneer, "Quality of care: the need for medical, contextual and policy evidence in primary care," *Journal of Evaluation in Clinical Practice*, vol. 11, no. 5, pp. 417–429, 2005.

[132] W. Schäfer, P. P. Groenewegen, J. Hansen, and N. Black, "Priorities for health services research in primary care," *Quality in Primary Care*, vol. 19, no. 2, pp. 77–83, 2011.

[133] M. W. Friedberg, P. S. Hussey, and E. C. Schneider, "Primary care: a critical review of the evidence on quality and costs of health care," *Health Affairs*, vol. 29, no. 5, pp. 766–772, 2010.

[134] R. H. Brook and R. T. Young, "The primary care physician and health care reform," *Journal of the American Medical Association*, vol. 303, no. 15, pp. 1535–1536, 2010.

[135] K. Grumbach and J. W. Mold, "A health care cooperative extension service: transforming primary care and community health," *Journal of the American Medical Association*, vol. 301, no. 24, pp. 2589–2591, 2009.

[136] A. Hill, C. Levitt, L. W. Chambers, M. Cohen, and J. Underwood, "Primary care and population health promotion. Collaboration between family physicians and public health units in Ontario," *Canadian Family Physician*, vol. 47, pp. 15–17, 22–25, 2001.

[137] M. Norbury, S. W. Mercer, J. Gillies, J. Furler, and G. C. M. Watt, "Time to care: tackling health inequalities through primary care," *Family Practice*, vol. 28, no. 1, pp. 1–3, 2011.

[138] J. E. Wennberg, D. C. Goodman, R. F. Nease, and R. B. Keller, "Finding equilibrium in U.S. physician supply," *Health Affairs*, vol. 12, no. 2, pp. 89–103, 1993.

[139] S. A. Schroeder and L. G. Sandy, "Specialty distribution of U.S. physicians—the invisible driver of health care costs," *New England Journal of Medicine*, vol. 328, no. 13, pp. 961–963, 1993.

[140] S. Greenfield, E. C. Nelson, M. Zubkoff et al., "Variations in resource utilization among medical specialties and systems of care: results from the Medical Outcomes Study," *Journal of the American Medical Association*, vol. 267, no. 12, pp. 1624–1630, 1992.

[141] R. A. Rosenblatt, "Specialists or generalists: on whom should we base the American health care system?" *Journal of the American Medical Association*, vol. 267, no. 12, pp. 1665–1666, 1992.

[142] K. Grumbach and P. R. Lee, "How many physicians can we afford?" *Journal of the American Medical Association*, vol. 265, no. 18, pp. 2369–2372, 1991.

[143] J. P. Leigh, "International comparisons of physicians' salaries," *International Journal of Health Services*, vol. 22, no. 2, pp. 217–220, 1992.

[144] D. A. Rublee and M. Schneider, "International Health spending: comparisons with the OECD," *Health Affairs*, vol. 10, no. 3, pp. 187–198, 1991.

[145] J. J. Escarce, "Explaining the association between surgeon supply and utilization," *Inquiry*, vol. 29, no. 4, pp. 403–415, 1992.

[146] J. P. Weiner, "The demand for physician services in a changing health care system: a synthesis," *Medical care review*, vol. 50, no. 4, pp. 411–449, 1993.

[147] S. A. Schroeder, "Physician supply and the U.S. medical marketplace," *Health Affairs*, vol. 11, no. 1, pp. 235–243, 1992.

[148] H. D. Banta and K. B. Kemp, " The management of health care technologies in ten countries," Background Paper 4, Congress Office of Technology Assessment, Washington, DC, USA, 1980.

[149] US Congressional House Subcommittee Oversight Investigation, *Cost and Quality of Health Care: Unnecessary Surgery*, GPO, Washington, DC,USA, 1976.

[150] L. L. Leape, "Unnecessary surgery," *Annual Review of Public Health*, vol. 13, pp. 363–383, 1992.

[151] S. Walker, A. R. Mason, K. Claxton et al., "Value for money and the quality and outcomes framework in primary care in the UK NHS," *British Journal of General Practice*, vol. 60, no. 574, pp. e213–e220, 2010.

[152] B. Friedman and J. Basu, "Health insurance, primary care, and preventable hospitalization of children in a large state," *American Journal of Managed Care*, vol. 7, no. 5, pp. 473–481, 2001.

[153] R. A. Deyo, "Cost-effectiveness of primary care," *Journal of the American Board of Family Practice*, vol. 13, no. 1, pp. 47–54, 2000.

[154] K. D. Frick, L. Shi, and D. J. Gaskin, "Level of evidence of the value of care in federally qualified health centers for policy making," *Progress in Community Health Partnerships*, vol. 1, no. 1, pp. 75–82, 2007.

[155] D. Gurewich, K. R. Tyo, J. Zhu, and D. S. Shepard, "Comparative performance of community health centers and other usual sources of primary care," *Journal of Ambulatory Care Management*, vol. 34, no. 4, pp. 380–390, 2011.

[156] C. Staub, "Primary care: building the health-care institutions of the future," *Connecticut Medicine*, vol. 74, no. 6, pp. 357–359, 2010.

[157] M. B. Rosenthal, H. B. Beckman, D. Dauser Forrest, E. S. Huang, B. E. Landon, and S. Lewis, "Will the patient-centered medical home improve efficiency and reduce costs of care? A measurement and research agenda," *Medical Care Research and Review*, vol. 67, no. 4, pp. 476–484, 2010.

[158] D. D. Maeng, J. Graham, T. R. Graf et al., "Reducing long-term cost by transforming primary care: evidence from Geisinger's medical home model," *American Journal of Managed Care*, vol. 18, no. 3, pp. 149–155, 2012.

[159] R. S. Hooker, "A cost analysis of physician assistants in primary care," *Journal of the American Academy of Physician Assistants*, vol. 15, no. 11, pp. 39–48, 2002.

[160] E. T. Momany, S. D. Flach, F. D. Nelson, and P. C. Damiano, "A cost analysis of the Iowa medicaid primary care case management program," *Health Services Research*, vol. 41, no. 4, part 1, pp. 1357–1371, 2006.

[161] M. E. Chernew, L. Sabik, A. Chandra, and J. P. Newhouse, "Would having more primary care doctors cut health spending growth?" *Health Affairs*, vol. 28, no. 5, pp. 1327–1335, 2009.

[162] S. J. Wang, B. Middleton, L. A. Prosser et al., "A cost-benefit analysis of electronic medical records in primary care," *American Journal of Medicine*, vol. 114, no. 5, pp. 397–403, 2003.

[163] J. Brown, N. J. Welton, C. Bankhead et al., "A Bayesian approach to analysing the cost-effectiveness of two primary care interventions aimed at improving attendance for breast screening," *Health Economics*, vol. 15, no. 5, pp. 435–445, 2006.

[164] C. A. Brownson, T. J. Hoerger, E. B. Fisher, and K. E. Kilpatrick, "Cost-effectiveness of diabetes self-management programs in community primary care settings," *Diabetes Educator*, vol. 35, no. 5, pp. 761–769, 2009.

[165] H. J. Salize, S. Merkel, I. Reinhard, D. Twardella, K. Mann, and H. Brenner, "Cost-effective primary care-based strategies to improve smoking cessation," *Archives of Internal Medicine*, vol. 169, no. 3, pp. 230–235, 2009.

[166] M. K. Eriksson, L. Hagberg, L. Lindholm, E. B. Malmgren-Olsson, J. Österlind, and M. Eliasson, "Quality of life and cost-effectiveness of a 3-year trial of lifestyle intervention in primary health care," *Archives of Internal Medicine*, vol. 170, no. 16, pp. 1470–1479, 2010.

[167] L. Shi, J. Macinko, B. Starfield, R. Politzer, J. Wulu, and J. Xu, "Primary care, social inequalities and all-cause, heart disease and cancer mortality in US counties: a comparison between urban and non-urban areas," *Public Health*, vol. 119, no. 8, pp. 699–710, 2005.

[168] L. Shi, J. Macinko, B. Starfield, R. Politzer, and J. Xu, "Primary care, race, and mortality in US states," *Social Science and Medicine*, vol. 61, no. 1, pp. 65–75, 2005.

[169] Agency for Healthcare Research and Quality, *2008 National Healthcare Disparities Report*, Department of Health and Human Services, Rockville, Md, USA, 2009.

[170] S. Siegel, E. Moy, and H. Burstin, "Assessing the nation's progress toward elimination of disparities in health care: the national healthcare disparities report," *Journal of General Internal Medicine*, vol. 19, no. 2, pp. 195–200, 2004.

[171] R. J. Campbell, A. M. Ramirez, K. Perez, and R. G. Roetzheim, "Cervical cancer rates and the supply of primary care physicians in Florida," *Family Medicine*, vol. 35, no. 1, pp. 60–64, 2003.

[172] L. Shi, C. B. Forrest, S. von Schrader, and J. Ng, "Vulnerability and the patient-practitioner relationship: the roles of gatekeeping and primary care performance," *American Journal of Public Health*, vol. 93, no. 1, pp. 138–144, 2003.

[173] L. Shi, J. Macinko, B. Starfield, J. Wulu, J. Regan, and R. Politzer, "The relationship between primary care, income inequality, and mortality in US States, 1980–1995," *Journal of the American Board of Family Practice*, vol. 16, no. 5, pp. 412–422, 2003.

[174] L. Shi, J. Macinko, B. Starfield, J. Xu, and R. Politzer, "Primary care, income inequality, and stroke mortality in the United States: a longitudinal analysis, 1985–1995," *Stroke*, vol. 34, no. 8, pp. 1958–1964, 2003.

[175] L. Shi, B. Starfield, J. Xu, R. Politzer, and J. Regan, "Primary care quality: community health center and health maintenance organization," *Southern Medical Journal*, vol. 96, no. 8, pp. 787–795, 2003.

[176] L. Shi, L. H. Green, and S. Kazakova, "Primary care experience and racial disparities in self-reported health status," *Journal*

of the American Board of Family Practice, vol. 17, no. 6, pp. 443–452, 2004.

[177] L. Shi, J. Macinko, B. Starfield et al., "Primary care, infant mortality, and low birth weight in the states of the USA," *Journal of Epidemiology and Community Health*, vol. 58, no. 5, pp. 374–380, 2004.

[178] L. Shi, G. D. Stevens, J. T. Wulu Jr., R. M. Politzer, and J. Xu, "America's health centers: reducing racial and ethnic disparities in perinatal care and birth outcomes," *Health Services Research*, vol. 39, no. 6, pp. 1881–1901, 2004.

[179] A. Lee, A. Kiyu, H. M. Milman, and J. Jimenez, "Improving health and building human capital through an effective primary care system," *Journal of Urban Health*, vol. 84, supplement 1, pp. i75–i85, 2007.

[180] L. Shi, B. Starfield, B. Kennedy, and I. Kawachi, "Income inequality, primary care, and health indicators," *Journal of Family Practice*, vol. 48, no. 4, pp. 275–284, 1999.

[181] L. Shi and B. Starfield, "Primary care, income inequality, and self-rated health in the United States: a mixed-level analysis," *International Journal of Health Services*, vol. 30, no. 3, pp. 541–555, 2000.

[182] L. Shi, B. Starfield, R. Politzer, and J. Regan, "Primary care, self-rated health, and reductions in social disparities in health," *Health Services Research*, vol. 37, no. 3, pp. 529–550, 2002.

[183] L. Shi and B. Starfield, "The effect of primary care physician supply and income inequality on mortality among Blacks and Whites in US metropolitan areas," *American Journal of Public Health*, vol. 91, no. 8, pp. 1246–1250, 2001.

[184] L. Shi, "Experience of primary care by racial and ethnic groups in the United States," *Medical Care*, vol. 37, no. 10, pp. 1068–1077, 1999.

[185] K. Fiscella and K. Holt, "Impact of primary care patient visits on racial and ethnic disparities in preventive care in the United States," *Journal of the American Board of Family Medicine*, vol. 20, no. 6, pp. 587–597, 2007.

[186] E. C. Strumpf, "Racial/ethnic disparities in primary care: the role of physician-patient concordance," *Medical Care*, vol. 49, no. 5, pp. 496–503, 2011.

[187] A. Beal, S. Hernandez, and M. Doty, "Latino access to the patient-centered medical home," *Journal of General Internal Medicine*, vol. 24, supplement 3, pp. S514–S520, 2009.

[188] G. D. Stevens and L. Shi, "Racial and ethnic disparities in the primary care experiences of children: a review of the literature," *Medical Care Research and Review*, vol. 60, no. 1, pp. 3–30, 2003.

[189] J. L. Raphael, B. A. Guadagnolo, A. C. Beal, and A. P. Giardino, "Racial and ethnic disparities in indicators of a primary care medical home for children," *Academic Pediatrics*, vol. 9, no. 4, pp. 221–227, 2009.

[190] S. Bauer and V. S. Kantayya, "Improving access to primary care and health outcomes in migrant farm worker populations: challenges and opportunities," *Disease-a-Month*, vol. 56, no. 12, pp. 706–718, 2010.

[191] M. Abrams, R. Nuzum, S. Mika, and G. Lawlor, "Realizing health reform's potential: how the Affordable Care Act will strengthen primary care and benefit patients, providers, and payers," *Issue Brief*, vol. 1, pp. 1–28, 2011.

[192] A. Dievler and T. Giovannini, "Community health centers: promise and performance," *Medical Care Research and Review*, vol. 55, no. 4, pp. 405–431, 1998.

[193] L. Shi, G. D. Stevens, and R. M. Politzer, "Access to care for U.S. health center patients and patients nationally: how do the most

vulnerable populations fare?" *Medical Care*, vol. 45, no. 3, pp. 206–213, 2007.

[194] Health Resources and Services Administration (HRSA), *Uniform Data System Results*, Rockville, Md, USA, 2011.

[195] National Association of Community Health Centers (NACHC), *Community Health Centers and Health Reform*, Washington, DC, USA, 2011.

[196] L. Shi, L. A. Lebrun, J. Tsai, and J. Zhu, "Characteristics of ambulatory care patients and services: a comparison of community health centers and physicians' offices," *Journal of Health Care for the Poor and Underserved*, vol. 21, no. 4, pp. 1169–1183, 2010.

[197] L. Shi, L. A. Lebrun, and J. Tsai, "Assessing the impact of the health center growth initiative on health center patients," *Public Health Reports*, vol. 125, no. 2, pp. 258–266, 2010.

[198] L. Shi, M. E. Samuels, C. R. Cochran, S. Glover, and D. A. Singh, "Physician practice characteristics and satisfaction: a rural-urban comparison of medical directors at U.S. Community and Migrant Health Centers," *Journal of Rural Health*, vol. 14, no. 4, pp. 346–356, 1998.

[199] L. Shi, K. D. Frick, B. Lefkowitz, and J. Tillman, "Managed care and community health centers," *Journal of Ambulatory Care Management*, vol. 23, no. 1, pp. 1–22, 2000.

[200] National Association of Community Health Centers (NACHC), "Studies on Health Centers Improving Access to Care," 2009, http://www.nachc.org/client/documents/HC_access_to_care_studies_11.094.pdf.

[201] National Association of Community Health Centers (NACHC), "Studies on Health Centers Quality of Care," 2009, http://www.nachc.org/client/documents/HC%20Quality%20 Studies%208.09.pdf.

[202] National Association of Community Health Centers (NACHC), "Studies on Health Centers Cost Effectiveness," 2009, http://www.nachc.org/client/documents/HC_Cost_Effectiveness_Studies_11.09.pdf.

[203] National Association of Community Health Centers (NACHC), "Studies on Health Centers and Disparities," 2009, http://www.nachc.org/client/documents/HC_Disparities_Studies_11.091.pdf.

[204] K. D. Frick and J. Regan, "Whether and where community health center users obtain screening services," *Journal of Health Care for the Poor and Underserved*, vol. 12, no. 4, pp. 429–445, 2001.

[205] L. Shi and G. D. Stevens, "The role of community health centers in delivering primary care to the underserved: experiences of the uninsured and medicaid insured," *Journal of Ambulatory Care Management*, vol. 30, no. 2, pp. 159–170, 2007.

[206] C. B. Forrest and E. M. Whelan, "Primary care safety-net delivery sites in the United States: a comparison of community health centers, hospital outpatient departments, physicians' offices," *Journal of the American Medical Association*, vol. 284, no. 16, pp. 2077–2083, 2000.

[207] R. M. Politzer, J. Yoon, L. Shi, R. G. Hughes, J. Regan, and M. H. Gaston, "Inequality in America: the contribution of health centers in reducing and eliminating disparities in access to care," *Medical Care Research and Review*, vol. 58, no. 2, pp. 234–248, 2001.

[208] L. Shi, J. Tsai, P. C. Higgins, and L. A. Lebrun, "Racial/ethnic and socioeconomic disparities in access to care and quality of care for us health center patients compared with non-health center patients," *Journal of Ambulatory Care Management*, vol. 32, no. 4, pp. 342–350, 2009.

22

[209] B. L. Carlson, J. Eden, D. O'Connor, and J. Regan, "Primary care of patients without insurance by community health centers," *Journal of Ambulatory Care Management*, vol. 24, no. 2, pp. 47–59, 2001.

[210] A. Tourigny, M. Aubin, J. Haggerty et al., "Patients' perceptions of the quality of care after primary care reform: family medicine groups in Quebec," *Canadian Family Physician*, vol. 56, no. 7, pp. e273–e282, 2010.

[211] S. M. Campbell, E. Kontopantelis, D. Reeves et al., "Changes in patient experiences of primary care during health service reforms in England between 2003 and 2007," *Annals of Family Medicine*, vol. 8, no. 6, pp. 499–506, 2010.

[212] K. S. Babiarz, G. Miller, H. Yi, L. Zhang, and S. Rozelle, "New evidence on the impact of China's New Rural Cooperative Medical Scheme and its implications for rural primary healthcare: multivariate difference-in-difference analysis," *British Medical Journal*, vol. 341, p. c5617, 2010.

CHAPTER 29

The art of doing nothing

Job Metsemakers

NOMINATED CLASSIC PAPER

Iona Heath. The art of doing nothing. *European Journal of General Practice*, 2012; 18: 242–46.

At first, I found the title of this paper provocative. Doctors normally want to help and do something. We are trained to act, sometimes very quickly. We follow guidelines and protocols that tell us what to do, sometimes step by step.

Reading the paper, it turns out that 'doing nothing' is actually not about 'doing nothing'. It describes a very active way of doing *other things*, such as listening, noticing, thinking, waiting, witnessing, and preventing harm. These activities are core elements in the interaction with each patient, but get lost or endangered by our active, sometimes even aggressive, style of helping.

Iona Heath links this approach to the works of philosophers, scientists and poets, setting it even more in a reflective frame. But she also makes clear that this listening or waiting approach does not mean we should sit and wait as a spectator. We should act and intervene when needed.

These concepts have been described before, but the combination and the title made me aware of the fact that we are at risk of forgetting the patient in our quest for providing the best evidence-based care. We are at risk of forgetting the individual and how we should interact at the personal level. We need to find out the personal preferences, and get into the art of doing what is needed most at that time for that particular patient.

It will not be easy to learn this, as we will have to get rid of our fears of not doing enough. We will have to explain to patients that listening, noticing, thinking, waiting, witnessing and preventing harm are strong and powerful activities in the hands of the family doctor.

ABOUT THE LEAD AUTHOR OF THIS PAPER

Iona Heath worked as a general practitioner from 1975 until 2010 at the Caversham Group in Kentish Town, in a socially deprived but wonderfully diverse inner-city area in London in the United Kingdom. Over nearly 35 years, she looked after three generations of many families.

Iona has been a nationally elected member of the Council of the Royal College of General Practitioners since 1989, chaired the College's Committee on Medical Ethics from 1998 to 2004, the International Committee from 2006 to 2009, and served as President of the Royal College of General Practitioners from 2009 to 2012.

From 1993 to 2001, Iona was an editorial adviser for the *British Medical Journal* and chaired the journal's ethics committee from 2004 to 2009. She was a member of the UK Human Genetics Commission from 2006 to 2009, and was a member-at-large of the World Organization of Family Doctors (WONCA) world executive from 2007 to 2013.

Iona has written many essays in medical journals. She has been particularly interested in exploring the nature of general practice, the importance of medical generalism, issues of justice and liberty in relation to healthcare, the corrosive influence of the medical industrial complex and the commercialisation of medicine, and the challenges posed by disease-mongering, the care of the dying, and violence within families.

ABOUT THE NOMINATOR OF THIS PAPER

Professor Job F.M. Metsemakers studied medicine at Maastricht University in the Netherlands. He has worked as a family doctor for more than 30 years, in a small community. In 2002, he became professor and chair of the Department of Family Medicine at Maastricht University in the Netherlands. He was elected President of WONCA Europe in 2013.

> 'To become a good and empathic family doctor, you need to be interested much more in the person you are encountering than in the complaint or disease. Furthermore, you need to continue to be curious, critical of yourself, and reflective.'

> *Professor Job F.M. Metsemakers, the Netherlands*

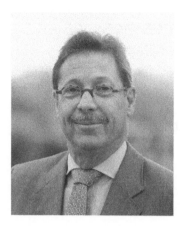

Attribution:

We attribute the original publication of *The art of doing nothing* to the *European Journal of General Practice*. With thanks to Alice Oven, and Taylor and Francis.

European Journal of General Practice, 2012; 18: 242–246

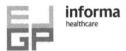

Background Paper

The art of doing nothing

Iona Heath

Royal College of General Practitioners, London, UK

THE WISDOM OF OTHERS

In his 1994 book *Alone again: Ethics after uncertainty,* the sociologist Zygmunt Bauman quotes the German psychiatrist and philosopher Karl Jaspers:

> Our time thinks in terms of "knowing how to do it," even where there is nothing to be done (1).

In her 2001 book, *Science and poetry,* the British philosopher Mary Midgley expanded on this point:

> Out of this fascination with new power there arises our current huge expansion of technology, much of it useful, much not, and the sheer size of it dangerously wasteful of resources. It is hard for us to break out of this circle of increasing needs because our age is remarkably preoccupied with the vision of continually improving means rather than saving ourselves trouble by reflecting on ends (2).

Ours has become the age of unthinking doing—keep doing, do not stop to think—there's no time! There's no time because we are too busy doing.

The American poet William Carlos Williams who was also a general practitioner understood very clearly how easy it is for doctors to succumb to this particular vicious circle. In his 1932 short story about 'Old Doc Rivers' he wrote:

> With this pressure upon us, we eventually do what all herded things do; we begin to hurry to escape it, then we break into a trot, finally into a mad run (watches in our hands), having no idea where we are going and having no time to find out (3).

I suspect that everyone who has worked in general practice recognises this phenomenon. Rushing around all day—no time to stop, to listen, to think, to notice—or even—to go to the toilet!

The Austrian Nobel Prize winning physicist Erwin Schrödinger, most famous for his cat, seems to have understood the importance and the power of the art of doing nothing:

> In an honest search for knowledge you quite often have to abide by ignorance for an indefinite period. ... The steadfastness in standing up to [this requirement], nay in appreciating it as a stimulus and a signpost to further quest, is a natural and indispensable disposition in the mind of a scientist (4).

He seems to me to be describing the importance of the pause for thought—especially in the conditions of ignorance and uncertainty so common in general practice.

Taking all this wisdom into account, my conclusion is that, perhaps counter intuitively, in medicine, the art of doing nothing is active, considered, and deliberate. It is an antidote to the pressure to DO and it takes many forms and these are just some of them:

- Listening, noticing
- Thinking
- Waiting
- Witnessing
- Preventing harm

Each is an art in its own right—requiring judgment, wisdom and even a sense of beauty.

LISTENING AND NOTICING

Doing nothing—but instead—listening and noticing. It is impossible to do and to listen intently and accurately at the same time. Anyone who has tried to listen to their

This paper was given as a keynote lecture 'Art' at the Wonca Europe Conference in Vienna on July 5 2012. I was given this marvellous title by Professor Manfred Maier and used it to explore the excess of doing within contemporary medical practice.
Correspondence: I. Heath, Royal College of General Practitioners, 1 Bow Churchyard, London EC4M 9DQ, UK. Fax: +44 (0)20 3188 7401. E-mail: iona.heath22@yahoo.co.uk

(Received 14 September 2012; accepted 21 September 2012)

ISSN 1381-4788 print/ISSN 1751-1402 online © 2012 Informa Healthcare
DOI: 10.3109/13814788.2012.733691

children while also trying to cook a dinner knows this to be true. William Carlos Williams describes the intensity of listening in general practice:

> It is actually there, in the life before us, every minute that we are listening, a rarest element—not in our imaginations but there, there in fact. It is that essence which is hidden in the very words which are going in at our ears and from which we must recover underlying meaning as realistically as we recover metal out of ore (5).

He describes this essence as the nearest most patients come to the poetry of their lives as they struggle to give expression to their deepest feelings and fears in the quiet privacy of the doctor's consulting room.

The Scottish poet Kathleen Jamie thinks that the necessary commitment and concentration of listening and noticing come close to the idea of prayer

> Isn't that a kind of prayer? The care and maintenance of the web of our noticing, the paying heed (6).

And when she describes her experience of birdwatching—it sounds so close to the kind of receptiveness that we need in general practice:

> This is what I want to learn: to notice, but not to analyse. To still the part of the brain that's yammering, "My god, what's that? A stork, a crane, an ibis?—don't be silly, it's just a weird heron." Sometimes we have to hush the frantic inner voice that says "Don't be stupid," and learn again to look, to listen. You can do the organizing and redrafting, the diagnosing and identifying later, but right now, just be open to it, see how it's tilting nervously into the wind, try to see the colour, the unchancy shape—hold it in your head, bring it home intact.

Right now—do nothing—just be open to the patient—notice them and hold them in your head. Do not start to analyse—to diagnose—too soon.

It is Zbigniew Herbert, the great Polish poet who reminds us of our responsibility to those who are sometimes the most difficult to pay attention to—to listen to—to notice:

> His only weapon was abuse, the rebellion of the helpless—without hope but precisely because of that, deserving admiration and respect (7).

THINKING

Do nothing—stop and think instead. Does this patient need a diagnostic label—will it really help them? What sort of care would be right for them—at this time and in this place?

The German philosopher Hans Georg Gadamer reminds us just how serious this task of thinking is:

> Thinking is the dialogue of the soul with itself. This is how Plato described thinking, and this means at the same time that thinking is listening to the answers that we give ourselves, and that are given to us, when we raise the question of the incomprehensible (8).

The legacy of the well-intentioned emphasis on the evidence base of medicine has been the proliferation of guidelines which were designed to provide guidance but, abetted by a multitude of subtle pressures and the indiscriminate, and distinctly unsubtle, incentives of performance-related pay, have been slowly transmogrified into tablets of law that make it all too easy to DO without pausing to think.

WAITING

Doing nothing, but having the courage sometimes to wait—to use time as both a diagnostic and a therapeutic tool—to see what nature does—to wait and see. These are essential skills of the art of doing nothing that are profoundly important if we are not to fall into the seductive traps of over diagnosis and overtreatment.

The importance of waiting is captured in one of the poems by the New Zealand doctor and poet Glen Colquhoun:

> *Increasingly sophisticated methods of divination*
> *used in the practice of medicine*
> *By observing a rooster pecking grain.*
> *By the various behaviours of birds.*
> *By balancing a stone on a red-hot axe.*
> *By the shape of molten wax dripped into water.*
>
> *By the pattern of shadows cast onto plastic.*
> *By the colour of paper dipped in urine.*
> *By the growing of fresh mould in round dishes.*
> *By the magnification of blood.*
>
> *By the alignment of electricity around the outside*
> *of the heart.*
> *By the rise in a column of mercury.*
> *By timing exactly the formation of clots.*
> *By the examination of excrement.*
>
> *By the placement of sharp needles underneath*
> *the skin.*
> *By tapping the knee with a hammer.*
> *By the bouncing of sound against a full bladder.*
> *By the interpretations of pus.*
>
> *By the attractions of the body to strong magnets.*
> *By the characteristics of sweat.*
> *By listening carefully to the directions of blood.*
> *By waiting to see what happens next (9).*

Waiting to see what happens next is indeed the most sophisticated method of diagnosis and, in the face of the ever increasing availability of expensive and intimidating technology; we would do well to remember this.

BEING PRESENT

Doing nothing but simply being present—there with the patient—and bearing witness so that the old adage is reversed and becomes: 'Don't just do something, stand there.'

In *A fortunate man*, which is for me the best book ever written about general practice, John Berger writes:

> He does more than treat them when they are ill;
> he is the objective witness of their lives (10).

John and Bogdana Carpenter, responsible for the English translations of many of Zbigniew Herbert's poems, write:

> Our own freedom and our very reality depend upon the accuracy with which we are able to perceive the suffering around us, to bear witness to it, and to revolt against it (11).

This doing nothing while witnessing suffering precedes the action of revolting against it and in general practice that action is our responsibility for advocacy. We have an obligation to speak out for those who have no voice and to describe to politicians and policy-makers, as often as we can, how their policies play out in the realities of daily life for those struggling with relative deprivation in an unequal society.

Inadequate housing, homelessness, and family poverty are structural issues but are no less amenable to intervention than the health conditions they engender. The way they differ is in the type of intervention required. ... *Advocacy is structural therapeutics* (12).

In June, I had the wonderful privilege and good fortune of attending a seminar in Rosendal in Norway entitled: The nature of humans and the goals of medicine. At the seminar, I met a young doctor working in interventional cardiology who I had first met when she was a medical student at a similar seminar eight years ago. She is also a brilliant musician and, for this seminar, she had written a piece of electronica music that she played for us. It had a repeating line in the manner of electronic: 'I know I can see you through this' (13).

As this phrase repeated in the music, I slowly realized how different this statement is from the more usual 'I know I can help you with this' and the difference is about witnessing and about being there when there is little help to be had. It is an offer of companionship, of solidarity and a promise not to run away. It is part of the art of doing nothing.

Arthur Kleinman, the American anthropologist and psychiatrist, says something similar:

> ... empathic witnessing ... is the existential commitment to be with the sick person and to facilitate his or her building of an illness narrative that will make sense of and give value to the experience. ... This I take to be the moral core of doctoring and of the experience of illness (14).

Charles Rosenberg, Professor of the History of Medicine at Harvard, asks:

> How does one manage death—which is not precisely a disease—when demands for technological ingenuity and activism are almost synonymous with public expectations of a scientific medicine (15)?

Pointing out the excess of doing in modern medical care and perhaps the deficiency of witnessing.

Samuel Beckett understood more about futile doing than most. He is described by the literary critic Christopher Ricks as:

> —The great writer of an age which has created new possibilities and impossibilities even in the matter of death. Of an age which has dilated longevity, until it is as much a nightmare as a blessing (16).

In *Malone dies*, Beckett writes:

> And when they cannot swallow any more someone rams a tube down their gullet, or up their rectum, and fills them full of vitaminized pap, so as not to be accused of murder (17).

This was written more than 60 years ago and it is frightening to consider how much truer it has become over the intervening years.

'I know I can see you through this' is the commitment doctors can make to the dying when doing has become futile and even cruel. Simply being there and bearing witness is never futile.

PREVENTING HARM

Finally—doing nothing and thereby preventing harm. The importance of this was emphasized in a paper published in the Archives of Internal Medicine earlier this year which came to a somewhat unexpected conclusion (18).

In a nationally representative sample, higher patient satisfaction was associated with less emergency department use but with greater inpatient use, higher overall health care and prescription drug expenditures, and increased mortality.

In a commentary on this research paper, Brenda Sirovich from the Dartmouth Institute for Health Policy and Clinical Practice noted that:

> Practicing physicians have learned—from reimbursement systems, the medical liability environment, and clinical performance score-keepers—that they will be rewarded for excess and penalized if they risk not doing enough (19).

She mentioned a study she had done with her colleagues Steve Woloshin and Lisa Schwarz in which they found that nearly half of US primary care physicians believed that their own patients were receiving too much medical care (20). This somehow exemplifies this statement from Vladimir Nabokov:

> The lovely thing about humanity is that at times one may be unaware of doing right, but one is always aware of doing wrong (21).

I do not think that we in Europe are quite as bad as the Americans in this but we are not far behind and we too know that we are doing too much.

Brenda Sirovich also tells the story of Joseph Epstein, an American essayist, short story writer, and editor. On his sixtieth birthday, feeling perfectly well, he promised his wife that he would go for a medical check-up. He felt perfectly well, was not overweight, ate a healthy diet, exercised regularly and had not smoked for 20 years. He went for his check-up, had a normal ECG and had blood taken. His total cholesterol was normal but his HDL level was low. This was the only abnormality. In short order he was referred for a stress test, an angiogram and a CABG. He went from feeling perfectly well to having a huge scar, feeling traumatized, vulnerable and weak and wondering whether he would ever recover his previous sense of well-being. We know all this because he wrote about it in the New Yorker in an article entitled 'Taking the bypass—a healthy man's nightmare' (22). The truly remarkable thing is his conclusion:

> In the long view, I know I have to count myself lucky.

He expresses himself grateful to his excellent doctors. As Sirovich points out, 'Satisfaction with seemingly adverse outcomes of potentially excessive medical care appears to be the norm.' But remember where we started this—higher patient satisfaction is correlated with increased mortality.

About 15 years ago, at a research conference, I heard a nurse reporting on a qualitative study of nurses' feelings when they are asked to try to persuade parents to accept infant vaccination. Her finding was a clear conclusion that the nurses thought that a crime of omission causing potential harm to an unvaccinated child was somehow less than a crime of commission—precipitating serious side effects by giving the vaccination. Doing nothing was felt to be less bad than doing something that went wrong. Active harm is worse than passive harm.

Joseph Epstein's story suggests that this has been turned completely upside down—as doctors, we seem to have persuaded ourselves that commission is now much less bad than omission.

We seem trapped in an uncontrolled positive feedback loop with doctors convinced they are doing the best for their patients and grateful and satisfied patients feeling that somehow their lives have been saved. It is surely time to step back and reconsider the virtues of doing nothing before the harms multiply and health care becomes exponentially more expensive than it already is.

CONCLUSION

Doing nothing is preferable to leaping to conclusions; applying inappropriate or premature labels; medicalizing ordinary human distress; and instigating futile or ineffective treatments. Yet, while aspiring to the undoubted benefits of the art of doing nothing, we must also take heed of the warning from Aimé Césaire, the great francophone poet from Martinique:

> Beware, my body and my soul, beware above all of crossing your arms and assuming the sterile attitude of the spectator, because life is not a spectacle, because a sea of sorrows is not a proscenium, because a man who cries out is not a dancing bear (23).

So let us cultivate the art of doing nothing but never allow ourselves to take refuge in the sterile attitude of the spectator.

ACKNOWLEDGEMENTS

I am grateful to Glen Colquhoun for allowing me to reproduce his poem.

Declaration of interest: The author reports no conflicts of interest. The author alone is responsible for the content and writing of the paper.

REFERENCES

1. Bauman Z. Alone again: Ethics after uncertainty. London: Demos; 1994.
2. Midgley M. Science and poetry. London: Routledge; 2001.
3. Williams WC. Old Doc Rivers, 1932. In: Williams WC. The doctor stories. New York: New Directions Books; 1984.

246   *I. Heath*

4. Schrödinger E. Nature and the Greeks. Cambridge: Cambridge University Press; 1954.

5. Williams WC. The practice. In: Williams WC. The doctor stories. New York: New Directions Books; 1984.

6. Jamie K. Findings. London: Sort of Books; 2005.

7. Herbert Z. King of the ants: Mythological essays. New York: WW Norton & Co.; 1999.

8. Gadamer H-G. The enigma of health. The art of healing in a scientific age. Stanford: Stanford University Press; 1996.

9. Colquhoun G. Playing God: Poems about medicine. London: Hammersmith Press Limited; 2007.

10. Berger J, Mohr J. A fortunate man. Harmondsworth: Allen Lane The Penguin Press; 1967.

11. Carpenter J, Carpenter B. Introduction to Herbert Z. Report from the besieged city and other poems. Oxford: Oxford University Press; 1987.

12. Roberts I. Deaths of children in house fires. Br Med J. 1995;311:1381–2.

13. Aase Schaufel M. Sick sinus. On CD Appearing, Ischaemia Records; 2009.

14. Kleinman A. The illness narratives: Suffering, healing and the human condition. New York: Basic Books; 1988.

15. Rosenberg CE. The tyranny of diagnosis: Specific entities and individual experience. The Milbank Quarterly 2002;80: 237–260.

16. Ricks C. Beckett's dying words. The Clarendon Lectures 1990. Oxford: Oxford University Press; 1995.

17. Beckett S. Malone dies. 1951. London: Penguin Books; 1962.

18. Fenton JJ, Jerant AF, Bertakis KD, Franks P. The cost of satisfaction: A national study of patient satisfaction, health care utilization, expenditures, and mortality. Arch Intern Med. 2012; 172:405–11.

19. Sirovich BE. How to feed and grow your health care system. Arch Int Med. 2012;172:411–3.

20. Sirovich BE, Woloshin S, Schwartz LM. Too little? Too much? Primary care physicians' views on US health care: A brief report. Arch Intern Med. 2011;171:1582–5.

21. Nabokov V. The assistant producer (1943). In: Nabokov V. Nabokov's dozen. London: Penguin Books; 1990.

22. Epstein J. Taking the bypass—a healthy man's nightmare. New Yorker, 12 April 1999.

23. Césaire A. Return to my native land, (1939, 1956). Harmondsworth: Allen Lane The Penguin Press; 1969.

CHAPTER 30

Family medicine development in China

Shanzhu Zhu and Donald K. T. Li

NOMINATED CLASSIC PAPER

Guidelines of the China State Council on the Establishment of a General Practitioner System. The State Council of the People's Republic of China, 2013 (published in Chinese).

In April 2009, the China Central Communist Party, along with the China State Council, announced a comprehensive healthcare reform initiative and issued a new healthcare reform plan named *Implementation Plan for Deepening Pharmaceutical and Health System Reform 2009–2011*.

This paper is a follow-up announcement, issued in 2011 by the State Department of the Chinese Government, and outlining plans to redevelop primary care across the nation and making a commitment to the training of competent general practitioners (GPs).

The paper reflects the intent of the Government of China to initiate healthcare reform through the establishment of a strong system of general practice, ensuring access and equitable outcomes for the population.

The effort to build up a reliable network of non-hospital-based primary care providers is a difficult and long-term process in China, since many patients have a well-founded distrust of the quality of many primary care providers. Before the reform, the large majority of doctors working in primary care had only received very brief postgraduate vocational training at best. This announcement declares that China aims to provide postgraduate training to an additional 300,000 GPs within 10 years, with a target of two to three trained GPs for every 10,000 urban and rural residents, and to promote the development of the primary healthcare system, strengthening the quality and funding for village clinics, township health centres and urban community health centres, and launching a new upskilling programme for GPs designed to bring barefoot doctors into the 21st century in terms of training and quality. This 2011 paper also introduces China's 5+3 GP training programme for new medical graduates, with three years of postgraduate GP training, following a five-year undergraduate medical course.

This announcement from the highest authority in China shows determination by this country to place resources and priority in the establishment of a strong national healthcare system based in primary care. It demonstrates commitment to the belief that good primary care will have a dramatic benefit by reducing both healthcare expenditure and health inequalities for the 1.3 billion people of China. It also has the potential to have profound influence over the development of family medicine in other parts of the world. As World Health Organization Director-General Dr Margaret Chan reminded us in 2015, 'Worldwide, healthcare workers are looking to China to see how it goes about achieving its desire to provide safe, effective, convenient and affordable healthcare services to its 1.3 billion citizens. ... This new system has the opportunity to be an example to the whole world.'

This paper serves as an encouragement to family doctors around the world, and sets an example for global healthcare leaders and the governments of other nations to follow suit in appreciating and recognising the value of quality primary care delivered by well-trained family doctors, and highlights the need to allocate appropriate resources to train specialist family doctors in each country.

ABOUT THE NOMINATORS OF THIS PAPER

Professor Shanzhu Zhu is Director of the General Practice Faculty of the Shanghai Medical College at Fudan University in China. She is Director of the National GP Teacher Training Centre of China, and Vice-director of the Shanghai GP Teacher Training Centre. She is a former Chairwoman of the General Practice Society of the Chinese Medical Association, a member of the Steering Committee of the Chinese Medical Doctor Association, and Chief Editor of *The Chinese Journal of General Practitioners*.

Professor Donald K.T. Li is a specialist in family medicine in private practice in Hong Kong. He is an adviser to the People's Republic of China on general practice development and enhancement. He is the current President of the Hong Kong Academy of Medicine, and also chairman of the governing committee of the Hong Kong Jockey Club Disaster Preparedness and Response Institute of the Academy of Medicine. He is Honorary Treasurer and member-at-large of the World Organization of Family Doctors (WONCA) and Censor of the Hong Kong College of Family

Physicians. In 2011 he was awarded the Silver Bauhinia Star by the Government of the Hong Kong Special Administrative Region for his long leadership in public affairs and voluntary work.

'General practice is the main way to solve the challenges of primary care in China. Initial development of general practice in the mainland of China has been difficult, but this document about general practice systems development, formulated by the government of China, indicates that the government is determined to strengthen primary care throughout the country.'

Professor Shanzhu Zhu, China

'Health is about people – beyond the glittering surface of modern technology, the core space of every health system is occupied by the unique encounter between people who need services and those entrusted to deliver them. Trust is earned through a special blend of technical competence and service orientation, steered by ethical commitment and social accountability, which forms the essence of our professional work.'

Professor Donald K.T. Li, Hong Kong

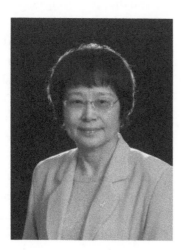 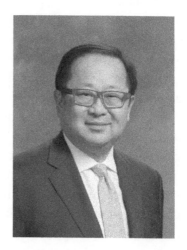

Attribution:

We attribute the original publication of *Guidelines of the State Council on the Establishment of a General Practitioner System* to the National Health and Family Commission of the People's Republic of China, and thank the commission for permission to reproduce this document and its English translation.

Guidelines of the State Council on the Establishment of a General Practitioner System

G.F. [2011] No. 23

People's government of provinces, autonomous regions, municipalities directly under the Central Government, ministries and commissions of, and organizations directly under the State Council:

Guidelines are hereby given on the establishment of a general practitioner system to thoroughly enhance reform of the medical and health system:

I. Fully understanding the significance and necessity of establishing a general practitioner system

(1) **It is an urgent need of ensuring and improving health of urban and rural residents to establish a general practitioner system.** China is a developing country with a population of over 1.3 billion citizens, and we witness an increasing demand for a higher standard of health of urban and rural residents due to economic growth and improvement of living standards. Industrialization, urbanization, and eco-environmental changes are exerting a greater impact on health. Meanwhile, aging of population combined with changes of spectrum of disease are commanding new requirements on medical and health services. General practitioners are medical talents with a more comprehensive knowledge providing an all-in-one service including prevention and health care, diagnosis and treatment as well as referral of common diseases and frequently-occurring diseases, rehabilitation, management of chronic diseases, and health care management. They are commonly referred to as 'gatekeeper' of residents' health. Establishment of a general practitioner system and proper functioning of general practitioners would help implement the policy of prevention and thus providing better medical service to people.

(2) **It is an objective requirement of improving primary medical and health service to establish a general practitioner system.** Operational improvement of primary medical and health service is the focal point of medical and health reform and a basic, fair, and feasible way of improving primary medical and health service; primary medical and health service depend on medical talents. Over the years, there is a lag in the organization of primary medical teams in China, with significantly insufficient quantity of qualified general practitioners, which greatly limits the improvement of primary medical and health service. Establishing and cultivating qualified

general practitioners who 'are willing to continuously work at and contribute effort to the primary level' is an objective requirement of and a necessity for improving primary medical and health service.

(3) **The establishment of a general practitioner system is a significant measure for promoting the transition of mode of medical and health service.** A hierarchical mode of diagnosis and treatment should be established; general practitioners shall individually have contractual agreement on the provision of medical service. It is the direction of medical and health service in China and also the common and successful practice in many countries. Establishing a proper general practitioner system based on the actual situation of China would help optimize the allocation of medical resources; develop a mode of diagnosis and treatment on the basis of reasonable division of duties among primary medical institutes and urban hospitals; provide continuous, harmonious, and convenient primary medical and health service for the mass; and thus solving the problem of 'great difficulties in and huge cost seeking for medical service'.

II. Guidelines on general rules and overall goals of the establishment of a general practitioner system

(4) **Guidelines.** Complying with the overall thought of enhancing reform of the medical system; taking into account economic and social development of China, and trends of residents' needs for health; sticking to the general ways of emphasizing fundamental measures; enhancing primary operation and establishing systems; following the rules of medical and health development, and cultivation of general practitioners; strengthening leading role of the government in primary medical and health service; making use of market system; focusing on basic realities of China; referring to international experience; facilitating system innovation; conducting pilot plans; gradually establishing and improving a system covering training; employing and motivating of Chinese general practitioners; and comprehensively improving standards of primary medical and health service.

(5) **General principles**. Highlighting practice and emphasizing quality; focusing on improvement of clinical practice; regulating mode of training; making general standards for training; developing strict admission criteria and qualification examinations, and practically improving quality of training of general practitioners; innovative systems and healthy service; reforming methods for practice of general practitioners; establishing and improving incentive mechanism; leading general practitioners to primary operation; gradually organizing primary medical and health teams mainly consisting general practitioners to provide safe, efficient, convenient, and low-cost primary medical and health service for the mass; designing step-by-step implementation; focusing on long-term development; strengthening the

overall design and gradually establishing a uniform and standard general practitioner system while at the same time; focusing on the current situation; and cultivating general practitioners via multiple channels and satisfying current needs of the primary level for general practitioners.

(6) **Overall goals**. By 2020, we aim to establish a vital and dynamic general practitioner system by developing a uniform and standard mode of general practitioner training and service mode of 'initial diagnosis at the primary level', establishing a stable service relation between general practitioners and urban and rural residents, realizing the goal of 2 to 3 qualified general practitioners for every ten thousand residents, raising the standards of service of general practitioners, and satisfying the needs of the mass for primary medical and health service.

III. Gradually establishing a uniform standard system of cultivating general practitioners

(7) **Regulating training mode of general practitioners**. A standard model of '5+3' years of training for general practitioners should be gradually developed, where general practitioners shall receive 5-year undergraduate education in clinical medicine (including traditional Chinese medicine) and 3-year standardized general practitioner training. During the transitional period, the 3-year standardized general practitioner training can be implemented in two ways such as 'standardized post-graduate training' and 'research education of clinical medicine'; specific method shall be determined by provinces (regions or municipalities).

Trainees receiving standardized post-graduate training shall be selected among graduates of clinical medicine with an undergraduate or higher degree. During the training period, trainees will receive standardized general practitioner training under the joint supervision of local authorities of health (including traditional Chinese medicine management authorities) and authorities of education in respective training ground. Research students of general clinical medicine shall be trained in accordance with uniform standardized general practitioner training; qualified students would obtain a qualification certificate upon passing of the assessment of such training. Postgraduate research degree of clinical medicine shall be mainly managed by authorities of education.

(8) **Standardizing methods for and details of standardized general practitioner training**. Standardized general practitioner training shall focus on improving practical capabilities of clinical service and public health, and shall be conducted on the basis of tutorial system and credit system in standardized general practitioner training grounds recognized by the government. Trainees shall be rotated among different departments in the training ground for different clinical and public health disciplines as well as practical exposure at the

community level. In principle, trainees shall receive training from departments in clinical training bases for at least two years in addition to service practice for a certain duration in primary practice bases and professional public health institutions. Upon assessment organized by training bases in accordance with national standards, trainees satisfying requirements for disease entities, case load and basic clinical abilities, practical abilities in public health and occupational quality and having acquired required credits shall obtain a qualification certificate of standardized general practitioner training. Details and standards of standardized training shall be formulated by the Ministry of Health, Ministry of Education and State Administration of Traditional Chinese Medicine.

(9) **Regulating management of trainees of standardized general practitioner training**. Trainees of standardized general practitioner training shall be part of resident physicians in the training ground and shall be treated as resident physicians during the training period. Financial subsidies should be provided based on different situations; postgraduate trainees shall be subject to relevant existing national regulations while for those trainees deployed by the employers, employment status and salaries for them shall remain unchanged. No training fees (tuition) will be charged for the standardized training, while training expenses for training beyond standard credits or specified duration shall be borne by individual trainees. Specific management methods shall be formulated by the Ministry of Human Resources and Social Security, Ministry of Health, Ministry of Education, and Ministry of Finance.

(10) **Developing uniform admission criteria for practice of general practitioners**. During standardized general practitioner training, trainees may be engaged in clinical operation such as medical examination, disease investigation and medical treatment, and work shifts in hospitals under tutorial guidance; they may take the national physician's qualification exam in accordance with relevant rules. A registered general practitioner must receive a 3-year standardized general practitioner training to obtain a qualification certificate and pass the national physician's qualification exam to obtain physician's qualification.

(11) **Developing uniform standards for degree awarding of general medicine degrees.** Corresponding professional degrees of clinical medicine (general medicine) shall be granted to persons who have received 5-year undergraduate education of clinical medicine or higher clinical medical education, have obtained qualification upon receiving standardized general practitioner training and satisfy national requirements for academic degree. Specific provisions shall be put forward by the Degree Committee of the State Council and the Ministry of Health.

(12) **Improving primary education of clinical medicine**. Undergraduate education of clinical medicine shall

focus on fundamental medical theories, fundamental knowledge of clinical medicine and preventive medicine, and training of basic skills; it shall at the same time strengthen theoretical and practical education of general medicine, emphasize skills in doctor-patient communication, use of basic drugs, and management of medical expenses.

(13) **Reforming postgraduate research education of clinical medicine (general medicine).** Starting from 2012, fresh postgraduate research students majoring in clinical medicine (general medicine) shall be regularized in accordance with requirements of standardized general practitioner training. Such education shall satisfy needs of positions of general practitioners and training of clinical medical graduate students shall be further enhanced, gradually enrolling more graduate students of clinical medicine oriented to general medicine.

(14) **Promoting continuing medical education of general practitioners.** Continuing medical education of general practitioners shall be enhanced based on frequent, targeted, and practical problems in general medicine, focusing on new knowledge and new skills in technical development of modern medicine. Assessment of continuing medical education of general practitioners shall be strengthened and taking continuing medical education as a significant factor for employment, promotion of technical positions and qualification of medical practice of general practitioners.

IV. Nurturing qualified general practitioners via multiple channels in the short run

To find a balance between great needs of the primary level for general practitioners and prolonged standardized general practitioner training, multiple measures shall be taken in the near future, striving to achieve the goal of qualified general practitioners in every urban community health service institution and every rural health center by 2012.

(15) **Adequately implementing training for existing doctors at the primary level for rotation of position.** Qualified physicians or assistant physicians practicing at the primary level shall be trained for 1 or 2 years for rotation of position. Training by rotation shall be conducted in standardized general practitioner training grounds recognized by the government and shall focus on improvement of skills in general medical service and public health service. After such training, trainees shall pass the uniform examination organized by provincial administrative authorities of health and obtain a qualification certificate; they may then register as a general practitioner or general practitioner assistant.

(16) **Enhancing directional skill training for general practitioners.** Training for clinical skills and public health shall be properly increased for the 5-year clinical medical trainees with the orientation to the primary level. For those 3-year postgraduates working in less developed rural areas may receive 2-year training in clinical skills and public health in training grounds

recognized by the government to obtain qualification of assistant physician and then register as an assistant general practitioner, provided that provincial (regional or municipal) administrative authorities of health shall strictly control the inflow of practitioners.

(17) **Enhancing academic level of existing doctors at the primary level**. Existing doctors at the primary level shall be encouraged to receive adult higher education to improve their academic standard and shall take corresponding qualification examination upon satisfying relevant requirements; having passed such examination, they may register as a general practitioner or assistant general practitioner.

(18) **Encourage hospital doctors to serve at the primary level**. The rule that doctors in urban hospitals awarded the title of attending physician or assisting attending physician shall have served at the primary level for at least 1 year and authorities of health shall duly organize, manage and assess. Targeted support system and two-way communication mechanism shall be established and improved between urban hospitals and primary medical and health institutions; hospitals of county level or higher levels shall enhance technical instruction and training for the primary level via distance medical learning. Administrative methods shall be put forward to facilitate doctors (including retired doctors) from hospitals to offer service to primary medical and health institutions (including private clinics and other medical institutions based on public efforts) and to receive reasonable remuneration.

V. Reforming mode of practice of general practitioners

(19) **Leading general practitioners to practice in various ways.** General practitioners with qualification for practice typically register at one site or register and practice at more sites based on actual needs. General practitioners may work full time or part time in medical and health institutions (hospitals) at the primary level and may as well independently operate a clinic or jointly operate a partnership clinic with others. Organization of general practitioner teams shall be encouraged consisting of general practitioners, community nurses, public health physicians, or rural doctors, and service shall be provided for residents based on divided zones. Human resources management methods of general practitioners shall be improved by primary medical and health institutions to regulate management of labor relation of employees of private clinics.

(20) **Government providing service platforms for general practitioners**. For general practitioners (including specialist physicians of large-scale hospitals) working at primary level, the government shall sign agreements with primary medical and health institutions to provide service platforms. Based on the existing resources, regional medical examination and test centers shall be established, community-based retail drugstores shall be

encouraged and regulated, so as to provide conditions for practice of general practitioners.

(21) **Facilitating the establishment of contractual service relation between general practitioners and residents.** Primary medical and health institutions or general practitioners shall sign a service agreement of a certain period with residents to establish a stable contractual service relationship and delegate the responsibility for medical and health service to individual practitioners. Insured patients may select a physician in local medical insurance service institutions or among general practitioners to sign an agreement at their discretion; upon expiration of such agreement, they may renew or sign an agreement with another physician. Administrative authorities of health and medical insurance handling institutions shall sign an agreement with such service institutions or physicians based on the independent choice of insured patients to ensure the implementation of service agreements between general practitioners and residents. With the improvement of a general practitioner system, each general practitioner shall sign agreements with about 2,000 patients with a certain percentage of special crowds such as the elderly, chronic disease patients, and the disabled.

(22) **Actively exploring the establishment of hierarchical medical service and bi-directional referral system.** System of initial diagnosis at the primary level and hierarchical medical management system shall be established, specifying admission criteria and bi-directional referral system of hospitals at different levels. Initial diagnosis of general practitioner shall be piloted in qualified areas and then gradually conducted. The Ministry of Human Resources and Social Security and Ministry of Health shall put forward relevant policies and measures to encourage bi-directional referral and define bi-directional referral and hierarchical medical service as indicators for assessment of directional medical institutions of medical insurance, attaching results of assessment to payment of medical insurance.

(23) **Enhancing regulation and supervision of service quality of general practitioners.** Administrative authorities of health shall enhance practice registration management and service quality supervision of general practitioners. Authorities of health and medical insurance handling institutions shall establish an assessment system based on key indicators of quantity, quality and satisfaction of residents, developing strict assessment of general practitioners. Results of such assessment shall be directly related to payment of medical insurance and granting of basic public health service funds.

VI. Establishing incentive mechanism of general practitioners

(24) **Charging service fees based on number of patients signing agreement.** General physicians shall provide basic medical and health service for signing residents as agreed and collect service fees on an annual basis. Such

service fees shall be borne by medical insurance funds, basic public health service funds, and individual signing residents; specific standards and coverage shall be determined by local institutions based on local medical and health service standards, structure of signing residents, and tolerance of basic medical insurance funds and public health funds. Different standards of service fees may be adopted for different crowds based on full consideration of acceptance by residents. Locally specified service details and standards of service fees of general practitioners shall be combined with coordination of medical insurance clinics and payment methods.

(25) **Regulating charges for other diagnosis and treatment of general practitioners**. General physicians shall not collect any fees other than service fees collected in accordance with relevant regulations for provision of basic medical and health service as agreed. General physicians may provide non-agreed medical and health service for signing residents and collect service fees in accordance with relevant regulations and may provide clinical service for non-signing residents and collect service fees such as general fees for diagnosis and treatment in accordance with relevant regulations. Clinical expenses of insured patients covered by policies may be paid in accordance with regulations on medical insurance. Standards for diagnosis and treatment service charges shall be gradually adjusted to reasonably realize technical value of general practitioners.

(26) **Reasonably determining remuneration of general practitioners**. General practitioners and team members who are official employees of primary medical and health institutions organized by the government shall achieve salaries in accordance with national regulations; other general practitioners shall achieve remuneration based on service contract with primary medical and health institutions and service agreement with residents, and may receive remuneration for clinical service provided for non-signing residents. Internal performance salaries of primary medical and health institutions may be distributed in the way of allowance to general practitioners, with a greater proportion to general practitioners and other persons fulfilling tier-1 clinical duties. Performance assessment shall take full consideration of quantity and constitution of signing residents, clinical workload, service quality, satisfaction of residents, and control of medical costs of residents.

(27) **Improving subsidiary and allowance policies that encourage general practitioners to work in remote and less developed areas.** General practitioners working at primary medical and health institutions in remote areas shall receive relevant subsidiaries in accordance with national regulations. General practitioners independently practicing in remote and less developed areas with a small population shall receive necessary allowance from local government based on privilege policies formulated thereby and the

central and provincial authorities of finance shall allocate properly greater funds upon making transfer payment.

(28) **Expanding career development channels of general practitioners**. Local government shall be encouraged to establish special positions in accordance with relevant regulations to enroll excellent professional technical talents for primary medical and health institutions. General practitioners having received standardized training may apply for title promotion 1 year in advance and shall be offered privileges in employment of general attending physician under the same conditions. Number of signing residents, clinical reception, service quality, and satisfaction of residents shall be taken as key factors for title promotion of general practitioners; title promotion of general practitioners in primary organizations may be less bound to requirements of foreign languages in accordance with relevant national regulations, with no strict regulation on thesis. A talent rotation mechanism shall be established for primary medical and health service to encourage bi-directional rotation of general practitioners between county hospitals and primary medical and health institutions. Specialist physician training bases shall offer privilege to general practitioners with experience of practicing at the primary level under the same conditions when enrolling trainees.

VII. Relevant protection measures

(29) **Improving relevant laws and regulations**. Revision to Law of the People's Republic of China on Medical Practitioners and other relevant laws and regulations shall be facilitated based on full argumentation and admission criteria of practice of physicians shall be improved, specifying practice scope, rights and responsibilities of general practitioners and protecting legal interest of general practitioners. Administrative rules shall be formulated on general practitioners practicing in more than one sites and occupational development policies for freelance practitioners shall be specified, leading doctors from hospitals to provide service at the primary level and encouraging retired doctors to practice in primary medical and health institutions.

(30) **Enhancing development of general practitioner training**. A general practitioner training and practice network including tier-3 general hospitals and qualified tier-2 hospitals as clinical training and qualified community health service centers, township health centers and professional public health institutions shall be developed, based on full use of existing resources and the principle of 'average allocation of resources'. The government shall offer necessary support to construction and education practice of general practitioner training bases and the Ministry of Finance shall grant subsidiaries to financially unfavorable areas. Relevant authorities including the Ministry of Health and Ministry of Education shall formulate standards and administrative rules for clinic and practice-based training. Establishment

of faulty teams of general practitioners shall be enhanced and standards shall be developed therefore, constructing regional general practitioner training with the assistance of qualified high education institutes and focusing on training of faculty of primary practice.

(31) **Reasonably planning training and deployment of general practitioners.** The state government shall make an overall plan for training and deployment of general practitioners and publish list and enrollment quotas of general practitioner training, with greater effort to central and western areas. Provincial (regional or municipal) administrative authorities of health shall make overall plans for demands of corresponding province (region or municipality) for general practitioners and publish positions of general practitioner based on the level of county (district). Such plans shall be made based on needs for medical positions and enrollment scale of clinical medicine shall be adjusted and controlled in a scientific way. The Ministry of Health shall make plans for national demands for medical positions and the Ministry of Education shall take into account such plans while making plans for enrollment of undergraduate and graduate clinical medical majors.

(32) **Making full use of relevant industrial associations (academies).** Capabilities of relevant associations (academies) shall be improved and such associations (academies) shall be fully made use of in self-regulation of the medical industry and formulation of details, standards and procedures of general practitioner training as well as qualification examination of general practitioners.

VIII. Actively and stably facilitating the establishment of general practitioner system

(33) **Concretely enhancing organizational leadership.** Provincial (regional or municipal) governments shall, in accordance with these Guidelines, put forward respective implementation plans of their own as soon as possible. Authorities of health, education, human resources and social security, finance, traditional Chinese medicine and law shall arrange for revision and improvement of existing regulations and policies as soon as possible and put forward relevant implementation rules.

(34) **Strictly conducting pilot implementation.** The establishment of general practitioner system is a significant reform of existing physician training system, practicing methods of physicians and medical and health service modes, strictly complying with relevant policies, covering various aspects and exerting a thorough influence. In respect to difficulties in the reform, local pilot operation shall be encouraged to ensure proactive exploration. Relevant authorities shall timely summarize practical experience to achieve gradual promotion. The establishment of general practitioner system shall properly comply with relevant policies and measures to timely study new cases and new problems, ensuring stable implementation of such system.

(35) **Properly directing public opinions**. Health education and public opinion promotion and other relevant methods shall be adopted to develop residents' awareness of prevention and health care and residents shall be instructed to renew traditional awareness and habits of seeking for medical service; contractual awareness among all social members shall be improved to create a favorable environment for implementation of reform.

State Council
July 1, 2011

- 騰讯微博微信QQ空间人人网开心网豆瓣网

【字體：大中小】打印本頁

分享

新華微博人民微博新浪微博

國務院關于建立全科醫生制度的指導意見

國發〔2011〕23號

各省、自治區、直轄市人民政府，國務院各部委、各直屬機構：

為深入貫徹醫藥衛生體制改革精神，現就建立全科醫生制度提出以下指導意見：

一、充分認識建立全科醫生制度的重要性和必要性

（一）建立全科醫生制度是保障和改善城鄉居民健康的迫切需要。我國是一個有13億多人口的發展中國家，隨著經濟發展和人民生活水平的提高，城鄉居民對提高健康水平的要求越來越高；同時，工業化、城鎮化和生態環境變化帶來的影響健康因素越來越多，人口老齡化和疾病譜變化也對醫療衛生服務提出新要求。全科醫生是綜合程度較高的醫學人才，主要在基層承擔預防保健、常見病多發病診療和轉診、病人康復和慢性病管理、健康管理等一體化服務，被稱為居民健康的"守門人"。建立全科醫生制度，發揮好全科醫生的作用，有利于充分落實預防為主方針，使醫療衛生更好地服務人民健康。

（二）建立全科醫生制度是提高基層醫療衛生服務水平的客觀要求。加強基層醫療衛生工作是醫藥衛生事業改革發展的重點，是提高基本醫療衛生服務的公平性、可及性的基本途徑；醫療衛生人才是決定基層醫療衛生服務水平的關鍵。多年來，我國基層醫療衛生人才隊伍建設相對滯後，合格的全科醫生數量嚴重不足，制約了基層醫

療衛生服務水平提高。建立全科醫生制度,為基層培養大批"下得去、留得住、用得好"的合格全科醫生,是提高基層醫療衛生服務水平的客觀要求和必由之路。

(三) 建立全科醫生制度是促進醫療衛生服務模式轉變的重要舉措。建立分級診療模式,實行全科醫生簽約服務,將醫療衛生服務責任落實到醫生個人,是我國醫療衛生服務的發展方向,也是許多國家的通行做法和成功經驗。建立適合我國國情的全科醫生制度,有利于優化醫療衛生資源配置、形成基層醫療衛生機構與城市醫院合理分工的診療模式,有利于為群眾提供連續協調、方便可及的基本醫療衛生服務,緩解群眾"看病難、看病貴"的狀況。

二、建立全科醫生制度的指導思想、基本原則和總體目標

(四) 指導思想。按照深化醫藥衛生體制改革的總體思路,適應我國經濟社會發展階段和居民健康需求變化趨勢,堅持保基本、強基層、建機制的基本路徑,遵循醫療衛生事業發展和全科醫生培養規律,強化政府在基本醫療衛生服務中的主導作用,注重發揮市場機制作用,立足基本國情,借鑒國際經驗,堅持制度創新,試點先行,逐步建立和完善中國特色全科醫生培養、使用和激勵制度,全面提高基層醫療衛生服務水平。

(五) 基本原則。堅持突出實踐、注重質量,以提高臨床實踐能力為重點,規范培養模式,統一培養標準,嚴格準入條件和資格考試,切實提高全科醫生培養質量。堅持創新機制、服務健康,改革全科醫生執業方式,建立健全激勵機制,引導全科醫生到基層執業,逐步形成以全科醫生為主體的基層醫療衛生隊伍,為群眾提供安全、有效、方便、價廉的基本醫療衛生服務。堅持整體設計、分步實施,既著眼長遠,加強總體設計,逐步建立統一規范的全科醫生制度;又立足當前,多渠道培養全科醫生,滿足現階段基層對全科醫生的需要。

(六) 總體目標。到2020年,在我國初步建立起充滿生機和活力的全科醫生制度,基本形成統一規范的全科醫生培養模式和"首診在基層"的服務模式,全科醫生與城鄉居民基本建立比較穩定的服務關係，基本實現城鄉每萬名居民有2-3名合格的全科醫生，全科醫生服務水平全面提高，基本適應人民群眾基本醫療衛生服務需求。

三、逐步建立統一規范的全科醫生培養制度

（七）規范全科醫生培養模式。將全科醫生培養逐步規范為"5+3"模式，即先接受5年的臨床醫學（含中醫學）本科教育，再接受3年的全科醫生規范化培養。在過渡期內，3年的全科醫生規范化培養可以實行"畢業後規范化培訓"和"臨床醫學研究生教育"兩種方式，具體方式由各省（區、市）確定。

參加畢業後規范化培訓的人員主要從具有本科及以上學歷的臨床醫學專業畢業生中招收，培訓期間由全科醫生規范化培養基地在衛生部門（含中醫藥管理部門）和教育部門共同指導下進行管理。全科方向的臨床醫學專業學位研究生按照統一的全科醫生規范化培養要求進行培養，培養結束考核合格者可獲得全科醫生規范化培養合格證書；臨床醫學專業學位研究生教育以教育部門為主管理。

（八）統一全科醫生規范化培養方法和內容。全科醫生規范化培養以提高臨床和公共衛生實踐能力為主，在國家認定的全科醫生規范化培養基地進行，實行導師制和學分制管理。參加培養人員在培養基地臨床各科及公共衛生、社區實踐平臺逐科（平臺）輪轉。在臨床培養基地規定的科室輪轉培訓時間原則上不少於2年，並另外安排一定時間在基層實踐基地和專業公共衛生機構進行服務鍛煉。經培養基地按照國家標準組織考核，達到病種、病例數和臨床基本能力、基本公共衛生實踐能力及職業素質要求並取得規定學分者，可取得全科醫生規范化培養合格證書。規范化培養的具體內容和標準由衛生部、教育部、國家中醫藥管理局制定。

（九）規范參加全科醫生規范化培養人員管理。參加全科醫生規范化培養人員是培養基地住院醫師的一部分，培養期間享受培養基地住院醫師待遇，財政根據不同情況給予補助，其中，具有研究生身份的，執行國家現行研究生教育有關規定；由工作單位選派的，人事工資關係不變。規范化培養期間不收取培訓（學）費，多于標準學

分和超過規定時間的培養費用由個人承擔。具體管理辦法由人力資源社會保障部、衛生部、教育部、財政部制定。

（十）統一全科醫生的執業準入條件。在全科醫生規范化培養階段，參加培養人員在導師指導下可從事醫學診查、疾病調查、醫學處置等臨床工作和參加醫院值班，並可按規定參加國家醫師資格考試。注冊全科醫師必須經過3年全科醫生規范化培養取得合格證書，並通過國家醫師資格考試取得醫師資格。

（十一）統一全科醫學專業學位授予標準。具有5年制臨床醫學本科及以上學歷者參加全科醫生規范化培養合格後，符合國家學位要求的授予臨床醫學（全科方向）相應專業學位。具體辦法由國務院學位委員會、衛生部制定。

（十二）完善臨床醫學基礎教育。臨床醫學本科教育要以醫學基礎理論和臨床醫學、預防醫學基本知識及基本能力培養為主，同時加強全科醫學理論和實踐教學，著重強化醫患溝通、基本藥物使用、醫藥費用管理等方面能力的培養。

（十三）改革臨床醫學（全科方向）專業學位研究生教育。從2012年起，新招收的臨床醫學專業學位研究生（全科方向）要按照全科醫生規范化培養的要求進行培養。要適應全科醫生崗位需求，進一步加強臨床醫學研究生培養能力建設，逐步擴大全科方向的臨床醫學專業學位研究生招生規模。

（十四）加強全科醫生的繼續教育。以現代醫學技術發展中的新知識和新技能為主要內容，加強全科醫生經常性和針對性、實用性強的繼續醫學教育。加強對全科醫生繼續醫學教育的考核，將參加繼續醫學教育情況作為全科醫生崗位聘用、技術職務晉升和執業資格再注冊的重要因素。

四、近期多渠道培養合格的全科醫生

為解決當前基層急需全科醫生與全科醫生規范化培養周期較長之間的矛盾，近期要採取多種措施加強全科醫生培養，力爭到2012年每個城市社區衛生服務機構和農村鄉鎮衛生院都有合格的全科醫生。

（十五）大力開展基層在崗醫生轉崗培訓。對符合條件的基層在崗執業醫師或執業助理醫師，按需進行1-2年的轉崗培訓。轉崗培訓以提升基本醫療和公共衛生服務能力為主，在國家認定的全科醫生規范化培養基地進行，培訓結束通過省級衛生行政部門組織的統一考試，獲得全科醫生轉崗培訓合格證書，可注冊為全科醫師或助理全科醫師。

（十六）強化定向培養全科醫生的技能培訓。適當增加為基層定向培養5年制臨床醫學專業學生的臨床技能和公共衛生實習時間。對到經濟欠發達的農村地區工作的3年制醫學專科畢業生，可在國家認定的培養基地經2年臨床技能和公共衛生培訓合格並取得執業助理醫師資格後，注冊為助理全科醫師，但各省（區、市）衛生行政部門要嚴格控制比例。

（十七）提升基層在崗醫生的學歷層次。鼓勵基層在崗醫生通過參加成人高等教育提升學歷層次，符合條件後參加相應執業醫師考試，考試合格可按程序注冊為全科醫師或助理全科醫師。

（十八）鼓勵醫院醫生到基層服務。嚴格執行城市醫院醫生在晉升主治醫師或副主任醫師職稱前到基層累計服務1年的規定，衛生部門要做好組織、管理和考核工作。建立健全城市醫院與基層醫療衛生機構的對口支援制度和雙向交流機制，縣級以上醫院要通過遠程醫療、遠程教學等方式加強對基層的技術指導和培訓。要制定管理辦法，支持醫院醫生（包括退休醫生）採取多種方式到基層醫療衛生機構（含私人診所等社會力量舉辦的醫療機構）提供服務，並可獲得合理報酬。

五、改革全科醫生執業方式

（十九）引導全科醫生以多種方式執業。取得執業資格的全科醫生一般注冊1個執業地點，也可以根據需要多點注冊執業。全科醫生可以在基層醫療衛生機構（或醫院）全職或兼職工作，也可以獨立開辦個體診所或與他人聯合開辦合夥制診所。鼓勵組建由全科醫生和社區護士、公共衛生醫生或鄉村醫生等人員組成的全科醫生團隊，劃片為居民提供服務。要健全基層醫療衛生機構對全科醫生的人力資源管理辦法，規范私人診所雇傭人員的勞動關係管理。

（二十）政府為全科醫生提供服務平臺。對到基層工作的全科醫生（包括大醫院專科醫生），政府舉辦的基層醫療衛生機構要通過簽訂協議的方式為其提供服務平臺。要充分依托現有資源組建區域性醫學檢查、檢驗中心，鼓勵和規范社會零售藥店發展，為全科醫生執業提供條件。

（二十一）推行全科醫生與居民建立契約服務關係。基層醫療衛生機構或全科醫生要與居民簽訂一定期限的服務協議，建立相對穩定的契約服務關係，服務責任落實到全科醫生個人。參保人員可在本縣（市、區）醫保定點服務機構或全科醫生范圍內自主選擇簽約醫生，期滿後可續約或另選簽約醫生。衛生行政部門和醫保經辦機構要根據參保人員的自主選擇與定點服務機構或醫生簽訂協議，確保全科醫生與居民服務協議的落實。隨著全科醫生制度的完善，逐步將每名全科醫生的簽約服務人數控制在2000人左右，其中老年人、慢性病人、殘疾人等特殊人群要有一定比例。

（二十二）積極探索建立分級醫療和雙向轉診機制。逐步建立基層首診和分級醫療管理制度，明確各級醫院出入院標準和雙向轉診機制。在有條件的地區先行開展全科醫生首診試點並逐步推行。人力資源社會保障部、衛生部要制定鼓勵雙向轉診的政策措施，將醫保定點醫療機構執行雙向轉診和分級醫療情況列為考核指標，並將考核結果與醫保支付掛鉤。

（二十三）加強全科醫生服務質量監管。衛生行政部門要加強對全科醫生執業注冊管理和服務質量監管。衛生部門和醫保經辦機構要建立以服務數量、服務質量、居民滿意度等為主要指標的考核體係，對全科醫生進行嚴格考核，考核結果定期公布並與醫保支付、基本公共衛生服務經費撥付掛鉤。

六、建立全科醫生的激勵機制

（二十四）按簽約服務人數收取服務費。全科醫生為簽約居民提供約定的基本醫療衛生服務，按年收取服務費。服務費由醫保基金、基本公共衛生服務經費和簽約居民個人分擔，具體標準和保障范圍由各地根據當地醫療衛生服務水平、簽約人群結構以及基本醫保基金和公共衛生經費承受能力等因素確定。在充分考慮居民接受程度的基礎上，可對不同人群實行不同的服務費標準。各地確定全科醫生簽約服務內容和服務費標準要與醫保門診統籌和付費方式改革相結合。

（二十五）規范全科醫生其他診療收費。全科醫生向簽約居民提供約定的基本醫療衛生服務，除按規定收取簽約服務費外，不得另行收取其他費用。全科醫生可根據簽約居民申請提供非約定的醫療衛生服務，並按規定收取費用；也可向非簽約居民提供門診服務，按規定收取一般診療費等服務費用。參保人員政策範圍內的門診費用可按醫保規定支付。逐步調整診療服務收費標準，合理體現全科醫生技術勞務價值。

（二十六）合理確定全科醫生的勞動報酬。全科醫生及其團隊成員屬于政府舉辦的基層醫療衛生機構正式工作人員的，執行國家規定的工資待遇；其他在基層工作的全科醫生按照與基層醫療衛生機構簽訂的服務合同和與居民簽訂的服務協議獲得報酬，也可通過向非簽約居民提供門診服務獲得報酬。基層醫療衛生機構內部績效工資分配可採取設立全科醫生津貼等方式，向全科醫生等承擔臨床一線任務的人員傾斜。績效考核要充分考慮全科醫生的簽約居民數量和構成、門診工作量、服務質量、居民滿意度以及居民醫藥費用控制情況等因素。

（二十七）完善鼓勵全科醫生到艱苦邊遠地區工作的津補貼政策。對到艱苦邊遠地區政府辦基層醫療衛生機構工作的全科醫生，按國家規定發放艱苦邊遠地區津貼。對在人口稀少、艱苦邊遠地區獨立執業的全科醫生，地方政府要制定優惠政策或給予必要補助，中央財政和省級財政在安排轉移支付時要予以適當傾斜。

（二十八）拓寬全科醫生的職業發展路徑。鼓勵地方按照有關規定設置特設崗位，招聘優秀的專業技術人才到基層醫療衛生機構工作。經過規范化培養的全科醫生到基層醫療衛生機構工作，可提前一年申請職稱晉升，並可在同等條件下優先聘用到全科主治醫師崗位。要將簽約居民數量、接診量、服務質量、群眾滿意度等作為全科醫生職稱晉升的重要因素，基層單位全科醫生職稱晉升按照國家有關規定可放寬外語要求，不對論文作硬性規定。建立基層醫療衛生人才流動機制，鼓勵全科醫生在縣級醫院與基層醫療衛生機構雙向流動。專科醫生培養基地招收學員時同等條件下優先錄取具有基層執業經驗的全科醫生。

七、相關保障措施

（二十九）完善相關法律法規。在充分論證的基礎上，推動修訂執業醫師法和相關法規，提高醫生執業資格準入條件，明確全科醫生的執業范圍和權利責任，保障全科醫生合法權益。研究制定醫生多點執業的管理辦法，明確自由執業者的職業發展政策，引導醫院醫生到基層提供服務，鼓勵退休醫生到基層醫療衛生機構執業。

（三十）加強全科醫生培養基地建設。在充分利用現有資源基礎上，按照"填平補齊"原則，建設以三級綜合醫院和有條件的二級醫院為臨床培養基地，以有條件的社區衛生服務中心、鄉鎮衛生院和專業公共衛生機構為實踐基地的全科醫生培養實訓網絡。政府對全科醫生規范化培養基地建設和教學實踐活動給予必要支持；中央財政對財政困難地區給予補助。衛生部會同教育部等有關部門制定臨床培養基地、實踐基地的建設標準和管理辦法。加強全科醫學師資隊伍建設，制定全科醫學師資標準，依托有條件的高等醫學院校建設區域性全科醫學師資培訓基地，重點支持基層實踐基地師資的培訓。

（三十一）合理規劃全科醫生的培養使用。國家統一規劃全科醫生培養工作，每年公布全科醫生培養基地名單及招生名額，招生向中西部地區傾斜。各省（區、市）衛生行政部門要統籌本省（區、市）全科醫生需求數量，以縣（區）為單位公布全科醫生崗位。以醫生崗位需求為導向，科學調控臨床醫學專業招生規模。衛生部要制定全國醫生崗位需求計劃，教育部在制定臨床醫學本科生和臨床醫學專業學位研究生招生計劃時要與醫生崗位需求計劃做好銜接。

（三十二）充分發揮相關行業協（學）會作用。加強相關行業協（學）會能力建設，在行業自律和制訂全科醫生培養內容、標準、流程及全科醫師資格考試等方面充分依托行業協（學）會，發揮其優勢和積極作用。

八、積極穩妥地推進全科醫生制度建設

（三十三）切實加強組織領導。各省（區、市）人民政府要按照本指導意見精神，盡快制定本省（區、市）的實施方案。衛生、教育、人力資源社會保障、財政、中醫藥、法制等部門要盡快組織修訂完善現行法規政策，制定出臺相關實施細則。

（三十四）認真開展試點推廣。建立全科醫生制度是對現行醫生培養制度、醫生執業方式、醫療衛生服務模式的重要改革，政策性強，涉及面廣，影響深遠。對改革中的難點問題，鼓勵地方先行試點，積極探索。有關部門要及時總結實踐經驗，逐步推廣。要強化政策措施的銜接，及時研究新情況、新問題，確保全科醫生制度穩步實施。

（三十五）做好輿論宣傳引導。通過健康教育、輿論宣傳等方式培養居民的預防保健觀念，引導居民轉變傳統就醫觀念和習慣，增強全社會的契約意識，為實施改革營造良好環境。

國　務　院

二〇一一年七月一日

CHAPTER 31

Family medicine transforming rural primary care in Nepal

Pratap Prasad

NOMINATED CLASSIC PAPER

Amogh Basnyat. Primary care in a rural set up in Nepal: perspectives of a generalist. *Journal of Family Medicine and Primary Care*, 2013; 2(3): 218–21.

Nepal is a developing country and due to its geography and economic constraints, many people of Nepal are denied proper healthcare. This also applies to other developing countries of this region where many people do not have access to basic primary healthcare. This article depicts the real-life healthcare scenario that exists in a part of our world that is practically living and breathing in a bygone age. Kalikot, in the Karnali region of Nepal, exists in a socioeconomic condition that must have been commonplace in the present-day first world almost a millennium ago, or perhaps even long before that. Even by third-world standards it could be called backwards. The point this article makes is that it is not any so-called 'cutting edge' specialty of the present-day modern medicine that is making (or rather would be able to make) any significant impact in a remote and inaccessible place like Kalikot. What does make a real impact is the generalist approach to the practice of medicine. Family medicine today is practised all over the world not just as a remnant, but as a direct and uninterrupted continuum of generalist practice. This article shows the real worth of our discipline of medical practice. Not just that, our discipline has actually and significantly contributed to the healthcare needs of the most far-flung populaces of the world. That's why the revelation of our real contributions is so important to global healthcare.

This paper shows how generalist medical practice cannot just exist, but how it can establish a strong foothold in the rural hinterlands of Nepal. This model is ongoing through the support of government, academic institutions and non-government organisations and also through the work of many independent general practitioners in Nepal. Today family medicine/general practice has a stronger and more resoundingly felt presence in rural healthcare delivery in Nepal than ever before. Nepal and other developing countries need much greater future efforts to bring about real improvements in the health status of the people of rural areas. The benefit of the depiction of this model of practice has been that it demonstrates an efficient way of achieving this end. And the model is relevant not just in Nepal, but in many low- and middle-income countries. Should the model depicted in this paper be adopted on a wider scale, it will result in a significant impact on healthcare service delivery to many disadvantaged people in rural communities around the world.

ABOUT THE AUTHOR OF THIS PAPER

Dr Amogh Bahadur Basnyat was born in Kathmandu, Nepal. His father was a government employee and his mother was a nurse. He completed his MBBS and MD at the Institute of Medicine at Tribhuvan University in Nepal. He was the Gold Medallist in his postgraduate general practitioner course. Currently, he works as a rural family doctor, serving as consultant generalist physician and hospital director of Sindhu Sadabahar Hospital in Khadichaur, Sindhupalchok, Nepal. This district is in a seriously disadvantaged area in Nepal and was one of the most severely affected regions in the devastating 2015 earthquakes. According to government figures, over 95% of homes in the region were destroyed by the earthquakes and over 3500 people lost their lives in the region where Amogh works.

ABOUT THE NOMINATOR OF THIS PAPER

Professor Pratap Narayan Prasad is head of the department of General Practice and Emergency Medicine at the Institute of Medicine of Tribhuvan University in Nepal. He also serves as the Regional President of the WONCA South Asia Region. He has twice received the 'Educational Award' from the Nepal Ministry of Education in recognition of his service to his country.

'In your career you will come across two drastically opposite points of view. There will be people saying that you are not required, as everything you do can be done "better" by "specialists". And then there will be the underserved, poverty-stricken people unable to afford care in high-end specialty hospitals.

Who do you choose to believe? Those who say that you are not required? Or those who need you much more than anybody else? I choose my patients.'

Professor Pratap Narayan Prasad, Nepal

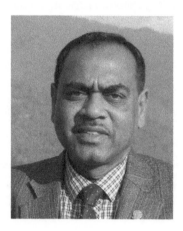

Attribution:

We attribute the original publication of *Primary care in a rural set up in Nepal: perspectives of a generalist* to *Journal of Family Medicine and Primary Care*. With thanks to the Academy of Family Physicians of India.

Rural Family Medicine

Primary Care in a Rural Set Up in Nepal: Perspectives of a Generalist

Amogh Basnyat

Clinical and Medical Education Coordinator, Nick Simons Institute, District Hospital of Kalikot, Nepal

Abstract

This article deals with the author's personal perspectives while having to serve as a generalist in a rural hospital in one of the most underdeveloped and far away regions of Nepal. Having been deputed in Kalikot District Hospital (KDH) through Nick Simons Institute's (NSI) Rural Staff Support Program (RSSP), the author mentions the technical hardships and resource constraints of the government hospital. Highlighting the improvement in the hospital profile after the arrival of the RSSP, the article cursorily mentions the modalities of primary care spanning the common clinical presentations. Particularly, the difficulties related to the provision of Comprehensive Emergency Obstetric Care (CEOC) services are highlighted. Also, a brief introduction as to the NSI, Kathmandu is provided.

Keywords: CEOC, Kalikot District Hospital, Nick Simons Institute, Rural Staff Support Program

Introduction

I have been serving in the Kalikot District Hospital (KDH), Manma, Nepal in the capacity of the Clinical and the Medical Education Coordinator through Nick Simons Institute's (NSI) Rural Staff Support Program (RSSP) for the last 6 months now. The purpose of this paper is to reflect up on my own personal experiences, in terms of the primary care management of various kinds of emergencies and other presentations in the emergency room (ER), outpatient department (OPD) and in-patient department (IPD) of the hospital.

Kalikot and the district hospital

Kalikot is a district located in the mid-western development region of Nepal and is one of the districts of the Karnali zone which is touted as the most backward and underdeveloped region of the whole country. Kalikot was placed in the 72nd position among the 75 districts in terms of its district health office performance in a report issued by the Ministry of Health this year. No doubt, the general health scenario and related public awareness in the area are abysmal.[1]

The district hospital is located in the district headquarter Manma. It has a three-bedded ER and a 15-bedded IPD. It caters to around 10-15 emergencies and 100-150 out-patients on any given working day. It also provides radiology and lab services during the office hours. Presently, besides the RSSP MD (General Practice) doctor, there is one more MBBS doctor who is working in the hospital under the Government's scholarship contract.

Although presently C-sections are regularly being conducted here, the Health ministry's Comprehensive Emergency Obstetric Care (CEOC) program is formally going to be operational soon and for the purpose a CEOC building is under construction. The two main hospital blocks housing the ER, OPD, lab, and the in-patients, however, are in dilapidated condition.

As in any other district hospital, lack of awareness as to its assets of all kinds and consequently the lack of their maintenance are rampant in this hospital too. Hence, the prevalence of "disuse atrophy" rather than wear and tear due to use is more visible regarding almost each and every biomedical equipment and other devices. It's indeed very disheartening to see the same tendency in terms of the government-supplied drugs as well.

The state of the cleanliness, orderliness, and the measures for the infection prevention are nominal even when described in the most optimistic term.

Access this article online	
Quick Response Code:	**Website:** www.jfmpc.com
	DOI: 10.4103/2249-4863.120714

Address for correspondence: Dr. Amogh Basnyat,
158 Padma Marg, Bhatbhateni, Kathmandu, Nepal
E-mail: dramoghbasnyat@hotmail.com

No need to mention that like any other district hospital it's understaffed, underresourced, and too often overexerted. The fact that it's linked to the rest of the country by a highway track that is meagrely a fair-weather road and remains clogged throughout the rainy season only makes the matters worse for it.

However, after the RSSP's inception about 2 years ago, things have slowly been improving. There has been a general trend of improvement and increase in terms of OPD, ER visits, and IPD admissions, major and minor procedures being undertaken in the hospital itself. If anything the Health Ministry's Health Management Information System data comparing the last 3 fiscal years' parameters show a positive trend for KDH [Table 1].

Clinical conditions

Regarding the conditions requiring primary emergency care that we mostly encounter in the KDH, to name a few would include:
1. Acute gastroenteritis (AGE),
2. Fever of unknown origin (FUO),
3. Fractures and trauma,
4. Chronic obstructive pulmonary disease (COPD),
5. Upper and lower respiratory tract infections (U and RTIs),
6. Abdominal pain (acute abdomen, biliary colic, renal colic, acid peptic disorder, and so on),
7. Obstetric (and gynecologic) emergencies.

Not many emergency presentations related to the lifestyle disorders such as hypertension, diabetes mellitus, stroke, renal failures, and so on are encountered. We do come across congestive cardiac failure once in a while, mostly secondary to rheumatic heart disease. Most of the emergencies are further complicated and overlapped by the presence of protein energy malnutrition, both in the paediatric and adult populations.

Once in a while we also come across poisonings, mostly organophosphates and other kinds of pesticides, insecticides. Once in a while burns also present in our ER. Foreign body ears and noses, particularly in the kids are also fairly common. Unlike in the OPD, not much in terms of dermatology is seen in the ER. Abscesses of all kinds alongside impetigo and other kinds of wound and skin infections are rampant, mostly in the OPD and also in the ER.

Management

Most of the common primary care conditions are managed in the local level itself. However, for a few of them, referral to the higher centre is opted for. Availability of a fairly wide variety of government-supplied drugs (KDH being a secondary level district hospital) and also due to the growth of privately owned drug stores due to opening of the Karnali highway track has made the practice of modern day medicine fairly easy in KDH.

The AGEs mainly present during the summer and rainy seasons and is equally common in the pediatric and the adult population. They are managed both on the OPD as well as the ER in-patient basis, depending up on the severity and degree of dehydration. The use of WHO's Integrated Management of Childhood Illness (IMCI) guidelines in the children by classifying the dehydration into no, some, and severe classes and use of plans A, B, and C help us medicos save more lives than any other modality and practice in medicine. Oral Rehydration Solution (ORS) is the blessing of modern day medicine — personally I have come to realize this fact only after working in this rural set up.

IMCI guidelines come equally handy for pneumonias in children. Use of respiratory rate along with other physical signs to classify pneumonia is another blessing of our age in medicine, particularly true for the rural set ups. Availability of nebulizers has made life easy for us in terms of managing pediatric URTIs, although nebulized racemic epinephrine is not available.

Lack of culture facilities and unavailability of all spectra of antibiotics particularly pose a challenge in terms of management of FUOs in the ER in-patient areas. Rampant and injudicious use of antibiotics, particularly the third generation cephalosporins and macrolides could pose some serious problems in the days to come but I suppose this is equally as much a problem in the tertiary set ups too. Now, they are being used even in the grass root levels such as subhealth posts and more concerning is the fact that they are even sold over the counter. The latter practice must be barred by the government's drug authority, and this holds equal truth in the hinterlands as it does in the center.

COPDs are again managed in much the same manner as in a tertiary set up as availability of beta agonists and anticholinergics along with corticosteroids have become fairly common now.

Mostly, the closed fractures are reduced and plastered (in casts or slabs) locally itself, except for the severely displaced varieties such

Table 1: Comparative hospital indicators for the last 3 fiscal years in Kalikot District Hospital, Nepal			
Indicators	FY2009/10	2010/11	2011/12
Number of sanctioned beds	15	15	15
Number of available beds	18	18	18
Total no. of OPD cases	14286	18304	15957
Total no. of emergency cases	1144	1354	1625
Total no. of OPD (OPD + Emergency) cases	15430	19658	17572
Total no. of inpatients discharged	628	954	1111
Total no. of preventive service provided	2319	3764	3203
Total no. of lab services provided	—	5266	8174
Total no. of hospital services provided	18719	25109	22340
Total no. of delivery conducted	189	213	304
Referral cases (in) total	0	0	0
Referral cases (out) total	43	60	64
Total maternal death	0	1	1
Total hospital death	4	11	9
Total minor procedures	60	41	109
Total major procedures	0	0	23

EMR: Emergency, OPD: Outpatient department. (Nick Simons Institute started the Rural Staff Support Program in this hospital in the fiscal year 2010/11. The major procedures were, however, started only in the year 2011/12 after the set up of operating room and other amenities)[2]

as gartland type 3 fractures of supracondylar region. Intravenous anesthesia (IVA) ketamine is used mostly for the reduction of fractures and dislocations. Open fractures are referred after primary wound cleaning and dressing. Similarly, minor traumas and wounds that need suturing are managed locally under local or intravenous (IV) anesthesia. For severe traumas that need referral, primary care is provided as much as possible before patient disposal.

IVA ketamine or local anesthesia is used also for the incision and drainage, lump excisions, foreign bodies of ear and nose removal, and so on depending up on the patient's age and condition.

Acute abdomen that need emergent surgical management such as the ones presenting with peritonism are referred quickly after initial analgesic, antibiotic doses, IV access and IV fluid placement, free nasogastric drainage placement and explanation of the need for nil per os status. Laparotomy in such situations has not been possible in KDH so far due to the unavailability of general anesthesia mainly. However, possibly due to better availability of Helicobacter *pylori* eradication therapy and other antibiotics, acute abdomen such as duodenal ulcer perforation, enteric perforation, and so on, are seen relatively less here. Acute appendicitis is operated in the KDH itself under subarachnoid block (SAB) [Table 2].

As of now a lack of trained ultrasonography (USG) operator has been a hindrance to its full use in terms of management of emergencies. However, after having undergone a USG training to be held shortly, I expect to use it much more properly and it should be of greater help in the timely and correct diagnosis of many emergencies.

Obstetric and gynecologic emergencies mainly present in the form of per vaginal bleeding, mostly either as a case of dysfunctional uterine bleeding or secondary to medical abortion pill consumption. Availability of postabortion care services along with the presence of complete abortion care trained staff has really made things simpler in these situations now. However, unavailability of blood storage services does pose a genuine threat in such circumstances. The concept of walking blood bank although very pleasant to hear is not much applicable in set ups like these, mostly due to the reason that people do not have awareness regarding the blood donation need. Hence, at times of dire need of blood we either have to look up to our own hospital staff or the police or military personnel for help [Figure 1].

The concept of CEOC is pretty much afloat now in the KDH. A separate hospital block is already under construction for the purpose. Regular cesarean sections are being undertaken in the hospital despite its own unique set of challenges and constraints. During my 4-month long tenure in KDH, I preformed 14 emergency C-sections. They were mostly conducted for either nonprogress of labour or fetal malposition, except two of them where fetal distress was the indication.

Table 2: Various surgical procedures in the Kalikot District Hospital (KDH) after the inception of Rural Staff Support Program	
Procedure	Number
Lower segment cesarean section	31
Appendectomy	3
Pelvic anterior/posterior floor repair	10
Circumcision	3
Vulvar hematoma release	2
Amputation of fingers (postcrush injury)	1
Inguinal hernia repair	2
Hydrocele sac eversion	2

The first lower segment cesarean section took place in Aug 2011. This table includes data from Aug 2011 to Feb 2013, a short period of 18 months in the many decades long history of KDH. Notable is the fact that routine performance of the procedures such as the following is exceedingly rare, not just in KDH but in any Government District Hospital in Nepal[5]

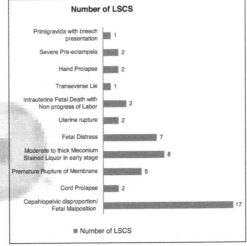

Figure 1: Breakdown of various indications present in the lower segment cesarean section performed in Kalikot District Hospital

Possibly due to timely referral from the health centers of the catchment areas and greater availability of safe obstetric services even in the grass root levels, not much in terms of severe complications in obstetrics such as ruptured uterus has been encountered so far.

In the majority of these procedures, I have myself provided the SAB. In a few of these, another doctor has done the job. But mostly, I prefer the junior doctor to be assisting me in the surgery rather than looking after the anesthetic part. Usually, a nurse stands by for the anesthetic monitoring. Sometimes, I would have to be operating entirely with the nursing personnel because the other doctor would be out of station.

Not forgettable at this point is the fact that operating without suction machine and cautery has become a norm here because neither the landline of electricity nor the generator (which is mostly out of order) is able to handle the extra load. Mostly, I do not even have the "luxury" (?) of having an oxygen concentrator by my patient's side. During bad days, I operate under quarter power solar lamps that look and work more like dinner lights in restaurants rather than properly focussed and powered operating theatre light.

Conclusion

Thus, being the only GP in the hospital and the senior most health staff not only in the KDH but in the entire district comes with a unique set of challenges as well as opportunities to me both as a clinician as well as a manager. Moreover, the roles played by a GP in our own Nepali context vary significantly from those in say a western set up. This too becomes more apparent than ever when one is able to serve in these capacities. Most important of all is the fact that one is able to play the role of a real, complete doctor for an entire community; this is one of the last remaining opportunities left out to be exercised by a quickly vanishing breed of health care providers in the present global scenario. One must feel blessed to be able to exercise all these privileges. Hence, despite whatever dismal conditions I am working under I also have my own reasons for solace.

A Brief Intro of NSI, Nepal

Nick Simons was 22 years old when he came to Nepal in 2002. He had worked with a nongovernment organization then for about a year. The next year when he went back home in the United States, he shared his dream to become a doctor and be able to help in places like Nepal with his parents, Jim and Marilyn Simons. Tragically, he drowned to death in Bali the same year before he could start his medical studies. In 2006, Jim and Marilyn Simons established the NSI in Kathmandu in memory of their son to provide quality health care to people in rural Nepal.[4]

The RSSP is run by the NSI to enhance the effectiveness of Nepal's government district hospitals, transforming them into institutions that can provide a range of services, including operations. Nepal's Ministry of Health and Population and the NSI began RSSP in 2007, and today seven government district hospitals are supported under this program. Before implementation of RSSP, all were poorly functioning hospitals located in underserved areas.

RSSP is a bundle of "enabling environment" supports which goes by the acronym, the eight Cs, namely
1. Communication,
2. Continuing medical education,
3. Community governance,
4. Clinical coordination by MD (General Practice) doctor,
5. Capital items,
6. Comfortable staff quarters,
7. Connection with district, and
8. Continuous quality improvement (source: nsi.edu.np).

References

1. Department of Health Services. 2012. Annual Report 2067/68 (2010/2011). Ministry of Health and Population, Government of Nepal.
2. District Health Office, Kalikot, Nepal. 2012. Annual Report 2068/69 (2011/2012). DoHS, Ministry of Health and Population, Government of Nepal.
3. Family Health Division. Survey of District Hospitals. 2011. Government of Nepal.
4. Nick Simons Institute. Available from: www.nsi.edu.np. 2013 [Last accessed date 23-02-2013].

How to cite this article: Basnyat A. Primary care in a rural set up in Nepal: Perspectives of a generalist. J Fam Med Primary Care 2013;2:218-21.

Source of Support: Nil. **Conflict of Interest:** None declared.

CHAPTER 32

Family medicine development in the nations of the Middle East

Faisal Alnasir

NOMINATED CLASSIC PAPER

Report on the regional consultation on strengthening service provision through the family practice approach (executive summary). World Health Organization Regional Office for the Eastern Mediterranean, 2014: 1–3.

This is a fascinating record distributed by the World Health Organization's Regional Office for the Eastern Mediterranean on strengthening health service provision through family practice. It includes a situational analysis of health systems in the Eastern Mediterranean Region, which comprises 23 nations stretching from Morocco in the west to Pakistan in the east, with an aggregate population of 630 million people. The health framework in each of these nations is portrayed in the full report, highlighting the issues and challenges that conflict with the generalisation of health service delivery to all members of each nation's population. The most vital challenge is the prevalence of communicable and noncommunicable diseases, which are affected by high levels of illiteracy and socioeconomic disadvantage in many of these nations. Such challenges constrain the capacity of nations to develop effective health services.

The report proposes the implementation of the family medicine concept as a solution for most health difficulties and recommends that this be the foundation of the health framework in each of these nations. It advocates for the foundation of departments of family medicine within the medical schools of each country, the development of postgraduate family medicine residency training programmes for medical graduates, and the establishment of accreditation bodies to certify the training and administration of family medicine.

Such strong promotion from the World Health Organization (WHO) not only encourages countries to consider family medicine as the foundation of their health systems, but supports those nations that have already started down this path. It highlights the need to confront challenges in encouraging more doctors to opt for a career as a family doctor. Frequently family doctors in this part of the world feel demoralised due to lack of appreciation of their skills and contributions. However, they should be encouraged by this strong backing from the WHO, and the possible improvements outlined in this paper, which should ultimately improve the health outcomes of the people of each nation of this region.

ABOUT THE AUTHOR OF THIS PAPER

This paper was developed under the leadership of WHO Regional-Director, Dr Ala Alwan, a strong supporter of family medicine. Dr Alwan was previously WHO Assistant Director-General for Noncommunicable Diseases and Mental Health, based in Geneva.

He graduated in medicine from the University of Alexandria in Egypt. He practised medicine in Scotland and obtained his postgraduate training and qualifications in the United Kingdom. Following his return to Iraq, his home country, he held several positions in clinical and academic medicine and public health. He was Professor and Dean of the Faculty of Medicine at Mustansiriya University in Baghdad. From 2003 to 2005, he was Minister of Education and Minister of Health in the Government of Iraq.

ABOUT THE NOMINATOR OF THIS PAPER

Professor Faisal Alnasir is Chairman of the Department of Family Medicine at the Arabian Gulf University in Bahrain. He is a former president of the Family Medicine Council of the Arab Board for Health Specialties and was the first Bahraini physician to obtain a PhD in family medicine. He has supported the development of family medicine in many Arab countries and around the world.

> 'Although it is hard, and occasionally you may feel burned out, working as a family physician offers you self-satisfaction, challenges, flexibility, tremendous diversity, and ensures that you are up to date in scientific knowledge in order to help your patients. The bond that develops between you and your patients is incredible. It is full of passion, empathy and care.'

> *Professor Faisal Alnasir, Bahrain*

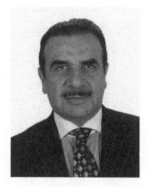

Attribution:

We attribute the original publication of *Report on the regional consultation on strengthening service provision through the family practice approach* to World Health Organization Regional Office for the Eastern Mediterranean copyright 2014. With thanks to the World Health Organization.

WHO-EM/PHC/165/E

Report on the

Regional consultation on strengthening service provision through the family practice approach

Cairo, Egypt
18–20 November 2014

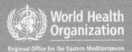

World Health Organization

Regional Office for the Eastern Mediterranean

WHO-EM/PHC/165/E

EXECUTIVE SUMMARY

The regional consultation on service provision through family practice (family practice) was held by the WHO Regional Office for the Eastern Mediterranean in Cairo, Egypt from 18 to 20 November 2014 in collaboration with the World Organization of Family Doctors (WONCA). Participants included international and regional experts on health system strengthening. The consultation also involved representatives from ministries of health, academia and health care delivery professionals from 20 countries of the Eastern Mediterranean Region as well as selected health system focal points from WHO country offices.

The objectives of the consultation were to: present the current status of family practice in the Eastern Mediterranean Region highlighting challenges, opportunities and priorities for moving towards universal health coverage; share regional and global good practices in implementing family practice programmes including aspects related to the integration of services, quality and safety of care, essential package of health services and alternative options to complement family practice approach and develop a road map and action framework for improved service provision as part of the commitments towards universal health coverage that is compatible for the three groups of countries of the Region.

The regional consultation was facilitated by WHO staff from the Regional Office and attended by regional experts from Afghanistan, Bahrain, Islamic Republic of Iran, Jordan, Lebanon, Pakistan, Palestine, Saudi Arabia and Somalia as well as international experts in family practice from Australia, Denmark, Malaysia, United Kingdom, Spain and Thailand. Participants discussed and presented family practice road map in support of universal health coverage for four groups of countries. Each group presented short term action plan and the WHO requested technical support for six main areas; governance and regulations (system absorption capacity); scaling up of family practice training programme; financing (strategic purchasing); vertical and horizontal integration of services; quality and accreditation process; community empowerment (demand, marketing and participation).

At the end of the consultation, the participants welcomed the scaling up of family practice programmes for moving towards universal health coverage and recognized the diversity in family practice implementation among the three groups of countries of the Region. During the working groups the participants discussed the challenges in accelerating family practice and came out with proposed actions to scale up implementation of family practice within countries the Region (see table below). They also emphasized the essential role that WHO can play in advocating family practice and guiding countries in adapting it as an overarching strategy for health care delivery.

WHO-EM/PHC/165/E
Page 2

Proposed family practice roadmap for universal health coverage in the Region

Major area	Short-term actions (2-year term)	WHO technical support
Governance/ regulations (system absorption capacity)	Advocate with policy-makers to adopt strengthening of family practice as a national health goal for universal health coverage Incorporate family practice as an overarching strategy for service provision within framework of universal health coverage (including projection of future needs for family physicians and other family practice team members) Establish public private partnership through contracting out mechanism with defined catchment population and defined package of services Establish/ strengthen a national high-level multisectoral commission for universal health coverage that sets goals, develop roadmap and oversee progress in scaling up family practice Assign and provide resources to the appropriate unit in the Ministry of Health to take responsibility for coordinating family practice activities Define/adapt the elements of family practice and identify family practice team members that suit the national context Update laws/ regulations for supporting implementation and expansion of family practice programme Establish standards for regulation of family practice programme (whether implemented through the public or private sector) Develop a health information and reporting system (manual/electronic) to monitor health facility (risk factors, health status, system) performance	Present an evidence informed case for family practice with policy-makers in high level forums, including the Regional Committee Assist in making rational projections for production of family physicians and family practice team members Provide terms of reference/roles and functions of the family practice unit within the Ministry of Health Frame a generic public health law/legislation in support of family practice, covering training and delivery aspects for adaption by countries Develop essential standards for family practice for adaptation by countries Build capacity in family practice facilities to report on core indicators agreed by Member States
Scaling up of family practice training programmes	Advocate with university presidents/chancellors and deans of Faculties of Medicine to establish, strengthen and expand family medicine departments and increase intake of family medicine trainees Develop and implement competency based short courses to orient general practitioners, nurses and allied health workers on principles and elements of family practice Introduce incentives for physicians to be enrolled in postgraduate family medicine programmes based on work experience in rural areas and primary health care services Develop continuous professional development programmes for recertification in family medicine Harmonize curricula, evaluation and standards of family medicine board certified programmes in countries of the Region Establish departments of family medicine in all medical schools and integrate a family medicine teaching programme into medical and nursing curricula	Prepare policy briefs and present before deans and chancellors of medical institutions the need to strengthen family medicine departments Collaborate with WONCA to develop short courses for orientation of general practitioners and nurses in family practice Develop a policy paper on options for incentives for health care professionals to participate in family practice training programmes Establish a group of regional experts to review and harmonize family medicine training programmes across the Region
Financing (strategic purchasing)	Introduce family practice financing as integral part of the national health financing strategy in a manner to ensure sufficient and sustainable funding for implementing expanding family practice Engage in strategic purchasing for family practice from	Update tools and guidelines for design and costing of essential health services packages and provide training in their use and implementation Synthesize and disseminate country experiences in financing family practice under

WHO-EM/PHC/165/E

Page 3

Major area	Short-term actions (2-year term)	WHO technical support
	public and private providers to achieve pre-set goals Design and cost essential health services packages to be implemented through family practice and identify target population to be covered Agree on implementation modalities of essential health services packages delivered by public, not-for-profit or for-profit private health care providers Build capacity to undertake contracting for family practice including outsourcing of services provision Decide and pilot provider payment modalities, e.g. capitation, case payment and necessary performance-based payment or their combinations	different health financing systems and provided related technical support to Member States Share and disseminate evidence on the advantages and limitations of different modalities of contracting (including outsourcing) and organize related capacity building activities Disseminate WHO guidelines as well as a organize a regional consultation on strategic purchasing and provider payment methods Provide evidence-based programme budgeting for financial sustainability
Vertical/ horizontal integration of services	Undertake an assessment of service delivery to review status of integration of priority programmes Develop and pilot a prototype referral system between primary, secondary and tertiary level including feedback and follow up (includes policies and procedures, instruments and staff training) Introduce functional integration of health services (preventive, curative, others) by multi-tasking and refresher training of staff Implement integration in all programmes in certain areas: training, supervision, health promotion, health information systems, drug supply and laboratories	Develop and update WHO guidelines, tools and policy papers on integration of health services Continue to share best practices and exchange experiences of successful integration of programmes within primary care Develop "integrated district health system based on family practice approach" assessment tool
Quality and safety/ standards/ accreditation process	Develop quality standards and indicators for family practice (inputs, process, outputs and outcomes) Develop training and continuous professional development programmes for primary health care workers on improving the quality of service delivery Strengthen supervision and monitoring functions including through interventions to improve the quality of care Introduce/institutionalize accreditation programmes to support higher primary health care performance Enforcing the accreditation of primary health care facilities	Develop framework for quality standards for primary care including those for family practice Pilot and validate assessment framework in countries Organize a regional consultation/workshop to develop consensus and build capacity in the use of framework Support countries in the monitoring quality of care using the endorsed framework Guide for set up monitoring tool to measure progress in family practice implementation with list of indicators
Community empowerment (demand, marketing and participation)	Establish a community health board to oversee the establishment of family practice Launch a community-wide campaign to encourage populations to register with reformed health facilities in the catchment population (including civil registration and vital statistics) Strengthen/initiate and support training of community health workers/outreach teams in scaling up home health care as integral part of the family practice approach Encourage the health volunteer approach as a bridge between households and health care facilities and train volunteers in the use of WHO manuals Organize orientation training for staff of health facilities on communication skills Develop multimedia educational campaigns	Update tools and guides for community engagement in family practice Provide technical support in developing a communication strategy for family practice programmes Exchange successful experiences of community volunteer programmes in support of family practice Provide technical support to increase access to primary health care services through community health workers, outreach teams and home health care strategies

CHAPTER 33

The challenge of assisting people in improving adherence to medications

Christos Lionis

NOMINATED CLASSIC PAPER

Roger Ruiz Moral, Luis Angel Pérula de Torres, Laura Pulido Ortega, Margarita Criado Larumbe, Ana Roldán Villalobos, Jose Angel Fernández García, Juan Manuel Parras Rejano. Effectiveness of motivational interviewing to improve therapeutic adherence in patients over 65 years old with chronic diseases: a cluster randomised clinical trial in primary care. *Patient Education and Counselling*, 2015; 98(8): 977–83.

This final paper addresses several of the current greatest global health challenges: the provision of healthcare to growing numbers of elderly people in each nation's population; the management of chronic (noncommunicable) diseases; the safe use of medicines in people with multimorbidity; and the need for more person-centred healthcare. It demonstrates the important role of family medicine in meeting each of these challenges and the importance of primary care research in finding solutions.

The paper tackles the challenging subject of therapeutic adherence in people aged over 65 years with chronic diseases. It is well documented that the cost of medications is rising at the same time that health inequalities are increasing in many settings. This especially affects many people over 65 years with multimorbidity who are among the most frequent visitors to the offices of family doctors. Medication prescribing is the most common intervention used by physicians. Inappropriate use of medications has many consequences in both cost of healthcare services and quality of care.

This paper describes the results of a cluster randomised clinical trial, which utilised motivational interviewing to improve therapeutic adherence in people over 65 years of age. The authors assessed the effectiveness of motivational interviewing on therapeutic adherence and the well-being of participants. Their main conclusion is that a 'face to face motivational approach in primary healthcare helps elderly patients with chronic diseases that are being treated by polypharmacy to achieve an improved level of treatment adherence', compared to traditional strategies of providing information and advice. The authors state that this relatively new intervention could change the traditional approach in general practice and could have an important impact on patients' adherence to treatment.

This paper introduces a new area of thinking to clinical medicine that may alter existing conventional and authoritative approaches to become more patient-centred with positive consequences on behaviour change.

ABOUT THE LEAD AUTHOR OF THIS PAPER

Professor Roger Ruiz Moral is Professor of Medicine and Clinical Communication at Francisco de Vitoria University in Madrid in Spain. He is a specialist in family medicine and has researched and published extensively in the fields of clinical communication and shared decision making. Prior to moving to Madrid, he was Associate Professor of Medicine at the University of Cordoba where he was in charge of the Residency Program for Family Medicine trainees. He received the 2002 Andalusia Ministry of Health Award for his pioneering study about the effectiveness of a 'National Training Program in Communication for Residents'.

In recent years he has led various research projects about different aspects of communication among specialists and primary care physicians with patients and their influence on clinical outcomes, and the effectiveness of different educational approaches for teaching clinical communication to students and residents. He has lectured extensively in Spain, Italy and countries of South America. He has published many papers and several books. He is the Chief Editor of '*doctutor*', a web Bulletin of Medical Education. He is also a short story writer.

ABOUT THE NOMINATOR OF THIS PAPER

Christos Lionis is Professor of General Practice and Primary Health Care at the School of Medicine at the University of Crete in Greece. Christos leads an active research team and is involved in several international collaborations. He is involved in the Executive Boards of various professional organisations and has published 282 papers in international journals.

'My advice to new doctors of family medicine is to explore the possibility of introducing the spirit of motivational interviewing into your clinical work by quitting authoritative or paternalistic therapeutic approaches. In this period of austerity taking the opportunity to introduce a "change talk" to support people to alter their behaviour is more important than ever.'

Professor Christos Lionis, Greece

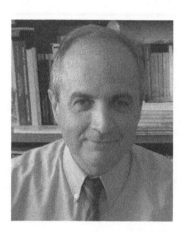

Attribution:

We attribute the original publication of *Effectiveness of motivational interviewing to improve therapeutic adherence in patients over 65 years old with chronic diseases: A cluster randomized clinical trial in primary care* to *Patient Education and Counselling.* With thanks to Lakshmi Priya at Elsevier.

Patient Education and Counseling 98 (2015) 977–983

Contents lists available at ScienceDirect

Patient Education and Counseling

journal homepage: www.elsevier.com/locate/pateducou

Intervention

Effectiveness of motivational interviewing to improve therapeutic adherence in patients over 65 years old with chronic diseases: A cluster randomized clinical trial in primary care

Roger Ruiz Moral [a], Luis Angel Pérula de Torres [b,*], Laura Pulido Ortega [b], Margarita Criado Larumbe [b], Ana Roldán Villalobos [b], Jose Angel Fernández García [c], Juan Manuel Parras Rejano [d] Collaborative Group ATEM-AP Study[1]

[a] Faculty of Medicine, Francisco de Vitoria University, Madrid, Spain
[b] Teaching Unit of Family and Community Medicine of Córdoba (Córdoba-Guadalquivir Health District), Maimonides Institute for Biomedical Research Córdoba (IMIBIC)/University of Cordoba, Reina Sofia University Hospital, Cordoba, Spain
[c] Villarrubia Health Center, UGC Occidente (Córdoba-Guadalquivir Health District), Maimonides Institute for Biomedical Research Córdoba (IMIBIC)/University of Córdoba/Reina Sofia University Hospital, Córdoba, Spain
[d] Villanueva del Rey Health Center, UGC-Pueblonuevo Penyarroya (Northern Córdoba Health District), Maimonides Institute for Biomedical Research Córdoba (IMIBIC)/University of Córdoba/Reina Sofia University Hospital, Córdoba, Spain

ARTICLE INFO

Article history:
Received 9 July 2014
Received in revised form 29 January 2015
Accepted 7 March 2015

Keywords:
Medication adherence
Communication
Geriatrics
General practice/family medicine
Treatment/intervention research
Patient involvement (empowerment, self-management)

ABSTRACT

Objective: To evaluate the effectiveness of motivational interviewing (MI) in improving medication adherence in older patients being treated by polypharmacy.
Methods: Cluster randomized clinical trial in 16 primary care centers with 27 health care providers and 154 patients. Thirty-two health care providers were assigned to an experimental (EG) or control group (CG). Interventions: MI training program and review of patient treatments. Providers in the EG carried out MI, whereas those in the CG used an "advice approach". Three follow-up visits were completed, at 15 days and at 3 and 6 months. Medication adherence in both groups was compared ($p < 0.05$).
Results: Patients recruited: 70/84 (EG/CG). Mean age: 76 years; female: 68.8%. The proportion of subjects changing to adherence was 7.6% higher in the EG ($p < 0.001$). Therapeutic adherence was higher for patients in the EG (OR = 2.84), women (OR = 0.24) and those with high educational levels (OR = 3.93).
Conclusion: A face-to-face motivational approach in primary care helps elderly patients with chronic diseases who are being treated by polypharmacy to achieve an improved level of treatment adherence than traditional strategies of providing information and advice.
Practice implications: MI is a patient-centered approach that can be used to improve medication adherence in primary care.
Trial registration: This trial is registered at ClinicalTrials.gov (NCT01291966)

© 2015 Elsevier Ireland Ltd. All rights reserved.

* Corresponding author at: Teaching Unit of Family and Community Medicine of Córdoba (Córdoba-Guadalquivir Health District), Maimonides Institute for Biomedical Research Córdoba (IMIBIC)/University of Cordoba, Reina Sofia University Hospital, C/Al-Andalus, 21. 14011 Cordoba, Spain. Tel.: +34 659681627; fax: +34 957354233.
E-mail addresses: r.ruiz.prof@ufv.es (R.R. Moral), luisangel.perula@gmail.com (L.A.P.d. Torres), laurapulidoortega@yahoo.es (L.P. Ortega), margarita.criado.exts@juntadeandalucia.es (M.C. Larumbe), anab.roldan.sspa@juntadeandalucia.es (A.R. Villalobos), joseangelfernandezgarcia@hotmail.com (J.A.F. García), juanprj@gmail.com (J.M.P. Rejano).
[1] Members listed in Appendix A.

http://dx.doi.org/10.1016/j.pec.2015.03.008
0738-3991/© 2015 Elsevier Ireland Ltd. All rights reserved.

1. Introduction

The most common intervention used by physicians is to prescribe medication. However, a problem often related to this intervention is that of poor medication adherence (MA). Medication adherence is defined as the patient's decision to accept and follow the instructions for taking the prescribed medication [1,2]. In the setting of chronic medical conditions such as hypertension and hypercholesterolemia, poor MA leads to worse medical treatment outcomes, higher hospitalization rates, and increased health care costs [3,4]. Because of this, adherence has been called "the key mediator between medical practice and patient outcomes" [5].

In people over 65 years of age, the prevalence of polypharmacy has been estimated at around 40% [6,7], and poor MA can have a negative health impact in this population group. Therefore, this subpopulation is considered a target for optimization of MA policies [8]. Different kinds of interventions have been tested to improve patient adherence, ranging from simple adjustments in the medication regimen to complex multidisciplinary interventions [9–13]. However, interventions to improve medication compliance for chronic conditions appear to be less effective and a combination of multifaceted interventions is considered the most effective strategy [14]. Given a lack of confidence in the prescriber and treatment, and concerns surrounding patient knowledge about prescribed medication [15], any strategy to improve medication adherence must include clear and tailored information [15,16]. Furthermore, most elderly patients frequently suffer from asymptomatic chronic diseases and many of them do not consider medication necessary, which frequently leads them to stop taking their medicine [17]. In these cases, communication strategies designed to promote patient self-empowerment and behavioral changes are particularly suitable [18].

Motivational Interviewing (MI) is an interview style designed to promote behavioral changes, and is defined as "a set of targeted communication skills to motivate patients to change their own behaviors in the interest of their health" [19]. In certain circumstances, MI has proven more effective than other strategies, such as the traditional informative strategy [20], and has been shown to be as equally effective as cognitive behavioral therapy, but with less time cost [21,22]. However, evidence of the effectiveness of MI in these areas remains scarce and further studies are required [23,24].

The objective of this study was to determine whether a face-to-face communicative strategy based on MI, used by health practitioners (family physicians and nurses) in a primary care setting and aimed at patients over 65 years old with a chronic disease who are being treated by polypharmacy and who have poor MA, can achieve better results than the usual approach based on an informative model of providing education and advice.

2. Methods

2.1. Study design

This two-arm trial, with experimental group (EG) and control group (CG), was conducted using a cluster randomized design, where two subpopulation levels were considered: (1) health professionals and (2) patients. Fig. 1 shows the CONSORT flow diagram with the cluster design features (25). The study took 18 months to complete, the patient recruitment period was from April 2009 to January 2010, and the follow-up period was 6 months.

2.2. Setting and subjects

The study was conducted in 16 health centers in Córdoba Province, Spain. One hundred health care providers (nurses and physicians from our Department of Family Medicine mailing list) were invited to participate, and 32 accepted. Allocation was based on clusters, and was stratified by profession (nurse or physician). We performed blinded randomization to one of the two study arms (C4-Study Design Pack; Glaxo S.A.).

Patients older than 65 who had chronic disease and were being treated by polypharmacy (taking 5 or more medicines or 12 or more daily doses for a period of no less than 6 months) [26], and who had a high probability for non-adherence to the prescribed treatment, were selected (consecutive sample) by health care

providers. An informed consent form was signed when each patient agreed to participate. Poor MA was assessed using the Haynes–Sackett [1] survey and the Morisky–Green test [27]. The former asks one question: "Most patients have difficulty taking all of their pills. Do you have any problems taking yours?" Because of its high specificity, this test is recommended in clinical practice as a first screening method to assess medication compliance [28]. The Morisky–Green scale comprises four yes/no questions: "Do you ever forget to take your medicines?"; "Are you careless at times about taking your medicine?"; "When you feel better, do you sometimes stop taking your medicine?"; and "Sometimes, if you feel worse when you take your medicine, do you stop taking it?" MA was considered to be poor when the patient answered affirmatively to the Haynes–Sackett question and answered inconsistently to at least one of the four Morisky–Green test questions.

Patients who were excluded from the study were those with serious psychiatric and neurological diseases, those who had difficulties coping with basic daily activities (Barthel Index below 60) [29], those who had cognitive impairment (Pfeiffer's test) [30], those admitted to hospital at least twice in the last year and patients under a carer's supervision.

2.3. Interventions

Before intervention, health care providers in both groups attended a 15-h workshop on patient safety and MA. Then providers from the EG attended an additional 20-hour-long workshop on MI. This training was conducted by two of the authors (JAFG; JMPR), who are both family physicians with experience in teaching physician-patient communication skills. The workshop was based on diverse interactive methodologies (trigger videos, discussions, role-playing alternative strategies, feedback and rehearsal).

To assess the effectiveness of specific training for acquisition of motivational skills, participants in both groups were videotaped in a simulated encounter, and two evaluators independently scored these interviews using the CICAA and EVEM tools. The CICAA is a rating scale designed to evaluate patient-centered generic skills [31], and the EVEM evaluates specific MI skills [32]. A previously published inter-rater reliability assessment was carried out, which produced a good reproducibility index (Cohen's kappa > 0.4 in all items, and intraclass correlation coefficient > 0.90). CICAA scale results were as follows: rater A = 30.57 points (EG) versus 16.56 points (CG), $p = 0.003$; rater B = 29.7 (EG) versus 17.7 (CG), $p = 0.04$. EVEM scale results were as follows: rater A = 21.1 (EG) versus 12.1 (CG), $p = 0.022$; rater B = 20 (EG) versus 12.6 (CG), $p = 0.01$.

Time between the training program and patient recruitment and intervention was about two weeks. Interventions in both groups included: (1) initial assessment of the status of each patient regarding medication; (2) detection of critical incidents and possible medication errors; (3) providing information (e.g., an informative pamphlet) that effectively describes prescribed medications (usefulness, indications, side effects, dosage, active formula, and other information) [33]; (4) developing a customized action plan; and (5) proposal for implementation of activities included in the plan. The latter two interventions were implemented using different approaches in each group: the CG based the interventions on informative, persuasive and advice strategies, while motivational strategies were used in the EG (see below).

2.4. Main features of motivational interviewing

MI is a counselling method that involves enhancing a patient's motivation to change behavior by means of four guiding principles,

R.R. Moral et al./Patient Education and Counseling 98 (2015) 977–983

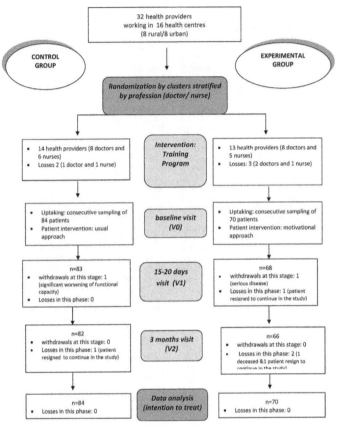

Fig. 1. Flow chart CONSORT.

represented by the acronym RULE: *Resist* the righting reflex; *Understand* the patient's own motivations; *Listen* with empathy; and *Empower* the patient. Conducting MI does not only involve applying a series of techniques, but also aims to create a spirit of collaboration and evoke a sense of personal resources, while respecting the patient's autonomy and personal freedom of choice [19].

Examination and resolution of ambivalence regarding treatment adherence is the main focus of this non-directive counselling, and the EG providers were trained to be intentionally directive in pursuing this goal. Intervention in the EG was more supportive than coercive and argumentative, with an overall goal to increase the patient's intrinsic motivation so that change could arise from within rather than being imposed from without. The EG providers followed these steps: (1) Assessment of ambivalence; (2) Exploration of patients' ideas and concerns about their lack of adherence; (3) Application of specific interviewing skills for reframing and promoting self-efficacy (using empathy, developing discrepancies, avoiding arguments, confronting barriers and problems, supporting the patient, and others). The CG providers used an informative approach reinforced by persuasive strategies and personal advice.

2.5. Measurements and outcomes

Scheduled visits were as follows: V0 or baseline visit (intake and initial assessment); V1 or second visit (at 15 to 20 days in patient's home); V2 or third visit (at 3 months in a health care setting); and V3 or final visit (at 6 months in patient's home). Office visits were about 15 minutes' duration, whereas home visits time were between 45 and 60 min, with no differences between the EG and CG.

Independent variables measured were: health center (urban or rural), provider (doctor or nurse), patient data (age, gender, marital status, educational level, occupation), chronic diseases, quality of life related to health, pharmacotherapeutic data, electronic prescription, treatment data (attendance at health center and hospital). Diseases were coded according to ICD-9 [34] classification, whereas drugs were classified by the ATC coding system [35]. Quality of life was measured by applying the COOP-WONCA charts [36].

Dependent variables measured were as follows. The primary outcome was MA, measured as average adherence percentage and calculated using the following formula: (Number of tablets presumably consumed/Number of tablets that should be consumed) × 100. An adherent patient was defined as having an average adherence >80% and <110% [1,36,27]. The method of MA assessment was similar at baseline and during the two follow-up home visits (V1 and V3), during which a review and medication count were taken.

2.6. Sample size

This study belongs to a wider study, the ATEM-AP study, which has the additional aim of assessing the effect of MI in preventing medication errors [38]. Therefore, "medication errors" was another principal end-point variable and was used to calculate the sample size of the study. For a one-tailed test, an alpha error of 5% and a power of 80%, based on the results obtained by Fernandez-Lisón [39] (average medication errors per patient: 1.8 and 1 SD), we expect to find an average of 1.0 medication errors in the EG and 1.6 in the CG. For 1.0 SD and 15% losses, the minimum number of patients to be studied would be 46 per group. Estimates of the intracluster correlation coefficient in cluster randomized trials in primary care are generally less than 0.05 [40]. These intracluster correlation coefficients are translated to a cluster size of 15 on a design effect that corresponds to a factor of 1.7. Therefore, the predetermined sample size was 78 patients in each group (46 × 1.7 = 78, that is, 156 patients). Because the main outcome variable of the present study is MA, and considering our previous results [38], with this sample size a difference of 10% in MA between both groups could be detected (alpha error = 5%, beta error = 20%, unilateral hypothesis).

2.7. Statistical analysis

The Student t-test and chi-squared test were used for analyzing differences between groups at baseline. McNemar's test was applied for assessing adherence. Absolute Risk Reduction (ARR = %MA in the EG − %MA in CG), Relative Risk Reduction (RRR = %MA in EG/%MA in CG) and Number Needed to Treat (NNT = 1/ARR) were also calculated (95% confidence interval (CI)). To control for a cluster effect, a multilevel logistic regression was performed, considering the presence or absence of patient MA at the end of the study as a dependent variable. The independent variables in the maximum model were: group, profession, age, gender, marital status, educational level, social class, family situation, type of clinical care received in the last year, number of chronic health problems, quality of life, amount of medication, and electronic prescription use. The MLwiN software package (Centre for Multilevel Modelling, Bristol, UK) was used. The study was approved by the Clinical Research Ethics Committee of Reina Sofia Hospital in Córdoba, Spain.

3. Results

3.1. Baseline characteristics

This study began with 154 patients (70 in the EG and 84 in CG) and ended with147 patients (66 in EG and 81 in CG) (Fig. 1). There were five losses (3/2 EG/CG) because they did not include any patient. There were 27 participating researchers (16 physicians and 11 nurses) in both groups: 11 males (4/7 EG/CG) and 16 females (8/8 EG/CG). None of the patients who were invited to participate refused to be included in the study.

Average participant age was 76 years, and 68.8% were women. The two groups were comparable at baseline and there were no significant differences in any of the prognostic variables (Table 1).

Table 1
Study population baseline characteristics.

Variables	Intervention ($n = 70$)	Control ($n = 84$)	P value
Sociodemographics:			
-**Age**: Mean (SD)	75.6 (5.9)	76.1 (5.8)	0.712
-**Gender**: Number (%)			
Females	49 (70.0)	57 (67.9)	0.775
Males	21 (30.0)	27 (32.1)	
-**Marital status**: Number (%)			
Marriage	44 (62.9)	50 (59.4)	
Widowed	21 (30.0)	30 (35.7)	0.413
Divorced	2 (2.9)	0 (0.0)	
Single	3 (4.3)	4 (4.8)	
-**Education**: Number (%)			
Illiterate	17 (24.3)	11 (13.1)	
No education	39 (55.7)	59 (70.2)	
Primary studies	11 (15.7)	12 (14.3)	0.185
High school	3 (4.3)	1 (1.2)	
University studies	0 (0.0)	1 (1.2)	
-**Family situation**: Number (%)			
Living with children	9 (12.9)	16 (19.0)	
Couple	37 (52.9)	42 (50.0)	0.533
Living with other relatives	4 (5.7)	1 (1.2)	
Living alone (children nearby)	9 (12.9)	14 (16.7)	
Living alone (children far away/no kids)	7 (10.0)	6 (7.1)	
Couple with children	4 (5.7)	5 (6.0)	
Chronic diseases: Mean (SD)	4.9 (2.1)	5.1 (2.6)	0.554
Self reported quality of life -COOP-WONCA Index-: Mean (SD)	27.4 (6.0)	28.8 (5.4)	0.122
Care related and medication:			
-Type of visit (last year): Mean (SD)			
Health centre visits:	25.7 (19.0)	27.3 (19.8)	0.519
Home visits:	2.1 (5.6)	2.1 (4.0)	0.918
-Electronic prescription: number (%)	65 (92.9)	75 (89.3)	0.443
-Medication consumption at the beginning of the study: Mean (SD)	8.7 (2.5)	9.0 (3.1)	0.576
-Medication Adherence at the beginning of the study: Mean % (SD)	86.05 (16.8)	80.9 (10.0)	0.053

SD: standard deviation.

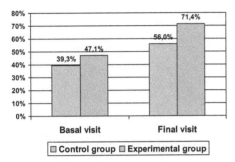

Fig. 2. Medication adherence (>80% or <110%) in both groups at baseline and at final of follow-up.

Table 2
Analysis of the variables related with medication adherence through logistic regression analysis.

Variables	OR	95% CI for OR	
		Lower	Upper
Group (EG vs. CG)	2.57	1.11	5.90
Gender (Male vs. Female)	0.16	0.05	0.50
Education (Yes vs. No)	5.67	1.37	23.41

EG: experimental group; CG: control group; OR: odds ratio; 95%CI: 95% confidence interval; Outcome (dependent variable): medication adherence (yes vs. non). Independent variables considered in the model up and ruled out for lacking statistical significance: Provider (doctor vs. nurse), age, marital status, family situation (single vs. accompanied), electronic prescription, health centre visits, home visits, health chronic problems, amount of medication at the end of the study, medication adherence at baseline, self reported quality of life (COOP-WONCA). $N = 154$; Hosmer & Lemeshow test = 0.840.

There was no significant difference between the groups regarding the number of medications taken at the first visit, medications stored at home, number of prescription or nonprescription medications, brand name or generic medication, and repeat or expired medication.

3.2. Proportional change in adherence category

Fig. 2 shows the percentage of patients classified as adherent in both groups at baseline and at the end of the study. The proportion of subjects changing to adherence in the EG was 24.3%, whereas it was 16.7% in the CG, i.e., 7.6% higher in the EG (McNemar's test; $p < 0.001$).

3.3. Factors related to medication adherence

Using multivariable analysis (Table 2) and after adjusting for other independent variables, those related to medication adherence were the following: motivational intervention (OR = 2.57; 95% CI: 1.12–5.90), female patient (OR = 0.16; 95% CI: 0.05–0.51), and high level of education (OR = 5.68; 95% CI: 1.38–23.41). Other results were: ARR: 15.6% (95% CI: 1.0–32%), RRR: 1.54 (95% CI: 0.99–2.40), and NNT: 7 (95% CI: 4–20.6).

4. Discussion and conclusion

4.1. Discussion

4.1.1. Main findings
In this study, MI showed a significant effect on improvement of MA in comparison with the usual intervention of providing patient information and advice. Providers who used a motivational strategy achieved an MA that was considered relevant to predetermined criteria (>80% and <110%) and that was 7.6% higher than for providers those who did not use this strategy. Furthermore, MI was one of the three variables (together with being female and having a high educational level) that were independently associated with MA. The effectiveness of the intervention was not related to the type of provider.

4.1.2. Interpretation of findings and comparison with existing literature
In this study, both groups of participants, those undergoing MI intervention and those receiving more traditional intervention, significantly increased their adherence to treatment during the follow-up period. This result showed the efficacy of both interventions; however, MI helped patients to further improve treatment adherence and to achieve a level of adherence considered relevant from a clinical standpoint [1,27,37], compared with a communicative approach based on only offering advice and information. Traditional MI has been mainly used in the treatment of various lifestyle problems and diseases, psychological as well as physiological. In the field of behavioral change, controversy still exists about the usefulness of advice and education in contrast to more (intensive) patient-centered approaches such as MI [21,41]. The findings of this study provide evidence to support the usefulness of both approaches in promoting medication adherence in elderly patients who are being treated by polypharmacy. However, the study also shows the advantages of a motivational strategy over a traditional one, and adds to other previous studies in the area of adherence, using more carefully selected populations and health problems [42–44].

In a primary care practice context, the practicability of any strategy is an important issue, and this is particularly true with respect to the application of MI counselling methods used to support the adherence efforts of patients taking medication [22]. This issue is closely related to other factors such as the provider, setting, timing of the intervention, and the number of sessions needed or duration of the effects. With respect to these practicability issues, our program characteristics (different providers, the number of visits, period between visits and duration of each visit) are in line with recommendations of the Spanish Primary Care Preventive Program (PAPPS) [45] and other Spanish regional health care programs [46]. Based on existing literature [41], one type of primary care practitioner (e.g., a physician) does not seem to be better equipped than another (e.g., a nurse) to provide face-to-face communication related to behavior change techniques. In our study, physicians and nurses were both trained in MI skills and delivered the intervention, providing evidence for the value of incorporating the MI communication style into clinical nursing practice, as other studies have also shown [43,47]. This is particularly important in a primary health care system, where the role of nurses is to a great extent, involved with the monitoring and follow-up of patients with chronic diseases. Thus, we consider the improvement in the main outcome as relevant not only because this kind of interventions are feasible in our setting (home visit programs) but also because they introduce a more respectful and patient-centered provider-patient relationship model. Although our motivational approach should be considered holistically, the role of some specific features stressed in our intervention can be highlighted here, particularly the specific evaluation of patient ambivalence and exploration of patient ideas and concerns about their lack of adherence, so as to apply specific interviewing skills. Carrying out any of these approaches specifically may be more feasible in a primary care context. Further research is needed to investigate the potential effect of these different interventions on MA in comparison with providing advice or information.

The percentage for participant lack of adherence recorded in this study was higher than that reported in other studies of polypharmacy in elderly patients. This low pattern of adherence at baseline could be owing to the fact that participants were chosen depending on their lack of adherence and the method used to identify this lack of adherence in the study (e.g., counting patients' pills). At the end of the period, participants in the EG increased their treatment adherence 24.3% whereas those in the CG increased 16.7%. Direct comparisons with other studies are difficult because of the varying time periods used to calculate adherence rates, the methods used to measure these rates and the type of patients and their health problems. Nevertheless, these figures can be considered comparable to those of other studies [43,47].

Finally, the success probability of MI interventions increases with the number of patient encounters, and a longer follow-up period increases the percentage of studies showing a positive effect. Ruback et al. [21] found this effect in 36% of studies with 3 months of follow-up, whereas this effect was found in 81% of studies with a follow-up period of 12 months or more, for any type of intervention. Our study found interventions effective with a follow-up period of 6 months, so we can assume that our program could have produced even better adherence rates with a longer follow-up period.

4.1.3. Strengths and limitations of the study

Our study has some limitations that should be noted. In line with what has been proposed by other authors [1,36,27], here we used a criterion of between 80% and 110% to define compliance as clinically significant. We consider this appropriate for the type of patients studied, the context of care in which the intervention was delivered and the characteristics of the intervention itself. However, it is certainly a subjective criterion, which may be considered inappropriate under different circumstances. This also represents a limitation in evaluating the real effectiveness of our intervention.

It was not possible to mask the intervention, either to patients or providers. This influences the performance and responsiveness of patients. Providers who chose to participate in the study may have had greater motivation for the study than those who declined. It is also possible that the CG providers conducted a more intensive intervention than usual (i.e., they might have been more friendly or pleasant with good performers and therefore more likely to improve patient compliance).

Participants were recruited by consecutive sampling from among patients who had medical consultations for any reason, so we can assume that they were representative of the population that regularly attends primary care centers that also met the inclusion criteria. The multicentric nature of the study gives greater external validity to the results. Obviously, the study could not be blind. Furthermore, we assume observer bias (Hawthorne effect), implicit in the behavior they may adopt when they are invited to participate in a clinical trial. However this is not a differential bias here, since patients in both the experimental and control groups received an intervention

On the other hand, some studies have shown that the very act of counting pills itself implies an increase in compliance that could mask any real effect. In any case, these factors could have produced a conservative effect on the results.

4.2. Conclusion

To promote adherence to treatments in elderly chronic patients who are being treated by polypharmacy, primary care physicians and nurses can effectively use both traditional informative and advice strategies and motivational approaches. Although MI seems to contribute more to acquiring levels of adherence considered

relevant, more research is needed to establish the efficacy of this counselling approach.

4.3. Practice implications

Motivational interviewing is a patient-centered method that can be used by physicians and nurses to improve medication adherence in primary care.

Conflict of interest statement

The authors have no conflict of interest to declare.

Acknowledgments

This study was supported by the Spanish Society of Family and Community Medicine (semFYC) and Andalusian Society of Family and Community Medicine "Isabel Fernández" research grant, and the Ministry of Health of the Government of Andalusia, Spain (PI-0101/2008).

Appendix A

Collaborative Group ATEM-AP Study

- Gabriel Romera, UGC Lucena (Córdoba, Spain)
- Antonio Hidalgo, UGC Lucena (Córdoba, Spain)
- Antonia Martínez Orozco, UGC Levante Norte (Córdoba, Spain)
- Santiago Cruz Velarde, UGC Bélmez (Córdoba, Spain)
- Juan Ignacio González, UGC Villanueva del Rey (Córdoba, Spain)
- Manuela Urbano Priego, UGC Huerta Reina (Córdoba, Spain)
- Maria Dolores Serrano Priego, UGC Huerta Reina (Córdoba, Spain)
- Caridad Dios Guerra, UGC Occidente (Córdoba, Spain)
- Maria Jesús Ocaña Jiménez, UGC Huerta Reina (Córdoba, Spain)
- Maria Reyes Martínez, UGC Fuensanta (Córdoba, Spain)
- Rafaela Muñoz Gómez, UGC Sector Sur (Córdoba, Spain)
- Estrella Castro Martin, UGC Occidente (Córdoba, Spain)
- Alicia Alvarez Limpo, UGC Lucena (Córdoba, Spain)
- María José Acosta García, Consultorio de Adamuz (Córdoba, Spain)
- Ana María Pérez Trujillo, UGC Santa Rosa (Córdoba, Spain)
- Isabel de Andrés Cara, UGC Levante sur (Córdoba, Spain)
- Antonio León Dugo, UGC Levante sur (Córdoba, Spain)
- Miriam Amian Novales, UGC Rute (Córdoba, Spain)
- Cristina Aguado Taberné, UGC Santa Rosa (Córdoba, Spain)
- Enrique Moreno Salas, UGC Santa Rosa (Córdoba, Spain)
- Adela Molina Luque, UGC Levante norte (Córdoba, Spain)
- Antonio José Valero Martín, Consultorio de Villafranca de Córdoba, UGC Bujalance (Córdoba, Spain)
- Rafael Bejarano Cielos, UGC Santa Rosa (Córdoba, Spain)
- Modesto Pérez Díaz, UGC Huerta de la Reina. Distrito Sanitario Córdoba y Guadalquivir/IMIBIC (Córdoba, Spain).
- Inmaculada Olaya Caro. Distrito Sanitario Córdoba y Guadalquivir/IMIBIC (Córdoba, Spain).
- Carlos José Pérula de Torres, Consultorio de Villaviciosa, UGC La Sierra (Córdoba, Spain)
- Jesús González Lama. UGC Cabra (Córdoba, Spain)
- Alfonsa Martín Cuesta. Distrito Sanitario Córdoba y Guadalquivir (Córdoba, Spain).

References

[1] Haynes RB, Taylor DW, Sackett DL. Compliance in health care. Baltimore, MD: Johns Hopkins University Press; 1979.

R.R. Moral et al. / Patient Education and Counseling 98 (2015) 977–983   983

[2] World Health Organization. Adherence to long-term therapies. Evidences for action. Geneva: WHO; 2003.

[3] DiMatteo MR, Giordani PJ, Lepper HS, Croghan TW. Patient adherence and medical treatment outcomes: a meta-analysis. Med Care 2002;40:794–811.

[4] Sokol MC, McGuigan KA, Verbrugge RR, Epstein RS. Impact of medication adherence on hospitalization risk and healthcare cost. Med Care 2005;43: 521–30.

[5] Kravitz RL, Melnikow J. Medical adherence research: time for a change in direction? Med Care 2004;42:197–9.

[6] Simon SR, Chan KA, Soumerai SB, Wagner AK, Andrade SE, Feldstein AC, et al. Potentially inappropriate medication use by elderly persons in U.S. health maintenance organizations, 2000–2001. J Am Geriatr Soc 2005;53:227–32.

[7] Fulton MM, Allen ER. Polypharmacy in the elderly: a literature review. J Am Acad Nurse Pract 2005;17:123–7.

[8] Simpson SH, Eurico DT, Majumdar SR, Padwal RS, Tsuyuki RT, Varney J, et al. A meta-analysis of the association between adherence to drug therapy and mortality. Brit Med J 2006;33:15–20.

[9] McDonald HP, Garg AX, Haynes RB. Interventions to enhance patient adherence to medication prescriptions: scientific review. J Amer Med Assoc 2002;288: 2868–79.

[10] Peterson AM, Takiya L, Finley R. Meta-analysis of trials of interventions to improve medication adherence. Am J Health Syst Pharm 2003;60:657–65.

[11] Roter DL, Hall JA, Merisca R, Nordstrom B, Cretin D, Svarstad B. Effectiveness of interventions to improve patient compliance: a meta-analysis. Med Care 1998;36:1138–61.

[12] Krueger KP, Felkey BG, Berger BA. Improving adherence and persistence: a review and assessment of interventions and description of steps toward a national adherence initiative. J Am Pharm Assoc 2003;43:668–78.

[13] Haynes RB, Yao X, Degani A, Kripalani S, Garg A, McDonald HP. Interventions to enhance medication adherence. Cochrane Database Syst Rev 2005;(4): CD000011.

[14] Schroeder K, Fahey T, Ebrahim S. How Can We Improve Adherence to blood pressure-lowering medication in ambulatory care? Systematic review of randomized controlled trials. Arch Intern Med 2004;164:722–32.

[15] Sabate E. Adherence meeting report. Geneva: WHO; 2001.

[16] Morisky DE, Green LE, Levine AM. Concurrent and predictor validity of selfreported measure of medication adherence. Med Care 1986;1:67–74.

[17] WHO. Adherence to long-term therapies: evidence for action. Geneva: WHO; 2003.

[18] Zolnierek CB, DiMatteo MR. Physician communication and patient adherence to treatment: a meta-analysis. Med Care 2009;47:826–34.

[19] Rollnick S, Miller WR, Butler CC. Motivational interviewing: principles and evidence in motivational interviewing in health care: helping patients change behavior. New York, NY: Gilford Press; 2008.

[20] Burke BL. The efficacy of Motivational Interviewing and Its Adaptations: What We Know So Far. In: Miller WR, Rollnick S, editors. Motivational interviewing: preparing people for change, vol. 2. New York, NY: Guilford Press; 2002.

[21] Rubak S, Sandbæk A, Lauritzen T, Christensen B. Motivational interviewing: a systematic review and meta-analysis. Br J Gen Pract 2005;55:305–12.

[22] Lundahl B, Burke BL. The effectiveness and applicability of motivational interviewing: a practice-friendly review of four meta-analyses. J Clin Psychol 2009;65:1232–45.

[23] Burke BL, Dunn CW, Atkins DC, Phelps JS. The emerging evidence base for motivational interviewing: a meta-analytic and qualitative inquiry. J Cogn Psychother 2004;18:309–22.

[24] Bóveda Fontán J, Pérula de Torres LA, Campíñez Navarro M, Bosch Fontcuberta JM, Barragán Brun N, Prados Castillejo JA. Current evidence on the motivational interview in the approach to health care problems in primary care. Aten Primaria 2013;45:486–95.

[26] [Portfolio of Services in Primary Care]. Sevilla: Servicio Andaluz de Salud. Dirección General de Asistencia Sanitaria. Subdirección de Programas y desarrollo, 2003. ⟨http://www.sas.junta-andalucia.es/contenidos/publicaciones/datos/97/pdf/CSAP_2003.pdf⟩.

[27] Rodríguez Chamorro MA, García-Jiménez E, Amariles P, Rodríguez Chamorro A, Faus MJ. Review of the test used for measuring therapeutic compliance in clinical practice. Aten Primaria 2008;40:413–7.

[28] Val A, Amorós G, Martínez P, Fernández Ferré ML, León Sanromà M. Descriptive study of adherence to antihypertensive drug treatment and validation of the Morisky and Green test. Aten Primaria 1992;10:767–70.

[29] Mahoney FI, Barthel D. Functional evaluation: the Barthel index. Md State Med J 1965;14:56–61.

[30] Martínez de la Iglesia J, Dueñas Herrero R, Onis Vilches MC, Dueñas Herrero R, Albert Colomer C, Aguado Taberné C, et al. Spanish adaptation and validation of the Pfeiffer questionnaire (SPMSQ) to detect the presence of cognitive impairment in people over 65. Med Clin (Barc) 2001;117:129–34.

[31] Gavilán E, Pérula de Torres LA, Ruiz Moral R. Assessing clinical patient-centered approach: analysis of the psychometric properties of CICAA scale. Aten Primaria 2010;42:162–8.

[32] Pérula LA, Campíñez M, Bosch JM, Barragán N, Arboniés JC, Bóveda J, et al. Validation of a scale for measuring motivational interviewing skills in primary care: EVEM study protocol. BMC Family Practice 2012;13:112.

[33] Instituto para el uso seguro de los medicamentos. OCU. [Pamphlet ISMP-OCU saftely How to use drugs ("How to use your medicine safely")]. ⟨http://www.ismp-espana.org/ficheros/ocu.pdf⟩.

[34] WHO. International Classification of Diseases, 9th revision. ⟨http://eciemaps.mspsi.es/ecieMaps-2010/basic_search/cie9mc_basic_search.html⟩.

[35] WHO. Collaborating centre for drug statistics methodology. Anatomical Therapeutic Chemical (ATC) classification index including defined daily doses (DDDs) for plain substances. ⟨http://www.whocc.no/atcddd/⟩.

[36] Lizán L, Reig A. Cross-cultural adaptation of a measure of quality of life related to health: the Spanish version of COOp/WONCA cartoons. Aten Primaria 1999;24:75–82.

[37] Márquez Contreras E, Casado Martínez JJ, Motero Carrasco J, Martín de Pablosa JL, Chaves González A, Losada Ruiz C, et al. Therapeutic compliance in dyslipidemias measured by electronic monitors. How effective is a reminder calendar to avoid forgetting? Aten Primaria 2007;39:639–47.

[38] Pérula de Torres LA, Pulido Ortega L, Pérula de Torres C, González Lama J, Olaya Caro I, Ruiz Moral R. Efficacy of motivational interviewing for reducing medication errors in chronic patients over 65 years with polypharmacy: Results of a cluster randomized trial. Med Clin (Barc) 2014;144. http://dx.doi.org/10.1016/j.medcli.2013.07.032.

[39] Fernández LC, Barón B, Vázquez B, Martínez T, Prendes JJ, Pujol E. Medication errors and failure therapy in elderly with polypharmacy. Farm Hosp (Madrid) 2006;30:2803.

[40] Campbell NC, Grimshaw J, Steen N. Sample size calculations for cluster randomised trials. J Health Serv Res Policy 2000;5:12–6.

[41] Noordman J, van der Weijden T, van Dulmen S. Communication-related behavior change techniques used in face-to-face lifestyle interventions in primary care: a systematic review of the literature. Pat Edu Couns 2012;89:227–44.

[42] Brown JM, Miller WR. Impact of motivational interviewing on participation and outcome in residential alcoholism treatment. Psychol Addict Behav 1993;7:211–8.

[43] Daley DC, Salloum IM, Suckoff A, Kirisci L, Thase ME. Increasing treatment adherence among outpatients with depression and cocaine dependence: results of a pilot study. Am J Psychiatry 1998;155:1611–3.

[44] Dilorio C, McCarty F, Resnicow K, McDonnell Holstad M, Soet J, Yeager K, et al. Using motivational interviewing to promote adherence to antiretroviral medications: a randomized controlled study. AIDS Care 2008;20:273–83.

[45] Luque A, del Canto AM, Gorroñogoitia A, Martín I, López-Torres JD, Baena JM: [Preventive activities in older]. semFYC: Update PAPPS. ⟨http://www.papps.org/upload/file/03%20PAPPS%20ACTUALIZACION%202009.pdf⟩.

[46] Bueno Dorado T, Carazo García M, Martos Cruz. Polymedicated elder care program. Madrid: Consejería de Salud de la Comunidad de Madrid; 2006 , ⟨http://www.madrid.org/cs/Satellite?blobcol=urldata&blobheader=application%2Fpdf&blobheadername1=Content-disposition&blobheadername2=cadena&blobheadervalue1=filename%3DMayor+polimedicado.pdf&blobheadervalue2=language%3Des%26site%3DPortalSalud&blobkey=id&blobtable=MungoBlobs&blobwhere=1220370012917&ssbinary=true⟩ Dirección General de Farmacia y Productos Sanitarios Consejería de Sanidad y Consumo.

[47] Harold E, Shinitzky H, Kub J. The art of motivating behavior change: the use of motivational interviewing to promote health public health. Public Health Nurs 2001;18:178–85.

Index

academic disciplines, defining, 77
accreditation systems, 317–18, 414
adherence, therapeutic, 421–2
Africa, family medicine in, 329–30, 347–8
Alder, Mortimer, 77
Alnasir, Faisal, 414
Alwan, Ala, 414
Al-Ansary, Lubna, 150–1
Anteyi, Kate, 347–9
antibiotics, overprescribing of, 249–50
anticipatory medicine, 37–9
The art of doing nothing, 373
at-risk groups, 337
Australia, rural, 57

barefoot doctors, 382
Barkley, Shannon, 191–3
Barnett, Karen, 338
Basnyat, Amogh, 406
Bazemore, Andrew, 307–8
Behind the Times, 1
Boelen, Charles, 318
Brazil, 259–60
Bridges-Webb, Charles, 57–8

Canada, accreditation standards in, 318
CEE (Central and Eastern Europe), 173–4
Ceitlin, Julio, 241–3
Chan, Margaret, 284, 382
China, general practice in, 381–2
Chochinov, Harvey, 275–6
Collings, Joe, 7–9
communities, defined, 330
community medicine, academic departments
  of, 46
comprehensiveness, 283
continuity of care, 1–2, 283
*Contribution of primary care to health systems
  and health*, 191
co-payments, *see* out-of-pocket payments

decision making, centrality of patients
  in, 69
Delamothe, Tony, 183
De Maeseneer, Jan, 92
Dignity and the essence of medicine, 275
dignity conserving care, 275
disease-focused approaches, 269
doctor–patient relationship, 8, 69, 141–2
'doing nothing', 373–4
Dool, Cees van den, 37–9
Doyle, Sir Arthur Conan, 2
Dutch College of General Practitioners,
  37–8

Eastern Mediterranean Region, 413
ecological fallacy, 307
*Effectiveness of motivational interviewing to
  improve therapeutic adherence*, 421
elderly people, 421–2
end-of-life care, 275–6
*Epidemiology of multimorbidity and
  implications for health care*, 337
*Evaluation of the impact of the Family Health
  Program on infant mortality in Brazil*, 259
evidence
  hierarchy of, 183–4
  secondary sources of, 149–50
  summaries of, 149
*Evidence based guidelines or collective
  constructed 'mindlines'?*, 183
evidence-based medicine (EBM)
  and GPs, 91, 149–50
  guidelines in, 183–4

family doctors
  advocacy role of, 329
  training of, 107–8, 242
  see also general practitioners; primary care
    physicians
Family Health Program (Brazil), 259–60

family medicine
  core principles of, 283
  decision making in, 69
  four themes of, 141–2
  global status of, 107–8, 269–70, 405–6
  intellectual respectability of, 77–8
  in Middle East, 413–14
  and other community services, 58
  recognition in Brazil, 260
  strategic sequence of developing, 241–2
  worldview of, 337
  see also general practice; primary care
family medicine research
  capacity building in, 157
  ecological fallacy in, 307
  importance and nature of, 250
  networks, 270
  value to policy-makers, 338
family practice, *see* family medicine

Gabbay, John, 183–4
generalist ambulatory care, 283
general practice
  academic departments of, 46
  in CEE, 173–4
  colleges and societies of, 8
General practice east of Eden, 173
*General practice in England today: a
  reconnaissance*, 7
general practitioners (GPs)
  and prevention, 37–8
  working conditions of, 7–8
*General practitioners' perceptions of the route
  to evidence based medicine*, 149
Global health, equity, and primary care, 269
globalisation, 242
Goal-oriented medical care, 91–2
Goodyear-Smith, Felicity, 250
Greenhalgh, Trisha, 184–5
Grossman, Carlos, 261
*Guidelines of the China State Council on the
  Establishment of a General Practitioner
  System*, 381
Gunn, Jane, 57–9
Gusso, Gustavo, 259–61
Guthrie, Bruce, 338

Haines, Andy, 46–7
Haq, Cynthia, 107–8
Hart, Julian Tudor, 39, 45–6

healthcare
  equity and quality in, 329
  expenditure on, 330
  universal access to, 329
health professionals, migration of, 317
health resources, equitable distribution of,
  191
health systems
  interface with population, 283
  reform of, 241
Heath, Iona, 102, 373–4
holistic approach, 284
Howe, Amanda, 338
human dimension, 284
humanity, 275
human resource development, global crisis
  in, 317

The impact of primary care, 347
The importance of being different, 141
Improving health care globally, 157
inequity, global *see* socioeconomic
  inequalities
integrated care, 276
integration, 283
The intellectual basis of family practice, 77
The Inverse Care Law, 45

judgement, clinical, 101

Kalikot, Nepal, 405
Kidd, Michael, 9
kindness, 275
Kumar, Raman, 78–9

La medicina familiar en América Latina, 241
Latin America, 241–2
le May, Andrée, 184
Li, Donald T. K., 382–3
Lionis, Christos, 422–3
Little, Paul, 249–50
*Longer term outcomes from a randomised
  trial of prescribing strategies in otitis media*,
  249

Macinko, James, 191, 259–60
managed care, 241
Manning, Garth, 276
Mash, Bob, 330
McCormick, James, 101–2

McWhinney, Ian, 69–70, 141–2
measurement
 patient-centred, 348
 perils of, 307
medical education
 accountability of, 317–18
 in Africa, 348
 in China, 382
 family medicine in, 242
 in Middle East, 414
medical professionalism, core values of, 275
medical students, recruitment of, 45
medications, costs of, 421–2
Mercer, Stewart, 338
Metsemakers, Job F. M., 374
Mold, James W., 91–2
Moosa, Shabir, 331
motivational interviewing, 422
multidisciplinary teams, 38
multimorbidity, 91–2, 337–8, 421

National Health Service (NHS), founding of, 8
needs-led services, 337
Nepal, 405–6
Norbury, Mike, 338

Osler, William, 142, 284
otitis media, 249–50
out-of-pocket payments, 45, 191

Padula Anderson, Maria Inez, 242–3
The paradox of primary care, 307
patient-centredness, 70, 330, 348
Perera, Antoinette, 284–5
performance measurement, 192
personal prevention, operationalisation of, 37–8
person-centeredness, 39, 276, 283, 421
Pettigrew, Luisa, 108–9
The place of judgement in medicine, 101
Policy on Training for Rural General Practice, 122
polypharmacy, 422
population-based approach, 39, 307–8
Prasad, Pratap, 406–7
preventive investigations, 38
primary care
 benefits of high-quality, 191–2
 characteristics of family medicine in, 242

in China, 382
chronic staff shortages in, 317
impact of, 347–8
paradox of, 307
rational systems of, 329
Primary care in a rural set up in Nepal, 405
primary care physicians
 importance of, 191–2
 supply of, 348
Primary care: putting people first, 283
primary care research, *see* family medicine research
primary healthcare, comprehensive, 107–8
Problem-solving and decision-making in family practice, 69
professional associations, 242, 269

Qidwai, Waris, 158

Reid, Steve, 330–1
Report on the regional consultation on strengthening service provision, 413
research-based knowledge, 183
respect, 275
Rosser, Walter, 158
Rouleau, Katherine, 270–1
Royal College of General Practitioners (RCGP), formation of, 8
Ruiz Moral, Roger, 422
rural areas, underserving of, 317
rural practice, 121–2

scepticism, 102
Scotland, 337–8
secondary prevention, 38
Seifert, Bohumil, 174–5
Semashko system, 173
Shi, Leiyu, 191, 347–8
social accountability, 317–18, 329
Social accountability and accreditation, 317
social determinants of health, 57–8, 338
socioeconomic inequalities, 329, 338, 413
South Asia, 283
specialties, inadequate proportions of, 317
specialty care, integration with primary care, 308
Stange, Kurt, 308
Starfield, Barbara, 192, 269–70
State Council of the People's Republic of China, 381

Stavdal, Anna, 2
Stephens, G. Gayle, 77–8
Strasser, Roger, 70, 122
subpopulation-focused approaches, 269
Surveillance van risicogroepen: anticiperende geneeskunde, 37
Švab, Igor, 173–4

team-based practice, 330
time, as diagnostic tool, 69
The Traralgon Health and Illness Survey, 57

universal health coverage (UHC), 46

van Weel, Chris, 39–40, 158

Walsh, Allyn, 318–19
Wessex Research Network, 150
Where there is no family doctor, 107

WHO (World Health Organization), 283–4, 413–14
whole-person care, 275, 308
Wilson, Ruth, 142
women, and global inequity, 329
WONCA (World Organization of Family Doctors)
   1998 conference of, 101–2
   as global voice, 270
   Guidebook of, 108
   member organisations of, 8
   Working Party on Rural Practice, 121
WONCA Europe, 174
Woollard, Bob, 318
Woudschoten Declaration, 37
Wyke, Sally, 338
Wynn-Jones, John, 122–3

Zhu, Shanzhu, 382–3